Multiple Sclerosis
and Related Disorders

Multiple Sclerosis and Related Disorders

Clinical Guide to Diagnosis, Medical Management, and Rehabilitation

Editors

Alexander D. Rae-Grant, MD, FRCP(C)
Staff Neurologist
Director of MS Education
Mellen Center for Multiple Sclerosis Treatment and Research
Cleveland Clinic Foundation
Cleveland, OH

Robert J. Fox, MD, MSc
Staff Neurologist
Mellen Center for Multiple Sclerosis Treatment and Research
Cleveland Clinic Foundation
Cleveland, OH

Francois Bethoux, MD
Director of Rehabilitation Services
Mellen Center for Multiple Sclerosis Treatment and Research
Cleveland Clinic Foundation
Cleveland, OH

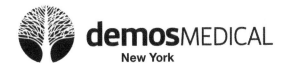

demosMEDICAL

New York

Visit our website at www.demosmedpub.com

ISBN: 9781936287758
e-book ISBN: 9781617051272

Acquisitions Editor: Beth Barry
Compositor: Exeter Premedia Services Private Ltd.

Medicine is an ever-changing science. Research and clinical experience are continually expanding our knowledge, in particular our understanding of proper treatment and drug therapy. The authors, editors, and publisher have made every effort to ensure that all information in this book is in accordance with the state of knowledge at the time of production of the book. Nevertheless, the authors, editors, and publisher are not responsible for errors or omissions or for any consequences from application of the information in this book and make no warranty, express or implied, with respect to the contents of the publication. Every reader should examine carefully the package inserts accompanying each drug and should carefully check whether the dosage schedules mentioned therein or the contraindications stated by the manufacturer differ from the statements made in this book. Such examination is particularly important with drugs that are either rarely used or have been newly released on the market.

Library of Congress Cataloging-in-Publication Data
Multiple sclerosis and related disorders : clinical guide to diagnosis, medical
management, and rehabilitation / Alex Rae-Grant, Robert Fox, François Béthoux, editors.
    p. ; cm.
  Includes bibliographical references.
    ISBN 978-1-936287-75-8—ISBN 978-1-61705-127-2 (e-book)
  I. Rae-Grant, Alexander.   II. Fox, Robert, 1969–   III. Béthoux, François.
  [DNLM: 1. Multiple Sclerosis—diagnosis.   2. Multiple Sclerosis—therapy. WL 360]
  RC377
  616.8′34—dc23
                                                                          2013002906

Special discounts on bulk quantities of Demos Medical Publishing books are available to corporations, professional associations, pharmaceutical companies, health care organizations, and other qualifying groups. For details, please contact:

Special Sales Department
Demos Medical Publishing, LLC
11 West 42nd Street, 15th Floor
New York, NY 10036
Phone: 800-532-8663 or 212-683-0072
Fax: 212-941-7842
E-mail: specialsales@demosmedpub.com

Printed in the United States of America by Courier.
14 15 16 17 / 5 4 3 2

Thanks to my wife, Mary Bruce, for her encouragement and support. Thanks to my children Michael, Tucker, George, and Sasha for making life complete. Thanks to my colleagues for their wisdom, and particularly, to my patients for their courage and extraordinary resilience.

Alexander D. Rae-Grant, MD, FRCP(C)

I appreciate my wife Barb's support and encouragement, Kevin always keeping me on my toes, and Brian reminding me to slow down and play catch in the yard. I also thank Amherst college's Al Sorenson, Steve George, and Richard Goldsby for introducing me to the neurosciences and immunology. Thanks also to the Mellen Center clinicians, research staff, and patients who teach me new things about multiple sclerosis every day.

Robert J. Fox, MD, MSc

With all my gratitude to my wife Sandrine for putting up with me and with my work commitments for 25 years; to my children Nicolas, Ambre, and Célina who keep me young in my head; to my brother Stéphane whose tragic destiny played a significant role in my career choices; and to the patients and families who have taught me what I didn't learn in medical school.

Francois Bethoux, MD

Contents

Contributors

Robert A. Bermel, MD
Staff Neurologist
Mellen Center for Multiple Sclerosis Treatment
and Research
Neurological Institute
Cleveland Clinic Foundation;
Assistant Professor
Cleveland Clinic Lerner College of Medicine
Cleveland, OH

Francois Bethoux, MD
Director of Rehabilitation Services
Mellen Center for Multiple Sclerosis Treatment
and Research
Cleveland Clinic Foundation
Cleveland, OH

Bridgette Jeanne Billioux, MD
Neurology Chief Resident Physician
Department of Neurology
Johns Hopkins University School of Medicine
Baltimore, MD

Allen C. Bowling, MD, PhD
Medical Director
Multiple Sclerosis Program and Complementary and
Alternative Medicine Service
Colorado Neurological Institute
Englewood, CO;
Clinical Professor of Neurology
Department of Neurology
University of Colorado
Aurora, CO

Aliye O. Bricker, MD
Clinical Associate
Department of Neuroradiology
Imaging Institute
Cleveland Clinic Foundation
Cleveland, OH

Peter A. Calabresi, MD
Professor of Neurology
Director of the Richard T. Johnson
Division of Neuroimmunology and
Neuroinfectious Diseases;

Director
Johns Hopkins Multiple Sclerosis Center
Johns Hopkins University School of Medicine
Baltimore, MD

Jeffrey A. Cohen, MD
Professor of Medicine (Neurology)
Cleveland Clinic Lerner College of Medicine;
Director of Experimental Therapeutics
Mellen Center for Multiple Sclerosis Treatment
and Research
Neurological Institute
Cleveland Clinic Foundation
Cleveland, OH

Devon S. Conway, MD, MSc
Staff Neurologist
Mellen Center for Multiple Sclerosis Treatment
and Research
Neurological Institute
Cleveland Clinic Foundation
Cleveland, OH

John R. Corboy, MD
Professor of Neurology
University of Colorado School of Medicine;
Co-Director
Rocky Mountain Multiple Sclerosis Center at
Anschutz Medical Campus
Aurora, CO

Elizabeth Crabtree-Hartman, MD
Associate Professor of Clinical Neurology
Director of Patient Education and Support
Department of Neurology
University of California, San Francisco
UCSF Multiple Sclerosis Center
San Francisco, CA

Bruce A. C. Cree, MD, PhD, MCR
Associate Professor of Clinical Neurology
Clinical Research Director
University of California, San Francisco
UCSF Multiple Sclerosis Center
San Francisco, CA

John F. Foley, MD
President
Rocky Mountain Multiple Sclerosis Clinic
Salt Lake City, UT

Susan Forwell, PhD, OT(C), FCAOT
Associate Professor
Department of Occupational Science
  and Occupational Therapy;
Research Associate
Multiple Sclerosis Clinic
Division of Neurology
University of British Columbia
Vancouver, British Columbia
Canada

Robert J. Fox, MD, MSc
Staff Neurologist
Department of Neurology
Mellen Center for Multiple Sclerosis Treatment
  and Research
Cleveland Clinic Foundation
Cleveland, OH

Steven Galetta, MD
Philip Moskowitz Professor and Chair
Department of Neurology
NYU Langone Medical Center
New York, NY

Kathleen Hawker, MD
Multiple Sclerosis Consultant
Cincinnati, OH

Margaret Henning, FNP-C, MSN, RN
Nurse Practitioner
Mellen Center for Multiple Sclerosis
  Treatment and Research
Neurological Institute
Cleveland Clinic Foundation
Cleveland, OH

Michael Hutchinson, FRCP, FRCPI
Consultant Neurologist
St. Vincent's University Hospital;
Newman Clinical Research Professor
University College Dublin
Dublin, Ireland

Megan H. Hyland, MD, MS
Assistant Professor
Department of Neurology
University of Rochester Medical Center
Rochester, NY

Stephen E. Jones, MD, PhD
Assistant Professor of Radiology
Cleveland Clinic Lerner College of Medicine;
Staff Neuroradiologist
Department of Neuroradiology
Cleveland Clinic Foundation
Cleveland, OH

Yuval Karmon, MD
Senior Attending Neurologist
Multiple Sclerosis Center
The Chaim Sheba Medical Center
Ramat Gan, Israel

Elias A. Khawam, MD
Psychiatrist
Department of Psychiatry and Psychology
Cleveland Clinic Foundation
Cleveland, OH

Marcus W. Koch, MD, PhD
Assistant Professor
Department of Clinical Neurosciences
University of Calgary;
Staff Neurologist
Calgary Multiple Sclerosis Clinic
Calgary, Alberta, Canada

Don Joseph Mahad, MBChB, MRCP, PhD
Senior Clinical Research Fellow
Centre for Neuroregeneration
University of Edinburgh
Edinburgh, Scotland

Sangeeta T. Mahajan, MD
Assistant Professor and Head
Division of Female Pelvic Medicine
  and Reconstructive Surgery
Departments of Obstetrics and Gynecology and Urology
University Hospitals Case Medical Center
Case Western Reserve University
Cleveland, OH

Collin McClelland, MD
Assistant Professor
Department of Ophthalmology and Visual Sciences
Washington University School of Medicine
St. Louis, MO

Keith McKee, MD
Associate Staff
Mellen Center for Multiple Sclerosis Treatment
  and Research
Cleveland Clinic Foundation
Cleveland, OH

Kara Menning, FNP-C, MSCN
Rocky Mountain Multiple Sclerosis Clinic
Salt Lake City, UT

Deborah Miller, PhD, MSSA
Associate Professor of Medicine
Mellen Center for Multiple Sclerosis Treatment
  and Research
Cleveland Clinic Foundation
Cleveland, OH

Ellen M. Mowry, MD, MCR
Assistant Professor
Department of Neurology
Johns Hopkins University School of Medicine
Baltimore, MD

T. Jock Murray, MD
Professor Emeritus
Division of Medical Education
Dalhouise University
Halifax, Nova Scotia
Canada

Jiwon Oh, MD
Clinical Fellow
Department of Neurology
Johns Hopkins Multiple Sclerosis Center
Johns Hopkins University School of Medicine
Baltimore, MD

Daniel Ontaneda, MD, MS
Staff Neurologist
Mellen Center for Multiple Sclerosis Treatment
    and Research
Cleveland Clinic Foundation
Cleveland, OH

Bogdan Orasanu, MD
Fellow
Division of Female Pelvic Medicine and
    Reconstructive Surgery
Departments of Obstetrics and Gynecology and Urology
University Hospitals Case Medical Center
Case Western Reserve University
Cleveland, OH

Alexander D. Rae-Grant, MD, FRCP(C)
Staff Neurologist
Director of MS Education
Mellen Center for Multiple Sclerosis
    Treatment and Research
Cleveland Clinic Foundation
Cleveland, OH

Sneha Ramesh, PhD
Research Coordinator
Mellen Center for Multiple Sclerosis Treatment
    and Research
Neurological Institute
Cleveland Clinic Foundation
Cleveland, OH

Richard M. Ransohoff, MD, PhD
Director
Neuroinflammation Research Center
Lerner Research Institute
Cleveland Clinic Foundation
Cleveland, OH

Stephen M. Rao, PhD
Director
Schey Center for Cognitive Neuroimaging;
Professor
Cleveland Clinic Lerner College of Medicine
Cleveland Clinic Foundation
Cleveland, OH

Mary R. Rensel, MD, ABIHM
Staff Neurologist
Mellen Center for Multiple Sclerosis Treatment
    and Research
Cleveland Clinic Foundation;
Associate Professor
Cleveland Clinic Lerner College of Medicine
Cleveland, OH

Cortnee Roman, MSN, FNP-C, MSCN
Rocky Mountain Multiple Sclerosis Clinic
Salt Lake City, UT

Richard Rudick, MD
Director
Mellen Center for Multiple Sclerosis
    Treatment and Research;
Vice Chairman, Research and Development
Neurological Institute
Cleveland Clinic Foundation
Cleveland, OH

Alessandro Serra, MD, PhD
Neuroimmunology Fellow
Department of Neurology
Mellen Center for Multiple Sclerosis Treatment
    and Research
Cleveland Clinic Foundation
Cleveland, OH

Lael A. Stone, MD
Staff Neurologist
Mellen Center for Multiple Sclerosis Treatment
    and Research
Cleveland Clinic Foundation
Cleveland, OH

Lindsey Stull, BA
Research Assistant
Children's Hospital of Philadelphia
Philadelphia, PA

Amy Burleson Sullivan, PsyD
Staff Clinical Health Psychologist
Mellen Center for Multiple Sclerosis
    Treatment and Research
Cleveland Clinic Foundation
Cleveland, OH

Amy T. Waldman, MD, MSCE
Co-Director, Inflammatory Brain Program
Children's Hospital of Philadelphia;
Assistant Professor of Neurology
Perelman School of Medicine at the University
    of Pennsylvania
Philadelphia, PA

Bianca Weinstock-Guttman, MD
Director
Baird MS Center and Pediatric MS Center
  of Excellence
Department of Neurology
Jacobs Neurological Institute;
Professor of Neurology
SMBS Department of Neurology
State University of New York at Buffalo
Buffalo, NY

Matthew S. West, MD
Assistant Professor of Neurology
University of Colorado School of Medicine
Aurora, CO

Timothy West, MD
Staff Neurologist and Director
Multiple Sclerosis Program
Lou Ruvo Center for Brain Health
Neurological Institute
Cleveland Clinic Foundation
Las Vegas, NV;
Staff Neurologist
Mellen Center for Multiple Sclerosis Treatment and Research
Neurological Institute
Cleveland Clinic Foundation
Cleveland, OH

Mary Alissa Willis, MD
Staff Neurologist
St. Dominic Hospital
Jackson, MS

Foreword

Alexander Rae-Grant, Robert Fox, and Francois Bethoux have put together a remarkably complete and up-to-date compendium entitled *Multiple Sclerosis and Related Disorders*. In 38 chapters, they have covered the field of MS from history and pathology through clinical presentation and disease course, to diagnosis and misdiagnosis, treatment, psychosocial issues, and related diseases. They have succeeded beautifully in their effort to put together, "in one easily readable volume, the core information that guides day-to-day care in an MS center." It is valuable as a single volume that, if read thoroughly, will bring one up-to-date on all the key advances of the last two decades. In addition, one of the features that makes the book particularly useful as a reference is the policy of outlining the key points of the chapters at the beginning, which makes the information easily accessible.

The book begins with a well written short history of MS by T. J. Murray chronicling MS from the earliest clinical cases and identification of the pathology by Carswell and by Cruveilhier to its clinical recognition and characterization, and proceeding up to the development of treatment. This is followed by an overview of MS by Drs. Rae-Grant and Fox in which they point out many of the changes in our understanding of the disease process. Drs. Mahad and Ransohoff then provide an outstanding up-to-date review of the pathology and immunology of MS, including much of the new information on the inflammatory response in MS that has been discovered in the past few years. This chapter is a must for anyone who wants to understand the current status of the pathology and immunology of the disease. In Chapter 4, Dr. Koch surveys the factors affecting the risk of MS and course of the disease. Chapter 5 by Dr. Cree, on the genetics of MS, makes sense out of the complicated study of genetic risk factors in a clear and meaningful way, which is useful both for physicians and patients.

Chapters 6 and 7 on signs and symptoms and diagnosis provide practical information on the diagnostic process and the problem of misdiagnosis. Dr. Stone includes information on signs and symptoms that are typical of MS, and signs and symptoms that are not usual. She includes a helpful table of "red flags," which should cause you to think very carefully before accepting a diagnosis of MS. Dr. Hutchison discusses the formal diagnostic criteria, which in recent years, have made it possible to diagnose the disease earlier, sometimes at the time of the first attack. Despite significant advances in our ability to diagnose the disease, misdiagnosis remains common and the rate of misdiagnosis in individuals referred to MS centers with a diagnosis of MS remains above 10 percent.

Drs. Bricker and Jones do an excellent job of describing the use of MRI in the diagnosis of MS and the associated pitfalls in Chapter 8. While MRI has become one of the most important tools for the early diagnosis of MS and for monitoring its progress, it has also become one of the most significant sources of misdiagnosis. This chapter summarizes both the value and hazards of MRI, and is followed by complementary chapters on establishing the diagnosis and testing to exclude alternative diagnoses.

Chapters 11 through 16 review treatment of acute attacks, relapsing forms of MS, primary and secondary progressive MS, and emerging new therapies. The latter is particularly important given the new therapies in trial—those recently added and those under FDA review for approval. Treatment and treatment goals have been changing rapidly, and with the added armamentarium, complete arrest of the disease is becoming a realistic goal.

The next two sections (Chapters 17–36) deal with specific issues involved in rehabilitation and management of symptoms such as fatigue, pain, cognitive and sleep disorders, spasticity, visual problems, nontraditional therapies, and rehabilitation and management of MS in particular subgroups such as pediatric patients, elderly patients, and women. These chapters offer essential guidance for clinicians who follow patients through the course of the disease and seek to preserve function and improve quality of life.

The book concludes with chapters devoted to neuromyelitis optica, the major MS mimic that has only been able to be more or less cleanly separated from MS with the discovery of NMO antibody and acute disseminated encephalomyelitis, the related acute demyelinating disease that is often managed in MS centers.

Overall, I find this to be an eminently readable and thorough compendium. All in all, it is an outstanding effort and provides an exceptionally valuable addition to the MS literature.

Robert Herndon, MD
Professor of Neurology
University of Mississippi Medical Center
Jackson, MS

Preface

Nearly half a million people in the United States are affected by multiple sclerosis (MS) and related disorders. These conditions, which include multiple sclerosis, neuromyelitis optica, acute disseminated encephalomyelitis, and other neuroimmunological conditions, are a leading cause of disability and work loss in young adults. In the past 25 years, advances in basic neuroimmunology, imaging, and clinical trials have led to a revolution in our understanding of these disorders and a dramatic change in the therapeutics available to patients. With these advances comes added complexity in managing MS patients.

In this book, we have focused on the key topics a health care practitioner working with these patients needs to know in the evaluation and long-term management of neuroimmunological disorders. Information on disease history, pathophysiology, and biology are included to provide clinicians with a framework for understanding current diagnosis, monitoring, and treatment strategies for these disorders. In addition to reviewing disease-modifying treatments, we have devoted significant focus to the symptoms that frequently manifest and their treatment options. Symptoms and functional limitations are the "face of the disease" for our patients and their loved ones, and present their own set of challenges. Assessment tools and treatment options for symptom management and rehabilitation have also evolved and become increasingly complex. In addition, there are chapters on neuromyelitis optica and acute disseminated encephalomyelitis, which are often treated in the same clinics. An interesting recent development is the contribution of comorbidities to MS-related disability and symptoms, and the need to prevent and address these comorbidities as part of a comprehensive management plan.

Our goal was to put together in one readily readable volume the core information that guides day-to-day care in a MS center. Each chapter is an amalgam of evidence-based data with experience-based guidance, combining the science and art of MS management. The authors have been encouraged to present the approaches to care that they use in their centers, with the hope that these strategies will be useful to practitioners working in other centers or clinicians who frequently see MS patients outside of established MS centers.

Where applicable, the authors provide lists of "Key Points" for clinicians as well as "Key Points" for patients and families. These highlights make the "gist" of each chapter clear and immediately available, and also provide a short summary that may be shared with patients. Critical-to-know information and management pearls are pulled out from the text and boxed for quick reference throughout the book. Illustrative cases are included in chapters where appropriate to amplify clinical recommendations.

We have made every effort to update the most recent medication changes, recognizing that this is a very fast-changing field and we anticipate new medications in the near future. We have tried to show the great changes in our understanding of these conditions, while noting the long and eventful history of MS research and the great debt we owe to our predecessors. We have specifically focused on topics in rehabilitation and symptom management for MS care as these become paramount when the patient progresses through the disease course, and there have been great advances in the past several years that provide many tools for clinicians to use to help patients.

We thank all of our authors for their generous gift of time and effort. Their chapters have been a great learning opportunity for the editors, and we hope this volume provides useful clinical guidance for the many clinicians caring for these neurological disorders. We thank the patients and their families for teaching us, case by case, what we need to know about their care, and for working with us in a collaborative way to guide the course of our future efforts.

Alexander D. Rae-Grant
Robert J. Fox
Francois Bethoux

Part I. Basics for Clinicians

1

History of Multiple Sclerosis

T. JOCK MURRAY

Multiple sclerosis (MS) is well known to the general public but was only defined as a separate disorder of the nervous system in the middle of the 19th century. Initially it was thought to be a rare disorder, but soon clinicians became aware that it was the most common serious neurological disorder that occurs in young adults. This brief introduction to the history of MS shows how ideas and knowledge developed and how it moved from a feeling of hopelessness to a now exciting and therapeutic era [1].

EARLY CASES OF MS

Perhaps the earliest case suggestive of MS was that of Saint Lidwina van Schiedam (1380–1433) who developed a relapsing and progressive neurological disease. She was documented by the Catholic Church when she was considered for canonization [1]. The best described and most convincing case is that of Augustus d'Esté (1794–1848), the grandson of George III, documented over decades in his diary [2]. It is a remarkable record of a man's struggle with the disease and the various therapies used by the physicians in the early 19th century. Margaret Gatty (1809–1873), a popular Victorian writer of children's books and a respected guide to British seaweeds, developed a "nervous disorder" at age 41, with weakness and incoordination in her hand, and intermittent and eventually progressive neurological illness, a painful facial tic, and leg weakness. Her physician described her case in *The Lancet* [3]. Dealing with a longstanding and disabling medical condition that alters one's feelings and attitudes about life, self, and the future is a struggle known to many patients of MS. One who endured the battles, winning some and losing others to this relentless foe, was B. F. Cummings (1889–1919). In his diary, he documented a progressive form of MS and died at age 28, 10 years after the onset of his first symptoms [4]. Cummings, who wrote under the pseudonym W. N. P. Barbellion, was referred to a well-known neurologist, "Dr. H.," undoubtedly Sir Henry Head, who "chased me around his consulting room with a drumstick tapping my tendons and cunningly working my reflexes." He thought he could sense his body deteriorating

and he always wanted music playing, or he would lie in bed whistling so he would not hear the paralysis creeping and the feeling of gnawing at his spinal cord. His journal, *The Journal of a Disappointed Man* [4], is still in print.

EARLY DESCRIPTIONS OF MS

The first case of MS in the medical literature is described in the textbook on spinal cord diseases by Ollivier d'Angers in 1824 [5]. Robert Carswell in 1838 and Jean Cruveilhier in 1842, working separately in the hospitals of Paris, prepared atlases of medical and neurological conditions and both illustrated examples of MS [6,7].

In 1849, Friedrich Theodor von Frerichs (1819–1885), a German clinician-pathologist, made the first clinical diagnosis in a living patient who presented with an acute spinal cord syndrome [8]. Although some questioned his diagnosis, he was proven right when his student, Valentiner, did autopsies on some of his cases, demonstrating "the brilliant correctness of the diagnosis" [9].

Frerichs described the characteristics of the disease: (a) The condition is gradual with exacerbations and remissions; (b) One side of the body is involved, then the other; (c) Paralysis of the legs occurs early and gets much worse; (d) Motor changes are greater than sensory changes; (e) The seat of the disease is in the medulla with disturbances of the ninth, tenth, and eleventh cranial nerves; (f) There are frequent psychic episodes and mental changes; (g) Sclerosis of the nervous system is more frequent in the young; and (h) General health remains normal for a long time. It is surprising that Frerichs is never given credit for describing the disease, usually accorded later to Charcot. Other early descriptions came from the pathological observations of Ludwig Turck, Carl Rokitansky, Eduard Rindfleisch, and E. Leyden.

Although the long shadow of Charcot was prominent in French neurology of the day and he is accorded appropriate credit for making the disease well known, his colleague Edme Felix Alfred Vulpian (1826–1887) collaborated with Charcot and was the first author of the initial paper he and Charcot published on MS. Vulpian first used the term *sclérose en plaque disseminé* for the disorder in 1866. His contributions have been overlooked as the attention has been focused on Charcot's 3 published lectures on MS in 1868 [10].

DESCRIPTION BY CHARCOT

Jean-Martin Charcot in the Salpêtrière hospital in Paris was an expert at documenting the clinical course of patients and correlating their condition with the pathology when they came to autopsy, a method he called the clinicopathological method, which enabled him to publish the initial descriptions of a number of conditions.

His Tuesday clinics and Friday lectures attracted admirers and students from abroad, enhancing the reputation of the Salpêtrière and French neurology. In 1868, he brought together all the clinical and pathological information that had been accumulated on MS by Vulpian and the 12 others who had made observations on the progressive neurological disease in young adults, and his own experience with cases, and gave 3 lectures on the clinical and pathological features of the condition, giving it a name. He showed the pathology with his own drawing of what he saw under the microscope. Once these were published, other clinicians around the world could recognize the disease and reports appeared in the medical literature of many countries over the next few decades. Charcot's observations were so complete that very little new information was added in the next few decades. Although he called it *sclérose en plaque*, in English-speaking countries it was called *insular sclerosis*, then *disseminated sclerosis*, and finally *multiple sclerosis*.

EARLY MONOGRAPHS

Although Charcot did not publish a great deal on MS—perhaps only 34 cases—his other views on the disease were probably expressed through the writings of his pupils Bourneville and Guérard [11] in the first monograph on the disease, and by Ordenstein [12]. Pierre Marie, another of Charcot's students, presented 25 cases of MS in his monograph "Insular sclerosis and the infectious diseases" [13]. Marie said the causes were well known—fever, overwork, exposure to cold, injury, and excess of every kind. But although these are common precipitants, he said he knew of another cause that is even more important—infection.

EARLY REPORTS

More and more cases of MS were being reported in the medical journals of the world. The first American report was presented by Dr. J. C. Morris in 1867 and published the next year, with the pathology by S. Weir Mitchell [14]. The patient was a young physician, Dr. Pennock, who had symptoms of heaviness and numbness of his left and later his right leg that progressed so that he could no longer practice medicine and he died in 1867. S. Weir Mitchell,

often referred to as the father of American neurology, commented on the irregular gray translucent spots in the cervical and dorsal spinal cord, mainly in the white matter, and mainly in the lateral columns. Under the microscope he saw a total absence of the nerve tubes and nerve cells in these lesions, and small globules of fat and numerous degenerated fibers. Morris and Mitchell were not aware that they were describing the same disease reported by Charcot that same year, and they suggested no cause for the disease and had no references to other literature on similar conditions.

The first English description of MS appeared in 4 brief reports in *The Lancet* between 1873 and 1875. These were case reports from Guy's Hospital, and, although they were anonymous, 3 of the 4 were said to be under the care of Dr. William Moxon. These same patients appeared in a later report by Moxon when he reported 8 cases of what he called insular sclerosis, although he knew he was describing the disease published by Charcot [15].

S. Weir Mitchell's colleague from the Civil War, William A. Hammond, the former surgeon general, published a textbook in 1871 that contained chapters on "Multiple cerebral sclerosis" and "Multiple cerebro-spinal sclerosis" with descriptions of the pathology and referred to Charcot and other French authors on the subject. In his discussion, he mentioned that he had cared for 11 cases [16]. Allan McLane Hamilton of New York City published a textbook on neurological conditions that described the picture of cerebrospinal sclerosis, referring to both Sclérose en Plaques Disséminées of Charcot and the insular sclerosis of Moxon [17]. With the clear reports of Morris, Hammond, and Hamilton, it is surprising that the credit for the first report of MS in the United States was for many years given to Sequin [18]. Other early reports came from Allan McLane in the United States, Samuel Wilks in England, H. MacLauren, Alfred K. Newman, and James Jamison in Australia, and William Osler in Canada [1].

THREE LANDMARK REVIEWS OF MS

Most advances in medicine are recorded by the date of publication of the discovery and remembered in association with the discoverer, but we normally do not recognize that the field can advance by an intelligent review of the state of the art by an expert or by a pivotal meeting. The understanding of MS was advanced significantly by the 1921 meeting of the Association for Research in Nervous and Mental Disease (ARNMD) [19], the reviews by Russell Brain in 1930 [20], and the monograph by McAlpine, Compston, and Lumsden in 1955 [21]. These clinicians had tremendous impact, and each clarified what was becoming a confusing state of affairs. Each stood back and looked at the array of ideas and observations and intelligently tried to put them in a reasonable context, emphasizing some views, questioning or discarding others.

The ARNMD Report of 1922 was a landmark in the understanding of MS [22]. It brought together individuals who summarized the state of knowledge at the time and consolidated views. The published report came from a meeting held in New York City, December 27 to 28, 1921. The many papers, some now classics, reviewed the pathology, epidemiology, etiology, and clinical features of the disease. In writing the conclusions to the meeting, the commissioners emphasized that MS was among the most common organic diseases that affected the nervous system. They concluded that there was no particular psychic disorder characteristic of the disease and euphoria was not present in most cases and mental deterioration was often absent. They concluded that there was no solid evidence for a bacteriological cause but expected further experiments on this. The commission took the middle road on the question of whether the disease was an inflammatory or degenerative disease and thought that it might be initially inflammatory and later degenerative.

Russell Brain's remarkable review of the state of understanding of the disease in 1930 brought clarity to an increasingly confused field [20]. This was not a consensus; this was the personal conclusion and perception of an outstanding physician about an increasingly confusing field.

Equally influential in summarizing the state of understanding of MS was the first major textbook of the disease, *Multiple Sclerosis* by McAlpine, Compston, and Lumsden in 1955 [21]. The book was based on 1,072 cases accumulated by McAlpine, collated painstakingly by Compston, who wrote the first draft. Lumsden wrote the pathology section. In the last half of the 20th century, this was the major single reference about the disease [23].

THEORIES ABOUT CAUSATION

In the initial descriptions of this disease by Ollivier, Frerichs, Turck, and others, there was limited speculation as to the cause, other than that it was sometimes associated with acute fevers or exposure to dampness and cold. Pierre Marie was adamant that this was due to infections. Lewellys F. Barker discussed the exogenous causes of MS at the 1921 ARNMD meeting and said that infection and heat were more likely aggravating factors rather than the cause. He added there was little support for Oppenheim's belief in an environmental toxin and he was skeptical about trauma as a cause.

By 1950, the list of possible etiological factors was narrowing. There was no longer a strong belief in factors such as stress, cold and dampness, trauma, heavy metal poisoning, or other external toxins. Reese summarized the thought in the midcentury by stating that there were 2 possibilities: a transmissible agent, either a virus or a chemical agent; or a particular reaction of the nervous system to many causes.

SEARCH FOR AN INFECTION

At the end of the 19th century, a belief in an infectious etiology of MS was widely held. Pierre Marie believed that the advances of Pasteur and Koch would eventually lead to a vaccine for the disease. Because there were limited specific medicines or therapies for infection at that time, general approaches to treatment were used. When the advances in therapy of syphilis were announced by Erlich, these approaches were applied to MS, not because physicians thought MS was syphilis (they would repeatedly point out that it was not) but both diseases affected wide areas of the central nervous system (CNS) so it seemed logical to apply one's therapy to the other. Antisyphilitic therapies would be used until World War II. Great discoveries were being made in the area of infectious disease around the turn of the century and many of the approaches were applied to MS.

One of the puzzling stories in MS research relates to transmission experiments, when attempts were made to transmit the disease to animals. Bullock, Kuhn and Steiner, Siemerling, Marinesco, and Petit, all reported transmitting neurological disease like MS to animals using brain tissue or cerebrospinal fluid (CSF) from MS patients. But each time a report was made, others were unsuccessful in reproducing the same results. Dr. Oscar Teague of the New York Neurological Institute summarized this work at the 1921 ARNMD meeting on MS [24]. At this point, 5 investigators concluded that it was an infectious transmissible disease, and 4 opposed this view on the basis of their negative findings. He concluded there was nothing convincing about the transmission experiments. Interest grew in a viral cause when 2 articles appeared in *The Lancet* in 1930. Kathleen Chevassut, who worked under the supervision of Sir James Purves-Stewart, claimed that she could recover a virus from 90% of MS patients [25]. A companion paper by her mentor, Purves-Stewart, named the virus *Spherula insularis* and he announced the production of an autogenous vaccine that he had already given to 128 people with MS, 70 of whom were followed up long enough to yield results. Of the 70 cases, 40 had demonstrated improvement [26]. It would seem that they had not only discovered the cause of MS but also had developed a vaccine that produced clinical improvement. There was widespread quiet skepticism by the neurological community, and it became more vocal as they presented their work at medical meetings. Carmichael [27] was asked to investigate the research methods and results in their laboratory. He concluded there was nothing of merit in this, and later it was apparent that Miss Chevassut had been faking the results.

The story did not end easily as transmission reports continued until the 1950s [28,29].

When Gajdusek and others [30] formulated the concept of a slow virus in neurological disease, one that could infect cells and after a very long incubation period of years cause disease, MS was considered a prime suspect. However, all transmission experiments failed. The neurological community was disturbed to read in 1994 that a prominent German neurologist had carried out unethical experiments that involved the transmission of MS materials to humans during World War II (the Schaltenbrand experiments) [31]. At present, many believe, as did Gowers a century earlier, that the virus, if present, is probably a triggering agent rather than the cause.

EPIDEMIOLOGY

It was apparent early on that the disease was not as rare as Charcot and others thought, as larger and larger numbers of patients were being accumulated in hospitals and clinics in Germany, France, Austria, and the United States. There was confusing information about gender distribution, as some investigators were reporting many more men, others equal numbers, and some more women. It is puzzling that a 1922 review of 26 studies of MS showed a consistent male predominance of 58% to 42% female [32]. Six of the studies showed a slight female predominance but most showed a male predominance. Although there had been suggestions of MS occurring more in some occupations and social classes, this was not borne out in subsequent studies. By midcentury, Kurland concluded after reviewing the studies that the numbers of men and women with MS were equal [33]. At present, we understand that the female to male ratio is 2.5:1 and in some recent studies 3:1. It remains to be determined if the early results are a reporting anomaly or if the demography is changing.

Bramwell [34] found a rate of 20 and later 32 per 1,000 neurological cases in Scotland. Rates varied from 27 per 1,000 patients in Manchester to 60 per 1,000 in a more rigidly selected group of neurological patients at the National Hospital for the Paralyzed and Epileptics in London. Repeatedly it was commented that MS was much less frequent in the United States than in Europe. It was clear that Scandinavians had a higher incidence in many of the studies and that blacks had a low rate, although they were not immune, and the disease was less common in Japan.

Charles B. Davenport gave an important review of geographical distribution in 1921 [32]. He noted high rates in adjacent northern U.S. states, and wondered if that could be related to the many Swedes and Finns who live in that part of the country. He found higher rates in urban communities and in those with higher white to black populations, and in those who lived near the sea rather than the mountains. Since the 1950s it has been known that MS has an unusual geographical distribution. It increases in frequency with geographical latitude, both in the Northern and Southern hemispheres. Alter noted that the geographical distribution above and below the equator had a parabolic gradient that increased sharply with latitude, and that although the curve dramatically increased at increasing latitudes, it appeared to be lower or absent in very far north and south latitudes [35]. In Europe, the incidence of MS was highest in the central European areas and lower both north and south of that area.

The highest rates have been recorded in the Shetland and Orkney Islands off the coast of Scotland. Perhaps the geographical distribution of MS in the world and the increasing prevalence farther away from the equator is related to where those with Nordic ancestry migrated. Those migrating from northern and central Europe were more likely to go to more temperate climes than warm or equatorial areas.

In all the studies, there was surprising uniformity in the clinical features of MS, regardless of the geography or the incidence of the area. Some variations were noticed, with a higher incidence of Devic's disease in India and Japan and higher rates of transverse myelopathy and optic neuropathy in the Orientals.

Whenever there are groups or clusters of MS cases, it is tempting to look for an association that might explain the occurrence. The Faroes are a small number of Danish islands between Iceland and Norway, settled by the Norse Vikings over a millennium ago. Intensive search for all cases on the Faroe Islands in the 1970s revealed 25 cases among native-born residents up to 1977 [36]. All had the onset between 1943 and 1960 except for 1 case that had an onset in 1970. The 24 cases met the criteria for a point-source epidemic. Kurtzke, in 1979, suggested that this constituted an epidemic related to the introduction of British troops (or their baggage) and wondered if this were so, then MS was a transmissible disease and infection, with only 1 in 500 of the exposed individuals being affected.

GENETICS OF MS

Virtually all the early authors noted familial cases but thought it was rare, and each downplayed the importance of these occasional cases. Convincing evidence of a genetic factor had been noted by Curtius in Germany in 1933, showing that MS was 10 times more common in families with MS than in the general population [37]. MacKay surveyed all such reports from 1896 to 1948 and demonstrated that this was not an occasional or unimportant factor [38]. He documented all familial cases reported from Eichdorst's report in 1896 to the literature in 1948. He later showed a concordance rate of 23% in monozygotic twins, clearly indicating a genetic factor, later confirmed by Canadian and British studies.

VASCULAR THEORY

Early investigators such as Reinfleisch noted the presence of a vessel in the middle of most plaques. Marie believed that the vascular change was secondary to an infection, but others speculated that a thrombotic or vasospastic change might be the primary cause of the plaque. Following the discovery of effective anticoagulants a few years earlier, anticoagulants were used as a treatment for MS but interest in this approach rapidly declined. Speculation on a vascular basis for MS would again arise when Swank and others postulated a dietary factor in MS related to high fat intake affecting vascular flow [39]. The treatment would logically be a diet low in animal fat (Swank diet). Putnam proposed anticoagulants for the treatment of MS on the basis of the possibility that there was a thrombosis in the vessel found in the center of a plaque. A vascular theory was again revived with the current interest in chronic cerebrospinal venous insufficiency (CCSVI) postulated by Dr. Paolo Zamboni in 2009.

THE IMMUNOLOGICAL THEORY

The possibility that MS could be due to a hypersensitivity reaction dates back to the observation of Glanzmann, who noted postinfectious CNS involvement in chickenpox, smallpox, and vaccinations [40]. The creation of a model of experimental allergic encephalomyelitis (EAE) in 1933 by Rivers, Sprunt, and Berry seemed to strongly support the possibility that a similar process could be operating in MS [41]. Variations on the EAE model are still used to assess possible changes and effects in MS and to assess the likelihood that drugs might be effective in the disease. For years there were arguments that EAE was not MS, but it has been an important and lasting model for the study of processes that probably occur in the human disease as well.

Research on the immunology of MS has been extensive over the years. Ebers, who recently reviewed the background and theory of immunology in MS, reported a comment of Helmut Bauer that more than 7,000 papers have been written on this topic. Much of the current therapy is based on modifying the immune system [42].

MS PLAQUE

Early writers speculated little on the nature of the gray softenings they saw and felt in the spinal cords of their patients and did not examine these areas with a microscope. Charcot, who used the microscope, believed that an overgrowth of glia was the specific abnormality and that the glia damaged the myelin sheaths and sometimes the axons. Local vascular changes were presumed to be secondary to the glial overgrowth and the breakdown of nerve tissue that was followed by macrophage removal of lipid products of myelin. His student Joseph Babinski also thought it was a demyelinating process, even though one of Charcot's drawings shows the appearance of remyelination, with thin layers of myelin surrounding the axon and fat granule cells removing the myelin debris. Dawson [43] believed that the process occurring in the shadow plaques was demyelination, but believed the vascular change shown earlier by Rindfleisch [44] was the primary pathology. Marie [13] admitted the importance of the vascular element but believed the cause to be an infection. Early on there was a significant focus on the glia; even Charcot considered the glia feature at first, with everything else being secondary to it. Rindfleisch [44] thought that the principal abnormality was a vascular abnormality, although he did acknowledge that the glia were involved. McDonald and his colleagues showed that the remyelinated axon had distinct morphological features and that these nerves had slowed conduction with a reduced safety factor [45]. Later diagnostic tests (evoked potential studies) capitalized on the slowing of remyelinated central nerve fibers.

Once it was understood that nerves could demyelinate in MS, but could remyelinate again, it begged the question of why the disease progressed. Even if nerves had thin myelin and conducted slowly, reasonable function should continue. There must be some other factor that limits the process and causes the disease to eventually, and sometimes primarily, progress. The reason, noted by Charcot and others, is that not only myelin is damaged, but axons are often damaged and lost.

INVESTIGATIONS

Despite the development of elegant investigative techniques for the confirmation of MS, the clinical history and examination continue to be the gold standard for the diagnosis. Early on, however, efforts were made to complement the clinical assessment. The first important advance was the identification of increased gamma globulin in the CSF of MS patients by Hinton in 1922 [46]. The most characteristic change was the gold chloride test, with 50% of the fluids showing a paretic curve and 20% a luetic curve. Elvin Kabat used electrophoresis to look at MS CSF and suggested that the increased proportion of gamma globulin probably indicated immunological process occurring in MS [47].

Ventricular enlargement and cortical atrophy could be seen on pneumoencephalography, and myelography could demonstrate expansion of the cord in an area of transverse myelitis, but these were not useful diagnostic tests in most cases. Radionuclide scans occasionally showed evidence of breakdown in the blood–brain barrier. Positron emission tomography (PET) scanning showed some variations from a normal group, but this is not a helpful diagnostic method in MS.

With the advent of CT scanning in the 1970s, efforts were made to use this technique in MS [48]. Studies showed that 9% to 75% of patients had enhancing lesions, depending on how selective the cases were, but the main advantage was the ability to rule out other conditions.

The major advance in diagnosis was made by the collaborative work of Isidor Rabi, Norman F. Ramsey, Edward M. Purcell, Felix Bloch, Nicholas Blomembergen, Richard R. Ernst, Raymond V. Damadian, and Paul C. Lauterbur who were the pioneers of MRI. Damadian and Lauterbur were responsible for applying the technique clinically. Although arguments continue about who made the major contributions and who was the foremost pioneer, in the end it is the nature of modern innovations to be made by many individuals from many disciplines who ultimately remain anonymous [49].

In 1981, Ian Young and his colleagues at the Hammersmith Postgraduate Hospital published the striking pictures of MS lesions seen by MRI [50]. They showed the difference between the picture of CT and MRI in the same patient. The CT scan was normal but 5 lesions were clearly demonstrable on the MRI. He predicted "The technique may also prove a measure of the severity of disease . . . and thus be used to monitor the effectiveness of therapeutic regimens." A further study compared the lesions seen in 10 patients (8 definite and 2 possible MS patients) and saw 19 lesions on CT but 112 additional lesions more on MRI. Since then the characteristics of the lesions in MS have been better defined and the technology of MRI has improved year by year.

In 1986, Robert Grossman showed that the enhancing agent gadolinium-DPTA caused some lesions to enhance while others did not [51]. He indicated that the enhancement identified the breakdown of the blood–brain barrier, which indicated areas of inflammation. It then became an important technique to demonstrate new and active MS lesions, effectively monitoring the disease activity, which became important in subsequent clinical trials of new drugs for MS. The technology of MRI continues to improve and the next few years will see further advances.

Based on the increasing knowledge of the slower conduction in demyelinated and remyelinated nerves, the evoked potential technology was developed for the visual system, the auditory–brainstem system and the sensory–cortical system [52]. These are useful, especially when they can demonstrate another area of involvement and confirm that there are lesions in different areas of the nervous system. In practice, only the visual evoked potential studies are of practical use, and are now infrequently used, replaced in many instances by ocular coherence tomography (OCT).

COGNITIVE CHANGES IN MS

Until recent times there was a tendency to suggest to MS patients that mental changes were not a feature of the disease, but cognitive and emotional changes have in fact been noted throughout the known history of the disease, noted by Cruveilhier, Vulpian, Frerichs, Valentiner, Charcot, Morris, Sequin, Wilks, Osler, Gowers, and others. There was controversy about how common this was, and whether it was a reaction to the emotional stress of the disease, due to the demyelinating lesions in the nervous system, or perhaps both.

S. S. Cottrel and S. A. Kinnear Wilson evaluated the mental and emotional changes in MS [53]. This was the first effort to address the methodology of performing such studies and used representative samples, successive cases, operational definitions, reliable data collection techniques, such as semistructured interviews, and data analysis. They did not specifically measure cognitive changes, although they discussed these features in their patients. They discussed "spes sclerotica," "eutonia sclerotica," "euphoria sclerotica," and emotional lability as characteristic of MS. They believed that 70% had some degree of euphoria due to organic changes, but cognitive change was said to be rare. Ombredane attempted a systematic assessment of MS patients in Paris hospitals for his MD thesis [54], and although influential in shaping the thinking about cognitive changes in MS, an analysis of his results suggests that there were too many hidden factors in his data to make any conclusions of correlation of emotional change and intellectual change [55]. In 1938, David Arbuse reviewed the literature on psychiatric aspects of MS and concluded that mild euphoria was present in most people with MS and that inappropriate laughter and crying was not infrequent [56]. Borberg and Zahle agreed that in their series of 330 patients "light euphoria" was the most common psychological symptom [57]. A number of reviews of euphoria have suggested that it is a reflection of organic change, probably in the periventricular areas, but occurring in only 10% of patients [58].

Although better neuropsychometric techniques were developed, it was difficult to compare studies as they reflected different approaches and different schools of thought, and often were not based on a solid epidemiological approach. Since Charcot's descriptions, the observations

about cognitive and emotional change have moved from broad case-based generalizations about the MS patient to detailed, specific studies of emotional trauma, memory, and depression. More recently, MRI has allowed speculation about the localization of specific mental changes.

Only in the last 3 decades have we seen more clarity of definition and approach in the use of various psychometric techniques, requiring specific tools which took into account timing of tasks and confounding factors such as depression and fatigue. Paradoxically, as we learn to separate and more effectively measure the cognitive changes and the affective changes, the separation has made it possible to learn how they are linked.

THERAPY

In a disease with fluctuation, recovery from attacks and spontaneous remissions, it is no surprise that any attempt at therapy might appear to work, when it may just be the natural history of the condition. In addition, there is a strong placebo effect in any chronic, distressing, threatening and unpredictable disease. Although 19th century physicians were gloomy in their conclusions about therapy, they all had a list of remedies that they tried, often the same ones they would use in any chronic or serious disease. Some treatments were those applied to any serious neurological disease, and others were based on the current theory of what might be causing the disease. To a great extent the belief changed with the major scientific medical interest at the time. In the late 19th century, it centered around the possibility of infection. Although this concept did not disappear, suspicion of a vascular cause, and later an immunological cause, and our current interest in a genetic cause, all reflect the major interest in medical science of the times.

The physician to Saint Lidwina in the 15th century thought the disease came from God so he advised against expensive therapies as it would just impoverish her father. Although his physicians were puzzled by his nervous condition, Augustus d'Esté in the early 19th century was treated with a continuing array of therapies such as leeches, purges, venesection, liniments, spa waters, and a long list of medications, including prescriptions containing mercury, silver, arsenic, iron, antimony, and quinine.

Charcot was similarly negative about the results of treating this disease. At the end of his lecture, when he came to the point of discussing therapy of MS, he said, "After what precedes need I detain you long . . . the time has not yet come when such a subject can be seriously considered." Marie used therapies that were suitable for sclerotics, such as iodide of potassium or sodium, and for infections, such as mercury.

The late 19th century was an era of polypharmacy and enthusiastic empirical therapies, so it is not surprising that a wide variety of treatments were aimed at improving people with MS. Sir William Gowers was not convinced that any treatment worked but still had a list of recommended nerve tonics such as arsenic, nitrate of silver, and quinine in his textbook. He also recommended hydrotherapy, electricity, maintenance of general health, avoidance of depressing influences, and avoidance of pregnancy [59].

Beevor recommended rest and avoidance of worry, and treatments with nerve tonics, strychnine, quinine, iron, cod liver oil, and increasing doses of liquor arsenacalis [60]. Risien Russell advocated silver and arsenic, avoidance of stress, cold, and mental and physical fatigue, and limitation of indulgence in "wine and venery" [17].

One of the continuing themes in the writings of the 19th century was the similarities and differences between MS and syphilis. Even though clinicians were aware that MS was not a form of syphilis, all the therapies for syphilis, such as mercury, silver and potassium iodide, were used on MS patients and in the early 20th century the new salvarsan for syphilis was added, especially when controversial transmission experiments reported a spirochete in the CSF of MS patients.

At the National Hospital, Queens Square, intravenous (IV) typhoid vaccine was given 3 times a week. If there were severe reactions, intramuscular milk injections were substituted. Denny-Brown said the results were poor and sometimes disastrous, which is not surprising [18]. Oppenheim argued that the cause of MS was a toxin such as lead, copper, and zinc, and some unknown factor so he recommended silver nitrate and potassium iodide, mild galvanic current to the back of the head, spa baths at Oeynhausen or Nauheim, and leeches [61]. Other therapies included iodides, colloidal silver preparations either by inunction or IV, and intramuscular injections of fibrolysin every 5 to 7 days.

In the 1930s, infection continued to be a primary concern, so tonsillectomy, adenoidectomy, and tooth extraction were commonly used. Tremor was treated with veronal and hyoscin. The most common treatment was arsenic given either by mouth or through injections of cacodylate of soda. Sodium nucleinate was considered helpful. Various spas, warm baths, massage, and methodical exercises were recommended. Constipation was treated with enemas, and incontinence with tincture of belladonna. Spasticity was treated with passive motion, warm baths, and baking, whereas ataxia was treated with Fraenkel exercises. For spastic contractures the Foerster operation was used, even though Foerster himself was not enthusiastic about it.

In the 1930s and 1940s, treatments for tuberculosis were also applied to MS. In the 1940s, immune globulins were used, and in the 1950s antibiotics, Russian vaccine (which appeared to be rabies vaccine), plasma and blood transfusions, and dietary changes were tried out. In the 1970s, antiviral agents and in the 1980s interferons were assessed as treatments, all on the basis that MS might be an infection.

As well as recommended therapies, there were things to avoid. The ARNMD (1922) meeting recommended avoiding detoxification therapy on the basis of the rejected theories of Oppenheim which argued against the syphilis therapies applied to MS [19]. Common recommendations were avoidance of extreme temperatures, stress and the use of iodides, silver, mercury, neoarsphenamine, and farradic

stimulation. Patients should also avoid pregnancy, stress, heavy exertion, and extremes of temperature.

Despite the array of possible treatments, Russell Brain came to one sobering conclusion in 1930: "No mode of therapy is successful enough to achieve, at the most, a greater improvement than might have occurred spontaneously" [20].

When anticoagulants were discovered, Putnam became enthusiastic about the possibility that MS was due to embolic ischemia after some experiments he performed. For the next 2 decades, he treated his patients with warfarin [62]. Denny-Brown said he was more impressed with the dangers of anticoagulants than with their benefits [18].

It is interesting to contemplate the approach to therapy of MS through the years. Therapy might be governed by the concept of etiology, the concept of pathology, the nature of the symptoms, or just the need to offer some kind of help. We also see intertwined the enthusiasm for anything new and the common tendency to extrapolate from a beneficial therapy to another disease.

Adrenocorticotropic Hormone (ACTH)

When steroids became available, they were tried in small doses in MS with unconvincing results, but the popularity of these wonder drugs caused them to persist as a therapy up to the present day. Oral steroids have been studied in repeated trials, without convincing results, since the early 1960s and only shown to have convincing benefit recently when the dosage paralleled the high intravenous dosage. One of the early proponents of ACTH therapy was Dr. Leo Alexander of New York [63]. Alexander was a prominent and widely published neurologist who had investigated Nazi medical experiments and helped draft the Nuremburg Code. The long-term therapy with ACTH, the "Alexander Regimen," was widely used even though the prolonged use of ACTH caused many steroid side effects.

ACTH was used extensively for acute attacks. One of the early well-controlled trials of this agent in MS was conducted in 1969 and demonstrated a positive but very modest improvement over placebo. Despite the marginal results, ACTH treatment became the standard for many years, replaced since the mid-1980s with high-dose IV methylprednisolone.

Immunosuppressant Therapy

It would seem logical in a disease that seems to be immunologically mediated to seek therapies that suppress the immune system, but inadequate understanding of the mechanisms led to empirical attempts with many treatments that affect the immune system, such as azathioprine, cyclophosphamide, cyclosporine, sulfinpyrazone, total lymphoid irradiation, and plasmapheresis. Except in very highly selected instances, these therapies have had more complications and side effects than benefit.

Interferons

The interferons were independently discovered by 2 groups in the 1950s, Issacs and Lindenmann [64] and Nagano and Kojima [65]. It had been noted that during a viral infection in tissue culture, a soluble substance was released into the surrounding milieu, and that this tissue culture fluid could be harvested and used to protect other cells. Because this protection "interfered" with the process of the viral infection of the cells, the substance was named *interferon*. Soon after, it was noted that the interferon had antiproliferative and immunomodulatory properties. Three types were recognized, named after the primary cells of their origin: leukocyte interferon, fibroblast interferon, and immune interferon. The first 2 shared many properties and were later classified as type 1, and the distinct immune interferon was classified as type 2. Later, the type 1 was renamed alpha and beta interferon, whereas type 2 was named gamma interferon. A number of other interferons have subsequently been identified.

The antiproliferative property of the interferons led to an interest in them as a potential anticancer agent. Efforts were made to develop variations by cloning and development of recombinant forms of interferons in the 1970s and early 1980s. The initial promise did not play out, but the work continues and interest in its use in diseases such as MS developed at the same time.

In the early 1980s, Fog, Knobler and his associates, and Jacobs and his associates began to use interferons in the treatment of patients with MS. The early studies were with the Cantell preparation of interferon alpha made from human leukocytes prepared from the Finnish Red Cross Blood Donor Program. The popular press began to talk about a "breakthrough" when word got out that MS treatment trials studies were beginning at the Scripps Clinic in La Jolla, California, and the University of California, San Francisco. The first reports were disappointing because they did not reach statistical significance even though some patients reported feeling better. A third study was carried out by Jacobs and his colleagues in Buffalo, New York, using intrathecal injections of interferon beta [66]. Although there were only 10 patients who received the drug and 10 placebo patients, there was a statistically significant reduction in exacerbations and disease severity [66]. Limitations were the side effects and the need for intrathecal injections, but it increased the interest in the role of interferons in MS.

A number of important lessons were learned from these 3 pioneering studies: interferons were not useful in treating acute attacks but were of benefit in reducing the attacks; the side effects might be reduced by more purified recombinant forms; and intravenous injection was an acceptable method. Studies of different interferons demonstrated that interferon gamma worsened the disease, but evidence accumulated that interferon beta-1a and interferon beta-1b were beneficial.

When sufficient supplies of beta-interferons became available, a multiple sclerosis collaborative research group (MSCRG) was formed by Jacobs using Betaseron in a dose of 8 MIU every second day injected subcutaneously. This resulted in a 30% reduction in the frequency of acute attacks and a 50% reduction in moderate and severe attacks over a period of almost 5 years [67]. Aside from the important clinical information, perhaps the most persuasive data came from the MRI data on these patients. Donald Paty had argued that the new technique of MRI should be a part of the study assessment, and this turned out to be the most convincing part of the study. There was a dramatic reduction both in new lesions and in the accumulated lesion burden, as confirmed by the frequent MRI subset analyses of 52 patients at the University of British Columbia.

A major event in the treatment of MS occurred on Friday, March 11, 1993 when the U.S. Food and Drug Administration met to approve Betaseron for marketing in the treatment of MS. Impressed by the clinical but particularly the MRI data, Betaseron was approved in August 1993 by a very rapid process. Berlex Laboratories, the company that produced Betaseron, decided to use a lottery to distribute the drug to those who wanted the new therapy because they initially could not meet the demand. This created a public relations disaster even though it did focus the therapy toward those who were expected to benefit from it. Treatment was initiated if patients had insurance to cover the high cost, or could afford it, and were selected by the lottery to receive it. Fortunately the supply soon was adequate and the lottery was abandoned.

As commonly occurs in pharmacological research, clinical results were obtained only after more than 4 decades of painstaking laboratory and then clinical steps over 4 decades, from the development of interferons to its current demonstration of use in relapsing-progressive MS.

Glatiramer Acetate

Ruth Arnon (1996) related the 27-year saga of "persistent research effort, perseverance, and tenacity of purpose" that brought copolymer I, later named Copaxone, to the market [22]. Following the production of random copolymers that resembled myelin basic protein in the laboratory of Professor Ephraim Katchalski at the Weitzman Institute in Israel, the team expected these agents to produce encephalitogenic activity, but were surprised that the drug had the capacity to protect against EAE. Dr. Oded Abramsky carried out the first clinical trial in MS patients, and Dr. Helmut Bauer and Dr. Murray Bornstein planned the others. Bornstein carried out 3 trials that showed a reduction of exacerbations of MS with remarkably few side effects. Production problems delayed availability of the drug but it was approved for the treatment of MS almost one-quarter of a century after the drug was produced, a "designer drug" for MS patients.

New Developments in Therapy

Therapies for MS have changed dramatically over the last decade with new agents and increased experience [68]. Mitoxantrone was approved for the treatment of MS but reserved for patients who progress rapidly or who fail on other medications. The risks of cardiac effects and leukemia have tempered initial hopes for this drug, and use must be accompanied by careful cardiac and hematological monitoring, and there is a limit to the amount of drug that can be given over the long term.

Natalizumab (Tysabri) has shown impressive results but, again, caution has increased because of cases of progressive multifocal leukoencephalopathy (PML), which has a risk of about 1 in 1,000 but increases if the person has previously been on an immunosuppressant therapy or is positive for JC virus (JCV). The risk also increases the longer the patient is on the drug. Use of the drug is now accompanied by testing for JCV and MRI monitoring.

Alternative Therapies: The Parallel System

Alternative medicine (complementary and alternative medicine [CAM]) has always been with us. Therapies that were once in the forefront of medical approaches to symptoms and diseases are now in the list of alternative or complementary therapies, and alternative therapies that are eventually shown to be beneficial enter the realm of medical therapy. Alternative medicine is a different system, based on belief and sometimes longstanding historical and cultural practices, rather than science.

Any chronic disease for which there is not an effective treatment tends to have a lot of alternative approaches to treatment, and MS is a good example. One need only consult the frequently updated *Therapeutic Claims in Multiple Sclerosis* [69] to see the long list of the most frequently used medical and alternative approaches to MS.

Many of these have a long history in conditions other than MS. For example, spa therapy, herbal preparations, stimulants, minerals, detoxification, and rest therapies have been used for over a century and a half in MS, and wax and wane in popularity. Therapy with hyperbaric oxygen was suggested by some early anecdotal reports and uncontrolled use of hyperbaric chambers occurred in many communities, even though subsequent trials showed no benefit in MS.

MULTIPLE SCLEROSIS SOCIETIES

An important impetus for change and encouragement for research in MS in the last half-century has been the formation of MS societies in each country. The first step was taken by Miss Sylvia Lawry, who was distressed about her brother who had been diagnosed with MS and she placed an advertisement in the *New York Times* on May 1, 1945 which stated:

> *Multiple Sclerosis. Will anyone recovered from it please communicate with the patient. T272 Times.*

From the responses it was apparent to Miss Lawry that there should be an organization to foster research into the cause, treatment, and eventual cure of MS. The organization was named the Association for the Advancement of Research into Multiple Sclerosis (AARMS) but a few months later it was changed to the Multiple Sclerosis Society. She then assisted in the organization of MS societies in Canada, Great Britain and Ireland, Australia, and other countries and then a Federation to link all these groups. Much of the research on MS over the last half-century has been sponsored by the MS societies.

REFERENCES

1. Murray YJ. *Multiple Sclerosis: The History of a Disease*. New York: Demos; 2005.

2. Firth D. *The Case of Augustus d'Esté*. Cambridge: Cambridge University Press; 1948.

3. Maxwell C. *Mrs. Gatty and Mrs. Ewing*. London: Constable and Company Limited; 1949.

4. Barbellion WNP (pseudonym for Cummings BF). *The Journal of a Disappointed Man*. London: Chatto & Windus; 1919.

5. Ollivier CP. *De La Moelle Epiniére et de ses maladies*. Paris: Crevot; 1824.

6. Carswell R. *Pathological Anatomy: Illustrations of the Elementary Forms of Disease*. London: Longman, Orme, Brown, Green and Longman; 1938.

7. Cruveilhier J. *Anatomie Pathologique du Corps Humain*. Paris: JB Bailière; 1829–1842.

8. Frerichs FT. Ueber Hirnsklerose. *Arch für die Gesamte Medizin*. 1849;10:334–350.

9. Valentiner W. Ueber die Sklerose des Gehirns und Rückenmarks. *Deutsche Klin*. 1856;147–151, 158–162, 167–169.

10. Charcot JM. *Lectures on Diseases of the Nervous System*. Translated by G. Sigerson. London: The New Sydenham Society; 1877:158–222 (p. 221).

11. Bourneville DM, Guérard L. *De la sclérose en plaques disseminées*. Paris: Delahayne; 1869.

12. Ordenstein L. *Sur la paralysie agitante et la sclérose en plaques generalisées*. Paris: Delahaye; 1868.

13. Marie P. *Lectures on Diseases of the Spinal Cord*. Translated by Lubbock M. London: New Sydenham Society; 1895, 153:134–136.

14. Morris JC. Case of the late Dr. CW Pennock. *Am J Med Sci*. 1868;56:138–144.

15. Moxon D. Case of insular sclerosis of brain and spinal cord. *Lancet*. 1873;1:236.

16. Hammond WA. Multiple cerebro-spinal sclerosis. In: *A Treatise on Diseases of the Nervous System*. New York: D. Appleton and Co.; 1871:637–653.

17. Russell JSR. Disseminate sclerosis. In: Albutt TC, ed. *A System of Medicine*. Vol. 7. London: Macmillan & Co.; 1899:52–53, 90.

18. Denny-Brown D. Multiple sclerosis: The clinical problem. *Am J Med*. 1952;12:501–509.

19. Association for Research in Nervous and Mental Disease. *Multiple Sclerosis (Disseminated Sclerosis)*. New York: Paul B Hoeber; 1922.

20. Brain WR. Critical review: Disseminated sclerosis. *Q J Med*. 1930; 23:343–391.

21. McAlpine D, Compston ND, Lumsden CE. *Multiple Sclerosis*. Edinburgh: E & S Livingstone; 1955.

22. Arnon R. The development of Cop I (Copaxone), an innovative drug for the treatment of multiple sclerosis: Personal reflections. *Immunol Lett*. 1996; 50:1–15.

23. Compston A. Reviewing multiple sclerosis. *Postgrad Med J.* 1992;68(801):507–515.

24. Teague O. Bacteriological investigation of multiple sclerosis. In: *Multiple Sclerosis: Association for Research in Nervous and Mental Diseases.* Vol. 2. New York: Paul B Hoeber; 1922:121–131.

25. Chevassut K. Aetiology of disseminated sclerosis. *Lancet.* 1930;1:522–560.

26. Purves-Stewart J. A specific vaccine treatment in disseminated sclerosis. *Lancet.* 1930;1:560–564.

27. Carmichael EA. The aetiology of disseminate sclerosis: Some criticisms of recent work especially with regard to the "Spherula insularis." *Proc R Soc Med.* 1931;34:591–599.

28. Steiner G, Kuhn L. Acute plaques in multiple sclerosis, their pathogenic significance and the role of spirochetes as etiological factors. *J Neuropath Exp Neurol.* 1952;11:343–373.

29. Ichelson RR. Cultivation of spirochetes from spinal fluids of multiple sclerosis cases and negative controls. *Proc Soc Exp Biol (NY).* 1957;95:57–58.

30. Gajdusek DC, Gibbs CJ Jr, Alpers M, eds. *Slow Latent and Temperature Virus Infections.* Washington, DC: U.S. Dept. of Health, Education and Welfare; 1965.

31. Shevell M, Evans BK. The "Schaltenbrand experiment"—Würzburg, 1940: Scientific, historical, and ethical perspectives. *Neurology.* 1944; 44:350–356.

32. Davenport C. Multiple sclerosis: From the standpoint of geographic distribution and race. *Arch Neur Psych.* 1922;8:51–58.

33. Kurland LT. Epidemiologic characteristics of multiple sclerosis. *Am J Med.* 1952;21:561–571.

34. Bramwell B. Disseminated sclerosis with special reference to the frequency and etiology of the disease. *Clin Stud.* 1904;2:193–210.

35. Alter M. Clues to the cause based on the epidemiology of multiple sclerosis. In: Field EJ, ed. *Multiple Sclerosis: A Clinical Conspectus.* Baltimore: University Park Press; 1977:35–82.

36. Kurtzke JF, Hyllested K. Multiple sclerosis in the Faroe Islands. 1. Clinical and epidemiological features. *Ann Neurol.* 1979;5:6–21.

37. Curtius F. *Multiple Sklerose and Erbanlage.* Leipzig: G. Thieme; 1933.

38. MacKay RP. *Multiple Sclerosis and the Demyelinating Diseases. The Familial Occurrence of Multiple Sclerosis and its Implications.* Baltimore: Williams & Wilkins; 1950.

39. Swank RL. Multiple sclerosis: A correlation of its incidence with dietary fat. *Am J Med Sci.* 1950;220:421–430.

40. Glanzmann FL. Die nervosen komplikationen von varizellen, Variole Vakzine. *Schweiz med Wschr.* 1927;57:145.

41. Rivers TM, Sprunt DH, Berry GP. Observations on attempts to produce acute disseminated encephalomyelitis in monkeys. *J Exp Med.* 1933;58:39–53.

42. Ebers G. Immunology of MS. In: Paty DW, Ebers GC, eds. *Multiple Sclerosis.* Philadelphia: FA Davis; 1999:403–426.

43. Dawson J. The history of disseminated sclerosis. *T Roy Soc Edin.* 1916;50:517–740.

44. Rindfleisch E. Histologische Detail zu der Grauen Degeneration von Gehirn and Rückenmark. *Virchow Arch Path Anat.* 1863;26:474–483.

45. McDonald WI. Pathophysiology of multiple sclerosis. *Brain.* 1974;97:179–196.

46. Hinton WA. CSF in MS. Studies in the cerebrospinal fluid and blood in multiple sclerosis. In: Ayer, JB, Foster HE. *Multiple sclerosis: Association for Research in Nervous and Mental Diseases.* Vol. 2. New York: Paul B Hoeber; 1922:113–121.

47. Kabat EA, Moore DH, Landow H. An electrophoretic study of the protein components in cerebrospinal fluid and their relationship to the serum proteins. *J Clin Invest.* 1942;21:571–577.

48. Cala LA, Mastaglia FL. Computerized axial tomography in multiple sclerosis. *Lancet.* 1976;1:689.

49. Mattson J, Merrill S. *The Pioneers of NMR and Magnetic Resonance in Medicine.* The story of MRI. Jericho, NJ: Bar-Ilan University Press/Dean Books Company; 1996.

50. Young IR, Hall AS, Pallis CA, et al. Nuclear magnetic resonance imaging of the brain in multiple sclerosis. *Lancet.* 1981;2:1063–1066.

51. Grossman RI, Conzales-Scarano F, Atlas SW, et al. Multiple sclerosis: Gadolinium enhancement in MR imaging. *Radiology.* 1986;161:721–725.

52. Halliday AM, McDonald WI, Mushin J. Delayed visual evoked response in optic neuritis. *Lancet.* 1972;299:982–985.

53. Cottrell SS, Wilson SAK. The affective symptomatology of disseminated sclerosis. *J Neurol Psychopath.* 1926;7:1–30.

54. Ombredane A. Sur les troubles mentaux de la sclérose en plaques. Thesis. Paris: Les Presses Universitaires de France; 1929.

55. Berrios GE, Quemada JI, Andre G. Ombredane and the psychiatry of multiple sclerosis: A conceptual and statistical history. *Compr Psychiatry.* 1990;31(5):438–446.

56. Arbuse DI. Psychotic manifestations in disseminated sclerosis. *J Mt Sinai Hosp.* 1938;Nov/Dec:403–410.

57. Borberg NC, Zahle V. On the psychopathology of disseminated sclerosis. *Acta Psychol Neurol.* 1946;21:75–89.

58. Rabins PV. Euphoria in multiple sclerosis. In: Jensen K, Knudsen L, Stenager LE, Grant I, eds. *Mental Disorders and Cognitive Deficits in Multiple Sclerosis.* London: John Libbey; 1989:119–120.

59. Gowers WR. *A Manual of Diseases of the Nervous System.* Vol. 2. 2nd ed. London: J & A Churchill; 1893:544, 557–558.

60. Beevor CE. *Diseases of the Nervous System.* London: H. K. Lewis; 1898:272–278.

61. Oppenheim H. *Textbook of Nervous Diseases for Physicians and Students.* Translated by Bruce A. Edinburgh: Otto Schulze & Co.; 1911:350 (translation of the 1908 German edition).

62. Putnam TJ, Chiavacci LV, Hoff H, et al. Results of treatment of multiple sclerosis with dicoumarin. *Arch Neurol.* 1947;57:1–13.

63. Alexander L. Minutes of the Medical Advisory Board, National Multiple Sclerosis Society, 1949.

64. Issacs A, Lindenmann J. Virus interference I: The interferon. *Proc Roy Soc Lond.* 1957;147:258–267.

65. Nagano Y, Kojima Y. Inhibition de l'infection vaccinale par un facteur liquide dans le tissu infect par le virus homologue. *C R Soc Biol.* 1958;152:1627–1627.

66. Jacobs L, O'Malley J, Freedman A, Ekes R. Intrathecal interferon reduces exacerbations of multiple sclerosis. *Science.* 1981;214:1026–1028.

67. The IFNB Multiple Sclerosis Study Group. Interferon beta-1b is effective in relapsing-remitting-multiple sclerosis. *Neurology.* 1993;43:655–661.

68. Polman CH, Thompson AJ, Murray TJ, et al. *Multiple Sclerosis: The Guide to Treatment and Management.* 6th ed. New York: Demos; 2006.

69. Sibley, WA. *Therapeutic Claims in Multiple Sclerosis.* 4th ed. New York. Demos Vermande; 1996.

2

Overview of Multiple Sclerosis

ALEXANDER D. RAE-GRANT
ROBERT J. FOX

KEY POINTS FOR CLINICIANS

- Multiple sclerosis (MS) is a continuously active disease with subclinical lesions occurring 5 to 10 times as often as clinical relapses.

- Gray matter demyelination occurs commonly and is an early component of MS pathology.

- New international criteria for diagnosis allow for a MS diagnosis at the time of the first clinical event in some patients.

- Monitoring of MS is becoming more important as we have more options for treatment for patients.

- Symptom management is critical in MS care.

In the past, students and trainees were taught that multiple sclerosis (MS) was a demyelinating white matter disease that spared the cortex and nerve axons, and had epochs of biological remission. Our concept of the disorder was one of episodes of activity (relapses) followed by disease quiescence. Relapses always resolved, so early treatment was not necessary. Even after the development of brain MRI, lesions correlated poorly with relapses so were frequently ignored. In terms of mechanism, we considered MS solely a disease of autoimmune T-cell activation. We did not think there were other diseases hiding under the umbrella of MS which might require substantially different treatment. Many thought that studying MS and ways of treating it was a waste of research time and effort.

Over the past 20 years, we have seen a revolution in our thinking about this disorder. This revolution has overturned the standard concepts of MS and has refocused our research and treatment approaches dramatically. Of any area in the neurosciences, the field of clinical neuroimmunology has seen the most dramatic change in terms of biological understanding, monitoring strategies, and

therapeutic approaches. For those entering the field, this is a time of great promise but also challenge as we balance increasingly powerful medications and treatment against safety, tolerability, and ultimately cost. Despite these advances there is much work to be done, particularly to understand and address the causation and treatment of the progressive components of this disease.

NEW DIRECTIONS IN UNDERSTANDING MS

Prior to the application of MRI in MS, the concept of MS was of a "punctuated equilibrium," that is, episodes of clinical worsening (relapses) interspersed with clinical and biological remission. Treatment was directed at relapse management, assuming that in between relapses the disease was quiescent. On this background, studies using sequential MRI in MS showed new MRI lesion formation 5 to 10 times as often as new clinical events. Progressive subclinical changes were observed in longitudinal studies, as shown by progressive brain and spinal cord atrophy, change in volume of T2 and T1 brain lesions, and other measures of brain degeneration. Clinical recovery after a relapse was therefore not due to resolution of the lesion per say, but based on a variety of factors including ion-channel redistribution, nitric oxide level modification, change in inflammatory cell populations, neural plasticity, and remyelination. The impact of these observations on our understanding of MS and our approach to its treatment cannot be overemphasized. The observation that much of MS was subclinical moved the philosophy of "treating for relapses" to a preventive strategy for ongoing disease management. Instead of, "treat the patient, not the MRI scan," we adopted "treat the disease, and use the MRI scan to understand the disease and its activity." In addition, the common observation that patients often had progression years after disease stability now made more sense, as new lesion formation would gradually erode the brain and spinal cord's ability to buffer injury.

Many other observations helped further our understanding of MS. For example, microscopic analysis of brain tissues in MS autopsy cases showed huge numbers of transected axons in acute MS lesions, averaging an astonishing 11,000 per cubic millimeter. Myelin and myelin-producing cells were reduced, too. Beyond focal lesions, axons were reduced in normal appearing white matter, indicating extensive injury beyond the visible lesion boundaries.

Observations from both autopsy and (more recently) brain biopsies have shown conclusively that the gray matter is targeted at least as much as the white matter in MS. While this observation had in fact been made on pathological specimens in the past, recent observations from biopsies of early MS cases emphasized the cortical component of MS and the concept that some immune activity may arise from the cerebrospinal fluid (CSF)/pial boundary into the brain, rather than as a purely blood-borne process. Conventional MRI sequences do not provide sufficient contrast to appreciate cortical demyelination, and so researchers are testing novel techniques to improve the characterization of cortical disease. The presence of early cortical disease may partially explain early cognitive dysfunction and the presence of seizures in a subset of patients with MS.

We have also seen the development of additional concepts regarding MS pathogenesis, among them a dying back oligodendrogliopathy, a complement mediated inflammatory response, and other pathological and immunological concepts. We have begun to appreciate the importance not only of T cells, but of other immune effector systems such as B cells, macrophages, microglia, and mast cells in the MS cascade of injuries. Whether these observations will be confirmed as truly separate disorders with different treatment paradigms is unclear, but it opens the door to potentially subsegment the group of patients we lump together as MS into more precise prognosis and treatment subsets. The development of robust testing measures to segregate neuromyelitis optica from other neuroimmunological disease is, perhaps, the first of many such changes which will refine our understanding, monitoring, and treatment approaches to our patient population. At the same time, these concepts are allowing us to recognize that the degeneration of progressive MS is likely ongoing during the early, relapsing stage of MS, active inflammation is occurring in some patients in the progressive stage of MS, and the primary and secondary progressive forms of MS may be more similar than different.

NEW DIRECTIONS IN DIAGNOSING MS

Prior to the advent of MRI, the diagnosis of MS was more difficult than it is today. Over the past 10 years, the criteria for the diagnosis of MS have been revised in an attempt to meet 2 countervailing needs: first, to effectively reduce the number of patients diagnosed as MS who do not have this condition (specificity), and second, to increase the number of patients identified as MS who have this disorder (sensitivity). In the past, we required either a second clinical event to occur after an initial demyelinating event (so called "dissemination in time") or a new MRI lesion to form (also "dissemination in time") before the diagnosis of MS was made. In addition, complex MRI diagnostic criteria were impossibly complex and not easily applied in daily practice. In the most recent iteration of the International Panel Criteria for MS (also known as the McDonald Criteria), patients with a single clinical event who have both enhancing and nonenhancing demyelinating lesions (implying "dissemination in time") as well as asymptomatic lesions in 2 or more central nervous system (CNS) regions (implying "dissemination in space") can meet the criteria for MS. Clearly, these new criteria have both sped up the time to diagnosis and reduced the waiting time to demonstrate dissemination in time, both of which are common sources of frustration and confusion for patients and clinicians alike. Without a single test for MS, clinicians continue to be challenged by patients who have conditions mimicking MS; MS remains a clinical diagnosis, requiring clinical judgment and ongoing surveillance regarding alternative and additional diagnoses.

Another collateral benefit of more robust MRI measures is that CSF testing, at the best of times a distasteful pursuit for patients, is deemphasized in relapsing patients. We are moving to a more noninvasive, but no less scientifically grounded, approach to the diagnosis and monitoring of MS in most patients.

NEW DIRECTIONS IN MONITORING MS

With the advent of multiple long-term therapies for MS, patient management has shifted toward methods to adequately monitor both the disease course and the treatment response. MRI provides a useful tool to monitor for new disease activity as indicated by new lesion formation and enhancing lesions. Conventional MRI also provides a general sense of brain atrophy, the end result of MS injury. As we shift to monitoring and testing treatments for the neurodegenerative component of MS, we will require more robust imaging measures that characterize smaller changes in brain volumes, lesion burden, and other tissue characteristics of both lesional and nonlesional brain tissue.

To this end, MRI appears to have promising utility. Volumetric lesion and atrophy measures are being used in clinical trials and longitudinal studies and show progressive brain atrophy. Measures such as magnetization transfer ratio (MTR) and MRI spectroscopy may characterize the longitudinal change in tissue injury within both focal lesions and other areas of the brain that appear normal using conventional imaging. Diffusion tensor imaging is sensitive to changes in certain white matter tracts and may differentially characterize demyelination and axonal degeneration. Each of these tools may be beneficial in measuring neuroprotective or neurorestorative strategies as we move into new areas of therapeutic development.

Ocular coherence tomography (OCT) is a new and powerful tool to monitor the result of optic neuritis. Newer generation OCT machines using spectral domain technology have shown a reduction in retinal nerve fiber layer after optic neuritis, as well as injury to other retinal structures. OCT may provide another way of monitoring inflammation, axonal injury, and later degeneration in a quick, convenient, noninvasive and relatively inexpensive fashion.

In the clinic, we are now using more quantitated measures to assist with the longitudinal monitoring of our patients. The timed 25 foot walk, 9 hole peg test, 6 minute walk, and the "up and go" test, all provide measurable continuous scales of function which can be charted over time. The future is likely to bring computer-based measurement tools to track disease activity and measure function, depression, and cognitive capacities.

NEW DIRECTIONS IN TREATMENT OF MS DISEASE ACTIVITY

Prior to 1993 there were no FDA-approved medicines for MS. Clinicians caring for patients with MS were often discouraged from "wasting their time" doing clinical trials in MS. At the time of this publication, there were 10 FDA-approved medicines for relapsing forms of MS, as well as FDA-approved medicines to increase walking speed in MS, bladder dysfunction, and emotional incontinence. Many more disease-modifying therapies and symptom therapies are currently in phase 2 and phase 3 trials. The astonishing development in pharmacological approaches to MS is notable in view of the fact that while 3 medicines for MS have been approved in the past 3 years, a similar total number has been approved for all other neurological disorders outside of pain and depression.

It has become clear that an increased efficacy as measured by reduced relapses, short-term measures of disability on exam, and MRI activity can be achieved with some of the newer agents. However higher efficacy may come with a price, as exemplified by our experience with progressive multifocal leukoencephalopathy and natalizumab. However, we are now becoming more adept at risk-stratifying patients for this drug by monitoring John Cunningham virus (JCV) antibody levels prior to and during therapy. Similar risk stratification is being used for the first oral agent available (fingolimod) by assessing for antibodies against varicella zoster and assessing cardiac rhythm disorders, medications, and baseline eye exam.

Newer agents such as alemtuzumab may have their own risk stratification procedure. Surprisingly, the goal of personalized treatment in MS has not been through personalizing efficacy, but through personalizing safety and risks of toxicity.

A recently emerging theme in relapsing MS is the recognition that a subset of patients treated in clinical trials appear to be free of disease activity, as defined by stable clinical exam, lack of relapses, and stable MRI without new lesions or gadolinium enhancement. The proportion of patients free of disease activity may become the new benchmark of success, both in clinical trials and in clinical populations. Of course, this simple definition begs the question of whether patients are truly free of disease activity or just have changes which escape current clinical and imaging monitoring methods. This will be a point of discussion particularly as we increase the number of trials in progressive MS, where robust measures of progression are urgently needed to guide treatment assessment and decision making.

NEW DIRECTIONS IN TREATMENT OF MS SYMPTOMS

While the search for newer disease-modifying therapies has been fruitful, other areas of MS management have also moved forward. We now have a new agent for pseudobulbar affect, a socially stigmatizing disorder seen in MS, amyotrophic lateral sclerosis, head injury, and some dementing disorders. A long-acting form of 4-aminopyridine is FDA-approved to increase walking speed in MS. Botulinum toxin has been approved for the management of spasticity and bladder dysfunction. Additional agents are available for the treatment of neurogenic bladder symptoms. Implanted lioresal pumps provide a management tool for patients with severe spasticity and have seen useful application to both ambulatory and nonambulatory patients. Now, the challenge may be who to treat with what and when, a challenge to be met with better training and a more thoughtful practice style.

GREATER RECOGNITION OF THE IMPORTANCE OF OTHER HEALTH MEASURES IN MS

In the past, neurologists typically confined themselves to the diagnosis and sometimes treatment of MS alone. They did not provide care for (or indeed cared about) other medical issues in their MS population. Over the past 5 years, we have come to recognize how comorbid conditions such as obesity, smoking, and vascular disease require attention in the MS population and how they accelerate progression of MS owing to secondary injury. We are seeing a greater focus on the potential role of vitamin D deficiency in the pathogenesis of MS and trials aimed at modifying vitamin D stores and assessing for clinical and MRI benefits. We are learning that depression, sleep disorders, and pain are not only common in MS, but drivers of health-related quality of life and even employment in affected patients. We need to treat the entire patient and attend to their social surroundings, rather than just seeing them as relapses and brain lesions.

EMBRACING A TEAM APPROACH TO MS

It has become crystal clear that a neurologist alone cannot meet the needs of this challenging patient population. A team approach, where many health care practitioners with different competencies aid the patient through their disease course, works better than a solo act. New research has supported the concept that wellness approaches, cognitive behavioral therapies, physical and occupational strategies, and a host of other interventions are not only beneficial but critical in improving function and improving the lot of patients and their families. As we move into newer health care systems, a more comprehensive approach to all the factors which go into MS care needs to be taken so that we can effectively and efficiently help this group of people through their long-term disease.

ONGOING CHALLENGES AND FUTURE PROMISE

Despite great successes in so many areas of MS—successes in understanding its pathogenesis, diagnosis, treatment, and monitoring—many challenges still remain. Perhaps no challenge is more prominent than that of treating progressive MS. Although symptomatic therapies in progressive MS have emerged, there still is a fundamental lack of understanding regarding progressive MS pathobiology, methods for phase 2 proof-of-concept trials, clinical outcomes for phase 3 trials. These holes in our understanding have inhibited the development of an effective therapy for progressive MS. We also need better clinical and imaging tools to monitor the evolution of MS disease beyond just foci of inflammation. These tools will better characterize disease progression over time and the potential impact of disease-modifying and symptomatic therapies.

At the present time, we are at crossroads in MS. If we catch patients early enough in their relapsing course, intervene, monitor treatment response, and alter treatment accordingly, then we feel we can substantively alter the course of their disease. Admittedly, definitive long-term evidence of this is still lacking, but preliminary clinical trial and innovative propensity-weighted virtual trials suggest this is the case. However, we would also like to be able to provide more protection from neurological worsening, and optimally to provide for improvement or restoration of function where it has been permanently injured in the past. The continued significant unmet needs and challenges in MS call for an active MS research enterprise, clinically astute and forward thinking treatment strategies, as well as targeted advocacy and fundraising. The last 2 decades of tremendous progress in MS need to be leveraged toward the remaining significant unmet needs of this disease.

KEY POINTS FOR PATIENTS AND FAMILIES

- Because MS is active even when you are not having symptoms, treatment is important to reduce the disease before you have major problems. Treating MS is like treating high blood pressure, in that treatment is preventive.

- Monitoring MS is important to tell us whether the medicines are working for you and whether we need to modify medications.

- The symptoms of MS are treatable and an important part of maintaining a good quality of life.

BIBLIOGRAPHY

Filippi M, Rocca MA, De Stefano N. Magnetic resonance techniques in multiple sclerosis: The present and the future. *Arch Neurol.* 2011;68(12):1514–1520.

Harris JO, Frank JA, Patronas N, et al. Serial gadolinium-enhanced magnetic resonance imaging scans in patients with early relapsing-remitting multiple sclerosis. Implications for clinical trials and natural history. *Ann Neurol.* 1991;29:548–555.

Krupp LB, Banwell B, Tenembaum S. Consensus definitions proposed for pediatric multiple sclerosis and related disorders *Neurology.* 2007;68(Suppl 2):S7–S12.

Miller DH, Weinshenker BG, Filippi M, et al. Differential diagnosis of suspected multiple sclerosis: A consensus approach. *Mult Scler.* 2008;14:1157–1174.

Morales Y, Parisi JE, Lucchinetti CF. The pathology of multiple sclerosis: Evidence for heterogeneity. *Adv Neurol.* 2006;98:27–45.

Polman CH, Reingold SC, Banwell B, et al. Diagnostic criteria for multiple sclerosis: 2010 revisions to the McDonald Criteria. *Ann Neurol.* 2011;69:292–302.

Scalfari A, Neuhaus A, Degenhardt A, et al. The natural history of multiple sclerosis: A geographically based study 10: Relapses and long-term disability. *Brain.* 2010;133:1914–1929.

3

Pathology and Pathophysiology of Multiple Sclerosis

DON JOSEPH MAHAD
RICHARD M. RANSOHOFF

KEY POINTS FOR CLINICIANS

- Demyelinating plaques are seen both in the white matter and in the gray matter and are now known to occur early in multiple sclerosis (MS) in the gray matter.
- Multiple cell types are involved in the inflammatory process in MS.
- Axon and neuron loss occur commonly in MS and can be early features of the disease.
- Axon loss may lead to later Wallerian degeneration.
- Entry of inflammatory cells appears to occur both via venules as well as through the pial surface from the subarachnoid space.

Recent studies have dramatically changed our thinking about the pathology and pathophysiology of multiple sclerosis (MS). MS is now regarded as both a gray matter (GM) and a white matter (WM) disease, where well-recognized components of WM pathology, demyelination, and inflammation are also seen the GM. In fact, lesions of the GM may be an early component of MS pathology as shown by pass through pathology at the time of early needle biopsy. Neurons as well as axons degenerate from an early stage in MS so that the pathology is just not demyelinating. Recent studies have shown a better correlation between GM atrophy and clinical disability in MS patients than WM atrophy [1]. This highlights the clinical relevance of GM pathology in MS.

> MS is both a gray matter and a white matter disease and lesions of the GM are now known to occur early in MS.

These observations not only extend the spectrum of MS pathology but also have important implications for understanding the pathophysiology of the disease, particularly disease progression and cognitive dysfunction in MS.

DEMYELINATION WITHIN GM AND WM IN MS

WM lesions, identified by the loss of myelin (demyelination) in autopsy tissue from MS cases, tend to be prevalent in the periventricular region, corpus callosum, and spinal cord. The WM lesions occur early in MS, as illustrated by diagnostic MRI, and increase in volume with longer disease duration. This may reflect ongoing demyelination and incomplete remyelination (restoration of myelin sheaths to axons). The lesions are considered as acute, chronic active, or slow expanding, and chronic inactive depending on the intensity of the inflammatory reaction and presence of myelin debris (indicating ongoing demyelination). In the cortex, however, MS lesions are subclassified into type 1 (leukocortical), type 2 (intracortical), and type 3 (subpial) on the basis of the anatomical location of GM demyelination, as the inflammatory activity in demyelinated cortex at autopsy is relatively uniform.

> In the cortex, MS lesions are subclassified into type 1 (leukocortical), type 2 (intracortical) and type 3 (subpial).

Until recently, GM demyelination was appreciated as a late feature of MS, partly because the detection of cortical lesions by conventional MRI at any point during the course of MS is challenging [2,3]. However, a biopsy study of GM from an early-stage MS patient with suspected tumors in the WM revealed that GM demyelination may occur at an early stage (type 1 lesions accounting for the majority) and GM inflammation may be florid compared with the findings at autopsy in cases with long-standing MS. MRI techniques such as double inversion recovery imaging have helped establish GM lesions as an early feature in MS. Interestingly, neuropathological findings at the end stage of MS suggest the genesis of cortical lesions as a process that is independent of WM lesions.

INFLAMMATION IN MS

The cellular components of the parenchymal inflammatory infiltrate in MS consist of T lymphocytes (cytotoxic [CD8], T-helper [CD4] type 1 and type 2), B lymphocytes, monocytes, macrophages, and activated microglia. Findings in premyelinating lesions from cases with fulminant MS suggest an early role for innate immunity (activated microglia and macrophages) in a subset of acute MS lesions, while complement and immunoglobulins appear to play a predominant role at the early stages of other lesions [4,5]. Besides the parenchymal inflammation in the WM and GM, there is a gathering body of evidence implicating both diffuse and organized inflammation in the form of B-cell follicles within the meninges in MS.

> Follicular aggregates containing B cells occur within the meninges in MS.

WM INFLAMMATION IN MS

In addition to the characterization of a cellular inflammatory component, cell adhesion molecules, integrins, chemokines, and chemokine receptors have been studied extensively in the WM of MS, as summarized here.

Adhesion Molecules and Integrins

Intercellular adhesion molecule 1 (ICAM-1), ICAM-3, and vascular cell adhesion molecule 1 (VCAM-1) are expressed with differing temporal and spatial patterns within lesional and nonlesional white matter (NLWM) in MS. ICAM-1 expression, which colocalized to the luminal surface of brain endothelial cells, was most prominent in MS lesions (81% of lesions). Thirty-seven percent of blood vessels in nonlesional WM MS expressed ICAM-1 compared to 10% in control brains. Within MS lesions, ICAM-1 expression was most prominent in acute lesions, although Cannella et al. [6] reported, using a somewhat subjective scoring system, maximum staining in chronic silent lesions. The upregulation of ICAM-2 was not detected in MS lesions. ICAM-3 is expressed mainly on lymphocytes and monocytes in perivascular cuffs and lesion edges. ICAM-3 expression on monocytes decreased during maturation into macrophages. Leukocyte function antigen 1 (LFA-1), which binds to ICAMs, was expressed on activated microglia in MS lesions. The coexpression of LFA-1 and ICAM-3 on majority of lymphocytes in MS lesions is consistent with the role of LFA-1/ICAM-3 interaction in lymphocyte recruitment. The LFA-1 expression on microglia and ICAM-3 on lymphocytes suggest a role in lymphocyte–microglial interaction as part of antigen presentation in MS.

Expression of VCAM-1 was most prominent at the border of active MS lesions. Based on morphology, VCAM-1+ cells were identified as lymphocytes and monocytes in the perivascular spaces, large lipid-filled macrophages in the cores and borders of active lesions, and activated microglia in association with oligodendrocyte somata in perilesional WM. Very late activation antigen 4 (VLA-4), which binds to VCAM-1, was seen on perivascular lymphocytes and monocytes in chronic active MS lesions. VCAM-1 and VLA-4 are also expressed in noninflammatory central nervous system (CNS) tissue, in diseases such as amyotrophic lateral sclerosis (ALS) and olivopontocerebellar degeneration (OPCD), but the expression in control brain tissue was minimal. Consistent with a pathogenic role of VLA-4 in MS, intravenous administration of a humanized monoclonal antibody against human alpha-4 integrin led to a significant reduction of new lesion formation, as defined by gadolinium-enhancing MRI.

Chemokines and Chemokine Receptors

Chemokine ligand 2 (CCL2), CCL3, CCL4, CCL5, and CXCL10 are expressed in MS lesions as summarized here. Monocyte chemoattractant protein-1 (MCP-1)/CCL2, a potent monocyte chemoattractant in vivo, is expressed in MS lesions with much greater intensity of staining in acute lesions compared to sections of control brain tissue or normal-appearing white matter (NAWM). CCL2 also chemo-attracts memory T lymphocytes, dendritic cells, natural killer cells, and microglia. Hypertrophic astrocytes are the main source of CCL2 in MS lesions and the intensity of CCL2 staining in the cytoplasm and processes of astrocytes reduced as the lesions became chronic.

Macrophage inflammatory protein 1-alpha (MIP 1-alpha)/CCL3 and MIP 1-beta/CCL4, RANTES/CCL5 are expressed within MS lesions and chemoattract CCR1-, CCR3-, and/or CCR5-bearing T cells and monocytes. In active MS lesions, CCL3 is expressed on microglia and macrophages, whereas CCL5 is expressed on perivascular cells, blood vessel endothelial cells, and to a lesser extent, on perivascular astrocytes.

CXCL10/IP-10, a potent lymphocyte chemoattractant, immunoreactivity is observed on cell bodies and foot processes of reactive astrocytes in active MS lesions and on the endothelium in NLWM [7,8]. CXCL10 was not expressed in silent/inactive MS lesions or in control brain tissue. Double staining for CXCL10 and CXCR3 showed a significant correlation between CXCL10+ cellular elements and CXCR3+ perivascular cells. CXCL10 levels in the cerebrospinal fluid (CSF) from patients with MS correlated with the clinical disease activity and the CSF leukocyte count [8,9]. While there is a degree of redundancy in the chemokine system, blockage of selective ligand/receptor interactions may offer therapeutic benefit by limiting the entry of inflammatory cells from the circulation into the brain.

GM INFLAMMATION IN MS

In established cortical lesions of MS, activated microglia are the most abundant component of cellular inflammatory infiltrate, and perivascular cuffs and CD3+ T cells were lacking compared to active WM lesions at autopsy. These consistent observations led to the consideration of the inflammatory component of cortical MS lesions as relatively homogeneous. The recent identification of perivascular cuffs with abundant CD3+ T cells (including cytotoxic T cells) in biopsy material from cases suspected to have a tumor and subsequently diagnosed with MS, raises the possibility that the GM at the early stages of "classical" MS may harbor florid inflammation akin to what has been described in the WM (Figure 3.1A,B). Given all the aspects relating to studying pathology in brain biopsy material and the recent discovery of florid GM inflammation, it is perhaps not surprising that the cellular inflammatory infiltrate as well as CAMs, chemokines, and chemokine receptors in the GM have not been studied to the same extent as the WM.

> GM at the early stages of "classical" MS may harbor florid inflammation.

NEURONAL AND AXONAL DEGENERATION IN MS

Axonal Loss

Using autopsy tissue from MS cases with long-standing MS (disease duration from 12 to 39 years and mean Expanded Disability Status Scale [EDSS] of 7.5) and a triangulation method of quantitation, Bjartmar et al. reported 68% loss of axonal numbers and 60% loss of axonal density in chronic inactive spinal cord MS lesions [10]. The extent of axonal loss correlated with neurological disability but not with disease duration or the degree of spinal cord atrophy, which was greater in the cervical than lumbar spine. The majority (7 out of 10) of the chronic lesions were atrophic (17%–45% loss of volume) and others were hypertrophic in comparison to site-matched control tissue. The lack of correlation between axonal loss and volume loss of spinal cord lesions may be due to other factors, such as axonal atrophy, demyelination, inflammation-related edema, and astrogliosis, which influence the volume of MS lesions. The proportion of WM and GM areas were similar in MS and control cervical and lumbar spinal cords, indicating that the loss of spinal cord volume in MS is due to a combination of both GM and WM loss. This study also validated the biological implications of the in vivo studies of axonal loss and injury using magnetic resonance spectroscopy (MRS) to detected levels of N-acetyl aspartate (NAA). NAA, localized primarily in the neurons and neuronal processes, is produced in the mitochondria and transported to the cytoplasm. Although the function of NAA is unknown, reduction of NAA levels represents either reversible neuronal and axonal dysfunction or irreversible axonal and neuronal loss. NAA levels detected by high performance liquid chromatography (HPLC) were reduced by 53% to 55% in whole spinal cord sections with inactive lesions compared to controls and reduction of NAA levels significantly correlated with the degree of axonal loss. Consistent with MRS findings, NAA levels were significantly reduced in demyelinated axons and myelinated axons in NLWM. Potentially reversible processes such as altered neuronal and axonal metabolism, demyelination, conduction block, and redistribution of axonal sodium channels may alter the NAA levels in demyelinated and myelinated axons. Further evidence for axonal loss as the cause of irreversible disability in MS is suggested by the studies of "clinically silent" cases with neuropathological features of MS at autopsy, where axons were well preserved.

In active MS lesions, Bitsch et al. reported 35% loss of axons [11]. Axonal loss, based on APP accumulation, in chronic active lesions was greater than in active lesions. The extent of axonal loss in NLWM would depend on whether or not the axons have been transected elsewhere owing to a proximal or a distal lesion [10,12].

Neuronal Loss

A number of MRI studies consistently indicated a decrease in GM volume (cortical atrophy), rate of which is fastest during progressive stage of MS, while the rate of WM atrophy appeared to remain steady throughout the course of MS. Besides, neocortical atrophy, deep GM nuclei (caudate, thalamus, and hypothalamus), and spinal cord GM are damaged in MS. Furthermore, mechanisms of GM atrophy have been suggested to differ between relapsing-remitting multiple sclerosis (RRMS) and secondary progressive multiple sclerosis (SPMS), as MRI parameters such as lesion volume changes and magnetization transfer ratio did not account for the variance in GM atrophy during progressive MS.

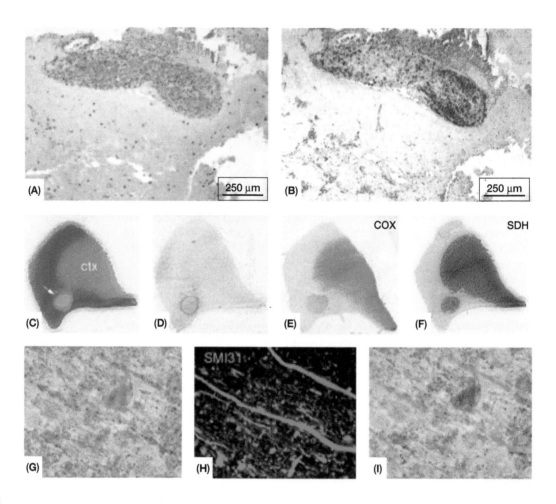

FIGURE 3.1

Pass through pathology at the time of early needle biopsy of selected cases with MS show focal meningeal infiltrates with T cells (CD3) (A) and B cells (CD20) (B). Adopted from [17]. Low magnification images of a chronic active MS lesion in the WM identified by luxol fast blue staining (C), and HLA immunoreactivity at the edge of the lesion (D). The mitochondrial respiratory chain complex IV activity (cytochrome c oxidase [COX], stained brown) and complex II activity (succinate dehydrogenase [SDH], stained blue) are increased within the chronic active MS lesion as judged by COX/SDH histochemistry (E–F). Sequential COX histochemistry (G) and immunofluorescent labeling of phosphorylated neurofilament (SMI31 in red) (H) in a chronic active MS lesion identified numerous complex IV active mitochondria within the demyelinated axons (I) illustrating part of the axonal mitochondrial response to demyelination.

Neuropathological estimates of percentage neuronal loss in MS GM vary depending on anatomical location and glial pathology (lesions): hippocampus (CA1, CA3-2, and CA4) approximately 23% loss with hippocampal GM lesions showing significantly more neuronal loss than those without lesions (36% vs. 28%) [13], neocortical lesions in frontal and temporal lobes have shown an average of 10% loss of neurons while the association with B-cell follicles within the meninges was linked to an approximate 40% and 50% pyramidal neuron loss (in layers III and V) [14]. In the thalamus, extent of neuron loss was reported to be around 35%. Neuronal loss in MS is also apparent in the spinal cord with 36%, 15%, and 23% loss in cervical, thoracic, and lumbar ventral horn neurons in one study and approximately 75% loss of neurons in thoracic and lumbar GM in another.

The damage to neurons and loss of synapses and apoptotic neurons provide further evidence of neuronal pathology in MS [15–17]. Synaptic loss in MS was apparent in type 3 or subpial lesions as well as hippocampal lesions.

In both actively demyelinating cortical lesions from biopsy material and GM tissue from autopsy cases, there was an association between neuronal injury and inflammation, either within the parenchyma or meninges [14,17,18].

PATHOPHYSIOLOGY OF NEURODEGENERATION IN MS

Fundamentally different concepts have been proposed for the mechanisms of neurodegeneration in MS: (a) as a direct result of inflammation, (b) related but independent of inflammation, or (c) MS as a primary neurodegenerative disorder where inflammation is secondary.

Mechanisms of Neuronal Degeneration

Neuronal loss in MS, at least in part, is because of the inflammation (cortical and meningeal), as evident in biopsy material containing active GM lesions and autopsy material from the end stage of the disease. In addition, there is robust evidence of a compromised bioenergetics status, judged by the mitochondria, within neurons in cortical lesions, as well as in nonlesional GM in MS.

Energy in the form of adenosine triphosphate (ATP) is most efficiently produced by the mitochondrial respiratory chain, which is encoded by both the nuclear genome and the mitochondrial DNA (mtDNA). The studies of nonlesional motor cortex from progressive MS cases identified a decrease in a number of nuclear DNA encoded subunits and an associated loss of respiratory chain enzyme activity (complex I and complex III) [19,20]. Furthermore, mtDNA deletions at high levels appear to render a proportion of cortical neurons biochemically deficient (devoid of the terminal complex of the electron transport chain or mitochondrial respiratory chain complex IV). The resulting impaired capacity to produce ATP is likely to compromise neuronal function and increase the susceptibility to further insult such as excitotoxicity. Furthermore, mitochondrial dysfunction is likely to imbalance calcium buffering in neurons and increase the production of reactive oxygen species and subsequent oxidative damage [21,22].

Mechanisms of Axonal Degeneration

Axonal damage or loss can be the result of several mechanisms: (a) inflammatory axonal transection (inflammatory neurodegeneration), (b) chronic demyelination-related axonal transection and degeneration, (c) Wallerian degeneration, (d) ischemia or pressure-related mechanical damage from surrounding edema.

Inflammatory Axonopathy

The correlation between the extent of axonal transection and the degree of inflammation suggests a causative role in MS [11,12,23], although direct evidence from clinical trials using anti-inflammatory agents is not yet available. In particular, CD8+ T lymphocytes, macrophages, and microglia have been implicated in inflammatory axonopathy. CD8 T lymphocytes may facilitate axonal damage through secretion of perforins resulting in pore formation on cell membranes and subsequent entry of ions. Further, nitric oxide, proteolytic enzymes, cytokines, and free radicals produced by macrophages in active and chronic active MS lesions may lead to axonopathy, particularly of demyelinated axons. Activated microglia surround axonal ovoids in the NLWM (likely owing to Wallerian degeneration) and damaged neuritis (non-phosphorylated NF+) in the GM lesions. Although microglia can mediate inflammation in neurodegenerative diseases, whether the association with ovoids and neuritis is deleterious or protective is unknown. Evidence for an immune response directed specifically against axons in the CNS is lacking.

Chronic Demyelination-Related Axonopathy

The presence of axonal ovoids (indicating recent transection) in chronically demyelinated axons in the center of chronic active lesions and inactive lesions suggests a pathogenic role for chronic demyelination in axonal damage [11,12,23].

Myelin gene defects in humans provide insight into the dependency of axons on myelin. Pelizaeus–Merzbacher disease (PMD) is a human neurodegenerative disease due to proteolipid protein (PLP) gene mutations, deletions, or duplications, which affects the CNS and causes spastic paraplegia, cerebellar ataxia, psychomotor developmental delay, and dystonia [24,25]. The pathological processes in myelin gene defects are likely to be due to the gain of toxic functions rather than due to loss of physiological functions.

The chronically demyelinated axons are at risk of further damage due to exposure to cytokines and other proinflammatory agents. Several studies have associated relapses or recurrence of symptoms associated with previous relapses, with upregulation of systemic cytokines. Although these inflammatory agents may not damage the demyelinated axons directly, they anatomically identify axons that are vulnerable (at risk) and subsequently may cause irreversible disability through chronic demyelination-related axonopathy.

Recent studies have defined the axonal mitochondrial response to demyelination: increase in mitochondrial content and activity within demyelinated axons, as well as increase in the size of stationary mitochondria and increase in speed of motile mitochondria (Figure 3.1C–I) [26]. This response appears to be homeostatic as the loss of mitochondrial activity and presence within demyelinated axons was associated with the degeneration of chronically demyelinated axons in MS.

Axonal Loss Secondary to Wallerian Degeneration

Wallerian degeneration, which follows axonal transection, entails the breakdown of the distal portion of the axon and the removal of the corresponding myelin sheath. The disintegration of the axonal cytoskeleton is thought to be due to the activation of proteases and the rise in intracellular calcium. Once transected, the axon may continue to conduct up to a week. In the CNS, axonal loss due to Wallerian degeneration may occur within days with immediate functional consequences, while the loss of myelin may occur over months or years following the initial axonal transection. Axonal loss of 22% in NLWM, in the absence of loss of myelin, was reported distal to a brain stem lesion of approximately 9 months duration since diagnosis.

SUMMARY

With the newly recognized GM pathology in MS, it is now clear that inflammation, demyelination, and neurodegeneration in MS are shared by both the WM and the GM. There is a gathering body of evidence implicating meningeal inflammation in the genesis of cortical pathology. Furthermore, accumulation of mitochondrial defects appear to compromise bioenergetics within the GM and WM in MS, which is likely to increase the susceptibility of neurons and axons to further insults such as excitotoxicity. It is hoped that a better understanding of mechanisms of neurodegeneration in MS will be an important step toward identifying effective therapy for progressive forms of MS.

REFERENCES

1. Fisher E, Lee JC, Nakamura K, et al. Gray matter atrophy in multiple sclerosis: A longitudinal study. *Ann Neurol.* 2008;64:255–265.

2. Geurts JJ, Bo L, Pouwels PJ, et al. Cortical lesions in multiple sclerosis: Combined postmortem MR imaging and histopathology. *AJNR Am J Neuroradiol.* 2005;26:572–577.

3. Tallantyre EC, Morgan PS, Dixon JE, et al. 3 Tesla and 7 Tesla MRI of multiple sclerosis cortical lesions. *J Magn Reson Imaging.* 2010;32:971–977.

4. Lucchinetti C, Bruck W, Parisi J, et al. Heterogeneity of multiple sclerosis lesions: Implications for the pathogenesis of demyelination. *Ann Neurol.* 2000;47:707–717.

5. Henderson AP, Barnett MH, Parratt JD, et al. Multiple sclerosis: Distribution of inflammatory cells in newly forming lesions. *Ann Neurol.* 2009;66:739–753.

6. Cannela B, Raine CS. The adhesion molecule and cytokine profile of multiple sclerosis lesions. *Ann Neurol.* 1995;37:424–435.

7. Simpson JE, Newcombe J, Cuzner ML, et al. Expression of the interferon-gamma-inducible chemokines IP-10 and Mig and their receptor, CXCR3, in multiple sclerosis lesions. *Neuropathol Appl Neurobiol.* 2000;26:133–142.

8. Sorensen TL, Tani M, Jensen J, et al. Expression of specific chemokines and chemokine receptors in the central nervous system of multiple sclerosis patients. *J Clin Invest.* 1999;103:807–815.

9. Mahad DJ, Howell SJ, Woodroofe MN. Expression of chemokines in the CSF and correlation with clinical disease activity in patients with multiple sclerosis. *J Neurol Neurosurg Psychiatry.* 2002;72:498–502.

10. Bjartmar C, Kinkel RP, Kidd G, et al. Axonal loss in normal-appearing white matter in a patient with acute MS. *Neurology.* 2001;57:1248–1252.

11. Bitsch A, Schuchardt J, Bunkowski S, et al. Acute axonal injury in multiple sclerosis. Correlation with demyelination and inflammation. *Brain.* 2000;123(Pt 6):1174–1183.

12. Trapp BD, Peterson J, Ransohoff RM, et al. Axonal transection in the lesions of multiple sclerosis. *N Engl J Med.* 1998;338:278–285.

13. Papadopoulos D, Dukes S, Patel R, et al. Substantial archaeocortical atrophy and neuronal loss in multiple sclerosis. *Brain Pathol.* 2009;19(2):238–253.

14. Magliozzi R, Howell OW, Reeves C, et al. A gradient of neuronal loss and meningeal inflammation in multiple sclerosis. *Ann Neurol.* 2010;68:477–493.

15. Peterson JW, Bo L, Mork S, et al. Transected neurites, apoptotic neurons, and reduced inflammation in cortical multiple sclerosis lesions. *Ann Neurol.* 2001;50:389–400.

16. Wegner C, Esiri MM, Chance SA, et al. Neocortical neuronal, synaptic, and glial loss in multiple sclerosis. *Neurology.* 2006;67:960–967.

17. Lucchinetti CF, Popescu BF, Bunyan RF, et al. Inflammatory cortical demyelination in early multiple sclerosis. *N Engl J Med.* 2011;365:2188–2197.

18. Vogt J, Paul F, Aktas O, et al. Lower motor neuron loss in multiple sclerosis and experimental autoimmune encephalomyelitis. *Ann Neurol.* 2009;66:310–322.

19. Broadwater L, Pandit A, Clements R, et al. Analysis of the mitochondrial proteome in multiple sclerosis cortex. *Biochim Biophys Acta.* 2011;1812:630–641.

20. Dutta R, McDonough J, Yin X, et al. Mitochondrial dysfunction as a cause of axonal degeneration in multiple sclerosis patients. *Ann Neurol.* 2006;59:478–489.

21. Fischer MT, Sharma R, Lim JL, et al. NADPH oxidase expression in active multiple sclerosis lesions in relation to oxidative tissue damage and mitochondrial injury. *Brain.* 2012;135:886–899.

22. Trevelyan AJ, Kirby DM, Smulders-Srinivasan TK, et al. Mitochondrial DNA mutations affect calcium handling in differentiated neurons. *Brain.* 2010;133:787–796.

23. Ferguson B, Matyszak MK, Esiri MM, et al. Axonal damage in acute multiple sclerosis lesions. *Brain.* 1997;120(Pt 3):393–399.

24. Garbern J, Cambi F, Shy M, et al. The molecular pathogenesis of Pelizaeus-Merzbacher disease. *Arch Neurol.* 1999;56:1210–1214.

25. Inoue K, Osaka H, Imaizumi K, et al. Proteolipid protein gene duplications causing Pelizaeus-Merzbacher disease: Molecular mechanism and phenotypic manifestations. *Ann Neurol.* 1999;45:624–632.

26. Mahad DJ, Ziabreva I, Campbell G, et al. Mitochondrial changes within axons in multiple sclerosis. *Brain.* 2009;132:1161–1174.

4

Epidemiology and Natural History of Multiple Sclerosis

MARCUS W. KOCH

KEY POINTS FOR CLINICIANS

- The incidence and prevalence of multiple sclerosis (MS) varies between different geographical regions and ethnicities.

- MS is a lifelong disease, the overall survival of patients with MS is about 6 years shorter than that of the general population.

- The environmental risk factors, vitamin D (deficiency), and smoking influence the risk of developing MS, as well as the disease course.

- Sex, age at onset, and onset symptoms cannot reliably predict the disease course.

- The times to landmark disability have recently been found to be longer than initially reported, with a time to expanded disability status scale (EDSS) 6.0 of about 30 years overall, and about 15 years in primary progressive MS. There is significant variation in time to reach this landmark.

- While the concept of benign MS has been challenged in recent years, a substantial number of patients have a mild long-term disease course.

EPIDEMIOLOGY, SURVIVAL, INCIDENCE, AND PREVALENCE OF MULTIPLE SCLEROSIS

In comparison to other diseases of the central nervous system such as stroke, epilepsy, and traumatic brain injury, multiple sclerosis (MS) is a relatively uncommon disease. MS has a protracted disease course, with often long periods of clinical stability, and can be viewed as a lifelong condition; the overall survival of patients with MS is about 6 years less than that of the general population [1].

> People with MS die about 6 years earlier than the general population.

MS is newly diagnosed in about 1 in 20,000 people per year (incidence) and affects about 1 in 1,000 people (prevalence) [2]. The incidence and prevalence of MS are, however, highly variable between different geographical areas. The prevalence of MS increases with latitude, such that the countries farthest from the equator have the highest prevalence of MS, while countries closer to the equator have a lower prevalence. For example, MS affects about 1 in 400 people in Canada [3], but only 1 in 5,000 people in Brazil [4]. Several factors are believed to contribute to this latitudinal difference. The influence of increased vitamin D production due to a greater exposure to sunlight in countries closer to the equator is an explaining factor (see following discussion on environmental risk factors). Ethnic differences between countries could also contribute.

It appears that people of European descent may be especially susceptible to MS, while those of Asian and African descent may be less susceptible. This is illustrated best by epidemiological studies from around the world which compare the prevalence of MS among different ethnical groups living together in the same area: one study in Israel, for instance, showed that Jews of European extraction had a much higher prevalence of MS (68 per 100,000) than Arabs (11 per 100,000). A South African study showed that whites had a much higher prevalence (26 per 100,000) than both Indians (8 per 100,000) and blacks (0.22 per 100,000) [5]. Similar findings were also seen in New Zealand, where the prevalence of MS among people of European descent was much higher (103 per 100,000) than that among the Maoris (16 per 100,000) [6]. MS is rare in Southeast Asia, with prevalence in the range of 1.4 per 100,000 in Shanghai, China [7] to 3.6 per 100,000 in South Korea [8]. The reason for the influence of ethnicity on MS prevalence is not understood.

> The prevalence of MS differs between geographical locations and ethnicities. For example, MS affects about 1 in 400 people in Canada, but only 1 in 5,000 people in Brazil.

In the vast majority of patients, MS presents with a relapse, and the subsequent disease course is characterized by relapses and remissions: relapsing-remitting MS (RRMS). In about 10% of all patients with MS, the disease begins with a slow and relentless accumulation of disability, usually without any relapses. This form of the disease is called primary progressive MS (PPMS). In the longer term, most patients with RRMS experience a change in their disease course from the period with relapses and remissions to a more uniform and slow worsening of symptoms. This is called secondary progressive MS (SPMS). SPMS patients may continue to have relapses or cease having relapses, but the relapse rate tends to be less later in the disease course.

The median age at disease onset is around 30 years in RRMS and around 40 years in PPMS, the conversion to SPMS also occurs around a median age of 40 years. Women have a slightly, up to several years, earlier onset than men.

RRMS occurs more commonly in women, with a female-to-male ratio that was classically given as about 2. Recently, it has been found that this sex ratio of MS has changed in the last decade, so that it is now even more common in women, with the ratio of women-to-men with MS increasing from 1.4 in 1955 to 2.3 in 2000 [9]. The reason for this increase is unknown. PPMS affects men and women equally.

> RRMS occurs about twice as often in women than in men. PPMS affects men and women equally.

ENVIRONMENTAL RISK FACTORS FOR MS

While research on environmental risk factors for MS is ongoing and many possible risk factors are being investigated, 3 environmental risk factors, vitamin D, Epstein–Barr virus (EBV) infection, and smoking, currently have the most convincing evidence to support them.

Vitamin D has recently been found to influence the risk of developing MS. The best evidence for this comes from an investigation of routine blood samples in U.S. military personnel. Routine medical examinations for U.S. military personnel include the drawing of a blood sample, which is then stored. One study investigated 25 hydroxy-vitamin D levels in these blood samples and related the vitamin D level to the subsequent risk of developing MS in a nested case-control study. This included 257 people who developed MS and 2 matched controls per case drawn from over 7 million people registered in the U.S. Department of Defense Serum Repository. In the study, it was found that the risk of developing MS decreases with rising serum vitamin D levels (odds ratio 0.59 per 50 nmol/L increase in vitamin D serum level) [10]. Further studies suggest an association of vitamin D levels and the risk of developing MS with exposure to ultraviolet light: a retrospective Australian study showed that actinic skin damage (which occurs as a consequence of too much exposure to ultraviolet light), as well as the (remembered) time spent in the sun during childhood were associated with a lower risk of developing MS [11]. The reason for the latitudinal variation in MS risk is most likely the lower exposure to ultraviolet light at higher latitudes, and the subsequent lower levels of vitamin D.

> A low serum level of vitamin D is a risk factor for MS.

Studies on the influence of infections with EBV on MS risk are made difficult by the fact that the great majority (around 95%) of adults is seropositive for EBV, which makes for large required sample sizes. A recent meta-analysis on EBV and MS risk including 1,779 people with MS and 2,526 control persons showed that seronegativity for EBV is associated with a very low risk of developing MS (odds ratio of 0.06) [12]. Another large meta-analysis showed that a history of infectious mononucleosis (symptomatic EBV) was associated with a roughly doubled risk of developing MS (relative risk 2.17) [13].

> The reason for the latitudinal variation in MS risk is most likely the exposure to ultraviolet light at higher latitudes, and the subsequent lower levels of vitamin D.

Good evidence for the influence of smoking on the risk of developing MS comes from the two Nurses' Health Studies, each including more than 100,000 women.

An analysis of these studies showed an increased risk of MS among current (relative incidence rate compared to non-smokers: 1.6) as well as former smokers (relative incidence rate: 1.2). There also was a suggestion of dose dependency, with the relative incidence increasing with increasing pack years [14]. Further studies have since shown that second-hand smoke is associated with a higher risk of MS among children [15] and adults [16].

> Smoking and secondhand smoke are risk factors for MS.

THE NATURAL HISTORY OF MS

Studies on the natural history of MS have usually investigated how certain risk factors are related to the arrival at certain landmark disability levels. Typically, the time to a landmark disability score (such as expanded disability status scale [EDSS] 6.0, when patients need a cane for walking) was measured from disease onset. Early studies reported a relatively quick progression from disease onset to EDSS 6.0, with a median time from disease onset of RRMS in the range of 15 [17] to 20 [18] years, but newer studies have corrected these estimates to a median time from onset of around 30 years [19,20]. Early studies on the natural history of PPMS reported very short median times to EDSS 6.0 of less than 10 years [17,18]. More recent studies have corrected these to a median time from disease onset of around 15 years [21]. It should be noted that there is a very wide interpersonal variation in the progression of MS. Even within PPMS, which is thought to be the most uniform of the disease courses, the time to EDSS 6.0 ranged from around 8 years in 25% of patients with the quickest progression to more than 25 years in the 25% with the slowest progression [21].

> The accumulation of disability in MS is slower than previously thought and varies widely between individuals.

The classical epidemiological studies on risk factors for disease progression suggested that factors such as female gender and an early age at disease onset were associated with a better prognosis, although more recent studies show that the influence of risk factors is more complex. In studies which measure the time from disease onset to landmark disability, women and patients with an early disease onset take longer to reach landmark disability scores, such as EDSS 6.0. If we consider the age at which a landmark disability score is reached, this changes: men and women reach an EDSS score of 6.0 at a similar age [19]. Patients with an early disease onset seem to be at an advantage, as their time to EDSS 6.0 is significantly longer than that of patients with a late disease onset. On the other hand, if the age at EDSS 6.0 is considered, these patients are actually at a considerable disadvantage as they reach this outcome at

a younger age [19,22]. These studies suggest that disability accumulation in MS is at least partly dependent on age, rather than on gender or the age at onset. Onset symptoms are not clearly and consistently related to the overall MS prognosis.

> Estimates of progression to EDSS 6.0 show a median time from onset of around 30 years.

Ethnic differences in MS are not well researched to date. There is some indication that ethnic differences are not only associated with the risk of developing MS (see earlier paragraph) but also with the disease course. Two retrospective studies showed that adult blacks required a cane at a shorter time from onset than whites [23], and that black children with MS had a higher relapse rate than white children [24].

> Disability accumulation in MS occurs in 2 phases.

Another important issue that can be learned from natural history studies is the fact that risk factors affect the early rather than the late disease phase. One large population-based study showed that the time from onset to the landmark disability scores of EDSS 4.0, 6.0 and 7.0 was influenced by such risk factors as sex, age at onset, and number of relapses in the first years from onset, but that none of these factors influences the time from EDSS 4.0 to EDSS 6.0 or 7.0 [25]. This suggests that these risk factors only exert their influence at disability levels below EDSS 4.0, but that beyond this point the disease follows a more uniform course independent of any of these factors. Another epidemiological study from a different cohort confirmed these findings, and showed that the influence of risk factors already ended at a disability level of EDSS 3.0 [26]. This last study also showed that the time between disease onset and the assignment of EDSS 3.0 was highly variable, while the time from EDSS 3.0 to EDSS 6.0 was much more uniform. Taken together, these studies suggest that MS is a disease with 2 phases of disability accumulation: an early phase of variable duration, which is partly influenced by such risk factors as sex and the age at onset, and a late phase with a more uniform duration, that proceeds independent of any of the known risk factors.

> Time to progress from EDSS 4.0 to 6.0 is consistent no matter what prior course or type of MS the patient has.

> The known risk factors influence the disease course only up to a disability level of EDSS 3.0 or 4.0

ENVIRONMENTAL RISK FACTORS AND THE NATURAL HISTORY OF MS

The previously discussed environmental risk factors for MS of smoking and vitamin D status not only influence the risk of developing MS, but also the disease course (the role of EBV infection in the course of MS is less clear). Smoking leads to an increase in EDSS scores in the short term [27], and is associated with a faster increase in T2 MRI lesions, and faster brain atrophy [28]. The role of smoking for the longer term outcomes, however, is less clear: one study suggested that smoking was neither associated with the risk of secondary progression, nor with that of reaching EDSS 4.0 or EDSS 6.0 [29], whereas other studies showed a greater risk of smokers to progress to secondary progression [28,30]. While more research is needed to determine the role of smoking in the different stages of MS, patients should clearly be encouraged to stop smoking, not only because of the general health benefits that will bring them, but also because of the particular negative influence smoking has on MS. Studies on vitamin D status and the disease course of MS showed that that lower vitamin D levels are associated with higher levels of disability [31] and that higher levels of vitamin D are associated with a lower risk of relapse in adults and children [32,33]. While evidence from randomized controlled trials is still lacking, it would appear wise to at least avoid vitamin D deficiency in patients with MS.

BENIGN MS

Several "rules of thumb" have been proposed to help advise patients about their prognosis. We have previously described that having a particular onset symptom, sex, or age at onset cannot be used to accurately predict the prognosis.

The concept of "benign MS" reflects the idea that people with a slow disease progression in the beginning of the disease often remain at a low level of disability later. It was proposed that a disability level of EDSS 3.0 or lower 10 years after disease onset were indicative of an overall mild disease course. Such patients with "benign MS" constitute about 20% of the MS population and were believed to have very little risk of further worsening in the later disease course. One study followed-up patients for up to 20 years and showed that patients with an EDSS score of 2.0 or lower at 10 years had more than a 90% chance of remaining below a score of EDSS 4.5 at 20 years [20]. Recently, this idea has been challenged by a larger study examining patients with a disability level of EDSS 3.0 or lower at 10 years. Of these patients, a little more than one-half had progressed beyond EDSS 3.0 at 20 years' follow-up, and about 20% had progressed beyond EDSS 6.0 [34]. However, with around 80% of the initial cohort still not requiring the use of a cane at 20 years follow-up, it would appear that the concept of benign MS still has some merit. While patients with a mild disease course in the first 10 years of the disease cannot be guaranteed a benign disease course, there is such a thing as mild disease, and patients may be somewhat reassured that a sudden change in their disease course would be unlikely.

KEY POINTS FOR PATIENTS AND FAMILIES

- The overall prognosis of MS is difficult to predict in individual patients.
- Patient characteristics such as sex, age at onset, or onset symptoms cannot reliably predict the future disease course.
- Recently, environmental risk factors, vitamin D (deficiency), and smoking have been shown to influence the risk of developing MS, as well as the disease course.
- Patients with MS should not smoke, not only because of the general ill health effects, but also because there is good evidence to support a negative influence of smoking on the disease course of MS.
- A low serum level of vitamin D is associated with a worse disease course of MS, and vitamin D supplementation should be considered if patients are found to be deficient.
- The overall prognosis of MS, as expressed in times to landmark disability, has recently been found to be better than initially reported, with a time to EDSS 6.0 of about 30 years overall, and about 15 years in PPMS.
- While the concept of benign MS has been challenged in recent years, a substantial number of patients have a mild long-term disease course.

REFERENCES

1. Kingwell E, van der Kop M, Zhao Y, et al. Relative mortality and survival in multiple sclerosis: Findings from British Columbia, Canada. *J Neurol Neurosurg Psychiatr.* 2012;83:61–66.

2. Koch-Henriksen N, Sørensen PS. The changing demographic pattern of multiple sclerosis epidemiology. *Lancet Neurol.* 2010;9:520–532.

3. Beck CA, Metz LM, Svenson LW, Patten SB. Regional variation of multiple sclerosis prevalence in Canada. *Mult Scler.* 2005;11:516–519.

4. Callegaro D, Goldbaum M, Morais L, et al. The prevalence of multiple sclerosis in the city of São Paulo, Brazil, 1997. *Acta Neurol Scand.* 2001;104:208–213.

5. Bhigjee AI, Moodley K, Ramkissoon K. Multiple sclerosis in KwaZulu Natal, South Africa: An epidemiological and clinical study. *Mult Scler.* 2007;13:1095–1099.

6. Taylor BV, Pearson JF, Clarke G, et al. MS prevalence in New Zealand, an ethnically and latitudinally diverse country. *Mult Scler.* 2010;16:1422–1431.

7. Cheng Q, Miao L, Zhang J, et al. A population-based survey of multiple sclerosis in Shanghai, China. *Neurology.* 2007;68:1495–1500.

8. Kim NH, Kim HJ, Cheong HK, et al. Prevalence of multiple sclerosis in Korea. *Neurology.* 2010;75:1432–1438.

9. Alonso A, Hernán MA. Temporal trends in the incidence of multiple sclerosis: A systematic review. *Neurology.* 2008;71:129–135.

10. Munger KL, Levin LI, Hollis BW, et al. Serum 25-hydroxyvitamin D levels and risk of multiple sclerosis. *JAMA.* 2006;296:2832–2838.

11. van der Mei IAF, Ponsonby AL, Dwyer T, et al. Past exposure to sun, skin phenotype, and risk of multiple sclerosis: Case-control study. *BMJ.* 2003;327:316.

12. Ascherio A, Munger KL. Environmental risk factors for multiple sclerosis. Part I: The role of infection. *Ann Neurol.* 2007;61:288–299.

13. Handel AE, Williamson AJ, Disanto G, et al. An updated meta-analysis of risk of multiple sclerosis following infectious mononucleosis. *PLoS One.* 2010;5:ii.

14. Hernán MA, Olek MJ, Ascherio A. Cigarette smoking and incidence of multiple sclerosis. *Am J Epidemiol.* 2001;154:69–74.

15. Mikaeloff Y, Caridade G, Tardieu M, Suissa S. Parental smoking at home and the risk of childhood-onset multiple sclerosis in children. *Brain.* 2007;130:2589–2595.

16. Hedström A, Bäärnhielm M, Olsson T, Alfredsson L. Exposure to environmental tobacco smoke is associated with increased risk for multiple sclerosis. *Mult Scler.* 2011;17:788–793.

17. Weinshenker BG, Bass B, Rice GP, et al. The natural history of multiple sclerosis: A geographically based study. I. Clinical course and disability. *Brain.* 1989;112(Pt 1):133–146.

18. Confavreux C, Vukusic S, Moreau T, Adeleine P. Relapses and progression of disability in multiple sclerosis. *N Engl J Med.* 2000;343:1430–1438.

19. Tremlett H, Paty D, Devonshire V. Disability progression in multiple sclerosis is slower than previously reported. *Neurology.* 2006;66:172–177.

20. Pittock SJ, Mayr WT, McClelland RL, et al. Change in MS-related disability in a population-based cohort: A 10-year follow-up study. *Neurology.* 2004;62:51–59.

21. Koch M, Kingwell E, Rieckmann P, Tremlett H. The natural history of primary progressive multiple sclerosis. *Neurology.* 2009;73:1996–2002.

22. Confavreux C, Vukusic S. Age at disability milestones in multiple sclerosis. *Brain.* 2006;129:595–605.

23. Cree BA, Khan O, Bourdette D, et al. Clinical characteristics of African Americans vs Caucasian Americans with multiple sclerosis. *Neurology.* 2004;63:2039–2045.

24. Boster AL, Endress CF, Hreha SA, et al. Pediatric-onset multiple sclerosis in African-American Black and European-origin White patients. *Pediatr Neurol.* 2009;40:31–33.

25. Confavreux C, Vukusic S, Adeleine P. Early clinical predictors and progression of irreversible disability in multiple sclerosis: An amnesic process. *Brain.* 2003;126:770–782.

26. Leray E, Yaouang J, Le Page E, et al. Evidence for a two-stage disability progression in multiple sclerosis. *Brain.* 2010;133:1900–1913.

27. Pittas F, Ponsonby AL, van der Mei IAF, et al. Smoking is associated with progressive disease course and increased progression in clinical disability in a prospective cohort of people with multiple sclerosis. *J Neurol.* 2009;256:577–585.

28. Healy BC, Ali EN, Guttmann CR, et al. Smoking and disease progression in multiple sclerosis. *Arch Neurol.* 2009;66:858–864.

29. Koch M, van Harten A, Uyttenboogaart M, De Keyser J. Cigarette smoking and progression in multiple sclerosis. *Neurology.* 2007;69:1515–1520.

30. Hernán MA, Jick SS, Logroscino G, et al. Cigarette smoking and the progression of multiple sclerosis. *Brain.* 2005;128:1461–1465.

31. Smolders J, Menheere P, Kessels A, et al. Association of vitamin D metabolite levels with relapse rate and disability in multiple sclerosis. *Mult Scler.* 2008;14:1220–1224.

32. Simpson S, Taylor B, Blizzard L, et al. Higher 25-hydroxyvitamin D is associated with lower relapse risk in multiple sclerosis. *Ann Neurol.* 2010;68:193–203.

33. Mowry EM, Krupp LB, Milazzo M, et al. Vitamin D status is associated with relapse rate in pediatric-onset multiple sclerosis. *Ann Neurol.* 2010;67:618–624.

34. Sayao AL, Devonshire V, Tremlett H. Longitudinal follow-up of "benign" multiple sclerosis at 20 years. *Neurology.* 2007;68:496–500.

5

Multiple Sclerosis Genetics

BRUCE A. C. CREE

KEY POINTS FOR CLINICIANS

- Family aggregation and the studies of twins indicate that heredity contributes to multiple sclerosis (MS) risk.

- The primary MS susceptibility locus is within the major histocompatibility complex and encodes a protein, HLA-DRB1*15, that has a critical function in presenting antigens to T cells.

- Over 50 other genetic loci throughout the genome contribute to MS susceptibility.

- Many of these loci are associated with other autoimmune diseases, which suggest one or more common biological pathways in autoimmunity.

- The majority of identified MS susceptibility loci thus far are polymorphisms (which are common genetic alleles also found in healthy individuals), although rare risk alleles have been identified in some families.

- Genetic variants in the vitamin D enzymatic pathway are associated with MS susceptibility and underscore the importance of vitamin D's role in MS.

- Approximately 15% to 20% of MS patients reported a family history of MS.

- Risk of MS in monozygotic twins is about 25%, in dizygotic twins is 5%, first-degree relatives of MS patients is 3% to 5%, and children of 2 parents with MS is 30%.

RACE AND GEOGRAPHY

Race and geography are known to influence the prevalence of multiple sclerosis (MS). This suggests that heritable factors may contribute to MS pathogenesis [1]. The risk of MS is much higher in populations of northern European ancestry than in other ethnic groups residing at the same latitudes [2–5]. It follows that this increased susceptibility might be due to genetic differences between ethnic groups. MS is approximately 50% less common in blacks compared to whites [6,7]. MS is still less common in both native Japanese and Japanese Americans (5 per 100,000) compared to northern European populations (100 to 150 per 100,000) [8]. Similarly, MS is relatively less common among Native

Americans in both the United States and Canada [9–12]. These observations lead to the hypothesis that genetic traits for MS risk may be enriched in certain populations and occur less frequently in others, thereby contributing to these racial patterns. However, despite a generally shared environment, ethnic factors that can track with race, such as diet, might also account for such differences.

FAMILIAL AGGREGATION

Although first described as a sporadic disease, the familial occurrence of MS was recognized in the late 19th century [13,14]. Systematic studies of familial aggregation in MS support a genetic contribution to the disease [15–21]. These studies found that approximately 15% to 20% of MS patients reported a family history of MS, a proportion that is significantly higher than what would be expected on the basis of the relatively low prevalence of MS in these populations. The ratio of the relative risk of disease in siblings of affected individuals compared to the relative risk of disease in the overall population is referred to as λ_s [22]. For MS, this risk ratio is approximately 15 to 40 indicating a moderately strong familial influence on MS risk [23]. To help place the relevance of this value in the context of other heritable complex diseases, the λ_s ratio for MS is higher than that of schizophrenia (9), similar to that of type 1 diabetes (15), and less than that for autism (60) [24]. However, commonly shared environmental factors might also explain such familial aggregation [25].

> Systematic studies of familial aggregation in MS support a genetic contribution to the disease.

Twin Studies

The most compelling observation indicating that MS susceptibility has a genetic component comes from twin studies that demonstrate concordance rates of approximately 30% in monozygotic twins and 3% to 5% in dizygotic twins [26–28]. The rate for fraternal twins is similar to that of first-degree relatives of MS patients. Conjugal pair studies also show that the risk of MS increases substantially if both parents are affected by MS, again implying a heritable component to MS susceptibility (Table 5.1) [29–31]. Taken together, familial and population-based studies indicate that some component of MS risk is heritable; however, that the majority of MS patients have no family history indicates either that environmental factors may outweigh genetic risks or that genetic risk can be attributed to the influence of multiple traits that by

themselves have low disease penetrance. The concept that MS risk may be inherited as a complex trait rather than following simple Mendelian inheritance patterns, as is the case for recessive mutations such as cystic fibrosis or dominant mutations like Huntington's disease, is essential for understanding the genetic contributions to MS risk (Figure 5.1).

> The most compelling observation indicating that MS susceptibility has a genetic component comes from twin studies that demonstrate concordance rates of approximately 30% in monozygotic twins and 3% to 5% in dizygotic twins.

THE FIRST MOLECULAR MARKERS FOR MS: HUMAN LEUKOCYTE ANTIGENS

The first studies that identified a link between MS heredity and genetic variation compared human leukocyte antigen (HLA) protein polymorphisms between MS cases and healthy controls. These early studies found that cell surface antigens present on the membranes of peripheral blood mononuclear cells were overrepresented in MS patients compared to unaffected controls. The first such antigens were HLA-A3 [34–36], followed by HLA-B7, and then HLA-DRw2 [37–41]. These HLA associations were in fact not independent, but rather reflected a common shared haplotype as a consequence of linkage disequilibrium. Linkage disequilibrium refers to the observation that alleles of certain neighboring genes tend to be inherited together as a consequence of natural selection, although the driving factors for such selection may be obscure. Thus the molecules HLA-A3, HLA-B7, and HLA-DRw2 are closely associated especially in populations of European descent. Further elucidation as to which, or possibly more than one, of these linked genes contributes to MS genetics required development of improved molecular techniques.

TABLE 5.1
Familial Risks for MS

RELATIONSHIP TO PATIENT	MS RISK (%)	RISK RELATIVE TO GENERAL POPULATION	PROPORTION OF GENETIC SHARING (%)
Adopted first-degree relative	0.2	Same as general population	0
Sibling with MS	3.0–5.0	15–25-fold increase	50
Dizygotic twin	3.0–5.0	15–25-fold increase	50
Monozygotic twin	34	170-fold increase	100
Child of 1 parent with MS	3.0–5.0	15–25-fold increase	50
Child of 2 parents with MS	6–10	30–50-fold increase	50% with each parent

Assumes lifetime population prevalence of 0.2% [30,32].
MS, multiple sclerosis.

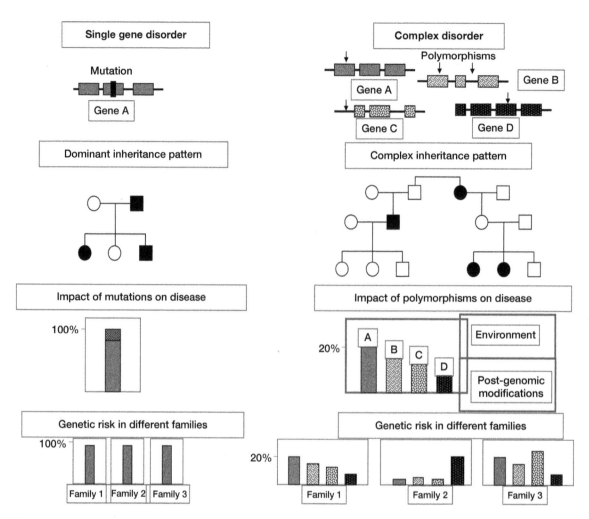

FIGURE 5.1

The inheritance pattern of a dominantly transmitted single gene mutation is contrasted with that of a complex polygenic disorder in which polymorphisms, as well as environmental factors and post-genomic modifications, contribute to the disease phenotype. Unlike the dominantly inherited trait that has high penetrance (the likelihood of developing the phenotype associated with the genotype) whose phenotype can be traced from one generation to the next, the inheritance pattern of a complex polygenic disorder may not be readily apparent from studying the family tree. Furthermore, unlike single gene disorders, polygenic traits could have different phenotypes across families. *Modified from [33].*

LINKAGE ANALYSIS

In the 1980s, new DNA-based technology was developed for studying Mendelian patterns of inheritance, first with restriction fragment length polymorphisms (RFLPs) followed by microsatellite repeats [42,43]. Using RFLPs to dissect the molecular contributions of the HLA locus to MS susceptibility, it became clear that alleles of HLA-DR2 are the major contributors to MS risk [44]. These new molecular techniques not only allowed for dissection of linked genes at HLA but also made possible the ability to screen for other associations with MS found at many other positions across the genome. By studying the linkage between an inherited trait and DNA markers in families with some members affected by a heritable disease, it was possible to identify the chromosomal location of disease-causing genes (Figure 5.2A,B). Markers that were physically near the disease-causing gene were likely to be inherited along with the disease trait because recombination between genetic loci occurs less frequently

between neighboring genes relative to genes at greater distances. Thus, the phenomenon of linkage disequilibrium that confounded efforts to discern between alleles of genes at HLA could be exploited to identify previously unknown disease-associated genes. These new techniques were first applied to Mendelian inherited diseases and culminated in the identification of many single-gene mutations, such as those for cystic fibrosis and Huntington's disease.

> Alleles of HLA-DR2 are the major contributors to MS risk.

MS AS A COMPLEX TRAIT

The linkage-based approach had the potential to also be applied not only to single-gene disorders but also to complex multigenic traits. However, the hurdles for identifying

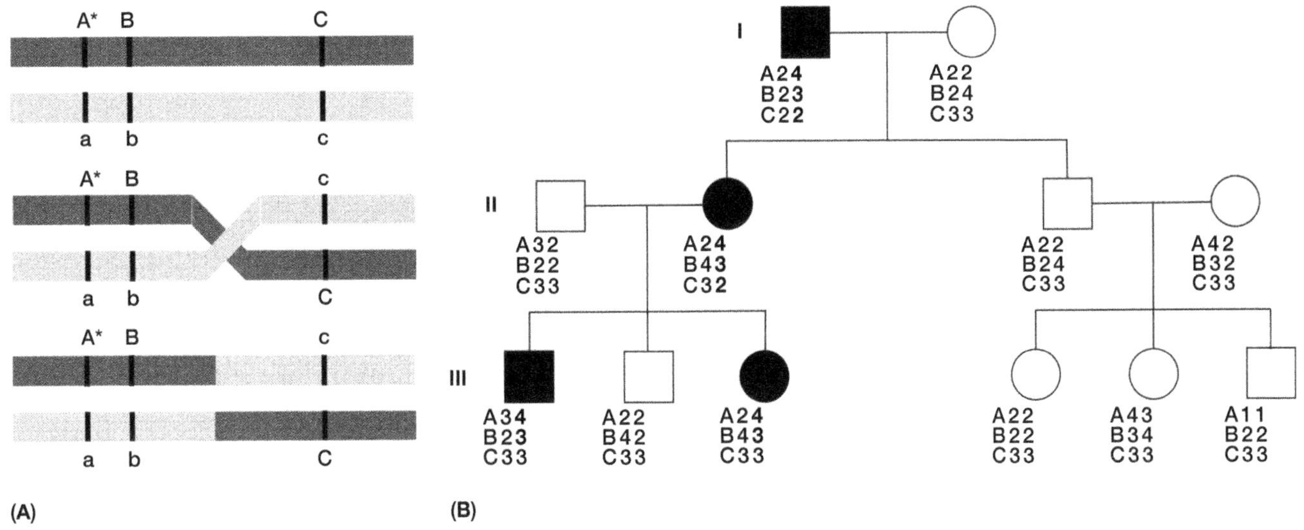

FIGURE 5.2

Meiotic recombination is the underlying genetic principle of linkage analysis. Paternal (dark gray) and maternal (light gray) chromosomes are aligned in a germ cell (cells that give rise to sperm or ova). Sequence A* is a disease-causing allele, whereas a is the normal allele. Alleles for nearby DNA sequences on the same chromosome are depicted as B and C. Paternal alleles are represented in capital letters and maternal alleles are represented in lower case. During meiotic recombination, paired chromosomal DNA strands cross over. The cross-over event results in a break in the paternal DNA strand that is recombined with the maternal DNA strand resulting in recombined chromosomes. The mixed chromosomes are passed to the sperm or ova. If the disease gene is A* then recombination is more likely to occur between the disease gene and alleles of C than alleles of B. By following the segregation of the disease gene in families along with the segregation of genetic markers, the disease causing gene A* can be mapped relative to the markers B and C (A). Pedigree analysis showing segregation of markers with a dominantly inherited trait. In the second generation, the marker combination A4 B3 C2 is inherited by the affected daughter. Owing to recombination between markers B and C, in the third generation affected individuals carry the marker combination A4 B3 C3 showing that the trait is linked to the A4 B3 haplotype. Although these markers are linked to the trait, they can also be found in the general population. Linkage analysis relies on segregation of markers that are linked to a trait taking into account family structure (B).

such traits would be considerably higher because the penetrance of each trait would be far less than for disease-causing mutations. Penetrance refers to the likelihood that a particular genotype will manifest as a phenotype. For Mendelian inherited mutations, such as those for dominant diseases such as Huntington's disease, the penetrance is very high, meaning that nearly all individuals who carry the disease-causing genotype will develop the disease. However, for complex traits, the penetrance is low and polymorphisms associated with the complex trait could be common in the overall population. This was clearly the case for the HLA locus. None of the HLA alleles associated with MS by themselves are disease-causing mutations. All these alleles were commonly found in healthy controls but were overrepresented among MS patients. The importance of this observation initially was perhaps not fully appreciated. Investigators assumed that because heritable MS risk could be found in families in whom the MS-associated HLA alleles were not carried, that other loci, perhaps with even stronger effects than that of HLA, must be present elsewhere in the genome. If this were the case, then systematic study of the genome in families affected by MS would surely identify these other loci.

GENOMIC LINKAGE SCREENS

The first series of genome-wide screens using several hundred microsatellite DNA markers across approximately 100 affected sib pairs was undertaken in the 1990s [45–47]. Assuming that other loci in the genome would have had similar effects on MS risk as that of, or even greater than, the major histocompatibility complex (MHC), these studies would have been expected to identify at least a few novel loci. However, no statistically significant additional loci were identified. Furthermore, one of these studies was unable to detect a signal from the MHC [45]. Follow-up studies using multiply affected families also failed to detect any convincing new MS susceptibility loci [48–52]. Adding more microsatellite markers to the initial genome screens also failed [32,53,54]. Pooling data for meta-analysis similarly failed to identify loci other than the MHC [55,56]. It became clear that identification of the effects of genetic variation on MS susceptibility would require not only better markers but substantially increased numbers of families for statistical power. The way forward required a much larger number of affected families to which any single group had access. The International Multiple Sclerosis Genetics Consortium (IMSGC) was thus founded in 2003 and brought together previously competing investigators in a collaborative effort to decode MS heritability [57] (www.neurodiscovery .harvard.edu/research/imsgc.html).

The first large-scale linkage study with sufficient statistical power to detect loci with effects similar to that of the MHC across the genome in populations from Australia, Scandinavia, the United Kingdom, and the United States identified a definite association between the MHC and MS

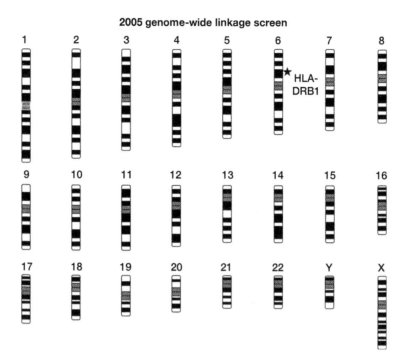

2005 genome-wide linkage screen

FIGURE 5.3
MS genomic regions of interest identified by linkage. *Source: [58].*

susceptibility (Figure 5.3) [58]. However, other loci whose associations with MS had been proposed from smaller studies were not replicated. This study was an important milestone in the study of MS genetics because for the first time an adequate number of markers and MS-affected families were brought together through an international collaborative effort. Furthermore, the markers used were sufficiently numerous and evenly spaced across the genome that there was confidence that the majority of the genome was adequately represented for linkage analysis. Perhaps most importantly, 730 families were studied, thus providing adequate power to detect genetic effects that increased the odds of MS risk by more than twofold. Only the MHC was found to increase risk of MS, which indicated that other possible loci that might influence MS risk must have more modest individual effects. Identification of such loci was effectively not possible using linkage analysis unless tens of thousands of families were analyzed [59]. This inherent limitation of linkage methodology potentially could be overcome by a different approach to genetic analysis: the genome-wide association screen (GWAS).

Genome-Wide Association Screen

Further technological innovation led to the identification of single nucleotide polymorphisms (SNPs). SNPs are genetic variants that occur at a single base pair position within the genome (Figure 5.4). The remarkable achievement of sequencing of the human genome in conjunction with mapping hundreds of thousands of these SNP variants led to the realization that 99.9% of the human genome is invariant [60,61]. Nevertheless, there are still billions of genetic

variations, many of which are exceedingly rare whereas others are more common. By focusing on the variants that are more commonly found, for example SNP alleles that are present in at least 5% of the overall population, it would be possible to map traits that are linked to common SNP variants. By coupling such potentially informative SNP variants with microchip-based miniaturization, it became possible to map hundreds of thousands of SNP variants from thousands of individuals (Figure 5.4). If heritable traits such as MS susceptibility are linked to commonly identified variants, then genotyping these common SNP variants could map the loci of the heritable trait. This hypothesis is referred to as the *common disease-common variant hypothesis.*

Unlike linkage analysis that required relatively large effect sizes for tracking heritable traits in families, the newer SNP-based technology was capable of detecting smaller individual genetic effects by increasing the numbers of affected individuals and unaffected controls. With a sufficiently large enough number of samples, association-testing that compares the prevalence of any given SNP marker between two populations has the capability to detect modest or small genetic effects as long as the numbers of affected and unaffected individuals are sufficient. Moreover, the samples for association screens did not necessarily require DNA from family members because although family structure could be taken into account in GWAS statistics, it did not have to be taken into account. In essence, this approach simply compares the prevalence of any given SNP marker in cases and controls, which is similar to a chi-square statistic. As long as the controls are from the same genetic background as the cases, then statistically significant differences in the prevalence of a particular SNP allele would presumably be due to a disease-related trait.

Case-control design compare single nucleotide
polymorphisms (SNPs) in two populations

Non-affected individuals
(controls)

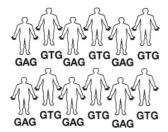

50% of controls carry the
GAG genotype and 50% carry
the GTG genotype (A→T SNP)

Affected individuals
(cases)

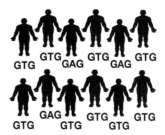

75% of cases carry the
GAG genotype and 25% carry
the GTG genotype (A→T SNP)

FIGURE 5.4

Association analysis compares the prevalence of markers in 2 populations. In this example, the marker of interest, an SNP at position 2, is present in 75% of cases and 25% of controls. The odds ratio for the association of this marker with the disease state is therefore 3.0.

GWAS Identifies the First Genes Outside the MHC

MS was one of the first diseases to be studied using this new GWAS technique. The IMSGC conducted the first GWAS in 2007 using over 334,923 SNPs in 930 MS trio families (a trio family is an MS patient and both parents) with a replication datasets consisting of another 609 family trios and an additional 2,322 case subjects and 789 unrelated controls [62]. It was hoped that this massive and costly effort would finally determine the genetic architecture of MS especially in regard to the much sought after non-MHC contributions. As anticipated, the MHC was definitively associated with MS susceptibility; however, beyond the MHC only 2 other loci were identified with a statistically significant level of confidence. These loci-encoded genes involved in immune regulation: the interleukin 2 receptor (IL2R-alpha) and the interleukin 7 receptor (IL7R-alpha). Associations with MS susceptibility for both loci were subsequently validated in other populations [63–68].

Alleles of the *IL2R-alpha* and the *IL7R-alpha* receptors were the first non-MHC loci that were definitively associated with MS risk.

> Alleles of the *IL2R-alpha* and the *IL7R-alpha* receptors were the first non-MHC loci that were definitively associated with MS risk.

The landmark achievement of identifying 2 non-HLA loci established that genes outside the MHC contributed to MS susceptibility. However, variations at these alleles, along with those of the MHC, could not account for all MS heritability. Moreover, the alleles identified were,

by definition, common alleles (the SNPs genotyped from GWAS are present in at least 5% of the population). However, the commonality of MS susceptibility-associated SNPs in both MS cases and controls were surprising. For example the *IL2R-alpha* variant was present in 85% of controls and 88% of cases. *IL7R-alpha* variant results were similar: the MS-associated variant was present in 78% of MS patients and 75% of controls. The presence of these variants in the majority of controls had 2 very important implications. First, these variants are not mutations but instead are the most common polymorphisms of each receptor. Therefore, the consequence to the protein associated with the polymorphism is normal function as opposed to loss of function or gain of an abnormal function associated with either recessive or dominant mutations, respectively. Second, because there was only a very slight overrepresentation of these polymorphisms in MS cases, the effect that this polymorphism has on MS risk is miniscule. Indeed, the odds ratios for these alleles were less than 1.5. If other non-HLA MS risk alleles were linked to common SNP variants, then sample size calculations showed that variants associated with a 1.1-fold or higher odds of MS risk would require at least 10,000 MS cases and a similar number of controls [69,70].

Although this GWAS identified only 2 non-HLA loci with a genome-wide level of statistical significance, there may be many other loci associated with MS susceptibility that missed the statistical cutoff for definite association. GWAS performed by other groups, as well as meta-analyses that combined GWAS data from different studies, identified multiple other MS susceptibility loci [71–79].

In order to expand the statistical power needed for the next round of GWAS, the IMSGC expanded its membership ultimately involving 23 research groups from 15 countries. The IMSGC also partnered with the Welcome Trust Case Control Consortium 2 (WTCCC2) to make use of the

TABLE 5.2
MS Risk Associated Non-MHC Common Genetic Variants

CHROMOSOME	SNP	GENE OF INTEREST	IMMUNE DISEASE	KNOWN IMMUNE FUNCTION	NEIGHBORING GENES	ODDS RATIO*	POPULATION FREQUENCY OF RISK ALLELE (%)
1	rs4648356	MMEL1	RA, CeD		7	1.16	66.8
1	rs11810217	EVI5			15	1.15	25.7
1	rs11581062	VCAM1		Yes	5	1.07	29.2
1	rs1335532	CD58		Yes	2	1.18	86.3
1	rs1323292	RGS1	CeD	Yes	1	1.12	80.1
1	rs7522462	KIF21B	UC, CeD, CrD		4	1.11	67.3
2	rs12466022	no gene			0	1.16	74.8
2	rs7595037	PLEK	CeD	Yes	4	1.15	54.9
2	rs17174870	MERTK		Yes	7	1.15	73.5
2	rs10201872	SP140	CLL		3	1.15	19.6
2	rs6718520**	THADA			5	1.17	48.0
3	rs11129295	EOMES		Yes	1	1.09	36.3
3	rs669607	no gene			0	1.15	48.7
3	rs2028597	CBLB		Yes	1	1.13	90.7
3	rs2293370	TMEM39A			7	1.16	85.0
3	rs9282641	CD86		Yes	5	1.20	90.2
3	rs2243123	IL12A	CeD	Yes	3	1.09	29.2
5	rs6897932	IL7RA	T1D	Yes	7	1.11	75.7
5	rs4613763	PTGER4	CrD	Yes	1	1.21	16.8
5	rs2546890	IL12B	PS, CrD	Yes	4	1.15	56.2
6	rs12212193	BACH2	CeD, T1D		1	1.08	47.8
6	rs802734	THEMIS	CeD		5	1.13	70.8
6	rs13192841	OLIG3				1.10	23.5
6	rs11154801	MYB			3	1.09	39.7
6	rs17066096	IL22RA2			3	1.14	18.1
6	rs1738074	TAGAP	CeD		2	1.14	53.5
7	rs354031	ZNF767			4	1.14	23.5
8	rs1520333	IL7		Yes	3	1.11	24.1
8	rs4410871	MYC			2	1.09	71.2
8	rs2019960	PVT1			1	1.16	24.3
9	rs2150702**	MLANA			10	1.16	49.0
10	rs3118470	IL2RA	RA	Yes	4	1.12	31.0
10	rs1250542	ZMIZ1	CeD, IBD		3	1.10	37.0
10	rs7923837	HHEX	T2D	Yes	3	1.09	63.3
11	rs650258	CD6			4	1.12	63.8
12	rs1800693	TNFRSF1A			4	1.12	48.2
12	rs10466829	CLECL1	T1D		9	1.12	46.9
12	rs12368653	CYP27B1	RA	Yes	33	1.11	44.7
12	rs949143	MPHOSPH9			13	1.08	33.2

(Continued)

TABLE 5.2
MS Risk Associated Non-MHC Common Genetic Variants (*Continued*)

CHROMOSOME	SNP	GENE OF INTEREST	IMMUNE DISEASE	KNOWN IMMUNE FUNCTION	NEIGHBORING GENES	ODDS RATIO*	POPULATION FREQUENCY OF RISK ALLELE (%)
14	rs4902647	ZFP36L1	CeD, T1D		3	1.13	56.2
14	rs2300603	BATF			3	1.08	70.4
14	rs2119704	GALC			3	1.12	93.2
16	rs7200786	CLEC16A	T1D		8	1.15	54.0
16	rs13333054	IRF8		Yes	1	1.12	20.8
17	rs9891119	STAT3	CrD	Yes	25	1.10	38.9
18	rs7238078	MALT1		Yes	2	1.14	79.6
19	rs1077667	TNFSF14		Yes	3	1.14	78.6
19	rs8112449	TYK2	T1D		12	1.10	69.5
19	rs874628	MPV17L2			11	1.07	71.7
19	rs2303759	DKKL1			9	1.11	29.6
20	rs2425752	CD40	RA	Yes	13	1.10	27.0
20	rs2248359	CYP24A1			2	1.11	58.8
22	rs2283792	MAPK1		Yes	9	1.12	52.7
22	rs140522	SCO2			15	1.12	34.5

*All P values associated with each odds ratio are less than 1×10^{-8}, the genomic level of significance, ie, Bonferroni correction for 1 million possible variants across the genome, a current estimate for all current genomic variants.
**These loci identified by recent meta-analysis [82].
CeD, celiac disease; CLL, chronic lymphocytic leukemia; CrD, Crohn's disease; PS, psoriasis; RA, rheumatoid arthritis; SNP, single nucleotide polymorphism; T1D, type 1 diabetes; T2D, type 2 diabetes; UC, ulcerative colitis.

most up-to-date GWAS technology [80]. Ultimately, 9,772 MS cases and 17,376 control DNA samples passed stringent quality control assessments. In the massive dataset, 441,547 autosomal SNPs were genotyped. During analysis it became clear that an important problem might bias the study: population stratification. Because this GWAS did not use a family-based approach, the comparison of cases to controls was predicated on the assumption that cases and controls shared a common genomic structure except at the MS susceptibility loci. However, if cases and controls had somewhat different genomic structures owing to differential sampling, then the differences identified between cases and controls could be due to either disease-causing loci or irrelevant differences in genomic structure introduced by sampling bias. When cases and controls from a single country, such as the United Kingdom, were compared there was no evidence of population stratification. However, because cases and controls were not perfectly matched by country of origin, the entire dataset showed evidence of genomic inflation, meaning that because cases and controls were not perfectly matched, there was a systematic difference for genomic markers between these 2 groups that would bias the GWAS results owing to population stratification. Several methods to control for genomic inflation were employed but ultimately a novel approach (variance component method) was able to effectively adjust for the genomic inflation bias.

The IMSGC and WTCCC2's MS GWAS identified 52 loci that were definitively associated with MS susceptibility (Table 5.2, Figure 5.5). This study not only replicated the known MHC, *IL2R-alpha* and *IL7R-alpha* associations, but also found 20 loci that had been implicated in MS risk through other GWAS studies as well as meta-analyses. Furthermore, 29 novel loci were identified. All non-MHC loci had minor influences on MS susceptibility with odds ratios ranging from 1.07 to 1.21. Perhaps the most important observation from this study was that the majority of SNPs identified were located near genes encoding immune functions. This observation supported the hypothesis that MS is indeed an autoimmune disease. Furthermore, many of the implicated genes share common pathways involved in immune regulation, providing important clues as to how normal immune function might become dysregulated in MS. Moreover, 23 of the identified loci are known to be involved in other autoimmune diseases indicating that common mechanisms, at least in part, underlie autoimmune diseases. However, the

> The IMSCG and WTCCC2's MS GWAS identified 52 loci that were definitively associated with MS susceptibility.

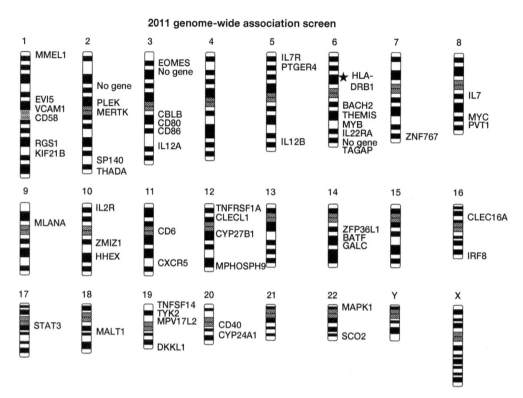

FIGURE 5.5

MS genomic regions of interest identified by GWAS. *Source: [80].*

identification of these common loci did not lead immediately to an understanding as to why the central nervous system (CNS) is the primary target of autoimmune injury, although several possible genes are expressed in the CNS and some, such as *GALC* encode proteins, were previously implicated in MS [81].

It is important to understand that for the majority of the loci, multiple neighboring genes are linked to the MS-associated SNP. Therefore, with the current level of resolution of this GWAS, the exact genetic variant involved in MS susceptibility cannot be determined. Although it is possible that the MS-associated variants are the SNPs identified by the GWAS, it is also possible that the identified SNPs are in linkage disequilibrium with the true MS-associated SNPs. Additional SNPs or resequencing of these regions of interest will be necessary to refine the map of the causal variant. Two SNP-identified loci do not have any neighboring genes. It is possible that these SNPs are false positive results, but it is more likely that these regions contain transcriptional regulatory elements such as promoters or enhancers for distant genes or even transcribed regulatory RNAs that are not translated into proteins. The recent Encyclopedia of DNA Elements (ENCODE) project's remarkable discovery that 80% of the human genome contains elements linked to biological processes underscores that DNA regions without open reading frames can be biologically important and, in fact, do not contain what previously had been disregarded as "junk" DNA [83,84].

MISSING HERITABILITY

Despite the remarkable achievement of the IMSGC–WTCC2 GWAS, the estimate of the total contribution to MS heritability by these the polymorphisms identified in this study was only 25%. MHC accounts for approximately 20% of MS heritability, and the other 51 genetic loci contribute only 5% to MS risk. This suggests that 75% of MS genetic risk will be accounted for by variants that cannot be identified using SNP chips, which are designed to test the common allele-common variant hypothesis. Identification of rare disease causative alleles that have individually weak or modest effects poses additional challenges for genetic analysis. First, the number of rare variants is much greater than the number of common variants. Second, the majority of rare variants have not yet been described in publicly available databases. Identifying and cataloguing these rare variants will require sequencing many more genomes. Finally, optimal methods for typing an individual's DNA for rare variants are still being developed.

> MHC accounts for approximately 20% of MS heritability, and the other 51 genetic loci contribute to only 5% to MS risk. This suggests that 75% of MS genetic risk will be accounted for by variants that cannot be identified using SNP chips.

VITAMIN D GENETICS

Vitamin D deficiency is a risk factor for MS susceptibility and likely accounts for some of the differences in MS's geographical prevalence. Multiple studies showed that 25-OH vitamin D levels are lower in MS cases compared to controls in both European descended and black populations [85–88]. The IMSGC–WTCC2 GWAS identified 2 genes involved in vitamin D metabolism as conferring increased susceptibility to MS. CYP27B1 encodes an enzyme that catalyzes the synthesis of 1,25-dihydroxyvitamin D (1,25 dihydroxyvitamin D is the biologically active form of the vitamin). CYP24A1 encodes an enzyme that degrades 1,25-dihydroxyvitamin D. Two genes that regulate vitamin D synthesis (CYP27B1) and degradation (CYP24A1) confer MS susceptibility. These genes may contribute to MS risk by decreasing the levels of active vitamin D and may link MS heritability with a known environmental risk factor. CYP27B1 was also shown to influence MS risk in MS families with multiply affected individuals [89]. By systematically sequencing all genomic protein-encoding regions in 43 MS patients from multiplex families, a nonsynonymous variant of CYP27B1 (R389H) was identified by segregating in one family with an incompletely penetrant dominant inheritance pattern. This variant leads to complete loss of CYP27B1 activity and therefore causes low levels of 1,25-dihydroxyvitamin D. The R389H CYP27B1 variant was genotyped in 3,000 parent-affected trios and was found to be transmitted from parent to affected offspring in 19 trios. These results underscore the important role of vitamin D in MS and show that not only environmental factors but also genetic factors influence vitamin D levels.

> Two genes that regulate vitamin D synthesis (CYP27B1) and degradation (CYP24A1) confer MS susceptibility. These genes may contribute to MS risk by decreasing the levels of active vitamin D and may link MS heritability with a known environmental risk factor.

Vitamin D itself has important regulatory roles in gene expression. RNA expression level of the major MS susceptibility gene HLA-DRB1*15:01 is regulated by vitamin D, albeit somewhat paradoxically (ie, expression of the allele is upregulated by vitamin D) [90]. Vitamin D receptor binding elements have been identified in the majority of MS-associated genes, implying that expression of many of these genes could also be controlled by vitamin D [91]. Although the details of the network of interactions between genes that regulate vitamin D synthesis and MS susceptibility genes, whose expression is in turn regulated by vitamin D, have yet to be established, these studies illustrate the

> RNA expression level of the major MS susceptibility gene HLA-DRB1*15:01 is regulated by vitamin D.

importance of vitamin D in MS pathogenesis. Low levels of vitamin D, either because of environmental factors such as decreased sunlight exposure or low dietary intake of vitamin D, or because of genetic traits that reduce levels of 1,25-dihydroxyvitamin D, clearly contribute to MS susceptibility and may also contribute to disease activity [92–95].

EXOME AND GENOME SEQUENCING

A second example of exome sequencing's power to detect rare alleles of MS susceptibility genes is the discovery of a missense mutation in the TYK2 gene [96]. An allele of the TYK2 gene was previously found to be protective in GWAS [73,97,98]. In contrast, the missense allele identified by exome sequencing modestly increases the risk of MS. Similar to the study of CYP27B1, the rare allele of TYK2 (rs557627444) was first identified in a multiply affected large MS pedigree and then replicated in 2,104 trios.

The studies of CYP27B1 and TYK2 showcase the powerful advantage of exome sequencing. Unlike the SNP chip-based technology that is restricted by the genetic variants imprinted on the chip, sequencing the exome has the potential to identify any variant present within an individual's coding DNA. Therefore, exome sequencing technology has the potential to identify rare coding variants that would not be present on SNP chips.

Individual genome sequencing is also now possible. The cost of high throughput sequencing has dramatically decreased since the first human genome was sequenced (about $1 billion) and currently runs at approximately $3500/genome. It is anticipated that in the next few years the price will fall further to less than $1000/genome. The advantage of genome sequencing over exome sequencing is that the entire genome is sequenced, which includes all the noncoding DNA that may contain important regulatory elements in addition to the sequences used to encode specific proteins. Not accounted for by the relatively low cost of sequencing is the added cost of data management and analysis for the additional noncoding sequences.

Although the technology for determining genetic sequences has rapidly progressed such that it will soon be commercially feasible to sequence any individual's entire genome, the analytical techniques for interpreting the massive amounts of data are still being developed. The technology for deriving the primary sequence has temporarily outpaced the technology for genomic data analysis. Both software and hardware computational technologies are being developed that will enable desktop analysis of the human genome's 3 billion base pairs.

Preliminary studies suggest that every individual's DNA contains over 50,000 SNP variants and over 5,000 insertion/deletion polymorphisms [99]. Importantly, 42% of the SNPs and 86% of the insertion/deletion polymorphisms are novel, meaning that they had not been previously recorded in publicly available databases. Given the very large numbers of rare polymorphisms contained in every individual's DNA, assigning disease causative roles for these variants poses considerable methodological

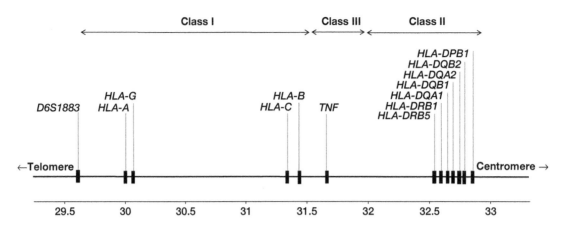

FIGURE 5.6
Chromosome 6 position in Mb.

challenges. The identification of the rare R389H *CYP27B1* allele was made possible by the additional information imparted by the multiplex family structure and was validated by large-scale trio analyses. It is likely that additional rare coding variants will be identified by this approach.

THE MHC AND MS SUSCEPTIBILITY

The MHC is 3.5 million bases (Mb) of DNA located on the short arm of chromosome 6. It is the most genetically dense area of the human genome and encodes over 3,000 genes. The HLA genes are grouped into 3 structurally related classes from the telomere to the centromere: class I, class III, and class II (Figure 5.6). The HLA genes encode for glycoproteins that are expressed on the cell surface and play critical roles in recognition of self-antigens by the immune system. Many of these genes are highly polymorphic, adding additional complexity of this locus. Multiple autoimmune diseases have risk alleles that map to this region, thereby underscoring its importance in the regulation of immune function [100].

As a consequence of selective pressures, the MHC is characterized by extensive linkage disequilibrium that can span the MHC and confound mapping studies. Thus, alleles of class I genes can be genetically linked to distant alleles of class II genes. Many of the HLA alleles were first identified serologically and gave rise to a complex and often inconsistent nomenclature. Recent extensive efforts were made at mapping the serological types to DNA sequences and the genetic architecture of the MHC is now much better understood [101–105]. As a consequence, the genetic basis of the serotypes is now understood and a consistent nomenclature has finally come into focus that will help advance further study of the MHC (hla.alleles.org).

As described, the first genetic associations identified in MS were found for HLA class I alleles using serological typing of HLA antigens on leukocytes [34–38]. When HLA class II alleles were also associated with MS susceptibility, it was proposed that the class I associations were accounted

for by linkage disequilibrium with the class II loci [39–41]. Clarifying the associations of HLA loci with MS susceptibility was ultimately made possible by DNA-based typing of HLA polymorphisms in multiple datasets.

It is now clear that the primary MS susceptibility signal at HLA stems from the MHC class II locus. In populations of European descent, the primary risk allele is *HLA-DRB1*15:01*, which is part of a haplotype: *DRB1*15:01, DQA1*01:02, DQB1*0602*. This haplotype encodes for a cell surface glycoprotein gene that can present antigens peptides to T cells. Together, these genes correspond to the serological markers known as HLA-DR2, DQ6.

Fine mapping studies indicate that the most important contributors to MS susceptibility are polymorphisms in the *DRB1* gene [106]. Neighboring polymorphisms in the *DQB1* gene, although tightly linked to *DRB1*, do not contribute to MS risk thus establishing a centromeric boundary for MS risk at *HLA-DRB1*.

> In populations of European descent, the primary risk allele is *HLA-DRB1*15:01*, which is part of a haplotype: *DRB1*15:01, DQA1*01:02, DQB*0602*.

Multiple polymorphisms within *HLA-DRB1* influence MS susceptibility in populations (Figure 5.6). *HLA-DRB1*15:01* contributes to MS susceptibility with a dominant, dose-dependent effect [107]. In populations of African descent, the closely related *HLA-DRB1*15:03* allele contributes to MS risk [106,108]. *HLA-DRB1*03* contributes to MS risk as a recessive trait [90]. *HLA-DRB1*13:03* also contributes to MS risk [80]. In the presence of *HLA-DRB1:15*, the *HLA-DRB1*08* allele further increases MS risk [108–111], whereas the *HLA-DRB1*14* and *HLA-DRB1*10* alleles attenuate the risk of MS transmitted by *HLA-DRB1*15* (Figure 5.7). To add to the complexity, certain alleles seem to contribute to MS in some, but not all, populations. In Sardinia, in addition to *HLA-DRB1*15* and *HLA-DRB1*03*, *HLA-DRB1*04* alleles contribute to MS susceptibility [112–115]. Although the allelic interactions at this class II

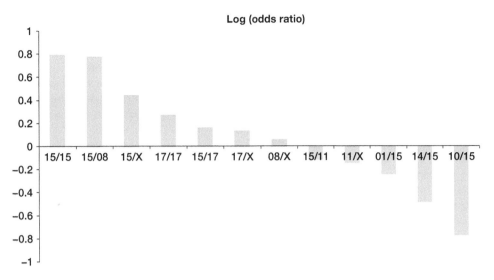

FIGURE 5.7

Combinations of *HLA-DRB1* alleles and risk of MS. Odds ratios for MS risk and various combinations of *HLA-DRB1* alleles are depicted graphically. The Y-axis shows the log of the odds ratio with positive values increasing the risk of MS and negative values decreasing the risk of MS. The highest odds ratios are for *HLA-DRB1*15* homozygotes and for *HLA-DRB1*15 / HLA-DRB1*08* heterozygotes. In contrast, *HLA-DRB1*14* and *HLA-DRB1*10* alleles are associated with a lower risk of MS in *HLA-DRB1*15* heterozygotes. The graph depicts that the impact of the *HLA-DRB1*08* allele on increasing MS risk is proportionally as strong as that of *HLA-DRB1*10* in lowering MS risk in *HLA-DRB1*15* heterozygotes. *Adapted from data presented in [109].*

MHC locus are remarkably complex, similar principals will likely apply to other risk loci.

Fine mapping studies of the telomeric boundary of MS susceptibility found that the MHC class I locus independently contributes to MS susceptibility, although the exact risk gene, or genes, in this region have not been precisely mapped [80,116–118]. Alleles of the class I gene *HLA-A* are proposed to have a protective effect for MS susceptibility. However, as with the class II locus, extensive linkage disequilibrium is present in the class I region and therefore the class I signal might stem from linked alleles of neighboring genes including *HLA-B* [119], *HLA-C* [117], and *HLA-G* [118]. Alleles of these genes form a linked haplotype that spans the MHC: *HLA-A*02:01–HLA-B*44:02–HLA-C*05:01–HLA-DRB1*04:01*. Thus far, no study to date has had a sufficiently large enough number of subjects to definitively establish the precise location of the class I MS susceptibility signal. MHC class I locus influences MS susceptibility, which implies a role for innate immune function in MS.

> Fine mapping studies of the telomeric boundary of MS susceptibility found that the MHC class I locus independently contributes to MS susceptibility.

In addition to influencing MS risk, HLA alleles may contribute to the MS phenotype. The most consistent effect of HLA on MS phenotype is for the *HLA-DRB1*15:01* allele on the age of onset. Several studies showed that this allele decreases the age of onset and does so in a dose-dependent manner [80,108,120–123]. *HLA-DRB1*15:01* may also contribute to the radiographic burden of disease on T2-weighted brain MRI and impact cognitive performance [124]. In contrast, the *HLA-B*44:02* allele, that is proposed to be protective for MS susceptibility, may reduce the radiographic burden of disease on T2-weighted brain MRI [119]. A consistent impact of HLA alleles on MS neurological impairments as measured by Expanded Disability Status Scale (EDSS) progression has not been found [112,125]. Interestingly, a spontaneously occurring null allele of the *HLA-DRB5* gene located telomeric to *HLA-DRB1* might contribute to MS severity [126].

CURRENT DIRECTIONS AND LIMITATIONS

Several genetic loci were identified in the recent IMSGC GWAS that narrowly missed the cutoffs for genome-wide levels of statistical significance (*NFKB1, CXCR5, SOX8, RPS6KB1*, and *TNFRSF6B*). A recent meta-analysis also found several candidate loci with suggestive evidence of association (*TBX21, EPS15L1, TNP2*, and an intergenic SNP rs9596270) [82]. One previously identified gene (*CXCR4*) may have been missed because of a genotyping error (false negative). Several of these genes have known functions in immune regulation (eg, *NFKB1, CXCR5, TNFRSF6B, CXCR4*, and *TBX21*) and efforts are underway using meta-analyses to establish whether these loci contribute to MS risk.

Saturated SNP studies are being performed to reduce the number of possible genes at each loci identified by the tagging SNPs. The results of the first large-scale targeted saturation SNP analysis (the IMMUNOCHIP) are expected soon.

Rare variants with low minor allele frequencies (MAFs) are being examined by GWAS and exome and genome sequencing studies in multiplex families to identify novel rare variants. The success of exome sequencing in identifying rare variants of *CYP27B1* and *TYK2* illustrates the limitations of the common variant hypothesis. These rare alleles may be the proverbial tip of the iceberg and many more rare MS variants might be found by exploiting this strategy. However, these rare variants were identified in families with multiply affected members. Multiply affected families are relatively uncommon in MS and not all such families have informative structures for identification of rare variants. Furthermore, risk alleles in multiply affected families might be expected to have stronger effect sizes than variants that contribute to sporadic MS. At this time, no solution is apparent that does not require extremely large sample sizes using the case-control approach.

In populations of non-European descent, studies have replicated some but not all non-MHC SNPs [127]. It is encouraging that at least some MS risk alleles identified in populations of European descent replicate in other racial groups and further substantiate that such risk alleles are genuine. Several explanations for lack of replication in diverse populations are possible and include relatively smaller sample sizes resulting in lack of power, inadequate control for population stratification, epistatic interactions, and differential gene–environment interactions. European descended alleles are present in the control groups for non-European populations, which indicates that genetic diversity alone does not account for the divergence in genotype to phenotype correlation.

As impressive as the advances in recent years have been for MS risk gene discovery, several limitations of genetic research in MS have become clear. First, it is highly unlikely that genotyping will yield clinically meaningful diagnostical tools. The effect sizes for genetic effects on MS risk are far too small to find application in diagnosing MS patients. Second, in as much as very large sample sizes became necessary for identifying the genetic differences between MS cases and controls, it seems likely that equally large sample sizes will become necessary for identifying genetic factors that influence the MS clinical phenotype, including rate of disease progression. As intriguing as the preliminary studies of MS risk genes on MRI and clinical correlates may be, the studies performed to date are underpowered and reported results carry a risk of being falsely positive (much as was the case for early studies of MS risk). Given that multiple factors influence the MS phenotype, including disease duration as well as widespread use of disease-modifying therapies, future studies of genotype–phenotype correlations may face even greater challenges than studies of MS risk. Similarly, although the use of genetics as a tool for individualizing treatment selection holds intrinsical appeal, proof that a genetic marker is associated with a particular outcome will require careful study of large populations given that the contribution of genetics to the overall effect of highly potent immune therapies is likely to be small. These daunting challenges raise the question as to whether genetic study in MS has value. Although MS genetics is unlikely to yield concrete clinical utility in the near future, genetics remains an invaluable tool for defining the key constituents underlying the complex biology of the disease. Only through identifying the genes involved in determining MS susceptibility can we hope to understand the role of heritability in the disease pathogenesis, which in turn may point to new therapeutic opportunities.

KEY POINTS FOR PATIENTS AND FAMILIES

- While most patients with MS do not have a family history, about 1 out of 5 patients will have family members who have MS.

- Children of a parent with MS have about a 3% to 5% lifetime risk of MS. Although this is higher than the general population, still they are unlikely to develop MS.

- There are no predictive genetic tests for MS.

REFERENCES

1. Davenport CB. Multiple sclerosis from the standpoint of geographic distribution and race. *Arch Neurol.* 1922;8(1):51–58.

2. Dean G, McLoughlin H, Brady R, et al. Multiple sclerosis among immigrants in Greater London. *Br Med J.* 1976;1(6014):861–864.

3. Pugliatti M, Sotgiu S, Rosati G. The worldwide prevalence of multiple sclerosis. *Clin Neurol Neurosurg.* 2002;104(3):182–191.

4. Alter M, Kahana E, Zilber N, Miller A. Multiple sclerosis frequency in Israel's diverse populations. *Neurology.* 2006; 66(7):1061–1066.

5. Smestad C, Sandvik L, Holmoy T, et al. Marked differences in prevalence of multiple sclerosis between ethnic groups in Oslo, Norway. *J Neurol.* 2008;255(1):49–55.

6. Kurtzke JF, Beebe GW, Nagler B, et al. Studies on the natural history of multiple sclerosis-8. Early prognostic features of the later course of the illness. *J Chronic Dis.* 1977;30(12):819–830.

7. Wallin MT, Page WF, Kurtzke JF. Multiple sclerosis in US veterans of the Vietnam era and later military service: Race, sex, and geography. *Ann Neurol.* 2004;55(1):65–71.

8. Detels R, Visscher BR, Malmgren RM, et al. Evidence for lower susceptibility to multiple sclerosis in Japanese-Americans. *Am J Epidemiol.* 1977;105(4):303–310.

9. Oger JF, Arnason BG, Wray SH, Kistler JP. A study of B and T cells in multiple sclerosis. *Neurology*. 1975;25(5):444–447.

10. Kurtzke JF, Beebe GW, Normal JE Jr. Epidemiology of multiple sclerosis in U.S. veterans: 1. Race, sex, and geographic distribution. *Neurology*. 1979;29(9 Pt 1):1228–1235.

11. Hader WJ. Prevalence of multiple sclerosis in Saskatoon. *Can Med Assoc J*. 1982;127(4):295–297.

12. Svenson LW, Woodhead SE, Platt GH. Regional variations in the prevalence rates of multiple sclerosis in the province of Alberta, Canada. *Neuroepidemiology*. 1994;13(1–2):8–13.

13. Gowers WR. *A Manual of Diseases of the Nervous System*, 2nd ed. London, England: Churchill; 1893.

14. Eichorst H. Über infantile und heriditare multiple Sklerose. *Virchow's Arch Pathologie Anat Berl*. 1896;146:173–192.

15. Curtius FSH. Multiple sklerose und erbanlage. *Zeitschrift fur die Gesamte Neurologie und Psychiatrie*. 1938;160(1):226–245.

16. McAlpine D. The problem of disseminated sclerosis. *Brain*. 1946;69:233–250.

17. Pratt RT, Compston ND, McAlpine D. The familial incidence of disseminated sclerosis and its significance. *Brain*. 1951; 74(2):191–232.

18. Millar JH, Allison RS. Familial incidence of disseminated sclerosis in Northern Ireland. *Ulster Med J*. 1954;23(Suppl 2):29–92.

19. Sadovnick AD, Baird PA, Ward RH. Multiple sclerosis: Updated risks for relatives. *Am J Med Genet*. 1998;29(3): 533–541.

20. Robertson NP, Fraser M, Deans J, et al. Age-adjusted recurrence risks for relatives of patients with multiple sclerosis. *Brain*. 1996;119(Pt 2):449–455.

21. Carton H, Vlietinck R, Debruyne J, et al. Risks of multiple sclerosis in relatives of patients in Flanders, Belgium. *J Neurol Neurosurg Psychiatry*. 1997;62(4):329–333.

22. Risch N. Linkage strategies for genetically complex traits. I. Multilocus models. *Am J Hum Genet*. 1990;46(2):222–228.

23. Compston A. Genetic epidemiology of multiple sclerosis. *J Neurol Neurosurg Psychiatry*. 1997;62(6):553–561.

24. Merikangas KR, Risch N. Genomic priorities and public health. *Science*. 2003;302(5645):599–601. doi: 10.1126/science .1091468

25. Guo SW. Sibling recurrence risk ratio as a measure of genetic effect: Caveat emptor! *Am J Hum Genet*. 2002;70(3):818–819.

26. Ebers GC, Bulman DE, Sadovnick AD, et al. A population-based study of multiple sclerosis in twins. *N Engl J Med*. 1986;315(26):1638–1642.

27. Mumford CJ, Wood NW, Kellar-Wood H, et al. The British Isles survey of multiple sclerosis in twins. *Neurology*. 1994; 44(1):11–15.

28. Willer CJ, Dyment DA, Risch NJ, et al. Twin concordance and sibling recurrence rates in multiple sclerosis. *Proc Natl Acad Sci USA*. 2003;100(22):12877–12882.

29. Robertson NP, O'Riordan JI, Chataway J, et al. Offspring recurrence rates and clinical characteristics of conjugal multiple sclerosis. *Lancet*. 1997;349(9065):1587–1590.

30. Ebers GC, Yee IM, Sadovnick AD, Duquette P. Conjugal multiple sclerosis: Population-based prevalence and recurrence risks in offspring. Canadian Collaborative Study Group. *Ann Neurol*. 2000;48(6):927–931.

31. Dyment DA, Ebers GC, Sadovnick AD. Genetics of multiple sclerosis. [Research Support, Non-U.S. Gov't Review]. *Lancet Neurol*. 2004;3(2):104–110.

32. Dyment DA, Sadovnick AD, Willer CJ, et al. An extended genome scan in 442 Canadian multiple sclerosis-affected sibships: A report from the Canadian Collaborative Study Group. *Hum Mol Genet*. 2004;13(10):1005–1015.

33. Peltonen L, McKusick VA. Dissecting human disease in the postgenomic era. *Science*. 2001;1224–1229.

34. Bertrams J, Kuwert E. HL-A antigen frequencies in multiple sclerosis. Significant increase of HL-A3, HL-A10 and W5, and decrease of HL-A12. *Eur Neurol*. 1972;7(1):74–78.

35. Bertrams J, Kuwert E, Liedtke U. HL-A antigens and multiple sclerosis. *Tissue Antigens*. 1972;2(5):405–408.

36. Naito S, Namerow N, Mickey MR, et al. Multiple sclerosis: Association with HL-A3. *Tissue Antigens*. 1972;2(1):1–4.

37. Jersild C, Svejgaard A, Fog T. HL-A antigens and multiple sclerosis. *Lancet*. 1972;1(7762):1240–1241.

38. Jersild C, Fog T, Hansen GS, et al. Histocompatibility determinants in multiple sclerosis, with special reference to clinical course. *Lancet*. 1973;2(7840):1221–1225.

39. Winchester R, Ebers G, Fu SM, et al. B-cell alloantigen Ag 7a in multiple sclerosis. *Lancet*. 1975;2(7939):814.

40. Compston DA, Batchelor JR, McDonald WI. B-lymphocyte alloantigens associated with multiple sclerosis. *Lancet*. 1976; 2(7998):1261–1265.

41. Terasaki PI, Park MS, Opelz G, Ting A. Multiple sclerosis and high incidence of a B lymphocyte antigen. *Science*. 1976;193(4259):1245–1247.

42. Botstein D, White RL, Skolnick M, Davis RW. Construction of a genetic linkage map in man using restriction fragment length polymorphisms. *Am J Hum Genet*. 1980;32(3):314–331.

43. Weber JL, May PE. Abundant class of human DNA polymorphisms which can be typed using the polymerase chain reaction. *Am J Hum Genet*. 1989;44(3):388–396.

44. Cohen D, Cohen O, Marcadet A, et al. Class II HLA-DC beta-chain DNA restriction fragments differentiate among HLA-DR2 individuals in insulin-dependent diabetes and multiple sclerosis. *Proc Natl Acad Sci USA*. 1984;81(6):1774–1778.

45. Ebers GC, Kukay K, Bulman DE, et al. A full genome search in multiple sclerosis. *Nat Genet*. 1996;13(4):472–476.

46. Haines JL, Ter-Minassian M, Bazyk A, et al. A complete genomic screen for multiple sclerosis underscores a role for the major histocompatability complex. The Multiple Sclerosis Genetics Group. *Nat Genet*. 1996;13(4):469–471.

47. Sawcer S, Jones HB, Feakes R, et al. A genome screen in multiple sclerosis reveals susceptibility loci on chromosome 6p21 and 17q22. *Nat Genet*. 1996;13(4):464–468.

48. Kuokkanen S, Gschwend M, Rioux JD, et al. Genomewide scan of multiple sclerosis in Finnish multiplex families. *Am J Hum Genet*. 1997;61(6):1379–1387.

49. Coraddu F, Sawcer S, D'Alfonso S, et al. A genome screen for multiple sclerosis in Sardinian multiplex families. *Eur J Hum Genet*. 2001;9(8):621–626.

50. Akesson E, Oturai A, Berg J, et al. A genome-wide screen for linkage in Nordic sib-pairs with multiple sclerosis. *Genes Immun*. 2002;3(5):279–285.

51. Ban M, Stewart GJ, Bennetts BH, et al. A genome screen for linkage in Australian sibling-pairs with multiple sclerosis. *Genes Immun*. 2002;3(8):464–469.

52. Eraksoy M, Hensiek A, Kurtuncu M, et al. A genome screen for linkage disequilibrium in Turkish multiple sclerosis. *J Neuroimmunol*. 2003;143(1–2):129–132.

53. Hensiek AE, Roxburgh R, Smilie B, et al. Updated results of the United Kingdom linkage-based genome screen in multiple sclerosis. *J Neuroimmunol.* 2003;143(1–2):25–30.

54. Kenealy SJ, Babron MC, Bradford Y, et al. A second-generation genomic screen for multiple sclerosis. *Am J Hum Genet.* 2004;75(6):1070–1078.

55. Ligers A, Dyment DA, Willer CJ, et al. Evidence of linkage with HLA-DR in DRB1*15-negative families with multiple sclerosis. *Am J Hum Genet.* 2001;69(4):900–903.

56. GAMES; Transatlantic Multiple Sclerosis Genetics Cooperative. A meta-analysis of whole genome linkage screens in multiple sclerosis. *J Neuroimmunol.* 2003;143(1–2):39–46.

57. Sawcer SJ, Maranian M, Singlehurst S, et al. Enhancing linkage analysis of complex disorders: An evaluation of high-density genotyping. *Hum Mol Genet.* 2004;13(17):1943–1949.

58. Sawcer S, Ban M, Maranian M, et al. A high-density screen for linkage in multiple sclerosis. *Am J Hum Genet.* 2005;77(3):454–467.

59. Risch N, Merikangas K. The future of genetic studies of complex human diseases. *Science.* 1996;273(5281):1516–1517.

60. International HapMap Consortium. The International HapMap Project. *Nature.* 2003;426(6968):789–796.

61. International Human Genome Sequencing Consortium. Finishing the euchromatic sequence of the human genome. *Nature.* 2004;431(7011):931–945.

62. International Multiple Sclerosis Genetics Consortium, Hafler DA, Compston A, et al. Risk alleles for multiple sclerosis identified by a genomewide study. *N Engl J Med.* 2007;357(9):851–862.

63. Matesanz F, Fedetz M, Collado-Romero M, et al. Allelic expression and interleukin-2 polymorphisms in multiple sclerosis. *J Neuroimmunol.* 2001;119(1):101–105.

64. Gregory SG, Schmidt S, Seth P, et al. Interleukin 7 receptor alpha chain (IL7R) shows allelic and functional association with multiple sclerosis. *Nat Genet.* 2007;39(9):1083–1091.

65. Lundmark F, Duvefelt K, Hillert J. Genetic association analysis of the interleukin 7 gene (IL7) in multiple sclerosis. *J Neuroimmunol.* 2007;192(1–2):171–173.

66. Lundmark F, Duvefelt K, Iacobaeus E, et al. Variation in interleukin 7 receptor alpha chain (IL7R) influences risk of multiple sclerosis. *Nat Genet.* 2007;39(9):1108–1113.

67. Rubio JP, Stankovich J, Field J, et al. Replication of KIAA0350, IL2RA, RPL5 and CD58 as multiple sclerosis susceptibility genes in Australians. *Genes Immun.* 2008;9(7):624–630.

68. Weber F, Fontaine B, Cournu-Rebeix I, et al. IL2RA and IL7RA genes confer susceptibility for multiple sclerosis in two independent European populations. *Genes Immun.* 2008;9(3):259–263.

69. Sawcer S. The complex genetics of multiple sclerosis: Pitfalls and prospects. *Brain.* 2008;131(Pt 12):3118–3131.

70. Sawcer S. Bayes factors in complex genetics. *Eur J Hum Genet.* 2010;18(7):746–750.

71. Wellcome Trust Case Control Consortium, Australo-Anglo-American Spondylitis Consortium (TASC), Burton PR, et al. Association scan of 14,500 nonsynonymous SNPs in four diseases identifies autoimmunity variants. *Nat Genet.* 2007;39(11):1329–1337.

72. Comabella M, Martin R. Genomics in multiple sclerosis—current state and future directions. *J Neuroimmunol.* 2007;187(1–2):1–8.

73. Australia and New Zealand Multiple Sclerosis Genetics Consortium (ANZgene). Genome-wide association study identifies new multiple sclerosis susceptibility loci on chromosomes 12 and 20. *Nat Genet.* 2009;41(7):824–828.

74. Baranzini SE, Wang J, Gibson RA, et al. Genome-wide association analysis of susceptibility and clinical phenotype in multiple sclerosis. *Hum Mol Genet.* 2009;18(4):767–778.

75. De Jager PL, Jia X, Wang J, et al. Meta-analysis of genome scans and replication identify CD6, IRF8 and TNFRSF1A as new multiple sclerosis susceptibility loci. *Nat Genet.* 2009;41(7):776–782.

76. Jakkula E, Leppä V, Sulonen AN, et al. Genome-wide association study in a high-risk isolate for multiple sclerosis reveals associated variants in STAT3 gene. *Am J Hum Genet.* 2010;86(2):285–291.

77. Nischwitz S, Cepok S, Kroner A, et al. Evidence for VAV2 and ZNF433 as susceptibility genes for multiple sclerosis. *J Neuroimmunol.* 2010;227(1–2):162–166.

78. Sanna S, Pitzalis M, et al. Variants within the immunoregulatory CBLB gene are associated with multiple sclerosis. *Nat Genet.* 2010;42(6):495–497.

79. IMSGC. Genome-wide association study of severity in multiple sclerosis. *Genes Immun.* 2011;12(8):615–625.

80. International Multiple Sclerosis Genetics Consortium, Wellcome Trust Case Control Consortium 2, Sawcer S, et al. Genetic risk and a primary role for cell-mediated immune mechanisms in multiple sclerosis. *Nature.* 2011;476(7359):214–219.

81. Menge T, Lalive PH, von Büdingen HC, et al. Antibody responses against galactocerebroside are potential stage-specific biomarkers in multiple sclerosis. *J Allergy Clin Immunol.* 2005;116(2):453–459.

82. Patsopoulos NA, Bayer Pharma MS Genetics Working Group, Steering Committees of Studies Evaluating IFNβ-1b and a CCR1-antagonist, et al. Genome-wide meta-analysis identifies novel multiple sclerosis susceptibility loci. *Ann Neurol.* 2011;70(6):897–912.

83. Djebali S, Davis CA, Merkel A, et al. Landscape of transcription in human cells. *Nature.* 2012;489(7414):101–108.

84. ENCODE Project Consortium, Dunham I, Kundaje A, et al. An integrated encyclopedia of DNA elements in the human genome. *Nature.* 2012;489(7414):57–74.

85. Munger KL, Levin LI, Hollis BW, et al. Serum 25-hydroxyvitamin D levels and risk of multiple sclerosis. *JAMA.* 2006;296(23):2832–2838.

86. Islam T, Gauderman WJ, Cozen W, Mack TM. Childhood sun exposure influences risk of multiple sclerosis in monozygotic twins. *Neurology.* 2007;69(4):381–388.

87. Gelfand JM, Cree BA, McElroy J, et al. Vitamin D in African Americans with multiple sclerosis. *Neurology.* 2011;76(21):1824–1830.

88. Ramagopalan SV, Handel AE, Giovannoni G, et al. Relationship of UV exposure to prevalence of multiple sclerosis in England. *Neurology.* 2011;76(16):1410–1414.

89. Ramagopalan SV, Dyment DA, Cader MZ, et al. Rare variants in the CYP27B1 gene are associated with multiple sclerosis. *Ann Neurol.* 2011;70(6):881–886.

90. Ramagopalan SV, Maugeri NJ, Handunnetthi L, et al. Expression of the multiple sclerosis-associated MHC class II allele HLA-DRB1*1501 is regulated by vitamin D. *PLoS Genet.* 2009;5(2):e1000369.

91. Ramagopalan SV, Heger A, Berlanga AJ, et al. A ChIP-seq defined genome-wide map of vitamin D receptor binding: Associations with disease and evolution. *Genome Res.* 2010;20(10):1352–1360.

92. Smolders J, Menheere P, Kessels A, et al. Association of vitamin D metabolite levels with relapse rate and disability in multiple sclerosis. *Mult Scler.* 2008;14(9):1220–1224.

93. Soilu-Hänninen M, Laaksonen M, Laitinen I, et al. A longitudinal study of serum 25-hydroxyvitamin D and intact parathyroid hormone levels indicate the importance of vitamin D and calcium homeostasis regulation in multiple sclerosis. *J Neurol Neurosurg Psychiatry.* 2008;79(2):152–157.

94. Mowry EM, Krupp LB, Milazzo M, et al. Vitamin D status is associated with relapse rate in pediatric-onset multiple sclerosis. *Ann Neurol.* 2010;67(5):618–624.

95. Simpson S Jr, Taylor B, Blizzard L, et al. Higher 25-hydroxyvitamin D is associated with lower relapse risk in multiple sclerosis. *Ann Neurol.* 2010;68(2):193–203.

96. Dyment DA, Cader MZ, Chao MJ, et al. Exome sequencing identifies a novel multiple sclerosis susceptibility variant in the TYK2 gene. *Neurology.* 2012;79(5):406–411.

97. Ban M, Goris A, Lorentzen AR, et al. Replication analysis identifies TYK2 as a multiple sclerosis susceptibility factor. *Eur J Hum Gen.* 2009;17(10):1309–1313.

98. Mero IL, Lorentzen AR, Ban M, et al. A rare variant of the TYK2 gene is confirmed to be associated with multiple sclerosis. *Eur J Hum Genet.* 2010;18(4):502–504.

99. Baranzini SE, Mudge J, van Velkinburgh JC, et al. Genome, epigenome and RNA sequences of monozygotic twins discordant for multiple sclerosis. *Nature.* 2010;464(7293): 1351–1356.

100. International MHC and Autoimmunity Genetics Network, Rioux JD, Goyette P, et al. Mapping of multiple susceptibility variants within the MHC region for 7 immune-mediated diseases. *Proc Natl Acad Sci USA.* 2009;106(44):18680–18685.

101. Allcock RJ, Atrazhev AM, Beck S, et al. The MHC haplotype project: A resource for HLA-linked association studies. *Tissue Antigens.* 2002;59(6):520–521.

102. Stewart CA, Horton R, Allcock RJ, et al. Complete MHC haplotype sequencing for common disease gene mapping. *Genome Res.* 2004;14(6):1176–1187.

103. Miretti MM, Walsh EC, Ke X, et al. A high-resolution linkage-disequilibrium map of the human major histocompatibility complex and first generation of tag single-nucleotide polymorphisms. *Am J Hum Gen.* 2005;76(4):634–646.

104. de Bakker PI, McVean G, Sabeti PC, et al. A high-resolution HLA and SNP haplotype map for disease association studies in the extended human MHC. *Nat Genet.* 2006;38(10): 1166–1172.

105. Horton R, Gibson R, Coggill P, et al. Variation analysis and gene annotation of eight MHC haplotypes: The MHC Haplotype Project. *Immunogenetics.* 2008;60(1):1–18.

106. Oksenberg JR, Barcellos LF, Cree BA, et al. Mapping multiple sclerosis susceptibility to the HLA-DR locus in African Americans. *Am J Hum Genet.* 2004;74(1):160–167.

107. Barcellos LF, Oksenberg JR, Begovich AB, et al. HLA-DR2 dose effect on susceptibility to multiple sclerosis and influence on disease course. *Am J Hum Genet.* 2003;72(3):710–716.

108. Cree BA, Reich DE, Khan O, et al. Modification of multiple sclerosis phenotypes by African ancestry at HLA. *Arch Neurol.* 2009;66(2):226–233.

109. Dyment DA, Herrera BM, Cader MZ, et al. Complex interactions among MHC haplotypes in multiple sclerosis: Susceptibility and resistance. *Hum Mol Genet.* 2005;14(14):2019–2026.

110. Barcellos LF, Sawcer S, Ramsay PP, et al. Heterogeneity at the HLA-DRB1 locus and risk for multiple sclerosis. *Hum Mol Genet.* 2006;15(18):2813–2824.

111. Chao MJ, Barnardo MC, Lui GZ, et al. Transmission of class I/II multi-locus MHC haplotypes and multiple sclerosis susceptibility: Accounting for linkage disequilibrium. *Hum Mol Genet.* 2007;16(16):1951–1958.

112. Marrosu MG, Muntoni F, Murru MR, et al. Sardinian multiple sclerosis is associated with HLA-DR4: A serologic and molecular analysis. *Neurology.* 1998;38(11):1749–1753.

113. Marrosu MG, Murru MR, Costa G, et al. DRB1-DQA1-DQB1 loci and multiple sclerosis predisposition in the Sardinian population. *Hum Mol Genet.* 1998;7(8):1235–1237.

114. Marrosu MG, Murru R, Murru MR, et al. Dissection of the HLA association with multiple sclerosis in the founder isolated population of Sardinia. *Hum Mol Genet.* 2001;10(25): 2907–2916.

115. Brassat D, Salemi G, Barcellos LF, et al. The HLA locus and multiple sclerosis in Sicily. *Neurology.* 2005;64(2):361–363.

116. Brynedal B, Duvefelt K, Jonasdottir G, et al. HLA-A confers an HLA-DRB1 independent influence on the risk of multiple sclerosis. *PLoS One.* 2007;2(7):e664.

117. Yeo TW, De Jager PL, Gregory SG, et al. A second major histocompatibility complex susceptibility locus for multiple sclerosis. *Ann Neurol.* 2007;61(3):228–236.

118. Cree BA, Rioux JD, McCauley JL, et al. A major histocompatibility class I locus contributes to multiple sclerosis susceptibility independently from HLA-DRB1*15:01. *PLoS One.* 2010;5(6):e11296.

119. Healy BC, Liguori M, Tran D, et al. HLA B*44: Protective effects in MS susceptibility and MRI outcome measures. *Neurology.* 2010;75(7):634–640.

120. Celius EG, Harbo HF, Egeland T, et al. Sex and age at diagnosis are correlated with the HLA-DR2, DQ6 haplotype in multiple sclerosis. *J Neurol Sci.* 2000;178(2):132–135.

121. Masterman T, Ligers A, Olsson T, et al. HLA-DR15 is associated with lower age at onset in multiple sclerosis. *Ann Neurol.* 2000;48(2):211–219.

122. Hensiek AE, Sawcer SJ, Feakes R, et al. HLA-DR 15 is associated with female sex and younger age at diagnosis in multiple sclerosis. *J Neurol Neurosurg Psychiatry.* 2002;72(2): 184–187.

123. Smestad C, Brynedal B, Jonasdottir G, et al. The impact of HLA-A and -DRB1 on age at onset, disease course and severity in Scandinavian multiple sclerosis patients. *Eur J Neurol.* 2007;14(8):835–840.

124. Okuda DT, Srinivasan R, Oksenberg JR, et al. Genotype-phenotype correlations in multiple sclerosis: HLA genes influence disease severity inferred by 1HMR spectroscopy and MRI measures. *Brain.* 2009;132(Pt 1):250–259.

125. Romero-Pinel L, Pujal JM, Martínez-Yélamos S, et al. HLA-DRB1: Genetic susceptibility and disability progression in a Spanish multiple sclerosis population. *Eur J Neurol.* 2011;18(2):337–342.

126. Caillier SJ, Briggs F, Cree BA, et al. Uncoupling the roles of HLA-DRB1 and HLA-DRB5 genes in multiple sclerosis. *J Immunol.* 2008;181(8):5473–5480.

127. Johnson BA, Wang J, Taylor EM, et al. Multiple sclerosis susceptibility alleles in African Americans. *Genes Immun.* 2010;11(4):343–350.

Part II. Diagnosis

6

Symptoms and Signs of Multiple Sclerosis

LAEL A. STONE

KEY POINTS FOR CLINICIANS

- Multiple sclerosis (MS) may present with a myriad of symptoms affecting the central nervous system (CNS).

- Careful history-taking is required to distinguish MS-related symptoms that are helpful for diagnosis from less specific complaints.

- It is important to look for confirmation of symptoms on neurological examination, eg, increased reflexes or tone on exam support a complaint of stiffness and/or cramping.

- Pattern recognition is important in distinguishing MS symptoms and signs.

- Specific symptoms of demyelinating events (eg, unilateral visual loss, diplopia, gait ataxia, motor weakness, focal paresthesias, Lhermitte's phenomenon) are useful in diagnosis. However nonspecific symptoms which are sometimes seen in MS (fatigue, headache, depression, back pain) are less helpful as they are seen in many conditions.

ILLUSTRATIVE CASE

Jenny Penny is a 23-year-old right-handed white female. Six months ago she developed a painful sensation behind her left eye which was worse with movement. Over 3 days she developed a progressive loss of central vision in that eye with impaired color vision and decreased light brightness. This spontaneously resolved over 3 weeks. Three months ago she noticed a tingling sensation in the toes of both feet which ascended to the bra line over 4 days. This was associated with some sense of unsteadiness with walking and also trouble initiating urination. She now notices that when she flexes her neck forward she gets a tingling sensation in both arms and legs. She has also been much more tired than usual since this all began.

INTRODUCTION

The Nature of the Problem

Multiple sclerosis (MS) may present in a multitude of ways and many times the initial symptom of MS is not recognized until the occurrence of a second symptom. The medical literature is replete with case reports of unusual presentations of MS, as lesions can be found in virtually any area of the central nervous system (CNS) and therefore cause a variety of symptoms [1–5]. This chapter confines itself to the so-called primary symptoms of MS, ie, those caused by direct damage to the CNS, whether it is acute and inflammatory or progressive and degenerative, or a combination of the 2, rather than secondary symptoms which may occur because of the primary symptom. Examples of primary symptoms causing secondary symptoms would be bladder dysfunction (primary) causing repeat urinary tract infections (secondary); increased motor tone, ie, spasticity (primary) causing fatigue due to sleep disturbance (secondary). A few symptoms can be both primary and secondary symptoms of MS such as depression and fatigue.

The most common presenting symptoms for MS are related to acute optic neuritis [6,7], usually visual loss and accompanying pain in 90% of cases. However, when lumped together in broader categories, the most common system affected is likely the somatosensory system, with over 70% of patients having sensory complaints at some point in their disease course [8,9]. Motor complaints would likely be the next most common with nearly the same percentage of patients affected, particularly allowing for complaints during some part of the disease course. While some symptoms are more common in younger, relapsing-remitting patients (eg, visual symptoms, paresthesias) and others are more common in older patients at a more progressive phase (eg, muscle weakness, spasticity), some symptoms can occur at any point in the disease course.

Because symptoms of MS can affect so many areas of the CNS, MS may present in a multitude of ways. Patients who have multiple or somewhat odd symptoms are frequently told by non-MS clinicians, as well as lay people or even internet search engines, that their symptoms "sound like MS." Differentiating true MS symptoms from a laundry list of complaints therefore, can be an exercise in fine-tuned pattern recognition. That is to say, a clinician who is attuned to and very familiar with typical descriptions of neurological symptoms by patients who turn out to have MS may hear and interpret symptoms somewhat differently from those who hear only a 1- or 2-word description from a list of possibly neurological symptoms particularly in the context of nonspecific white matter changes on cranial MRI. Vague symptoms appear to take on more import to the patient and primary care clinician in this context as discussed by Corboy's study of this phenomenon [10]. This chapter attempts to lead the history-taker through the steps that MS clinicians take in sorting out the symptoms which are most likely to be MS, from those which are least likely to be MS, and then turn to how one can find confirmation for these symptoms on neurological examination. More detailed information on the pathophysiology, consequences, and treatment of the most common and disabling MS symptoms can be found in other chapters.

EVALUATION OF SYMPTOMS

Part 1: History

The first pieces of information that we learn about a patient are the demographics, which are only moderately useful in the decision-making process to decide if symptoms are MS-related or not. While MS is certainly most common in white females from 20 to 50 years old, classic symptoms can occur in any age group and ethnic group. The main exception to this would be unilateral visual loss, where age is a distinguishing factor in helping to decide if this symptom is MS, ie, optic neuritis, or not MS [6,7]. A second exception may be progressive myelopathy (more likely due to MS in younger individuals and cervical spondylosis in older ones). Speaking in broad generalization, history-takers should attempt to place demographical information at the back of their mind when listening to histories of possibly MS symptoms.

Probably the most important piece to deciphering if a symptom is MS-related or not would be the quality of the symptom combined with the location. Localization should clearly match the CNS only, eg, hemibody, or band around the torso, or unilateral visual loss; or alternatively be so peculiar sounding that the patient often prefaces the description with "I know this sounds crazy but..." as in a patch of skin which feels wet or itching in the absence of any apparent skin change. Sensory or motor symptoms involving the whole body, or just hands and feet, are rarely related to MS. See Tables 6.1 and 6.2 for symptoms which are suggestive of CNS syndromes that can occur in MS.

Timing of the occurrence of symptoms is critical. For example, symptoms may occur a few days after a known trigger of demyelination, such as infection, or during the postpartum period (a time of increased relapse activity). Timing in the sense of how long the symptom lasts is also critical, as MS-related symptoms tend to occur in 2 types: longer lasting, ie, at least 48 to 72 hours up to several weeks, and brief repetitive symptoms known as transient neurological events or paroxysmal symptoms, lasting few seconds to minutes, but occurring in a stereotypical manner. Paroxysmal symptoms can occur frequently in MS patients and are often mistaken for seizures although alteration in consciousness is rare. These generally involve transient face, arm, and leg, or only arm and leg sensory and/or motor symptoms. Most MS symptoms though, last greater

TABLE 6.1

Some Symptom Descriptions Which Suggest MS Due to CNS Symptomatology

"I woke up with loss of vision in 1 eye and pain with moving that eye"

"When I bend my neck down I get an electric feeling through my body"

"I developed tingling in both feet which over a couple of days went up to just under the bra line on both sides"

"I developed double vision with 2 images one above the other"

"I got a patch of itching over my shoulder blade with no rash"

"I notice that when I exercise or take a hot shower my leg gets weaker"

"I find I now have to go to the bathroom right away when I get the signal" than 48 to 72 hours, and many, such as those consistent with progressive myelopathy, may take years to become apparent. On occasion, this chronicity makes clinicians think of orthopedic causes such as ankle or knee injuries which are actually the result rather than the cause of the gait abnormality before they consider CNS disorders.

Another important clue is to find out if heat and exertion worsen symptoms. Heat is a well-known trigger for temporary worsening of MS symptoms, but this should again be approached with caution in taking the history, as descriptions of complete exhaustion or generalized heat intolerance may be due to many things. More useful are individual symptoms worsening in the heat such as graying of vision with heat or exertion, ie, Uhthoff's phenomenon (increased symptoms occurring with increased body temperature). Very typical of CNS dysfunction related to MS would be descriptions of foot drop, sometimes described as making a slapping sound, after long walks, particularly if the distance needed to bring out the foot drop decreases with the passage of years, eg, the description that "2 years ago I was able to walk 1 mile before the foot drop occurred, but now I can only walk 2 blocks before it occurs." Some MS patients have no heat sensitivity at all, and many become stiffer in cold weather, or have increased bladder urgency upon encountering cold air. Worsening with change in position is rarely typical for MS symptoms. The main exceptions would be Lhermitte's phenomenon and severe spasticity when change of position causes spasms. While Lhermitte's may be caused by many abnormalities affecting the cervical spine, patients who describe a "zinging" electrical sensation down their back with neck flexion should undergo cervical cord imaging. Spasticity generally worsens with prolonged sitting and may present with complaint of calf tightness or pain, or toe/foot cramps at night or legs jerking/flexing involuntarily.

Part 2: Confirming the Symptoms With Signs on Examination

After completing the history, the examination should be geared toward strengthening the evidence that MS is the cause of the symptoms, or discovering alternative explanations. For example, if the patient complains of pain in the legs, increased reflexes and/or Hoffman or Babinski sign may confirm the suspicion that this is spasticity. Questionable histories of visual loss may be corroborated by red desaturation, altered visual acuity or contrast sensitivity, and/or pale optical discs. Whenever possible, the examination of the possible MS patient should begin with the evaluation of gait. Ideally, the patient should walk far enough to see subtle changes consistent with foot drop or decreased arm swing. Having the patient stand and hop on 1 foot will help confirm complaints of decreased strength on 1 side of the body, and also elicit these complaints from individuals who may have not noticed, or were reluctant to mention weakness. Spasticity and ataxia can also be ascertained with observation of gait. The presence of various sorts of functional gaits

TABLE 6.2
Red Flags of MS Symptoms and Signs

- Age of patient greater than 60
- Total body complaints, eg, total body weakness or numbness
- Excessive fatigue or depression
- Absence of visual complaints other than presbyopia
- Absence of bladder complaints other than cough and sneeze incontinence
- Diarrhea rather than constipation
- Sudden, ie, seconds to minutes onset of symptoms
- Positional symptoms other than Lhermitte's phenomenon
- Absence of investigation of comorbidities such as diabetes, sleep apnea, depression, and cervical spondylosis
- Prominent systemic manifestations (fever, weight loss, rash, arthritis, etc.)

such as astasia-abasia can also be evaluated. In proceeding through the rest of the neurological exam, it is interesting to note that eye signs may not produce symptoms noticeable to the patient although they are classic for MS, such as an intranuclear opthalmoplegia (INO) [11]. Alternative explanations for symptoms may be found on examination such as dystonia, muscle fasciculations or cogwheeling, all leading to other diagnoses. Unfortunately, some patients, even those with MS, may elaborate their symptoms, with inconsistent or nonphysiological exam features.

SYMPTOM REVIEW BY SYSTEM

Cognition

Changes in cognition and affect are common in MS, although generally not as the presenting symptom. Before invoking MS as the potential cause for memory change or cognitive change, it is critical to distinguish this from delirium or acute worsening in mental functioning due to infection, such as an indolent urinary tract infection, or side effect of medication. Particularly, if the mental decline is less than a month in duration and there are any symptoms referable to the urinary tract such as retention/hesitation, a urinalysis should be obtained. Similarly, a careful review of the medications both prescribed and over-the-counter supplements should be conducted, and potentially cognitively altering medications, such as statins, benzodiazepines, and narcotics, should be eliminated wherever possible.

Poorly controlled diabetes as well as hypothyroidism and low vitamin B_{12} are remarkably common in the same population that is susceptible to MS and should therefore be screened for as part of the cognitive evaluation. Cognitive changes due to MS must also be distinguished from general overload, as when individuals are trying to do too much, or are fatigued because of poor sleep quantity or quality. Anxiety and depression can similarly adversely affect both mood and fatigue, and many patients with depression say that their memory is impaired [12,13]. MS patients may suffer from cognitive changes at any time during the disease course and statistics regarding incidence range from 20% to 50% [14,15]. On formal neuropsychological testing, domains of verbal memory and attention/speed of information processing are most affected. Neuropsychological testing can assist with both distinguishing cognitive change in patients suspected of having MS from anxiety and depression and also assist individuals with knowing which areas of cognition are relatively retained and thus can be utilized more fully [16].

Mood

Depression and anxiety can be primary symptoms of MS, or secondary symptoms. Depression as a comorbidity has been noted to be associated with more rapid decline of MS [17]. Because the MS population also has a high risk for suicide, rapid identification of depression as well as aggressive treatment and follow-up is recommended. There is likely an increased incidence of bipolar disease in MS patients. Mania has been reported as well as frank psychosis [1–20]. Steroid-induced affective changes are common in MS patients and should be considered when using these medicines. Pseudobulbar affect or emotional incontinence is likely an underrecognized symptom in MS as well [21,22].

Cranial Nerves

Visual System
As previously stated, the most common, single presenting symptom in MS is optic neuritis, which generally involves unilateral visual loss [6,11]. Ninety percent of patients present with pain on moving the eye, and often describe their visual loss as "like looking through a screen or petroleum jelly." Decreased color vision is common, and patients may be checked for red desaturation possibly indicating a previous asymptomatic optic neuritis as well. INO, which is due to a disturbance in the medial longitudinal fasciculus of the brainstem, may present as double vision, or may be completely asymptomatic for reasons that are unclear given the significant nature of the disturbance. Since MS is the most common cause of INO, imaging should be obtained in these cases unless MS is known to be present. Nystagmus is also common in MS, and patients may complain of jumpy vision, particularly if they are tired or overheated. Various types of nystagmus and ocular movements have been reported and depend on which location or locations in the central neuraxis are affected.

Other cranial nerves may also show evidence of dysfunction in MS. Disturbances of facial sensation are common with or without pain. Trigeminal neuralgia, in particular, can be troubling to patients, and MS should certainly be considered as a potential cause in young female patients presenting with this condition, particularly if it is bilateral [23]. Atypical facial pains as well as ear pain may occur as well, but it is useful to have patients seen for dental evaluation to exclude temporomandibular joint (TMJ) disorders and other pathologies, as well as ears, nose, and throat (ENT) evaluation. Hearing loss may also occur in MS, although it is recommended to exclude other causes of hearing loss. Vertigo and dizziness may be seen in MS patients, but in the vast majority of the time MS is not the sole cause for the dizziness, given the significant number of patients who have cervicogenic dizziness which responds to effective physical therapy. Recent reports have indicated that many patients with MS and vertigo actually have benign positional vertigo which is readily treated with exercises such as the modified Epley [24].

Likewise, while swallowing problems certainly can occur in later stages of MS, ambulatory patients with MS who complain of swallowing problems generally point to the lower throat as the sticking point, and swallowing evaluation and gastrointestinal (GI) work-up reveals other more treatable causes of the difficulty. Dysfunction in articulation may occur in MS, usually in association with other lower cranial nerve difficulties. The staccato rhythms of cerebellar speech are occasionally seen in MS patients as well.

Somatosensory Pathways

As mentioned above, disturbances in sensory pathways in MS patients are very common, and most often involve hemibody complaints. Other typical complaints are patches of odd sensations, particularly the feeling of wetness or itching or something crawling (formication) in the absence of anything being on the skin. Spinal cord lesions may present with the so-called "MS hug," which is a band or belt like sensation often involving the thoracic region. Hemibanding sensations can also occur, and may lead to superfluous cardiac work-ups. Severe abdominal girdling sensation can occur as well, often associated with difficult-to-manage constipation. Patients may or may not have evidence of sensory dysfunction on examination, although loss of vibratory sensation is common in MS patients.

While many physicians are taught in training that pain does not occur in MS, unfortunately this is not true, and many of the sensory symptoms in MS are indeed painful, particularly those generated from spinal cord lesions as well as trigeminal neuralgia [25]. However, complaints of total body pain, like total body weakness, are not typical of MS. A distribution of the pain in an area consistent with CNS localization, as opposed to radicular or joint or fibromyalgia type pain would be the most reliable way of distinguishing MS-related pain from other causes. Paroxysmal symptoms may also cause brief but excruciating pain, usually involving the face, arm, and leg, or only the arm and the leg in a repetitive manner. Other head pains may be found in MS, for example in optic neuritis, particularly when bilateral, or severely swollen cervical cord lesions which may cause pain in the back of the head and upper neck associated with stiffness and difficulty with movement. Increases in tone, such as that found with spasticity or spasms, may also be perceived as painful, particularly in the calf, but sometimes also in the thigh and/or toes.

Motor Pathways

The dysfunction of motor pathways in MS follows an upper motor neuron distribution. Face, arm, and leg, or just arm and leg distribution of weakness is typical, although the patient may or may not be aware of the arm weakness particularly if it is on the nondominant side. Patients may not complain of spasticity per se, but complaints of calf or toe cramping at night, particularly unilateral or asymmetrical, may be related to MS, particularly in the context of increased reflexes on examination. Cold or prolonged inactivity such as sitting may worsen spasticity. Muscle weakness associated with MS occurs with increased tone and would only be associated with muscle atrophy in very late stages. Weakness from MS is often accompanied by altered autonomic function in the affected limb, causing swelling and dependent cyanosis which may lead to a fruitless search for deep vein thrombosis or arterial insufficiency. Foot dragging can occur frequently, and is often brought out by heat or exertion. Pattern of progression of weakness of 1 foot, which then progresses to weakness on the corresponding rest of the body is relatively common and may occur over days, weeks, or even years or decades. Sudden or acute onset of weakness would be much more likely to indicate a vascular cause rather than MS.

Cerebellum and Cerebellar Connections

Limb and gait ataxia are some of the most disabling symptoms that can occur in MS. Unfortunately, once the cerebellum and its connections are involved, symptoms tend to progress through time. Patients rarely complain of the scanning pattern which can occur with cerebellar speech, but family members will acknowledge the change in speech on questioning. Patients, however, are very much aware of and troubled by dysmetria and cerebellar tremors, when they occur, as well as truncal ataxia when present.

Bowel and Bladder Pathways

MS patients frequently complain of bowel and bladder issues. Constipation is the most common bowel complaint, and bowel incontinence is often overflow incontinence.

Constipation may be relatively mild to begin with, but is then exacerbated by symptomatic medications, and the tendency of MS patients to consciously or unconsciously reduce fluid intake in an attempt to control bladder problems. Diarrhea is not typically associated with MS, and if not medication- or food-related, should be investigated. Bladder complaints are also common in MS [26], and certainly are exacerbated by constipation as well as medications used for symptom management. MS patients may also have structural or non-MS-related bladder complaints, such as cough and sneeze (stress) incontinence, but the true complaints consistent with neurogenic bladder are more likely to be difficulty emptying (hesitancy), increased urge to void (urgency), and urge or overflow incontinence. History is very helpful in distinguishing structural and functional bladder complaints, but it is necessary to perform a post-void residual volume measurement or more extensive urological testing to diagnose and recommend treatment for the various types of neurogenic bladder dysfunction.

NONSPECIFIC VERSUS SPECIFIC SYMPTOMS

Frequently, patients are sent for MS evaluation because of nonspecific symptoms. These include fatigue, myalgias, headache, memory impairment, depression, and diffuse paresthesias. These symptoms are seen commonly in a variety of syndromes (eg, rheumatic disorders, somatization disorders, fibromyalgia, depression) and are not helpful in the diagnosis of MS. When taking a history of the symptoms of MS, focusing on more specific symptoms that suggest demyelination may be key. These include symptoms such as the Lhermitte's phenomenon (electrical feelings when flexing the neck), unilateral visual loss suggesting optic neuritis, focal paresthesias in a CNS distribution, diplopia particularly vertical, and spinal cord symptoms such as a combination of paresthesias below a level, motor weakness below a level, and bowel and bladder disruption. When we diagnose MS, we use the specific symptoms for diagnosis. When we treat MS, we also need to attend to the nonspecific symptoms in terms of management.

CONCLUSION-FINDING PATTERNS WHICH FIT TOGETHER

As illustrated, MS has truly protean manifestations, which can affect virtually every area controlled by the CNS. Distinguishing MS symptoms can often be best done by history, and then confirmed on examination, and then focused testing, as covered in other chapters. Pattern recognition, and the abilities to listen carefully and observe are key in this endeavor.

KEY POINTS FOR PATIENTS AND FAMILIES

- While the list of potential MS symptoms is long, actual MS symptoms can and must be distinguished from generic categories such as "bladder problems" or "visual symptoms."

- It is often more important to distinguish what is not due to MS, ie, a symptom is due to MS only if all other possibilities have been eliminated.

- Symptoms involving the entire body, eg, total body pain or weakness or fatigue severe enough to cause someone to actually fall asleep while sitting, are unlikely to be due to MS.

- MS symptoms can cause pain in some circumstances, much of which can be improved with appropriate diagnosis and management.

- MS symptoms often worsen with increased body temperature from fever or exercise, but may worsen with inactivity or cold in some cases.

- The symptoms of MS vary from patient to patient. Most people with MS have 1 or more of the following during their course: numbness or tingling, weakness, double vision, loss of vision in 1 eye, bladder difficulty, trouble with walking or balance.

- Not all symptoms are due to MS even when you have MS, and you may need to check with your primary doctor or neurologist whether new symptoms are due to something else.

- The symptoms help diagnose MS. However, the diagnosis of MS is not based solely on symptoms as they may have many causes.

REFERENCES

1. Sponsler JL, Kendrick-Adey AC. Seizures as a manifestation of multiple sclerosis. *Epileptic Disord.* 2011;13:401–410.

2. Chanson JB, Kremer S, Blanc F, et al. Foreign accent syndrome as a first sign of multiple sclerosis. *Mult Scler.* 2009;15:1123–1125.

3. Aguirregomozcorta M, Ramió-Torrentà L, Gich J, et al. Paroxysmal dystonia and pathological laughter as a first manifestation of multiple sclerosis. *Mult Scler.* 2008;14:262–265.

4. Ozünlü A, Mus N, Gulhan M. Multiple sclerosis: A cause of sudden hearing loss. *Audiology.* 1998;37:52–58.

5. De Santi L, Annunziata P. Symptomatic cranial neuralgias in multiple sclerosis: Clinical features and treatment. *Clin Neurol Neurosurg.* 2012;114:101–107.

6. Chan JW. Early diagnosis, monitoring, and treatment of optic neuritis. *Neurologist.* 2012;18:23–31.

7. Sakai RE, Feller DJ, Galetta KM, et al. Vision in multiple sclerosis: The story, structure-function correlations, and models for neuroprotection. *J Neuroophthalmol.* 2011;31:362–373.

8. Rae-Grant AD, Eckert NJ, Bartz S, Reed JF. Sensory symptoms of multiple sclerosis: A hidden reservoir of morbidity. *Mult Scler.* 1999;5:179–183.

9. Osterberg A, Boivie J. Central pain in multiple sclerosis – sensory abnormalities. *Eur J Pain.* 2010;14:104–110.

10. Carmosino MJ, Brousseau KM. Arciniegas DB, Corboy JF. Initial evaluations for multiple sclerosis in a university multiple sclerosis center: Outcomes and role of magnetic resonance imaging in referral. *Arch Neurol.* 2005;62:585–590.

11. Pula JH, Reder AT. Multiple sclerosis. Part I: Neuro-ophthalmic manifestations. *Curr Opin Ophthalmol.* 2009;20:467–475.

12. Mills RJ, Young CA. The relationship between fatigue and other clinical features of multiple sclerosis. *Mult Scler.* 2011;17:604–612.

13. Brown RF, Valpiani EM, Tennant CC, et al. Longitudinal assessment of anxiety, depression, and fatigue in people with multiple sclerosis. *Psychol Psychother.* 2009;82(Pt 1):41–56.

14. Staff NP, Lucchinetti CF, Keegan BM. Multiple sclerosis with predominant, severe cognitive impairment. *Arch Neurol.* 2009;66:1139–1143.

15. Langdon DW. Cognition in multiple sclerosis. *Curr Opin Neurol.* 2011;24:244–249.

16. Foley R, Benedict R, Gromisch E, Deluca J. The need for screening, assessment, and treatment for cognitive dysfunction in MS: Results of a multidisciplinary CMSC consensus conference, September 24, 2010. *Int J MS Care.* 2012;14:58–64.

17. Marrie RA, Horwitz R, Cutter G, et al. The burden of mental comorbidity in multiple sclerosis: Frequent, underdiagnosed, and undertreated. *Mult Scler.* 2009;15:385–392.

18. Feinstein A. Neuropsychiatric syndromes associated with multiple sclerosis. *J Neurol.* 2007;254(Suppl 2):II73–II76.

19. Agan K, Gunal DI, Afsar N, et al. Psychotic depression: A peculiar presentation for multiple sclerosis. *Int J Neurosci.* 2009;119:2124–2130.

20. Iacovides A, Andreoulakis E. Bipolar disorder and resembling special psychopathological manifestations in multiple sclerosis: A review. *Curr Opin Psychiatry.* 2011;24:336–340.

21. Work SS, Colamonico JA, Bradley WG, Kaye RE. Pseudobulbar affect: An under-recognized and under-treated neurological disorder. *Adv Ther.* 2011;28:586–601.

22. Ghaffar O, Chamelian L, Feinstein A. Neuroanatomy of pseudobulbar affect: A quantitative MRI study in multiple sclerosis. *J Neurol.* 2008;255:406–412.

23. Cruccu G, Biasiotta A, Di Rezze S, et al. Trigeminal neuralgia and pain related to multiple sclerosis. *Pain.* 2009;143:186–191.

24. Frohman EM, Kramer PD, Dewey RB, et al. Benign paroxysmal positioning vertigo in multiple sclerosis: Diagnosis, pathophysiology and therapeutic techniques. *Mult Scler.* 2003;9: 250–255.

25. Nurmikko TJ, Gupta S, Maclver K. Multiple sclerosis-related central pain disorders. *Curr Pain Headache Rep.* 2010;14:189–195.

26. Stoffel JT. Contemporary management of the neurogenic bladder for multiple sclerosis patients. *Urol Clin North Am.* 2010;37:547–557.

7

Diagnosis of Multiple Sclerosis

MICHAEL HUTCHINSON

KEY POINTS FOR CLINICIANS

- The diagnostic criteria for multiple sclerosis (MS) have changed. A diagnosis of MS may now sometimes be made when the patient has a first attack of MS. MRI criteria for dissemination in space have also been changed.

- Spinal fluid testing is no longer required for the diagnosis of relapsing MS. However, there may be cases where it is helpful in the diagnosis. It still is a part of diagnosis for some cases of primary progressive MS.

- The 3 principles of diagnosis remain dissemination in space, dissemination in time, and no better explanation.

The diagnosis of multiple sclerosis (MS) and the *giving* of that diagnosis is the responsibility of clinical neurologists. The diagnostic process, both in accuracy and in the manner in which it is conveyed, is crucial to the future management of the patient. While in many patients the diagnosis may be straightforward from the clinical presentation and investigations, a substantial proportion (one-third of patients referred to neurologists with suspected MS) do not have MS, but another disorder [1,2].

Our ability to diagnose MS earlier and more accurately than before is because of the more sensitive diagnostic criteria and the ubiquity of MRI scanning. The concept that therapy should be begun as soon as possible in the disease course has increased both the pressure for an early diagnosis and the possibility of misdiagnosis. A not infrequent clinical scenario is the misinterpretation by a general radiologist of an MRI brain scan showing nonspecific white matter lesions as indicative of demyelinating disease; such calamitous misdiagnosis may be conveyed to the primary physician and thus to the patient.

Diagnostic criteria for MS are needed because, unlike many other diseases, a single gold standard diagnostic test for MS is lacking. It is the aim of this chapter to describe the process of diagnosis of MS, using currently accepted criteria. The pitfalls, which are there for the unwary, are described in Chapter 10; almost every neurologist has, at some stage in their career, made a diagnosis of MS only for it to be later overturned.

DIAGNOSTIC CRITERIA: A VERY SHORT HISTORY

Up until 1983, diagnostic criteria for MS were based on the clinical history and neurological examination combined with the results of the paraclinical investigations, cerebrospinal fluid (CSF), and evoked response studies [3]. With the advent of MRI scanning in the early 1980s, demyelinating lesions in the brain could be visualized and a number of investigators proposed MRI criteria for diagnosis [4]. The need to include such information in the diagnosis of MS was recognized by the U.S. National MS Society and the International Federation of MS Societies who convened an expert group of experienced neurologists. They met in London in 2000 under the chairmanship of Professor Ian McDonald and devised a set of diagnostic criteria, subsequently called the McDonald Criteria [5] (see Figure 7.1).

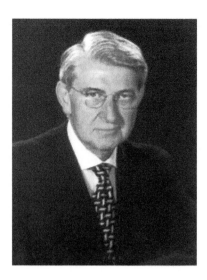

FIGURE 7.1
Professor William Ian McDonald (1933–2006) was born in
Wellington, New Zealand; his undergraduate and early
postgraduate studies were at the University of Otago,
Dunedin. His doctoral and initial postdoctoral research
delineated the pathology and physiology of demyelination
and remyelination in the peripheral and, later, the central
nervous system. He came to the National Hospital for
Neurology and Neurosurgery, Queen Square, London, United
Kingdom in the early 1960s; subsequently he was appointed
a consultant neurologist and a personal chair was established
in 1974. From the mid-1980s he led a team of world reknown
researchers examining the clinical, pathological, and natural
history features of multiple sclerosis as revealed by MRI
scanning. He had a long-time interest in the diagnosis of
MS and chaired the first meeting of a group of international
experts to update MS diagnostic criteria in 2000; the original
criteria and revisions were named the McDonald Criteria in
his honor. *(The author had the pleasure of working with him in
the 1970s.) (Photograph courtesy Institute of Neurology, London,
United Kingdom.)*

Subsequent reassessment of the McDonald Criteria
in patient cohorts, an increased understanding of the natural history of MS revealed by the MRI, and improved MRI
techniques led to revisions in 2005 in Amsterdam [6] and
in 2010 in Dublin [7]. The latest version has simplified the
diagnostic process, allowing MS to be diagnosed earlier,
making the criteria easier to use in everyday clinical practice, and more relevant for use in randomized controlled trials. The overall aim of the groups of international experts
from 2000 to 2010 has been to improve the sensitivity of the
criteria (and their utility) without sacrificing specificity. The
overwhelming benefit of incorporating MRI with clinical
data in diagnostic criteria is that one may diagnose MS with
confidence much earlier in the course of the illness than by
clinical grounds alone.

> The latest version of the McDonald Criteria (2010) has
> simplified the diagnostic process, allowing MS to be
> diagnosed earlier.

DIAGNOSING MS: THE MCDONALD CRITERIA (2010)

Three basic principles underlie and ensure the integrity of the criteria. All 3 must be fulfilled to diagnose MS
(Table 7.1) [7].

1. The principle of dissemination in space (DIS). This
   principle requires that there are lesions typical of MS
   present in 2 or more different sites within the central
   nervous system (CNS). DIS can be determined on clinical
   grounds alone or by clinical and MRI criteria combined.
2. The principle of dissemination in time (DIT). The principle of DIT requires that 2 attacks separated by more than
   30 days have occurred in different parts of the CNS. DIT
   can be defined on clinical grounds alone or by a combination of clinical and MRI criteria.
3. The principle of no better explanation. Even if the clinical and MRI findings are strongly indicative of MS, there
   is no better explanation for these abnormalities than MS
   for a secure diagnosis to be made. This is, in many ways,
   the most difficult principle to apply; many diseases
   mimic MS in that they demonstrate both DIT and DIS.

DEFINING THE PHENOMENOLOGY OF MS

A number of features of the clinical presentation of MS are
critical to the diagnosis and need strict definition.

The Clinical Course of MS

An international survey initiated by the National MS Society
(USA) resulted in an important publication defining, by
consensus, the various clinical subtypes of MS [8]. The subtype definitions agreed to were:

Relapsing-remitting MS (RRMS): Clearly defined
relapses (described subsequently) with full recovery
or with sequelae and residual deficit upon recovery;
periods between disease relapses are characterized
by a lack of disease progression.

Secondary progressive MS (SPMS): Initial RR disease
course followed by gradual clinical progression with
or without occasional relapses, minor remissions,
and plateaus.

Primary progressive MS (PPMS): Gradual clinical
disease progression from onset with occasional plateaus and temporary minor improvements allowed.

Progressive-relapsing MS (PRMS): Progressive disease
from onset, with clear acute relapses, with or without
full recovery; periods between relapses characterized
by continuing progression.

Relapse (Synonyms: Attack, Exacerbation)
Since approximately 85% of people with MS have an initially
relapsing course, it is of crucial importance to define a relapse

TABLE 7.1
A Summary of the Structure and Essential Features of the Scheme for the Diagnosis of Multiple Sclerosis Using the McDonald Criteria (2010) [7]. The Demonstration of DIS and DIT Can be Made by Clinical Features Alone or by a Combination of Clinical and MRI Features

CLINICAL FINDINGS AT PRESENTATION		ADDITIONAL DATA NEEDED FROM MRI OR CLINICAL FOLLOW-UP
EPISODES FROM HISTORY	OBJECTIVE CLINICAL SIGNS	
2 attacks	2 lesions	None
2 attacks	1 lesion	Evidence of DIS
1 attack	2 lesions	Evidence of DIT
1 attack	1 lesion	Evidence of both DIS and DIT
Progressive course over 1 year		DIS demonstrated by 2 of: a) MRI brain b) MRI cord c) CSF oligoclonal bands

In all cases ensure that there is no better explanation for the clinical presentation than that of multiple sclerosis.
CSF, cerebrospinal fluid; DIS, dissemination in space; DIT, dissemination in time.

accurately. The McDonald Criteria (quoted here because it is so elegantly and precisely stated) defined a relapse as

...patient-reported symptoms or objectively observed signs typical of an acute inflammatory demyelinating event in the CNS, current or historical, with duration of at least 24 hours, in the absence of fever or infection. Although a new attack should be documented by contemporaneous neurological examination, in the appropriate context, some historical events with symptoms and evolution characteristic for MS, but for which no objective neurological findings are documented, can provide reasonable evidence of a prior demyelinating event.

Reports of paroxysmal symptoms (historical or current) should consist of multiple episodes occurring over not less than 24 hours. Before a definite diagnosis of MS can be made, at least one attack must be corroborated by findings on neurological examination, visual evoked potential response in patients reporting prior visual disturbance, or MRI consistent with demyelination in the area of the CNS implicated in the historical report of neurological symptom.

> A relapse is defined as *...patient-reported symptoms or objectively observed signs typical of an acute inflammatory demyelinating event in the CNS, current or historical, with duration of at least 24 hours, in the absence of fever or infection.*

In summary, a relapse/exacerbation lasts at least 24 hours and must consist of symptoms typical (to a trained neurologist) of demyelination. If, as is not uncommon, one sees a patient with new symptoms and signs of a spinal cord lesion and he or she describes an event many years ago consistent with an optic neuritis, then one may accept the history as indicating a previous attack of MS and which often defines the time of symptom onset of MS. Ideally, one should confirm the true nature of the previous event by some neurological sign such as diminished visual acuity in

that eye, a relative afferent pupillary defect, optic atrophy or more definitively by a delayed visual evoked response in that eye (Figure 7.2 for another example).

Pseudorelapse
The caveat in the definition provided of a relapse, in relation to "absence of fever or infection" refers to the effect of a rise in body temperature in people with MS. Patients, usually with established MS, may have an intercurrent infection causing a rise in body temperature. Because an increase in body temperature, even by 0.5 degrees, causes conduction block in axons demyelinated in a previous (often forgotten) attack, new symptoms may appear and may last more than 24 hours. With resolution of the fever, the symptoms clear and neurological function returns to the state prior to the fever. This phenomenon does not represent a true relapse. When a fever (or rise in body temperature due to a hot bath or exercise) occurs in the setting of a previous optic neuritis, from which there had been a full recovery, then the patient may experience transient blurring of vision in the previously affected eye (Uhthoff's phenomenon).

The Interval Between Relapses—The 30-Day Rule
It is well recognized that a small proportion of patients experiencing a relapse may have multifocal symptoms indicating multiple lesions occurring almost simultaneously within the CNS. It has been accepted since the original McDonald Criteria (2000) that relapses can only be regarded as being separate in time (in order to satisfy criteria for dissemination in time) when there are at least 30 days separating the onset of the 2 episodes (Figure 7.2). For example, if a patient develops an optic neuritis and 2 weeks later numbness in their legs, that clinical scenario is a single multifocal relapse and, although satisfying the criterion for DIS, does not satisfy the criterion for dissemination in time. On the other hand, if these 2 symptoms are separated by an interval of 30 days or more, then they are regarded as representing 2 distinct relapses and satisfy both criteria (DIS and DIT).

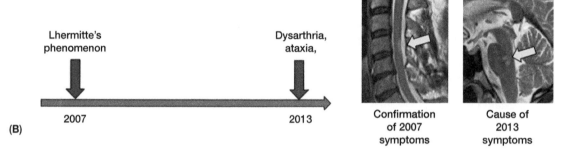

Features of a Relapse

Neurological disturbance of kind seen in MS indicating inflammatory/demyelinating pathology.

Subjective report *or* objective observation 24 hours duration minimum.

Excludes pseudorelapses and single paroxysmal episodes.

(A) Separate relapses: at least 30 days between *onset* of event 1 and *onset* of event 2.

30 days +

Relapse 1
duration > 24 hrs

Relapse 2
duration > 24 hrs

If a historical event and no abnormal clinical signs of that event:

Example (below): patient presenting now (2013) with brainstem symptoms/signs and history of Lhermitte's phenomenon lasting > 24 hours, 6 years ago.

Corroborate 2007 symptoms, if possible, by MRI cervical cord (see arrowed lesions).

Lhermitte's
phenomenon

Dysarthria,
ataxia,

2007

2013

(B)

Confirmation
of 2007
symptoms

Cause of
2013
symptoms

FIGURE 7.2

Clinical features defining a relapse. In particular: (A) for 2 episodes to be considered distinct relapses, there must be at least 30 days between the onset of the first relapse and the onset of the second relapse; (B) for relapses reported on history taking, attempt to define the historical relapse by MRI (in this particular example the true nature of the history of Lhermitte's symptom was confirmed by MRI of the cervical cord which showed a posterior column lesion [arrowed]).

PUTTING THE MCDONALD CRITERIA (2010) INTO PRACTICE

Diagnosing MS by Clinical Criteria Alone

Evidence for both DIT and DIS may be obtained from the clinical history and examination alone and thus MS may be diagnosed on clinical grounds alone (but see the following caveat).

Clinical Criteria for DIS

In a patient presenting with symptoms typical of an MS attack, such as double vision with signs of an internuclear ophthalmoplegia indicating a tectal brain stem lesion, other clinical signs may be present indicating a lesion or lesions elsewhere in the CNS. Such signs might include optic atrophy with a central scotoma or signs of a spinal cord lesion such as extensor plantar responses, loss of vibration sensation or a clumsy hand with proprioceptive loss. These signs, indicating lesions in at least 2 separate sites in the neuraxis, satisfy DIS by clinical grounds alone.

Clinical Criteria for DIT

Not uncommonly, a patient presenting with a symptom characteristic of an MS attack will, on careful history taking, give a story of an episode some years previously indicating an episode of demyelination. For example, a patient

presenting with unilateral optic neuritis may describe an episode of Lhermitte's symptom. By the definition of an attack (described earlier), such paroxysmal symptoms must have been recurrent and have lasted longer than 24 hours. Also, the clinical neurologist should attempt to confirm the nature of the history of Lhermitte's symptom by a paraclinical examination—most commonly an MRI scan of the cervical cord will show a plaque of posterior column demyelination (Figure 7.2). Some of these historical accounts may be vague and leave one uncertain whether they represent a previous episode of demyelination. Clinical judgment should be employed in the interpretation of these historical events.

> Some of these historical accounts may be vague or uncertain whether they represent a previous episode of demyelination.

Caveat

Despite the foregoing paragraph, and although symptoms and signs are essential to the MS diagnosis, it is unsafe to rely on clinical history and signs alone. In particular, in order to satisfy the third principle, *"no better explanation,"* because many diseases demonstrate both DIT and DIS, it is necessary to exclude these MS mimics by an MRI scan of the brain (and at times spinal cord). Such mimics might include the

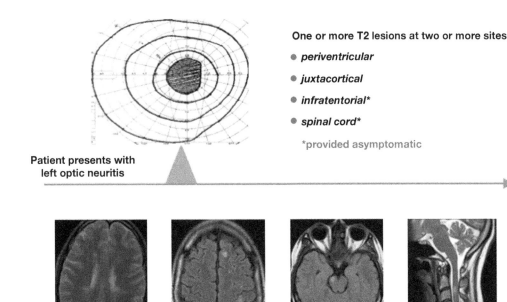

One or more T2 lesions at two or more sites

● *periventricular*

● *juxtacortical*

● *infratentorial**

● *spinal cord**

*provided asymptomatic

Patient presents with
left optic neuritis

Periventricular   Juxtacortical   Infratentorial   Spinal cord

FIGURE 7.3
Illustrating the McDonald (2010) MRI Criteria for determining dissemination in space (DIS).

anti-phospholipid syndrome which on history and signs might suggest MS but which has distinct MRI characteristics; these MS mimics are fully described in Chapter 10.

DIAGNOSING MS BY COMBINED CLINICAL AND MRI CRITERIA

MRI Evidence of DIS

Since the initial criteria in 2000, the MRI requirements to satisfy DIS have been reassessed by prospective longitudinal studies of patients presenting with the clinically isolated syndrome (see Table 7.1) [9,10].

The most recent revision has altered the MRI characteristics required to satisfy DIS:

DIS can be demonstrated with at least one T2 lesion in at least 2 of 4 locations considered characteristic for MS (juxtacortical, periventricular, infratentorial, and spinal cord), with lesions within the symptomatic region excluded in patients with brainstem or spinal cord syndromes. (Figure 7.3)

These criteria were shown to be more sensitive than the original McDonald Criteria without compromising specificity or accuracy [10].

Clinical example: In a patient presenting with, for example, an optic neuritis, in order to satisfy the criteria of DIS, it is now only necessary to have 2 other asymptomatic T2 lesions on MRI scanning as long as (a) they are considered

> DIS can be demonstrated with at least one T2 lesion in at least 2 of 4 locations considered characteristic for MS (juxtacortical, periventricular, infratentorial, and spinal cord), with lesions within the symptomatic region excluded in patients with brainstem or spinal cord syndromes.

to be typical of demyelination and (b) there is at least 1 T2 lesion situated in 2 of the 4 designated sites (juxtacortical, periventricular, infratentorial, or spinal cord) (see Figure 7.3).

MRI Evidence of DIT

The requirements for demonstration of DIT were simplified in the 2010 revisions (see Table 7.2). DIT can now be demonstrated in 2 ways:

1. A new T2 lesion and/or a gadolinium-enhancing lesion *at any time* on a follow-up scan compared to the baseline scan qualifies as DIT (Figure 7.4).
2. A single MRI scan with intravenous gadolinium which demonstrates the simultaneous presence of 1 or more T2 lesion(s) (which were nonenhancing on T1) and at least 1 gadolinium-enhancing T1 lesion, shows evidence of DIT (Figure 7.5). Thus, if the baseline scan shows both nonenhancing T2 lesions and gadolinium-enhancing lesions, then this qualifies as DIT, which is supported by empirical data [11].

TABLE 7.2

McDonald (2010) MRI Criteria for the Demonstration of DIS and DIT in Patients Being Considered for the Diagnosis of RRMS [7]

DISSEMINATION IN SPACE	DISSEMINATION IN TIME

One or more T2 lesions in at least 2 of 4 CNS regions:
  : periventricular
  : juxtacortical
  : infratentorial*
  : spinal cord*
	Either
	1) A new T2 and/or gadolinium-enhancing lesion at follow-up MRI (at any time) with reference to a baseline MRI.
	or
	2) Simultaneous presence of asymptomatic gadolinium-enhancing and nonenhancing lesions at any time.

*If the patient has a spinal cord or brain stem presentation then the symptomatic lesions are excluded from the lesion count.

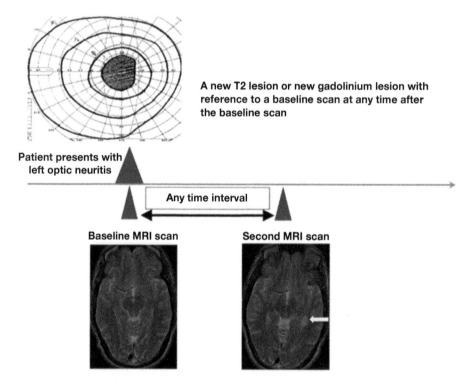

A new T2 lesion or new gadolinium lesion with reference to a baseline scan at any time after the baseline scan

Patient presents with left optic neuritis

Any time interval

Baseline MRI scan   Second MRI scan

FIGURE 7.4

McDonald (2010) MRI Criteria for DIT. Illustrating the first of 2 methods of determining DIT. A new T2 lesion (arrow) or gadolinium-enhancing lesion at any time period after a baseline scan.

Primary Progressive Multiple Sclerosis (PPMS)

In the most recent revisions of the McDonald Criteria [7], the MRI requirements for DIS in PPMS were revised (see Table 7.3 and Figure 7.6). It is now necessary to have:

1. At least 1 year of disease progression, and
2. Satisfy 2 of the following 3 requirements:
   A. Evidence of DIS in the brain by 1 or more lesions in at least one area (periventricular, juxtacortical, or infratentorial) characteristic for MS.
   B. Two or more asymptomatic spinal cord T2 lesions.
   C. An abnormal CSF characterized by CSF oligoclonal bands (CSFOBs) on isoelectric focusing or elevated IgG index.

Importantly, it must be noted that if the patient has a brain stem or spinal cord syndrome (as is most likely in PPMS), then all symptomatic lesions are excluded from the criteria. Determining the symptomatic lesion is not easy in practice, but if a patient has a progressive spastic paraparesis, it is clear that 1 spinal cord lesion must be symptomatic and, in order to satisfy spinal cord criteria for DIS, then there need to be at least 3 spinal cord T2 lesions, 1 of which is presumed to be causing the spastic paraparesis.

TABLE 7.3

McDonald 2010 Criteria for Diagnosing PPMS [7]. DIT is Represented by the History of 1 Year of Disease Progression. The Utility of Demonstrating CSF Immunoglobulin Abnormalities in PPMS is Recognized by According This the Same Value as the Demonstration of DIS Criteria in the Brain and Cord

1) One year of disease progression
   (prospectively or retrospectively determined)

and

2) Two of three criteria:
   a) Evidence for DIS in the brain by 1 or more T2 lesions in at least 1 area characteristic for MS (periventricular, juxtacortical, or infratentorial*).
   b) Evidence for DIS in the spinal cord based on 2 or more T2 lesions in the cord*.
   c) Positive CSF (oligoclonal bands on isoelectric focusing and/or elevated IgG index).

*If the patient has a symptomatic cord or brain stem presentation all symptomatic lesions are excluded from the lesion count.

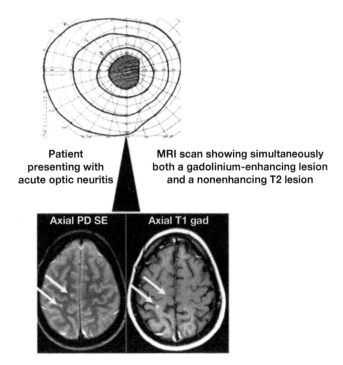

FIGURE 7.5

McDonald (2010) MRI Criteria for DIT. Illustrating the second of 2 methods of determining DIT. MRI scan showing simultaneous enhancing T1 and T2 nonenhancing lesions (arrows).

THE UTILITY OF CEREBROSPINAL FLUID EXAMINATION IN THE DIAGNOSIS OF MS: WHY DO A LUMBAR PUNCTURE?

Many patients with RRMS are diagnosed using MRI criteria alone and, in many neurological practices, CSF examination is not performed. In the case of PPMS, it is valuable to examine the CSF because the presence of CSFOBs forms 1 of the 3 criteria for DIS in the diagnostic criteria. However, not all PPMS patients have CSFOBs; of the 943 PPMS patients in the PROMiSe trial, 22% had negative CSFOBs despite fulfilling all other criteria for the diagnosis as determined by a patient eligibility committee [12].

Another reason to perform CSF analysis is to demonstrate an immunological abnormality consistent with MS. Although a normal CSF examination is consistent with both RRMS and PPMS and CSFOBs are found in MS mimics, the absence of CSFOBs serves to alert the clinician to other possible diagnoses and for that reason may help the clinician search for another (better) explanation for the clinical presentation [13].

- One year of progressive neurological deterioration
- PLUS TWO of the following
  - DIS in brain: one or more T2 lesions in two areas of: periventricular, juxtacortical or infratentorial*
  - DIS in cord: two or more T2 lesions in spinal cord*
  - CSF oligoclonal bands and/or increased IgG index

  *provided asymptomatic

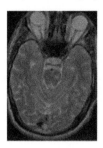 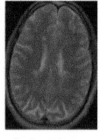 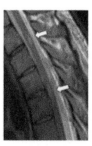 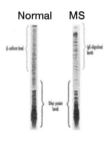

Infratentorial　　*Periventricular*　　*Spinal cord*　　*CSF oligoclonal bands*

FIGURE 7.6
McDonald (2010) Criteria for diagnosing PPMS. The arrows indicate 2 spinal cord plaques.

DIAGNOSTIC CATEGORIES RESULTING FROM APPLYING THE MCDONALD CRITERIA

After applying the 3 basic principles in any 1 patient as described, the clinician should arrive at the conclusion that the patient has 1 of 3 possible diagnoses:

a. **Multiple Sclerosis:** If the clinical and MRI features satisfy the McDonald Criteria.

or

b. **Possible Multiple Sclerosis:** If the clinical features are persuasive but not all criteria are fulfilled. Most commonly, this occurs when a patient has symptoms and clinical signs of only 1 lesion (for example, optic neuritis) and MRI of the brain satisfies criteria for DIS without evidence of DIT. This is called the *clinically isolated syndrome* (CIS) and such patients are at high risk of future events satisfying the requirement for DIT, confirming the diagnosis of multiple sclerosis. Other examples of "possible MS" include patients with a progressive myelopathy and CSF oligoclonal bands but insufficient MRI lesions in the brain or spinal cord to satisfy criteria for DIS. These patients need careful clinical and radiological follow-up.

or

c. **Not MS:** The patient has some other disorder.

"Clinically Definite Multiple Sclerosis"

The term *clinically definite multiple sclerosis* (CDMS) is not a diagnostic subgroup of the McDonald (2010) Criteria but is often used to indicate patients who have satisfied the criteria for DIS and DIT on clinical grounds (as opposed to patients who have demonstrated DIT or DIS by MRI criteria). The term CDMS has been used in studies of the CIS to indicate patients who subsequently have had a further clinically symptomatic attack (first relapse).

Possible MS, the CIS

The CIS refers to the first presentation with neurological symptoms and signs consistent with CNS demyelination. Such typical presentations include spinal cord symptoms such as a numb clumsy hand due to a plaque in a posterior column of the cervical cord, and double vision with an internuclear ophthalmoplegia due to a brain stem plaque. MRI scanning in CIS patients may reveal asymptomatic lesions, which increase the likelihood of further episodes. The 2010 McDonald Criteria made it possible to diagnose MS at the onset of the disease (ie, at the time of CIS presentation), if MRI scanning showed lesions consistent with DIS and DIT. Prior to the 2010 criteria, it was always necessary to repeat MRI scanning to show DIT. Now a patient with a CIS presentation may satisfy criteria for DIS and DIT (and thus be diagnosed as having MS) by a single first scan if the MRI scan shows both gadolinium-enhancing and nonenhancing lesions (Figure 7.5) and also lesions satisfying criteria for DIS (Figure 7.3).

LIMITATIONS OF THE MCDONALD (2010) CRITERIA

How Generalizable Are the Criteria?

The diagnostic criteria are evidence-based but much of that evidence comes from the examination of cohorts of white adult patients in Europe and North America. Thus, whether such criteria can be applied to the pediatric population or to Asian and Latin American patients has yet to be established by studies in those patient groups.

> Whether such criteria can be applied to the pediatric population or to Asian and Latin American patients has yet to be established.

Radiologically Isolated Syndrome

With the increased use of MRI scanning, neurologists not infrequently encounter patients with white matter CNS pathology typical for demyelination and who have no symptoms or signs of neurological disease. When further investigated, these patients often have CSFOBs and abnormal evoked responses. The panel of experts framing the McDonald Criteria (2010) concluded that in the absence of symptoms and signs one could not diagnose these patients as having MS. These patients are diagnosed as having radiologically isolated syndrome (RIS).

There have been several follow-up studies of radiologically isolated syndrome (RIS) cohorts indicating that such patients are at high risk of symptom development. The management of RIS patients is the subject of ongoing debate. It has been suggested that RIS patients should be regarded as having preclinical CIS, and might be treated with disease-modifying therapies [14–16].

FUTURE DIRECTIONS IN THE DIAGNOSIS OF MS

There have been significant changes in MS diagnostic criteria in the last 10 years and undoubtedly there will be more in the next decade.

One should expect McDonald Criteria (2015) and McDonald Criteria (2020). Why?

The changes in criteria in the last 10 years have been driven by research findings examining the utility of MRI in the natural history of MS. The main thrust has been to simplify and speed the process of diagnosis without sacrificing specificity. New MRI techniques including double inversion recovery sequences and the use of higher-powered MRI (3T) scanners may improve the detection of cortical lesions and thus affect the deliberations of future panels. Lastly, although biomarkers have not been established outside the research sphere, one may anticipate that a biomarker will be incorporated as a diagnostic tool in the next 10 years.

KEY POINTS FOR PATIENTS AND FAMILIES

- While the diagnosis of MS can sometimes be made on the basis of a history and neurological examination, MR imaging and possibly other testing is usually required to make this diagnosis.

- Other conditions can cause symptoms like MS and need to be considered when making a diagnosis of MS.

- New criteria for diagnosing MS mean that the diagnosis can be made earlier and with more confidence than in the past.

- Sometimes, continued follow-up and MR imaging may be necessary before a diagnosis of MS can be made.

REFERENCES

1. Carmosino MJ, Brousseau KM, Arciniegas DB, et al. Initial evaluations for multiple sclerosis in a university multiple sclerosis center. *Arch Neurol.* 2005;62:585–590.

2. Kelly SB, Chaila E, Duggan M, et al. Using atypical symptoms and red flags to identify non-demyelinating disease. *J Neurol Neurosurg Psychiatry.* 2012;83:44–48.

3. Poser CM, Paty DW, Scheinberg LC, et al. New diagnostic criteria for multiple sclerosis: Guidelines for research protocols. *Ann Neurol.* 1983;1:227–231.

4. Barkhof F, Filippi M, Miller DH, et al. Comparison of MR imaging criteria at first presentation to predict conversion to clinically definite MS. *Brain.* 1997;120:2059–2069.

5. McDonald WI, Compston A, Edan G, et al. Recommended diagnostic criteria for multiple sclerosis: Guidelines from the International Panel on the diagnosis of multiple sclerosis. *Ann Neurol.* 2001;50:121–127.

6. Polman CH, Reingold SC, Edan G, et al. Diagnostic criteria for multiple sclerosis: 2005 revisions to the "McDonald Criteria." *Ann Neurol.* 2005;58:840–846.

7. Polman CH, Reingold SC, Banwell B, et al. Diagnostic criteria for multiple sclerosis: 2010 revisions to the "McDonald Criteria." *Ann Neurol.* 2011;69:292–302.

8. Lublin FD, Reingold SC. Defining the clinical course of multiple sclerosis: Results of an international survey. National Multiple Sclerosis Society (USA) Advisory Committee on Clinical Trials of New Agents in Multiple Sclerosis. *Neurology.* 1996;46:907–911.

9. Swanton JK, Fernando K, Dalton CM, et al. Modification of MRI criteria for multiple sclerosis in patients with clinically isolated syndromes. *J Neurol Neurosurg Psychiatry.* 2006;77:830–833.

10. Swanton JK, Rovira A, Tintoré M, et al. MRI criteria for multiple sclerosis in patients presenting with clinically isolated syndromes: A multicentre retrospective study. *Lancet Neurol.* 2007;6:677–686.

11. Rovira A, Swanton JK, Tintoré M, et al. A single, early magnetic resonance imaging study in the diagnosis of multiple sclerosis. *Arch Neurol.* 2009;5:287–292.

12. Wolinsky JS, Narayana PA, O'Connor P, et al. Glatiramer acetate in primary progressive multiple sclerosis: Results of a multicenter, double-blind, placebo-controlled trial. *Ann Neurol.* 2007;61:14–24.

13. Miller D, Weinshenker B, Filippi M, et al. Differential diagnosis of suspected multiple sclerosis: A consensus approach. *Mult Scler.* 2008;14:1157–1174.

14. Lebrun C, Bensa C, Debouverie M, et al. Association between clinical conversion to multiple sclerosis in radiologically isolated syndrome and magnetic resonance imaging, cerebrospinal fluid, and visual evoked potential: Follow-up of 70 patients. *Arch Neurol.* 2009;66:841–846.

15. Okuda DT, Mowry EM, Beheshtian A, et al. Incidental MRI anomalies suggestive of multiple sclerosis: The radiologically isolated syndrome. *Neurology.* 2009;72:800–805.

16. Okuda DT, Mowry EM, Cree BA, et al. Asymptomatic spinal cord lesions predict disease progression in radiologically isolated syndrome. *Neurology.* 2011;76:686–692.

8

Magnetic Resonance Imaging in Multiple Sclerosis

ALIYE O. BRICKER
STEPHEN E. JONES

Like many diseases, multiple sclerosis (MS) was well known long before the introduction of MRI in the late 1970s. Although MS is fundamentally a clinical diagnosis supported by detailed history, careful neurological examination, and often additional bloodwork and sometimes cerebrospinal fluid (CSF) assessment, MRI has had a growing impact on accurate and early diagnosis, and is now an integral part of monitoring disease activity [1,2]. For example, as determined by the most recent International Panel on Diagnosis of Multiple Sclerosis, MRI of the central nervous system (CNS) can support, supplement, or even replace some clinical criteria necessary for the diagnosis [3–6]. MRI can clearly demonstrate multiple aspects of known MS pathology, such as dissemination in time (DIT) and space (DIS). The former is shown by changes in serial MRI imaging, or the simultaneous appearance of lesions with different ages. The latter is shown by multiple and widespread lesions. For example, estimates show more than 95% of patients with clinically definite MS having multifocal cerebral white matter lesions on brain MR imaging [1]. MS is known to have an early inflammatory phase, which is shown by enhancement after intravenous administration of gadolinium contrast, resulting from breakdown of the blood–brain barrier. Subsequent to the acute phase, localized loss of oligodendrocytes and axonal fibers manifests on MRI as chronic white matter lesions, which slowly accumulate over time. Although MS is classically considered a demyelinating disease involving white matter of the brain and spinal cord, gray matter involvement is also prevalent but more difficult to image. Newer imaging techniques such as high field strength imaging may help in demonstrating this involvement.

RELEVANT MRI PHYSICS

The strong magnetic field created by an MRI scanner causes hydrogen nuclei throughout the body's water molecules to align. By perturbing the magnetic field using the application of magnetic field gradients and radiofrequency electromagnetic radiation, whose orchestration is termed a "sequence," the alignments of these hydrogen nuclei can be altered in subtle ways to produce a detectable signal. Sophisticated analysis algorithms can use these signals to reconstruct images, where the grayscale contrast takes on different meanings depending on the details of the sequence. Furthermore, different tissue types such as fat, fluid, muscle, and the gray and white matter in the brain, all have different hydrogen nuclei concentrations and relaxation properties. These influence the depicted MRI image, for example, ranging from dark to bright signal intensity. In summary, MRI is extremely sensitive to the details of water concentration and is an exquisitely sensitive modality for detecting focal abnormalities, particularly in the white matter.

Different MRI sequences have been developed to best emphasize certain tissue characteristics. For example, T1-weighted sequences cause water to be dark, or have low signal intensity, while fat demonstrates bright signal. Conversely, T2-weighted sequences cause water and tissues with high water concentration to show bright signal intensity. The fluid-attenuated inversion recovery (FLAIR) sequence is a variant of a T2-weighted sequence in which free water, such as CSF, is suppressed and becomes dark. The FLAIR technique is invaluable for increasing the visibility of T2 bright lesions located near bright CSF structures, such as sulci and ventricles. Proton density (PD) sequences display a grayscale that is directly proportional to the concentration of hydrogen nuclei (the higher the number of protons in a given unit of tissue, the brighter the signal). This allows for excellent contrast between the central deep gray nuclei of the brain and brain stem (which have fewer protons and therefore darker signal) and inflammatory lesions containing higher proton content and therefore bright signal. Proton density sequence images are also particularly valuable in evaluating the cerebellum.

CHARACTERIZATION OF MS ON CONVENTIONAL MRI

The standard MR imaging protocol for detection of MS lesions and disease activity includes axial T2-weighted and axial PD images, as well as both axial and sagittal FLAIR images to better identify callosal and pericallosal lesions. Precontrast T1-weighted images (usually axial) are necessary to quantify the number of T1 dark signal intensity lesions or "black holes," followed by corresponding postcontrast T1-weighted images to identify areas

of enhancement thought to correspond to areas of active demyelination. The typical MR imaging protocol for MS is summarized in Table 8.1, and an example is shown in Figure 8.1. Although this imaging protocol utilizes imaging sequences available and is relatively consistent across all MRI machines, FLAIR and fast spin echo sequence parameters can nevertheless vary slightly between MRI vendors, thus varying specific lesion characteristics. For this reason, it is best, if possible, to consistently perform follow-up imaging on the same MRI machine to allow the most accurate comparison.

Central to the clinical diagnosis of MS is the concept of lesions *disseminated in both space and time*. The imaging correlate is a visualization of multiple MRI lesions with different ages (or evidence of a new lesion added to old lesions). Lesions can be located anywhere throughout the brain and spinal cord. Since MRI lesions can be nonspecific, or rather that many non-MS forms of neuropathology also produce similar lesions, it is important to classify lesions in terms of their signal characteristics, location, and morphology. Imaging criteria for MS diagnosis using recent guidelines are seen in Table 8.2. Note that older criteria requiring lesion counting are no longer used and criteria for DIT and DIS have both been simplified.

TABLE 8.1
Standard "MS Protocol" MR Imaging Sequences

SEQUENCE	PLANE	FEATURES
FLAIR	Axial	Workhorse: Best supratentorially
FLAIR	Sagittal	Best for callosal/pericallosal regions
T2	Axial	Best infratentorially
PD	Axial	Best infratentorially
T1 precontrast	Sagittal or Axial	Black holes; necessary to compare with post contrast
T1 postcontrast	Axial	Active lesions

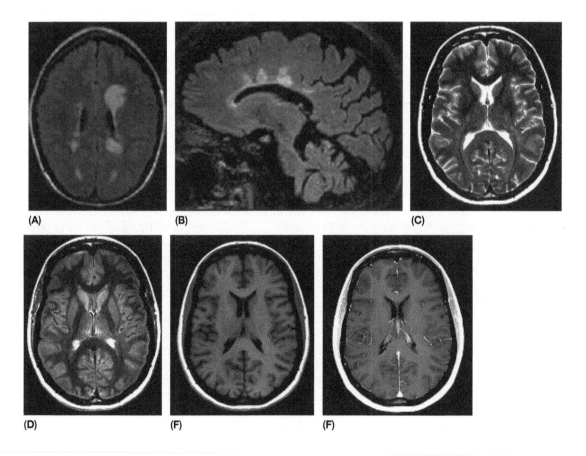

(A)   (B)   (C)

(D)   (F)   (F)

FIGURE 8.1
Example of typical MS protocol. Axial FLAIR (A) and sagittal FLAIR (B) images both demonstrate callosal and pericallosal with a perpendicular orientation along the callososeptal margin more conspicuous on the sagittal plane image (B). Axial T2-weighted image (C) demonstrates additional periventricular and deep white matter lesions in both hemispheres—slightly less obvious than on the FLAIR. Bottom row axial PD image (D) is useful to identify central deep white matter lesions. Axial precontrast T1-weighted (E) and axial postcontrast T1-weighted (F) images are used to identify areas of enhancement correlating to areas of active demyelination.

TABLE 8.2
2010 International MRI Criteria for Demonstration of DIS [5]

DIS can be demonstrated by 1 or more T2 lesions in at least 2 of 4 areas of the CNS:

Periventricular
Juxtacortical
Infratentorial
Spinal cord

Gadolinium enhancement of lesions is not required for DIS

If a patient has a brain stem or spinal cord syndrome, the symptomatic lesions are excluded from the criteria and do not contribute to the lesion count.

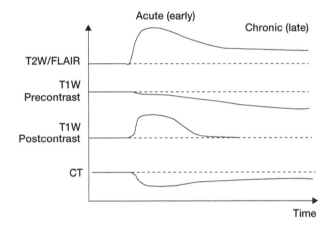

FIGURE 8.2
Time course of MRI change in MS lesion. Note early development of contrast enhancement and T2-weighted change and later development of T1 "black hole" changes.

MRI Signal Characteristics and Morphology

Lesions within the brain are generally small, 5 to 10 mm, with a rounded or ovoid shape. Signal characteristics of the lesions can be divided into early or acute, and late or chronic (see Figure 8.2).

Acute lesions have borders that are somewhat fluffy and ill defined on T2 and FLAIR sequences (Figure 8.3), while chronic lesions have sharply defined borders (Figure 8.4). For both acute and chronic lesions, the signal intensity is bright on T2, FLAIR, and PD sequences. Regarding T1 sequences, acute lesions may be the same or darker than the adjacent normal white matter. Occasionally, hyperacute lesions may even show a thin rim of bright signal on T1 images. Chronic lesions on T1 sequences show well-defined dark regions (so-called "black holes") with associated volume loss (Figure 8.5), likely representing long-standing disease with axonal destruction, and show some correlation with overall disease progression or disability [7,8].

In the acute setting, an actively demyelinating lesion typically enhances following intravenous contrast administration, reflecting inflammation-related localized breakdown of the blood–brain barrier. Enhancement patterns are often initially solid, subsequently enlarging radially and developing a classic, "incomplete ring" pattern (Figure 8.6), before dissipating after 2 to 6 weeks. The natural time course of enhancement of an acute MS lesion can be rapidly altered with treatment by steroids or immunosuppressants, specifically with the rapid resolution of enhancement, often within days [7]. These acute, actively demyelinating lesions are often bright on diffusion weighted images (DWI), likely reflecting high cellularity due to infiltrative inflammatory cells. Typically, MS lesions show minimal mass effect on the adjacent brain, or at least the degree of mass effect is disproportionately low compared to the size of the lesions,

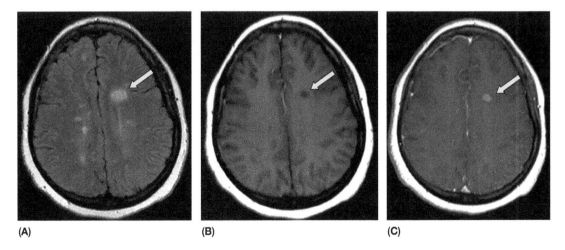

(A)   (B)   (C)

FIGURE 8.3
A 39-year-old woman with moderate disease burden MS. Axial FLAIR image (A) shows numerous patchy foci of FLAIR bright signal throughout the deep periventricular and pericallosal white matter of both hemispheres. The largest lesion in the left frontal lobe shows relatively fluffy, ill-defined margins on the FLAIR image (arrow, A), corresponding dark signal on precontrast T1 image (arrow, B), and avid enhancement following contrast administration (arrow, C) consistent with a new or acute lesion with active demyelination.

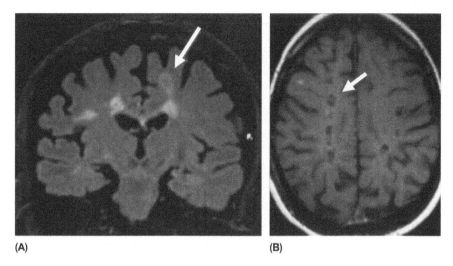

FIGURE 8.4
Coronal FLAIR (A) and axial T1 (B) images in this patient with known, long-standing MS show bilateral deep white matter lesions with sharp, well-defined margins and corresponding profoundly dark T1 signal consistent with late or chronic lesions. These T1 dark foci are commonly referred to as "black holes."

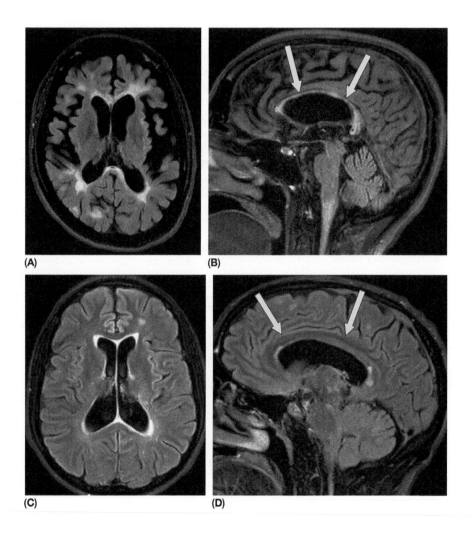

FIGURE 8.5
Upper row axial FLAIR (A) and sagittal FLAIR (B) images from a middle-aged woman with advanced MS demonstrate severe burden, patchy and near confluent bright signal abnormality throughout the periventricular and subcortical white matter with marked associated thinning of the corpus callosum (arrows, B) and marked generalized brain parenchymal volume loss greater than expected for age. Axial FLAIR (C) and sagittal FLAIR (D) images from a young, newly diagnosed patient with MS demonstrate relatively fewer white matter lesions with volume of the corpus callosum and overall brain parenchymal volume intact.

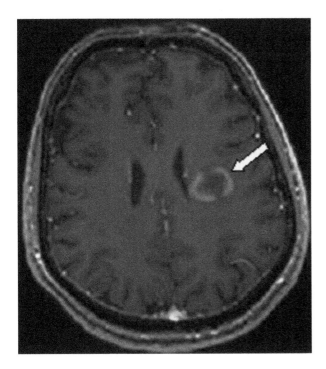

FIGURE 8.6
Lesion (arrow) within the deep white matter of the left cerebral hemisphere of this patient with known MS demonstrates incomplete ring of enhancement characteristic for acute demyelination. In patients not yet diagnosed with MS who present for the first time with neurological symptoms, identifying this "incomplete ring" pattern of enhancement on MR imaging of the brain can be an important clue to suggest underlying demyelinating disease.

as might be expected for a glioma, for example. Note that large "mass-like" lesions can also occur, although infrequently, with an imaging appearance termed *tumefactive MS* (Figure 8.7).

Location

The classical pattern of MS disease shows multiple lesions that are bilaterally scattered along periventricular margins, mostly elongated and oriented perpendicular to the ventricles (Figure 8.8). Lesions are commonly located within the corpus callosum or at the "callososeptal junction" along the midline at the septum pelucidum. The elongated periventricular lesions correspond to the classic description of "Dawson's fingers" representing collections of inflammatory cells clustered around perpendicularly oriented small veins or venules [9]. When viewed in the sagittal plain, the characteristic appearance of rounded and ovoid white matter lesions scattered along the ependymal margin or "under-surface" of the corpus callosum and extending into the pericallosal white matter and calloseptal junction has been coined as the "dot-dash" sign, shown to have 90% to 95% sensitivity and specificity for the diagnosis of MS [10,11] (see Figures 8.1 and 8.8). Other common lesion

locations in the brain include the juxtacortical white matter, anterior temporal lobes, brachium pontis, and cerebellum (Figure 8.8).

Although the typical MS patient will have relatively fewer lesions in the spinal cord compared to the brain, likely reflecting the relatively large volume of the brain compared to the cord volume, spinal cord lesions are usually more symptomatic. In fact, as many brain lesions can be clinically silent, cord lesions often cause the initial symptoms that persuade a patient to seek medical care. Thus, any cervical MRI demonstrating a spinal cord lesion with features suspicious for MS should prompt follow-up imaging of the brain. As in the brain, these lesions are bright on T2 or PD images, often located in the periphery of the cord, are generally less than 2 vertebral body segments in length, and encompass less than one-half of the cross-sectional area of the cord (Figure 8.8I). Also similar to the brain, acute or actively demyelinating lesions typically show enhancement following contrast administration. In addition, acute cord lesions can be mildly to moderately expansile, enlarging the overall diameter of the spinal cord at that level. In distinction, chronic cord lesions are associated with focal volume loss, or myelomalacia. This may impart a scalloped shape to the surface of the cord visible on sagittal images. In addition, cord lesions not uncommonly disappear entirely on imaging after months or years.

DIS

According to the most recent International Panel criteria, dissemination of lesions in space can be demonstrated on MR imaging by identifying 1 or more T2 bright lesions in at least 2 of 4 locations considered characteristic for MS: periventricular white matter, juxtacortical white matter, posterior fossa, or in the spinal cord [5] (see Figure 8.8).

DIT

DIT can be demonstrated in its simplest form by identifying new lesions on consecutive follow-up MRI (see Figure 8.9). A recent additional International Panel criterion to fulfill DIT on a single MRI examination is the simultaneous presence of lesions of different ages. Specifically, the criterion requires the presence of an asymptomatic gadolinium-enhancing (or lesions with an acute pattern of imaging characteristics) *and* nonenhancing lesions (or lesions with chronic imaging pattern) simultaneously on a single MRI study in a patient with typical clinical presentation, provided there is no non-MS pathology [5,12,13].

With progression of disease, there is an accumulation and coalescence of chronic lesions, many containing frank axonal destruction. Long-standing MS patients typically demonstrate a pattern of brain parenchymal volume loss that bears the stigmata of recurrent inflammatory damage. For example, given the preferential distribution of MS lesions throughout the corpus callosum and callososeptal junction, chronic MS patients eventually develop striking callosal volume loss. Deep white matter lesions and periventricular lesions lead to marked enlargement of the ventricles (see Figures 8.5, 8.10, and 8.11). The degenerative phase of MS leads to cortical volume loss with apparent widening of the sulci.

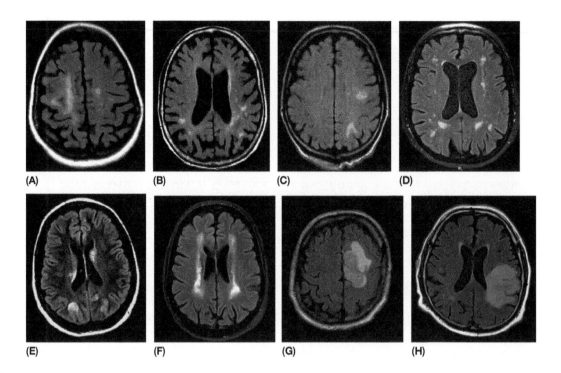

FIGURE 8.7
Examples of mimics and potential look-alikes based on imaging alone: Several axial FLAIR images from patients with entirely different diagnoses. Image A is a patient with lymphoma. Image B is an older patient with hypertension and nonspecific chronic microvascular white matter changes. Image C is a patient with progressive multifocal leukoencephalopathy from reactivation of the JC virus. Image D is a patient with giant cell arteritis demonstrating changes secondary to recurrent inflammation involving the cerebrovascular blood vessels. Image E is a patient with progressive reversible encephalopathy syndrome. Image F is a patient with Fahr's disease, an inherited neurological disorder of abnormal calcium deposition within the brain. Images G and H both demonstrate mass-like areas of signal abnormality with image G from a patient with malignant brain tumor (glioblastoma multiforme) and image H from a patient with the tumefactive mass-like presentation of MS.

Variations in Appearance and Potential Look-Alikes

Like many tissues, when subjected to pathological insult, the brain can only respond macroscopically in several ways. Since MRI typically images a tissue's macroscopic response rather than the pathology itself, many different pathologies or diseases can have a similar appearance. Specifically, MRI exquisitely measures water concentration within tissues, which can be altered in two ways: (a) vasogenic edema which allows excess water to enter the brain parenchyma from leaky vessels, or (b) the destruction or alteration of myelin (which is hydrophobic) which allows excess water to enter the now more-hydrophilic lesion. Thus, although extremely sensitive in the detection of white matter pathology, unfortunately many MRI abnormalities common in MS are nonspecific and can be seen in a variety of other disease processes, which are difficult to distinguish by imaging alone (see Figure 8.7). An additional difficulty is that the number, size, and overall burden of brain and spinal cord disease can vary dramatically depending on the stage at which an MS patient is imaged and the severity of their disease.

Nonspecific White Matter Disease

The most common differential diagnostic consideration for multiple nonenhancing foci of bright T2 or FLAIR signal in the supratentorial white matter without associated mass effect is nonspecific white matter disease (NSWMD), which are multiple small foci of white matter injury thought secondary to the sequelae of chronic, clinically silent, microvascular ischemia. These white matter changes are often associated with generalized, diffuse brain parenchymal volume loss frequently noted in patients over 50 years old [14], and can be accentuated in patients with chronic hypertension or diabetes. An example of nonspecific, likely chronic microvascular ischemic changes is included in Figure 8.7.

Though the imaging appearance of early or mild MS and mild chronic microvascular ischemic change can be nearly identical, nonimaging factors such as age, gender, other disease, and clinical presentation may help distinguish them. Several imaging features may favor MS over NSWMD. The distribution of lesions can be a distinguishing factor. Lesions involving the corpus callosum and along the callososeptal junction are more common in MS while relatively rare in chronic microvascular disease. The degree of volume loss specifically involving the corpus callosum is also generally greater in MS than in a patient with chronic microvascular ischemic change, which is more often associated with generalized volume loss involving the entirety of the brain and manifested by prominence of the cortical

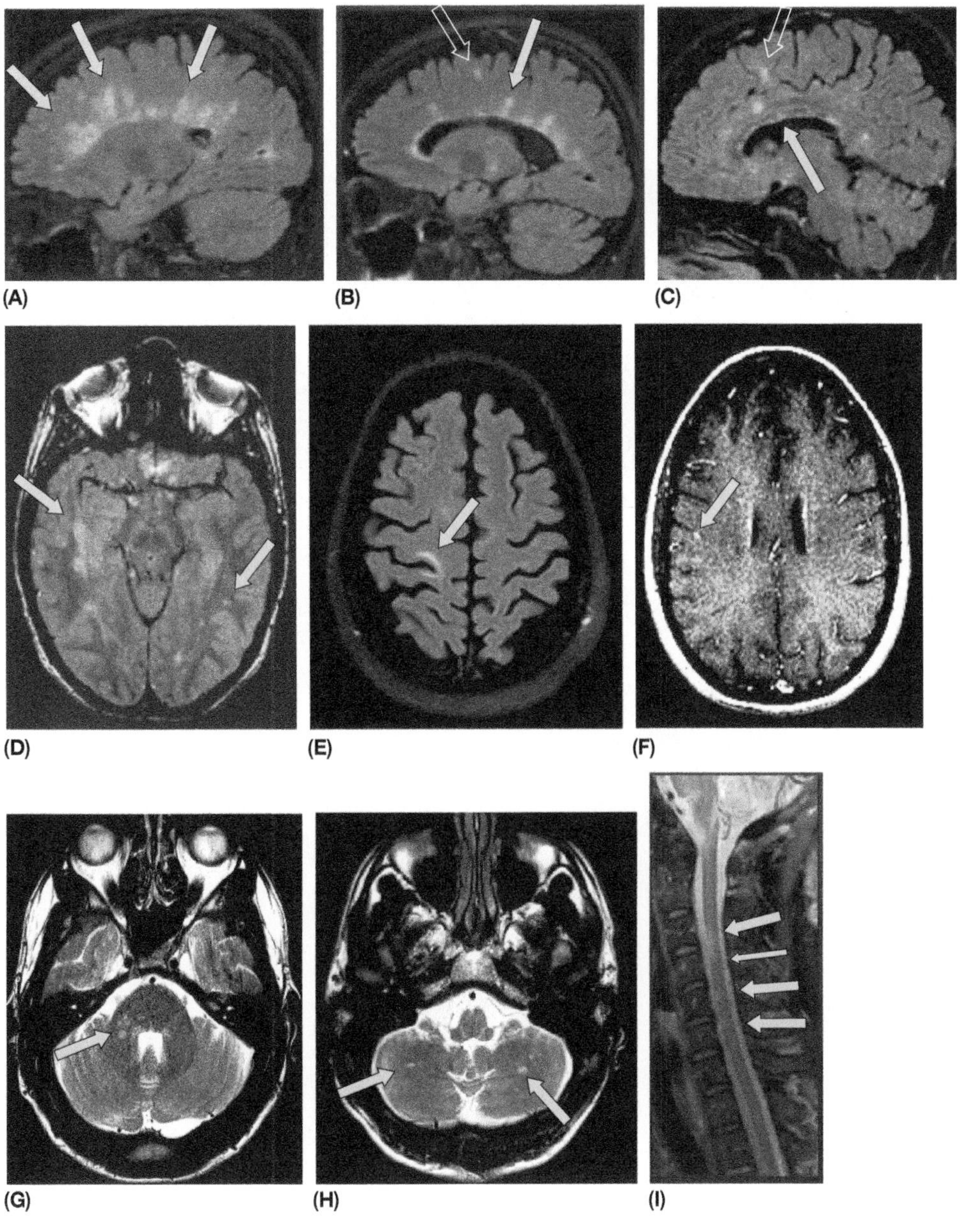

FIGURE 8.8

Examples of MS demyelinating lesions in characteristic locations pertinent to the new McDonald Criteria as included in Table 8.2. Sagittal FLAIR images (A–C) demonstrate perpendicularly oriented periventricular lesions along the callososeptal margins and corpus callosum (arrow, C) in a "dot-dash" pattern classic for MS. Additional juxtacortical or subcortical white matter lesions are seen on sagittal FLAIR images (B, C, open arrows) and in the temporal lobes on axial FLAIR image (D). Axial FLAIR image (E) demonstrates juxtacortical lesion spanning the subcortical white matter and portions of the overlying cortex (arrow), with postcontrast T1-weighted axial image (F) demonstrating small enhancing cortical lesion (arrow) consistent with a tiny focus of active demyelination. Axial T2-weighted images (G, H) demonstrate infratentorial lesions within the right brachium pontis (arrow, G) and both cerebellar hemispheres (arrows, H), with several spinal cord lesions designated by the arrows on sagittal PD image (I).

sulci. NSWMD also infrequently affects the anterior temporal lobes and the cerebellum. Since the cortex and subcortical U-fibers are hyperperfused from an abundant capillary network, NSWMD is rarely seen in those locations. White matter lesions of long-standing MS more commonly demonstrate corresponding T1 hypointensity [15] whereas those of chronic microvascular ischemia are often T1 isointense.

Finally, although enhancement is common with acute MS, it is extremely atypical for lesions of chronic microvascular ischemia.

Neuromyelitis Optica

Neuromyelitis Optica (NMO; formally known as Devic's syndrome) is a relapsing, inflammatory, demyelinating

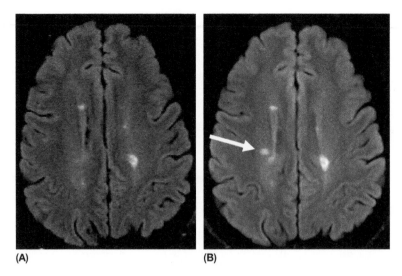

(A) (B)

FIGURE 8.9
DIT. Careful side-by-side comparison of 2 axial FLAIR images acquired 15 months apart demonstrates interval appearance of a new lesion within the deep, right frontoparietal white matter (arrow, B).

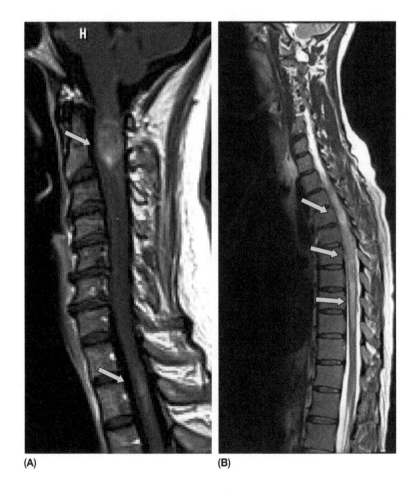

(A) (B)

FIGURE 8.10
Sagittal images from 2 different patients with demyelinating lesions of the spinal cord. T1-weighted postcontrast image (A) from a known MS patient demonstrates 2 short segment enhancing lesions (arrows). While the superior most enhancing lesion is somewhat expansile and also involves the central cord, the more inferior lesion involves the periphery of the cord and both are relatively short in length, less than 2 vertebral segments, and typical of MS. In contrast, sagittal T2-weighted image (B) from a patient with neuromyelitis optica (NMO) demonstrates expansile abnormal T2 bright signal (arrows) throughout a much larger or longer portion of the central cervical and thoracic cord.

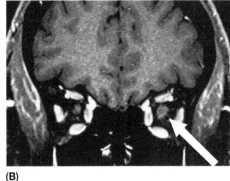

FIGURE 8.11
Fat-saturated coronal T2-weighted images (A) and fat-saturated postcontrast coronal T1-weighted MR images from 2 different patients with optic neuritis. Both patients (A and B) demonstrate asymmetric enlargement and enhancement of the left optic nerve (arrows) consistent with optic neuritis. Patient B also demonstrates somewhat fuzzy, ill-defined T2 bright signal surrounding the left optic nerve consistent with inflammatory fat stranding.

disorder of the CNS with imaging features occasionally similar to those of conventional MS. Unlike MS, however, NMO characteristically preferentially involves the spinal cord and optic nerves with relative sparing of the brain parenchyma. Moreover, to be able to suggest a diagnosis of NMO, the MRI appearance of the brain must be either normal or not meet diagnostic criteria for MS [16].

The classic, imaging appearance of the spine in NMO consists of a prominent cord lesion, often enhancing and expansile, with T2 hyperintensity, at least 3 vertebral segments in length, and primarily involving the central part of the spinal cord [16] (Figure 8.10). Although as many as 25% of MS cases have been documented to involve only the spinal cord [7,17,18], most MS spinal cord lesions (or foci of T2 hyperintensity) tend to be substantially smaller than those of NMO, measuring less than 2 vertebral body segments in length, and tend to be located along the periphery of the cord [18] (Figure 8.8). In contrast, the cord lesions of NMO tend to be larger or longer in length, and involve the central cord (Figure 8.10). In the acute phase, the cord lesions of both NMO and MS can be associated with focal cord expansion and enhancement. In both diseases, chronic lesions are eventually associated with volume loss.

In both MS and NMO, optic neuritis is characterized by a swollen optic nerve or chiasm lesion associated with abnormal T2 signal and inflammatory changes of the adjacent retro-orbital fat planes (Figure 8.11). A relationship between optic neuritis and MS has been well documented, with an overall risk of developing MS approximated at 50% within 15 years following initial presentation with optic neuritis [19]. Among patients with a normal brain MRI during documented optic neuritis, the risk of developing MS is nearly 3 times higher for females, and more than twice as likely to develop when the retrobulbar portion of the optic nerve was involved as opposed to the anterior optic nerve [19].

TECHNICAL CONSIDERATIONS AND PITFALLS

FLAIR images provide excellent contrast between the normal white matter and the bright signal intensity of demyelinating plaques, and are thus fundamental to the evaluation of any patient with suspected MS. Although FLAIR images are very sensitive to white matter injury, they are unfortunately also very prone to artifact, or the presence of signal abnormality not secondary to the actual disease but something extraneous. The most common causes of MRI artifact are patient motion and "pulsation" artifact, or pulsations from an adjacent vascular structure causing the overlay of abnormal signal across the image (see Figure 8.12). For this reason, T2-weighted and PD imaging sequences are often more reliable in assessing for demyelinating plaques or lesions in the brain stem and cerebellum, or for confirming the presence of a lesion that may be suspected on FLAIR.

While the FLAIR imaging sequence is particularly vulnerable to many types of artifacts, all MRI sequences will be degraded by patient motion (Figure 8.13). Thus, for certain patients unable to stay still within the scanner because of claustrophobia, anxiety, or other clinical disability, anesthesia or sedation may be required to obtain an optimally diagnostic MRI exam. The presence of various types of hardware can also limit the diagnostic utility of MRI. For example, dental braces cause loss of signal throughout the anterior-most portions of the brain, and mascara on eyelashes may cause localized loss of signal along the anterior orbits. Problems inherent with the MRI scanner such as inhomogeneity of the magnetic field or magnetic coils can also cause signal abnormalities limiting lesion detection.

The ability to detect lesions depends not only on the pulse sequence and imaging parameters, but also on the field strength of the MRI machine [20,21]. In 1 series studying 15 patients definitively diagnosed with MS, those imaged on a 4-Tesla (T) strength MRI machine had nearly one-third more lesions detected when compared with imaging performed on a 1.5 T strength MRI machine [20]. In a similar study comparing known MS patients imaged on a 3 T strength MRI machine versus a 1.5 T strength MRI machine, overall lesion volume was higher by 12% when imaged on the higher field strength MRI machine [21]. Although 3 T strength MRI machines are now more and more common in the everyday clinical practice setting, the use of ultra-high magnetic field strength MR imaging at field strengths of 7 T or more is primarily limited to research [23].

CLINICAL APPLICATIONS IN DISEASE MONITORING

MR imaging has become instrumental in monitoring patients already diagnosed with definitive MS, and allows

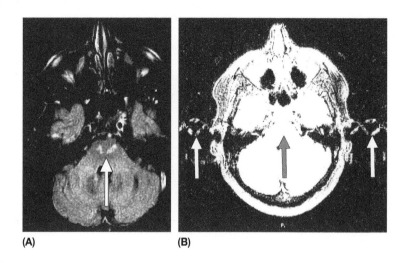

(A) (B)

FIGURE 8.12
Axial FLAIR image (A) demonstrates 2 areas of bright signal within the brain stem of this patient with known MS (arrow). This same image with parameters adjusted to highlight subtle differences (B) reveals that these apparent bright spots are secondary to pulsation artifact extending throughout the image (arrows) rather than secondary to actual new lesions within the brain stem. Though FLAIR sequences are fundamental to any imaging protocol to evaluate for MS, FLAIR sequences are unfortunately prone to artifact.

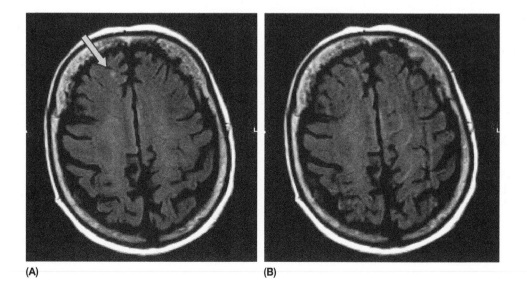

(A) (B)

FIGURE 8.13
Axial FLAIR images at the same level from a patient being evaluated for MS demonstrate a FLAIR bright lesion in the subcortical white matter of the right frontal lobe (arrow) seen when the patient is holding still (A), but virtually undetectable when the patient is moving within the MRI scanner (B).

for the objective assessment of disease severity, disease activity, and disease progression—specifically important in assessing responsiveness to therapy. Since its introduction into mainstream medicine in the 1980s, MR imaging has been estimated by some authors to detect MS disease activity 5 to 10 times more frequently than the clinical evaluation alone would suggest [22]—implying that many lesions found on MR imaging may be clinically silent. For this reason, MRI findings are often correlated with additional patient report measures when making clinical decisions regarding any potential changes in therapy.

Although no standardized guidelines exist, generally an MRI of the brain (with potential additional imaging of the cervical and thoracic spine) is performed at least once during course of disease to obtain further diagnostic confirmation. Follow-up imaging is often obtained if new diagnostic questions should arise or new neurological symptoms develop potentially suggesting comorbid conditions other than MS. Furthermore, most clinical practices will obtain imaging prior to starting new treatment, and then 6 months and 1 year into the treatment to assess response. In general, for those patients who develop 3 or more active lesions on subsequent MRI scans and demonstrate clinically active disease manifested by relapses and progression of disability, a change in treatment strategy is usually recommended.

MRI SAFETY

MRI examination with 1.5 to 3 T strength MRI scanners has now become the standard of care across much of the United States. While MRI is safe for the majority of the population, each patient must be screened prior to undergoing an MRI exam or coming too close to the MRI scanner, and general access to the public is restricted in areas having magnetic fields above 0.5 mT [24].

One of the greatest potential hazards around an MRI machine is the missile effect from ferromagnetic objects such as oxygen cylinders, scissors, pens, or other common metallic objects. When in proximity to the magnetic field created by the MRI scanner, these objects will rapidly accelerate toward the bore of the MRI scanner, potentially damaging those objects or injuring people in their path. For this reason, all patients and health care workers are scanned with metal detectors prior to entering the MRI suite, and are required to remove any and all ferromagnetic metallic objects beforehand. Likewise, all metallic objects in and around the MRI scanner must be constructed from specialized MRI-safe materials. Those patients with bullet fragments, shrapnel or other forms of metal embedded into their body may require additional imaging and clinical evaluation to ascertain whether or not it would be safe for them to undergo an MRI examination.

Patients with implantable devices must also be screened prior to undergoing MRI examination. Certain implantable devices, such as pacemakers, may be deactivated by a magnetic field, and those patients with certain cardiac conditions requiring constant cardiac pacing may require specialized examination in a closely monitored setting with their electro physiologist or cardiology staff nearby. Certain metallic devices may absorb energy and increase in temperature when exposed to radiofrequency pulses within the magnetic field. Moreover, because of the torque produced by the magnetic field, ferromagnetic devices such as certain aneurysm clips, implanted electrodes, cochlear implants or internal drug infusion pumps may also move or migrate during the MRI exam, potentially posing significant hazard. It is thus important for all patients to make their MRI technician aware of the make and model of any and all implanted medical devices they may have prior to entering the MRI scanner.

Though the U.S. Food and Drug Administration has not established guidelines with respect to the safety of MRI in pregnant women, according to the Policies, Guidelines, and Recommendations for MR Imaging Safety and Patient Management issued by the Safety Committee of the Society for Magnetic Resonance Imaging in 1991, "MR imaging may be used in pregnant women if other non-ionizing forms of diagnostic imaging are inadequate or if the examination provides important information that would otherwise require exposure to ionizing radiation such as fluoroscopy or computed tomography (CT)." When possible, MRI is commonly delayed until the second or third trimester owing to the theoretical concern over tissue heating caused by the radiofrequency pulses. Intravenous contrast agents are generally not recommended, as they are known to cross the placenta and their long-term effects are not yet well known.

REFERENCES

1. Inglese M. Multiple sclerosis: New insights and trends. *AJNR.* 2006;27:954–957.

2. Rocca MA, Anzalone N, Falini A, Filippi M. Contribution of magnetic resonance imaging to the diagnosis and monitoring of multiple sclerosis. *Radiol Med.* 2012: Epub ahead of print.

3. McDonald WI, Compston A, Edan G, et al. Recommended diagnostic criteria for multiple sclerosis: Guidelines from the International Panel on the diagnosis of multiple sclerosis. *Ann Neurol.* 2001;50:121–127.

4. Polman CH, Reingold SC, Edan G, et al. Diagnositc criteria for multiple sclerosis: 2005 revisions to the "McDonald Criteria." *Ann Neurol.* 2005;58:840–846.

5. Polman CH, Reingold SC, Banwell B, et al. Diagnostic criteria for multiple sclerosis: 2010 revisions to the McDonald Criteria. *Ann Neurol.* 2011;69:292–302.

6. Barkof F, Filippi M, Miller DH, et al. Comparison of MR imaging criteria at first presentation to predict conversion to clinically definite MS. *Brain.* 1997;120:2059–2069.

7. Ge Y. Multiple sclerosis: The role of MR imaging. *AJNR.* 2006;27:1165–1176.

8. Truyen L, van Waesberghe JH, van Walderveen MA, et al. Accumulation of hypointense lesions ("black holes") on T1 spin-echo MRI correlates with disease progression in multiple sclerosis. *Neurology.* 1996;47:1469–1476.

9. Adams CW, Abdulla YH, Torres EM, Poston RN. Periventricular lesions in multiple sclerosis: Their perivenous origin and relationship to granular ependymitis. *Neuropathol Appl Neurobiol.* 1987;13:141–152.

10. Lisanti CJ, Asbach P, Bradley WG. The ependymal "dot-dash" sign: An MR imaging finding of early multiple sclerosis. *AJNR.* 2005;26:2033–2036.

11. Gean-Marton AD, Vezina LG, Marton KI, et al. Abnormal corpus callosum: A sensitive and specific indicator of multiple sclerosis. *Radiology.* 1991;180:215–221.

12. Rovira A, Swanton J, Tintore M, et al. A single, early magnetic resonance imaging study in the diagnosis of multiple sclerosis. *Arch Neurol.* 2009;5:287–292.

13. Montalban X, Tintore M, Swanton J, et al. MRI criteria for MS in patients with clinically isolated syndromes. *Neurology.* 2010;74:427–434.

14. Fazekas F, Chawluk JB, Alavi A, et al. MR Signal abnormalities at 1.5T in Alzheimer's dementia and normal aging. *AJNR.* 1987;8:421–426.

15. Wallace CJ, Seland TP, Fong TC. Multiple sclerosis: The impact of MR imaging. *AJR.* 1992;158:849–857.

16. Wingerchuk DM, Lennon VA, Pittock SJ, et al. Revised diagnostic criteria for Neuromyelitis optica. *Neurology.* 2006;66(10):1485–1489.

17. Ikuta F, Zimmerman HM. Distribution of plaques in seventy autopsy cases of multiple sclerosis in the United States. *Neurology.* 1976;26:26–28.

18. Tartaglino LM, Friedman DP, Flanders AE, et al. Multiple sclerosis in the spinal cord: MR appearance and correlation with clinical parameters. *Radiology.* 1995;195:725–732.

19. Optic Neuritis Study Group. Multiple sclerosis risk after optic neuritis: Final optic neuritis treatment trial follow-up. *Arch Neurol.* 2008;65(6):727–732.

20. Keiper MD, Grossman RI, Hirsch JA, et al. MR identification of white matter abnormalities in multiple-sclerosis: A comparison between 1.5T and 4T. *AJNR.* 1998;19:1489–1493.

21. Sicotte NL, Voskuhl RR, Bouvier S, et al. Comparison of multiple sclerosis lesions at 1.5 and 3.0 Tesla. *Invest Radiol.* 2003;38:423–427.

22. Barkhof F, Scheltens P, Frequin ST, et al. Relapsing-remitting multiple sclerosis: Sequential enhanced MR imaging vs clinical findings in determining disease activity. *AJR.* 1992;159:1041–1047.

23. Kolia K, Maderwald S, Putzki N, et al. First clinical study on ultra-high-field MR imaging in patients with multiple sclerosis: Comparison of 1.5T and 7T. *AJNR.* 2009;30:699–702.

24. Bushberg JT, Seibert SA, Leidholdt EM Jr, Boone JM. *The Essential Physics of Medical Imaging.* Philadelphia: Lippincott Williams & Wilkins; 2002.

9

Tools and Tests for Multiple Sclerosis

ROBERT A. BERMEL

KEY POINTS FOR CLINICIANS

- Blood tests play an important role in excluding mimics of multiple sclerosis (MS).

- Spinal fluid analysis can help establish an inflammatory basis for abnormal imaging findings and help exclude mimics of MS in atypical situations, but is not routinely required to make the diagnosis of MS.

- Evoked potentials can help to establish dissemination in space consistent with the diagnosis of MS, but are not specific for MS.

- Biomarker blood tests exist to help establish the diagnosis of neuromyelitis optica and assess individual risk for complications associated with natalizumab.

- Biomarkers are not yet available to predict an individual patient's response to a specific therapy.

- Optical coherence tomography is a new technology that can track retinal neurodegeneration and monitor for macular edema in patients on fingolimod therapy for MS.

The diagnosis of multiple sclerosis (MS) is made clinically on the basis of a synthesis of the history, examination, imaging, and paraclinical testing where necessary [1]. No single paraclinical test can confirm or exclude MS with certainty. The brain MRI has emerged as the foremost test suggesting the diagnosis of MS if abnormal with typical features, or excluding the diagnosis of MS if normal. Paraclinical testing can be used to support the diagnosis of MS by fulfilling the criteria for dissemination in space (usually evoked potentials or optical coherence tomography [OCT]) and verifying an inflammatory etiology for the neurological disorder (spinal fluid analysis). The ubiquitous availability of MRI and its utility in diagnosing MS makes it a test that is now commonly performed early in the course of neurological symptoms. When the brain MRI is definitively abnormal but not classic for MS, it raises the possibility of an alternative neurological diagnosis, and blood and spinal fluid tests can be used to exclude "mimics" of MS at the time of diagnosis. When the brain MRI is mildly abnormal and the clinician views the diagnosis of MS as unlikely, testing such as evoked potentials and spinal fluid analysis can be utilized to show a lack of central nervous system (CNS) pathology, in order to more definitively exclude the diagnosis of MS.

BLOOD TESTS

The differential diagnosis of MS (discussed in detail in Chapter 10) is broad, and multiple alternative disease entities can cause similar symptoms and a similar imaging appearance to MS. When atypical clinical features make the exclusion of mimics essential, blood tests play a key role [2]. Even when the diagnosis of MS is secure, blood tests are indicated in order to exclude the presence of comorbid conditions which can occur at high frequency. Finally, there are also blood tests which can be used to help guide therapeutic decision making.

> When atypical clinical features make the exclusion of mimics essential, blood tests play a key role.

Testing to exclude mimics of MS is performed if prompted by red flags on the history or exam. The specific tests sent are guided by the specific clinical scenario. Some of the most commonly ordered tests are for rheumatological or autoimmune diseases which can cause CNS demyelination (Table 9.1). Many of these possibilities can be reliably distinguished from MS on the basis of clinical features, imaging findings, or lab results. Other organ-specific autoimmune diseases, such as thyroid autoimmunity and pernicious anemia, occur with higher frequency in patients with MS, have some symptomatic overlap with MS, and therefore justify screening (Table 9.1). Prior to initiating disease-modifying therapy for MS, it is often prudent to send tests of liver and kidney function, given the effect of some MS treatments on these organs. With the growing emphasis on vitamin D supplementation in patients with MS, some clinicians choose to check vitamin D levels to guide the dosage of vitamin D [3]. Immunity to varicella zoster virus is required (whether by exposure or vaccination) prior to utilizing some immunosuppressive therapies to treat MS, so this status is also often evaluated.

There are reports that antiglycan antibodies occur with increased frequency in MS, and serological tests for those have been proposed as a tool aiding in the diagnosis of MS at early stages or to help distinguish patients who are more likely to experience disability progression [4]. Although these serological tests are commercially available, they have limited specificity and sensitivity and have not been independently replicated. At this point, they are not commonly utilized in clinical practice. MRI and in some cases spinal fluid results are used preferentially to inform diagnosis and prognosis in MS, and it is not clear that antiglycan antibody testing would significantly affect treatment decisions even in cases where the MRI and other testing are equivocal.

The neuromyelitis optica IgG antibody (NMO-IgG) is a blood test that has approximately a 76% sensitivity and 94% specificity for neuromyelitis optica (NMO), and is now a key asset in making the diagnosis of NMO [5]. NMO-IgG is an autoantibody directed against the aquaporin-4 water channel on astrocyte foot processes, and is now recognized as the pathogenic autoantibody responsible for the manifestations of NMO [6]. The discovery of this autoantibody has solidified NMO as a unique pathological entity distinct from MS and requiring a different treatment regimen. NMO-IgG should be tested if inflammatory demyelination is suspected as a mechanism

> The neuromyelitis optica IgG antibody is now a key asset in making the diagnosis of NMO.

and clinical or imaging features are suggestive of NMO or atypical for MS. Testing in the blood is sufficiently sensitive in most cases, but on rare occasions this test will be positive in the cerebrospinal fluid (CSF) when it is negative in the blood.

Although there are not currently any predictive biomarker tests that help to guide choice of therapy on the basis of efficacy in individuals, there are some tests which can guide choice of MS therapy on the basis of risk of a therapeutic complication. A 2-step serological assay for antibodies to the JC virus (JCV) in the blood was developed

TABLE 9.1
Common Blood Tests Sent at the Time of MS Diagnosis

TESTS WHICH MAY HELP TO IDENTIFY MIMICS OF MS OR COMORBID CONDITIONS	TESTS WHICH MAY IMPACT OR HELP TO GUIDE MS TREATMENT
Erythrocyte sedimentation rate	Complete blood count
Antinuclear antibody	Renal and liver function tests
Thyroid stimulating hormone level	JC virus antibody status
Vitamin B$_{12}$ level	Varicella antibody status
Copper level	Vitamin D level
Antineutrophil cytoplasmic antibodies	
Rheumatoid factor	
SSA/SSB (Sjogren's antibodies)	
Extractable nuclear antigen antibodies	
Antiphospholipid antibodies	
Aquaporin-4 antibody (neuromyelitis optica IgG)	
Lyme titers	

and is currently utilized to help determine risk of progressive multifocal leukoencephalopathy (PML), a complication associated with natalizumab therapy for MS [7]. The pathogenesis of PML is thought to require multiple steps, beginning with acquisition of the JCV and requiring time for the virus harbored in individuals regardless of immune status, to become neurotropic. Only then, in immunocompromised hosts, can the virus cause PML. The prevalence of anti-JCV antibodies is approximately 56% in the MS population [8], and the current recommendation is to check JCV antibody status every 6 months in patients who initially test negative and are being treated with natalizumab. Thus, testing for JCV antibody status allows lower-risk utilization of natalizumab for at least limited and sometimes long periods of time in patients who have not been previously exposed to the virus. Other tests for risk stratification include EKG for cardiac risks and retinal examination for ophthalmological risks related to fingolimod.

> Testing for JCV antibody status allows lower-risk utilization of natalizumab in patients who have not been previously exposed to the virus.

Blood tests to either predict the response to therapy (predictive biomarkers) or prognosis in MS (prognostic biomarkers) would be helpful to guide therapeutic decision making, but are not currently available. In their absence, MRI remains the primary means for measuring MS disease burden, degree of disease activity, and assessing response to therapy.

> Blood tests to either predict the response to therapy or prognosis in MS would be helpful to guide therapeutic decision making, but are not currently available.

LUMBAR PUNCTURE/SPINAL FLUID ANALYSIS

Lumbar puncture often has a reputation with patients as a painful procedure and with clinicians as a requirement to establish the diagnosis of MS. Both of those represent unnecessary generalizations. In most cases, if the clinical history, examination, and imaging are typical for MS,

> If the clinical history, examination, and imaging are typical for MS, spinal fluid analysis is not a requirement in order to make the diagnosis of MS.

spinal fluid analysis is not a requirement in order to make the diagnosis of MS. Some situations in which spinal fluid analysis is useful in supporting a diagnosis of MS include:

1. Exclusion of other alternative etiologies (infectious, inflammatory, granulomatous disorders) if atypical features are present
2. Diagnosis of some cases of primary progressive MS (PPMS) (especially to distinguish PPMS from neurodegenerative disorders)
3. Diagnosis of MS in older individuals or those with vascular risk factors, where white matter lesions on MRI may have a vascular or other non-MS etiology
4. In patients with pacemakers or other reasons precluding MRI, if the diagnosis of MS is suspected
5. In situations where disease-modifying therapy is being considered (such as after a clinically isolated syndrome) but imaging and evoked potentials alone provide insufficient evidence to support a diagnosis of MS.

The brain MRI is the most predictive test for determining the risk of future attacks after a clinically isolated syndrome [9]. However, CSF studies do add additional predictive value, with the presence of oligoclonal bands in the CSF conferring almost double the risk of a second attack, independent of brain MRI [10]. If CSF analysis is being considered in this situation for risk estimation, it is generally only if the brain MRI is equivocal and the patient or physician would change their decision to start disease-modifying therapy on the basis of the result.

> The brain MRI is the most predictive test for determining the risk of future attacks after a clinically isolated syndrome.

When CSF is sent for analysis, multiple tests on the fluid are generally requested, guided by the clinical scenario (Table 9.2). The core findings from CSF analysis that support a diagnosis of MS are qualitative or quantitative evidence

TABLE 9.2
CSF Tests Commonly Sent When Evaluating for MS

ALWAYS SHOULD BE ORDERED IF CONSIDERING MS	SOMETIMES MAY BE ORDERED ON THE BASIS OF CLINICAL SUSPICION AND LABORATORY RELIABILITY
Cell count and differential	Cytology and/or flow cytometry (if clinical suspicion for lymphoma or other malignancy)
Total protein quantification	
Glucose quantification	Borrelia antibody titers (if clinical suspicion for lyme disease)
Oligoclonal bands evaluation (CSF and serum electrophoresis)	VDRL (if clinical suspicion for syphilis)
IgG index and IgG synthesis rate	Culture and other infectious antigen tests
	Free kappa light chains

VDRL, venereal disease research laboratory.

$$\text{IgG index} = \frac{(\text{CSF IgG} / \text{CSF albumin})}{(\text{Serum IgG} / \text{Serum albumin})}$$

FIGURE 9.1
CSF IgG index derivation.

of intrathecal antibody synthesis, in the form of oligoclonal bands or elevated IgG index. Oligoclonal bands are identified by electrophoresis of proteins present in CSF compared to the patient's own serum, and generally defined as present if there are 2 or more bands present in the CSF that are not present in the serum. It is a qualitative test that evaluates for unique immunoglobulins in the CSF that are not present in the serum [11]. The IgG index (Figure 9.1) is a quantitative representation of the amount of intrathecal IgG present, controlling for both the amount of albumin present in the CSF and the ratio of IgG to CSF in the blood. The IgG index is compared to a fraction derived from a reference population, and is interpreted as high if it exceeds the level defined as abnormal on the basis of the reference used for the individual laboratory. The IgG synthesis rate is another quantitative marker of intrathecal antibody synthesis. It is the calculated amount (in mg per 24 hours) of de novo IgG being produced in the CSF compartment based on measured serum and CSF values of albumin and IgG, plus constants derived from a normal reference population [12]. Its value parallels that of the IgG index.

> The core findings from CSF analysis that support a diagnosis of MS are qualitative or quantitative evidence of intrathecal antibody synthesis, in the form of oligoclonal bands or elevated IgG index.

Though evidence of oligoclonal bands or elevation of IgG index is supportive of the diagnosis, these tests are not the most specific tests for MS. Oligoclonal bands and elevated IgG index can be found in many neurological disorders. Other CSF tests commonly associated with MS are even less specific. If CSF protein is high then the IgG synthesis rate may be falsely elevated. Detection of myelin basic protein in the CSF occurs in many neurological and nonneurological disorders and should not be used in isolation to support a diagnosis of MS.

> Detection of myelin basic protein in the CSF occurs in many neurological and nonneurological disorders and should not be used in isolation to support a diagnosis of MS.

The performance characteristics of CSF laboratory measures can vary substantially on the basis of the methodology used. Electrophoresis using isoelectric focusing is increasingly becoming the standard method used to evaluate for oligoclonal bands, because of its sensitivity [11]. Assays for free kappa light chains may augment the diagnostic specificity for MS in some situations, but currently have low utility because of the wide methodological variability. Knowing the analytical method used and normative values associated with the individual laboratory where CSF testing was performed is essential for proper interpretation of the test results.

> Knowing the analytical method used and normative values associated with the individual laboratory where CSF testing was performed is essential for proper interpretation of the test results.

Neither oligoclonal bands nor IgG index can be utilized as a marker of response to disease-modifying therapy in MS. Even after immunoablation and hematopoetic stem

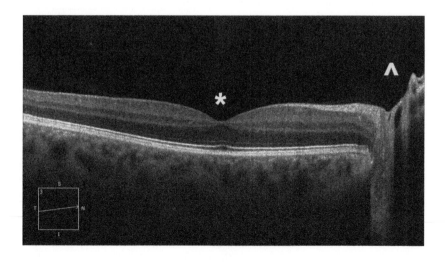

FIGURE 9.2
High resolution OCT image including both the macula (white star) and optic nerve head (caret symbol), demonstrating the ability to resolve individual retinal layers.

cell transplantation in patients with MS, CSF findings of oligoclonal bands and elevated IgG index remain abnormal [13]. Assays for the presence of neuron-specific markers in the CSF have been proposed as a measure of disease activity or neuroaxonal damage in MS, but none are currently utilized in widespread clinical practice. N-acetyl aspartate and CSF neurofilament heavy or light chains have all received recent attention as potential candidates [14], although the clinical utility remains uncertain and certainly feasibility of incorporating CSF testing into the routine monitoring of MS would present a challenge.

EVOKED POTENTIALS

Evoked potentials (EP) are an electrophysiological test where the delay is measured between the presentation of a sensory stimulus (whether visual, somatosensory, or auditory) and its low voltage evoked cortical potential. By averaging multiple stimulus presentations and responses, the timing of the cortical potential of interest can be measured with high accuracy, and compared to a known reference interval. A delay in the peak occurrence of the evoked potential (ie, an increased latency in the P100 peak) is evidence for dysfunction in the pathway of interest, with demyelination being a common cause. However, increased latency is nonspecific and can be caused by a number of different conditions.

Visual evoked potentials and somatosensory evoked potentials are the most commonly utilized evoked potentials, and are sensitive tests for demyelination in those respective pathways. Brain stem (auditory) evoked potentials are less commonly utilized. Evoked potentials are most useful for demonstration of dissemination in space, ie, they may be useful in the situation of a patient with a single lesion, if it would be helpful to demonstrate an asymptomatic slowing of evoked potentials in a different part of the neuraxis consistent with a second lesion [15]. In the setting of neurological symptoms of uncertain etiology, evoked potentials can be useful to demonstrate the presence or lack of CNS pathology, though a positive result is not specific for a primary demyelinating etiology. The sensitivity of visual evoked potentials at the time of a clinically isolated syndrome for predicting the development of clinically definite MS has been estimated at between 25% and 85%, with specificity between 63% and 78% [16,17]. The wide range of values is testament to the variability of yield based on the characteristics of patients put forth for EP testing, variability in methodology and quality control, and the definition of the outcome of interest.

> In the setting of neurological symptoms of uncertain etiology, evoked potentials can be useful to demonstrate the presence or lack of CNS pathology, though a positive result is not specific for a primary demyelinating etiology.

Evoked potentials now play a limited role in making the diagnosis of MS, as they have been generally superceded by more disease-specific studies including MRI of the brain and spinal cord and CSF studies.

OCT

OCT is an office-based imaging method that uses near-infrared light to generate high resolution cross-sectional images (in this case of the retina), analogous to B-mode ultrasound [18]. Two areas of the retina are currently imaged using OCT: the peripapillary region and the macular region. The peripapillary region is useful for measuring the thickness of the retinal nerve fiber layer (RNFL—measured circumferentially around the optic nerve head), at the point just before these developmentally unmyelinated axons coalesce to form the optic nerve. Volume or thickness of the macula can also be measured, and abnormal pathology including macular edema (a possible complication of fingolimod therapy for MS) can be sensitively detected. Newer OCT analysis techniques focus on segmentation of individual retinal layers, permitted by the high resolution spectral domain OCT instruments currently in use (Figure 9.2). One such measure of emerging interest is the thickness of the retinal ganglion cell layer (GCL). Measured at the macula, it is a way to assess the integrity of a layer of first-order sensory neurons. Thus, the 3 measures most commonly in use to monitor MS using OCT are the peripapillary RNFL thickness, total macular volume, and the GCL thickness.

> OCT is an office-based imaging method that uses near-infrared light to generate high resolution cross-sectional images (in this case of the retina), analogus to B-mode ultrasound.

Though OCT has been used for a number of years by ophthalmologists to monitor nerve fiber layer thinning in glaucoma, applications for neurological diseases, especially MS which commonly affects the optic nerves, are being explored. From large cross-sectional and some longitudinal studies, it is known that the RNFL (and also macular volume and GCL) becomes thinned most dramatically after optic neuritis, but also during the course of MS in the absence of classic optic neuritis [19]. OCT has also helped to elucidate the time course of axon loss after optic neuritis. By 3 months after the event, RNFL loss becomes apparent (Figure 9.3), and is largely complete by 6 months [20].

For these reasons, OCT has been proposed to have a role in the following clinical situations:

1. Evaluating for macular edema prior to starting and while on fingolimod therapy for MS
2. During recovery from acute optic neuritis, to quantify axon loss relative to visual deficits
3. On a yearly or biyearly basis, for monitoring longitudinal neurodegeneration in MS
4. To identify RNFL thinning to demonstrate a history of remote optic neuritis.

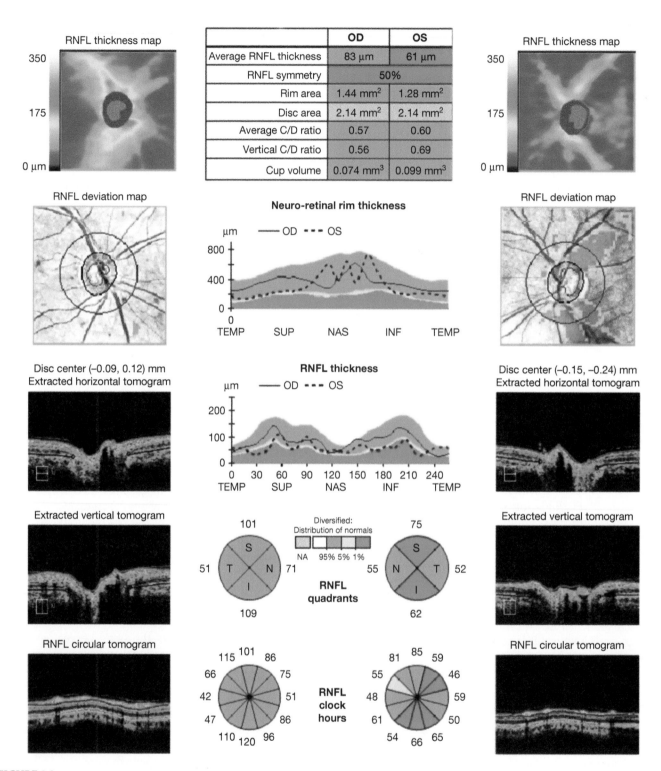

FIGURE 9.3

Example of a spectral domain peripapillary OCT. The left half of the figure shows images and measurements from the right eye (OD) of a patient with MS who previously experienced optic neuritis in the left eye (OS). The average RNFL thickness is normal OD (83 uM), and significantly thinned OS (61 uM). Images from top to bottom of the figure show a heat map of RNFL thickness (blue = thinner, red = thicker), fundus photo demarcating the optic nerve head (outlined in black) and peripapillary circle where the RNFL is measured (purple circle). Colorized images of the RNFL show the actual cross-sectional tomograms taken from the mid-horizontal slice, mid-vertical slice, and peripapillary circle. All boxes containing numerical measurements are shaded green, yellow, or red corresponding to the top 95%, top 99%, and bottom 1% compared to a normative database.

Spectral domain (high definition) OCT has emerged as the test of choice to screen for macular edema prior to and after starting fingolimod therapy for MS.

In certain circumstances, if a patient with optic neuritis has a persistent severe deficit despite a standard course

> Spectral domain (high definition) OCT has emerged as the test of choice to screen for macular edema prior to and after starting fingolimod therapy for MS.

of intravenous methylprednisolone, an OCT showing preserved axonal integrity may prompt additional immunotherapy, whether a second course of intravenous methylprednisolone (IVMP), plasma exchange, or intravenous immunoglobulin G (IVIG) [21].

Though OCT has the potential to become useful as a tool to monitor longitudinal neurodegeneration or axon loss, neuroprotective therapies do not yet exist to intervene on that process. Some physicians will still request OCT for longitudinal monitoring, to establish a patient's baseline in anticipation of an effective neuroprotective therapy in the future.

Paraclinical tests are used less frequently owing to the increased reliance on MRI to establish the diagnosis of MS and monitor its treatment; they still play a vital role in some clinical situations. OCT is an emerging technology that is useful for exploring the mechanisms and time course of damage and recovery in MS, while also serving as a tool in the clinic to monitor retinal neurodegeneration and screen for macular edema. Current research efforts are focused on developing biomarker tests to inform prognosis or response to specific therapies in MS.

ACKNOWLEDGMENT

Supported by RG 4449A1/T from the National Multiple Sclerosis Society (USA).

KEY POINTS FOR PATIENTS AND FAMILIES

- Accurately establishing the diagnosis of MS is important, and in most cases that can be done using a combination of the medical history, neurological examination, and MRI. If any of those components expose atypical features or are inconclusive, additional testing may be required to establish the correct diagnosis.

- Even if we are certain that MS is the correct diagnosis, blood tests are often helpful to evaluate for other conditions that are common in patients with MS and may contribute to symptoms, or other tests which guide how we treat MS.

- A "spinal tap" tests for abnormal immune activation around the brain and spinal cord, and in some (but not all) cases is necessary to correctly diagnose or exclude MS. Hearing of the need for a "spinal tap" often provokes anxiety. This is a safe test if done by an experienced practitioner, and is not as uncomfortable as its reputation would suggest.

REFERENCES

1. Polman CH, Reingold SC, Banwell B, et al. Diagnostic criteria for multiple sclerosis: 2010 revisions to the McDonald Criteria. *Ann Neurol.* 2011;69:292–302.

2. Miller DH, Weinshenker BG, Filippi M, et al. Differential diagnosis of suspected multiple sclerosis: A consensus approach. *Mult Scler.* 2008;14:1157–1174.

3. Mowry EM. Vitamin D: Evidence for its role as a prognostic factor in multiple sclerosis. *J Neurol Sci.* 2011;311:19–22.

4. Schwarz M, Spector L, Gortler M, et al. Serum anti-Glc(α1,4) Glc(α) antibodies as a biomarker for relapsing-remitting multiple sclerosis. *J Neurol Sci.* 2006;244:59–68.

5. Wingerchuk DM, Lennon VA, Pittock SJ, et al. Revised diagnostic criteria for neuromyelitis optica. *Neurology.* 2006;66:1485–1489.

6. Takahashi T, Fujihara K, Nakashima I, et al. Anti-aquaporin-4 antibody is involved in the pathogenesis of NMO: A study on antibody titre. *Brain.* 2007;130:1235–1243.

7. Gorelik L, Lerner M, Bixler S, et al. Anti-JC virus antibodies: Implications for PML risk stratification. *Ann Neurol.* 2010;68:295–303.

8. Bozic C, Richman S, Plavina T, et al. Anti-John Cunningham virus antibody prevalence in multiple sclerosis patients: Baseline results of STRATIFY-1. *Ann Neurol.* 2011;70:742–750.

9. Fisniku LK, Brex PA, Altmann DR, et al. Disability and T2 MRI lesions: A 20-year follow-up of patients with relapse onset of multiple sclerosis. *Brain.* 2008;131:808–817.

10. Tintoré M, Rovira A, Río J, et al. Do oligoclonal bands add information to MRI in first attacks of multiple sclerosis? *Neurology.* 2008;70:1079–1083.

11. Freedman MS, Thompson EJ, Deisenhammer F, et al. Recommended standard of cerebrospinal fluid analysis in the diagnosis of multiple sclerosis: A consensus statement. *Arch Neurol.* 2005;62:865–870.

12. Tourtellotte WW, Potvin AR, Fleming JO, et al. Multiple sclerosis: Measurement and validation of central nervous system IgG synthesis rate. *Neurology.* 1980;30:240–244.

13. Saiz A, Carreras E, Berenguer J, et al. MRI and CSF oligoclonal bands after autologous hematopoietic stem cell transplantation in MS. *Neurology.* 2001;56:1084–1089.

14. Teunissen CE, Iacobaeus E, Khademi M, et al. Combination of CSF N-acetylaspartate and neurofilaments in multiple sclerosis. *Neurology.* 2009;72:1322–1329.

15. Gronseth GS, Ashman EJ. Practice parameter: The usefulness of evoked potentials in identifying clinically silent lesions in patients with suspected multiple sclerosis (an evidence-based review): Report of the Quality Standards Subcommittee of the American Academy of Neurology. *Neurology.* 2000;54:1720–1725.

16. Hume AL, Waxman SG. Evoked potentials in suspected multiple sclerosis: Diagnostic value and prediction of clinical course. *J Neurol Sci.* 1988;83:191–210.

17. Filippini G, Comi GC, Cosi V, et al. Sensitivities and predictive values of paraclinical tests for diagnosing multiple sclerosis. *J Neurol.* 1994;241:132–137.

18. Frohman EM, Fujimoto JG, Frohman TC, et al. Optical coherence tomography: A window into the mechanisms of multiple sclerosis. *Nat Clin Pract Neurol.* 2008;4:664–675.

19. Pulicken M, Gordon-Lipkin E, Balcer LJ, et al. Optical coherence tomography and disease subtype in multiple sclerosis. *Neurology.* 2007;69:2085–2092.

20. Henderson APD, Altmann DR, Trip AS, et al. A serial study of retinal changes following optic neuritis with sample size estimates for acute neuroprotection trials. *Brain.* 2010;133:2592–2602.

21. Costello F. Evaluating the use of optical coherence tomography in optic neuritis. *Mult Scler Int.* 2011;2011:148394.

10

Differential Diagnosis of Multiple Sclerosis

MEGAN H. HYLAND
JEFFREY A. COHEN

KEY POINTS FOR CLINICIANS

- In patients with a "classic" multiple sclerosis (MS) presentation where MRI is consistent with the diagnosis, consideration of a broad differential diagnosis is unnecessary as the likelihood of an alternative diagnosis is low.

- Nonspecific white matter abnormalities and small vessel ischemic disease are the 2 most common alternative diagnoses in patients incorrectly labeled with MS.

- While it is important to diagnose MS early on in the disease course so that treatment may be initiated, it is also necessary to prevent mislabeling patients.

- Watch for "red flags" which may point to other diagnoses than MS.

- Be ready to rethink the diagnosis of MS if the course or response to therapy do not fit the usual MS pattern.

Because the differential diagnosis of multiple sclerosis (MS) is broad, distinguishing MS from other possible diseases can be challenging at times. The difficulty is illustrated in a recent survey of MS specialists, which showed that nearly all respondents (over 95%) reported seeing a patient within the past year who had been incorrectly diagnosed with MS [1]. Evaluation of potential MS is complicated by the lack of a single, definitive diagnostic test. Attempts to design a blood test for the diagnosis of MS have shown limited success thus far, often demonstrating either suboptimal sensitivity or specificity [2]. The role of potential blood tests is still unclear as the results of current tests do not clearly change diagnosis or management in the setting of more well-established clinical and paraclinical information. The currently accepted formal diagnostic criteria are outlined in Chapter 7. In general, MS is diagnosed by weighing data from clinical history, neurological exam, MRI, and, in some cases, evoked potentials or cerebrospinal fluid (CSF) tests. Historically, all of the diagnostic criteria for MS stipulate that the diagnosis cannot be made if an alternative etiology for the symptoms and test results is more plausible [3], making identification of other potential diagnoses crucial.

MULTIPLE SCLEROSIS OR NOT MULTIPLE SCLEROSIS?

The typical MS patient presents with focal neurological symptoms indicating a central nervous system (CNS) process, eg, weakness, positive sensory symptoms or sensory loss, monocular vision loss, diplopia, or ataxia. These symptoms typically evolve over several days and usually improve or resolve fully after several weeks or months. Objective findings on neurological examination reflect the site(s) of CNS involvement. The neurological manifestations typically are steroid responsive but also can remit spontaneously. Characteristic MRI findings include ovoid T2 hyperintense lesions in the brain and/or spinal cord, some of which enhance on post-gadolinium (Gd) T1 images. CSF typically shows normal or mildly elevated protein and mononuclear cell count, and evidence of intrathecal antibody production (oligoclonal bands and/or an elevated IgG index). In such patients, consideration of a broad different diagnosis is unnecessary as the likelihood of an alternative diagnosis is low. However, a relatively high percentage of patients referred to MS subspecialty clinics for the possibility of MS do not fit this "classic" phenotype and have a higher probability of having a different diagnosis. Important tools for differentiating MS from other diseases include additional focused history taking, laboratory studies, and close examination of MRI lesion patterns, focusing on findings that would be atypical for MS.

> In patients with a very typical MS presentation, consideration of a broad differential diagnosis is unnecessary as the likelihood of an alternative diagnosis is low.

Ideally, a uniform diagnostic algorithm could be applied to all patients. Potential diagnostic algorithms have been proposed [4] but are difficult to apply in practice because patients with possible MS come to medical attention for a variety of reasons. Patients may fall into several categories. First, some patients have symptoms and test results consistent with the broad range of potential MS manifestations but with features suggestive of another disease. These are the patients for whom it is most important to keep in mind the full spectrum of potential MS mimics (Table 10.1). Attention to "red flags"—features atypical for MS or indicative of another disease process—is the basis of avoiding misdiagnosis.

A second category of patients with "possible MS" has become common with the increasing use of MRI. These patients often have nonspecific symptoms suggestive of MS or may be asymptomatic but are primarily assessed for MS because of white matter abnormalities on brain MRI. Up to one-third of new diagnostic referrals to an MS center are estimated to be due to an abnormal brain MRI, with one MS center finding that only 11% of those patients ultimately had MS [5]. In addition, the recent survey of MS subspecialists regarding misdiagnosis cited MRI-based diagnoses—nonspecific white matter abnormalities and small vessel ischemic disease—as the 2 most common alternative diagnoses in patients incorrectly labeled with MS [1]. In this category of patients, particular focus must be placed on patient history and MRI patterns in order to make a correct diagnosis.

A third category of patients includes those with numerous symptoms, often overlapping with those of MS but lacking the classic time course, who frequently have normal neurological exams and test results. These patients may have underlying medical or psychiatric issues, such as fibromyalgia, depression, sleep disorders or conversion disorder—and may or may not have superimposed MS. Although it is important to diagnose MS early on in the disease course so that treatment may be initiated, it is also necessary to prevent mislabeling patients. Ethical concerns with misdiagnosing MS include the difficulty in "undiagnosing" a chronic disease, unnecessary use of long-term, costly medications, and the risk of other medical conditions being attributed to "MS" and subsequently not being treated adequately [6].

This chapter attempts to strike a balance between making readers aware of the many red flags and potential alternative diagnoses to MS and highlighting a practical approach to the most commonly seen "possible MS" patient.

TABLE 10.1
Differential Diagnosis of Multiple Sclerosis by Disease Category

Inflammatory demyelinating	Acute disseminated encephalomyelitis, neuromyelitis optica
Infection	Lyme disease, syphilis, PML, AIDS, HTLV-1, Herpes zoster
Inflammatory/autoimmune	SLE, Sjogren's syndrome, vasculitis, neurosarcoidosis, Behçet's disease, Susac's syndrome, celiac disease, thyroid disease
Vascular	Multiple embolic infarcts, small vessel ischemia, migraine
Metabolic	Vitamin B_{12} deficiency, copper deficiency
Genetic	Lysosomal disorders, adrenoleukodystrophy, mitochondrial disorders, Fragile X-associated tremor/ataxia syndrome, other genetic disorders, CADASIL, hereditary spastic paraparesis, hereditary ataxias
Neoplastic	Central nervous system lymphoma, primary or metastatic tumor, paraneoplastic syndrome
Neurodegenerative	Motor neuron disease
Spine disease	Vascular malformations, degenerative spine disease

CADASIL, cerebral autosomal dominant arteriopathy with subcortical infarcts and leukoencephalopathy; HTLV-1, human T-lymphotropic virus, type 1; PML, progressive multifocal leukoencephalopathy; SLE, systemic lupus erythematosus.

DIAGNOSTIC RED FLAGS

Clinical Red Flags

Certain symptom characteristics—either the type of symptom or time course over which it develops—may strongly support or argue against an MS diagnosis. For example, although pain is common in MS, it would be unlikely for MS to cause certain types of pain directly. Joint pain typically points more toward rheumatological mimics of MS. Headaches in the setting of MRI white matter changes raise suspicion for cerebral autosomal dominant arteriopathy with subcortical infarcts and leukoencephalopathy (CADASIL) or CNS vasculitis but more often may reflect common headache syndromes such as migraine. Although neck pain may occur with acute MS lesions in the cervical cord, chronic cervicalgia suggests a structural cause such as disc herniation or spinal stenosis. Fever warrants consideration of an infectious or rheumatological etiology. Although cognitive changes are seen in MS, they generally develop gradually later in the disease process, and usually affect processing speed, memory, and executive function, while language is rarely impacted. Acute mental status changes would be more typical for acute disseminated encephalomyelitis (ADEM) or an inflammatory etiology such as CNS lupus erythematosus. Symptoms and exam findings consistent with multiple cranial neuropathies raise suspicion for Lyme disease, neurosarcoidosis, or malignancy. Marked fatigue is a common but relatively nonspecific MS symptom, which usually warrants evaluation of other possible causes, such as sleep apnea, thyroid disease, or vitamin deficiencies. Migrating numbness and/or weakness are common symptoms prompting referral to an MS clinic, but the fluctuating nature typically prompts further investigation for other etiologies. A thorough review of systems for other organ system involvement (eg, pulmonary disease which may point to neurosarcoidosis) is recommended during the process of diagnosing MS.

The symptoms of MS are varied, making symptom evolution a critical consideration in the diagnostic process. An important red flag is a history of symptoms that do not follow a pattern of the typical MS relapse (evolution over hours to days, persistence over days to weeks, and resolution over weeks to months). Symptoms that only last hours at a time, frequently change location or severity, develop abruptly, or become rapidly cumulative, point away from MS. Other symptom patterns atypical for MS are summarized in Table 10.2. Of note is that primary progressive MS has a disease course that differs from the more common relapsing forms, typically characterized by weakness and spasticity that develop insidiously and worsen slowly over years. Painless progressive difficulty walking often is initially attributed by the patient to knee or back problems, causing the diagnosis of progressive MS to be delayed. Conversely, symptoms of progressive myelopathy should include consideration of mechanical etiologies (ie, disc herniation) or, more rarely, diseases such as human T-lymphotropic virus, type 1 (HTLV-1) or hereditary spastic paraparesis.

> Marked fatigue is a common but relatively nonspecific MS symptom.

Other aspects of patient history that may identify red flags include age of onset and family history. MS is most commonly diagnosed in patients ages 20 to 50 years; younger patients may be more likely to have ADEM or a leukodystrophy while older patients are more likely to have arthritic spine changes or vascular etiologies such as small vessel ischemia, particularly with a history of vascular risk factors. MS has only a relatively minor hereditary component, so a strong family history, particularly of

TABLE 10.2

Clinical Red Flags for the Potential Misdiagnosis of Multiple Sclerosis

Onset of symptoms before age 20 years or after 50 years

Very prominent family history of stereotyped manifestations

Atypical course
- Gradually progressive course from onset particularly in a young patient or with manifestations other than a myelopathy
- Abrupt development of symptoms

Unifocal manifestations (even if relapsing)

Neurological manifestations unusual for MS

Associated systemic manifestations

Missing features, particularly in long-standing or severe disease
- Lack of oculomotor, optic nerve, sensory, or bladder involvement

Atypical response to treatment
- Lack of any response to corticosteroids
- Exceptionally rapid or dramatic response to corticosteroids or disease-modifying treatments
- Lack of any response to potent disease therapies such as natalizumab

stereotypical manifestations, would be more concerning for a leukodystrophy, mitochondrial disease, hereditary ataxia, or other genetic disorder.

An atypical response to therapy is another red flag suggesting other potential diagnoses. Improvement in symptoms in response to steroid treatment is not specific for MS; it may occur, for example, in other inflammatory disorders, malignancy, and spinal vascular malformations or mechanical compression. However, MS symptoms typically do not respond immediately when steroids are initiated or worsen acutely after cessation of steroid treatment; this pattern would be suggestive of a steroid-responsive mimic. Additionally, lack of any response to potent MS disease-modifying therapy, such as natalizumab, particularly in the absence of anti-natalizumab neutralizing antibodies, should lead to reconsideration of the MS diagnosis.

> Lack of any response to a potent MS disease-modifying therapy should lead to reconsideration of the MS diagnosis.

Imaging Red Flags

MRI is an increasingly important diagnostic tool in MS, and as noted earlier, an "abnormal brain MRI" is a common reason for referral to neurologists, in particular MS subspecialists. White matter hyperintensities on T2-weighted and fluid-attenuated inversion recovery (FLAIR) MRI are a typical finding in MS, but the size, shape, and location of the lesions are vital in differentiating MS from other etiologies. A summary of MRI findings that may help differentiate MS from other diseases is shown in Table 10.3.

MS lesions may be punctate (less than 3 mm), making them harder to distinguish from lesions due to small vessel ischemic disease including migraine, but in MS, patients often have a combination of larger (greater than 6 mm) and smaller lesions. MS lesions can be a variety of shapes, but typical lesions are ovoid or "flame-shaped." Although lack of classically shaped lesions is not necessarily a red flag, the expectation of such lesions increases in patients with a larger lesion burden. The location of lesions is also important in the differential diagnosis. MS lesions are characteristically seen in periventricular and juxtacortical locations when located

TABLE 10.3
Distinguishing MRI Features of Selected Multiple Sclerosis Mimics

PML	Confluent posterior cerebral T2 lesions with decreased signal on T1-weighted images, gradual enlargement, absent Gd-enhancement or faint enhancement of the leading edge
HTLV-1 associated myelopathy	Thoracic spinal cord atrophy, sparse cerebral lesions
SLE and Sjogren's syndrome	Lesions predominantly in the subcortical white matter, gray matter involvement
Vasculitis	Ischemic lesions or cerebral infarcts, gray matter involvement, vascular or meningeal Gd-enhancement
Neurosarcoidosis	Parenchymal mass lesions with persistent Gd-enhancement, vascular or meningeal Gd-enhancement
Behçet's disease	Predominantly brain stem involvement
Susac's syndrome	Gray matter involvement or atypical callosal lesions
Vitamin B$_{12}$ deficiency	Abnormal signal limited to the dorsal cervical spinal cord
Leukodystrophies	Diffuse white matter abnormality
Adrenomyeloneuropathy	Symmetric lesions in posterior cerebral white matter
Mitochondrial disorders	Multifocal gray or white matter lesions, basal ganglia calcifications
Spinocerebellar degenerations	Brain stem or cerebellar atrophy without signal abnormality
Motor neuron disease	Typically normal MRI, or symmetrical atrophy or abnormal T2 hyperintensity in the pyramidal tracts
CADASIL	Lack of involvement of corpus callosum, cerebellum, optic nerves, or spinal cord; temporal lobe predominance; involvement of deep gray structures Presence of lacunar infarcts
CNS lymphoma	Unifocal or multifocal lesions with gradual enlargement or mass effect, gray matter involvement, persistent Gd-enhancement, vascular enhancement
Spinal vascular malformation	Patchy increased T2 signal in the spinal cord with faint Gd-enhancement or cord enlargement, possibly visible draining veins, absent or nonspecific cerebral lesions
Fragile X syndrome	Confluent white matter involvement; basal ganglia, brain stem, and cerebellar lesions; symmetric middle cerebellar peduncle involvement

CADASIL, cerebral autosomal dominant arteriopathy with subcortical infarcts and leukoencephalopathy; CNS, central nervous system; Gd, gadolinium; HTLV-1, human T-lymphotropic virus, type 1; PML, progressive multifocal leukoencephalopathy; SLE, systemic lupus erythematosus.

supratentorially, while small vessel ischemic lesions typically spare the immediate periventricular and callosal regions. Sagittal images are helpful when an MS diagnosis is being considered because they best demonstrate callosal lesions. One location red flag to consider is a predominance of temporal lesions—although MS lesions often occur around the temporal horn, a high proportion of temporal lobe lesions is potentially suggestive of CADASIL. MS lesions frequently involve the cerebellum and brain stem, but a predominance of brain stem lesions suggests a possibility of neurosarcoidosis or Behçet's disease.

> Sagittal images are helpful when an MS diagnosis is being considered because they best demonstrate callosal lesions.

Other imaging sequences are often helpful in distinguishing MS from other etiologies. In MS, T2 hyperintense lesions may be hypointense on T1-weighted images, representing areas of increased axonal loss following prior inflammation. Diffusion weighted imaging may occasionally present a "reverse" red-flag: the presence of restricted diffusion is a common finding in acute stroke but is also possible in acute MS lesions and should be considered with an appropriately corresponding history.

The pattern of Gd-enhancement often is useful in distinguishing MS lesions from another pathology. MS lesions often show either uniform Gd-enhancement or an open-ring pattern, with the presence of additional nonenhancing lesions. The Gd-enhancement typically resolves within 1 to 2 months. Closed ring lesions, enhancement of all lesions, or enhancement lasting more than 2 months raise the possibility of malignancy, infection, or other inflammatory conditions, such as neurosarcoidosis. PML may look similar to MS lesions on T2-weighted imaging initially, but classically is distinguished by gradual enlargement without enhancement or with only faint enhancement limited to the leading edge. Of note, natalizumab-associated PML may have an increased incidence of enhancement and has been seen in up to one-third of patients. Meningeal or vascular enhancement raises concern for neurosarcoidosis or CNS vasculitis.

> Typically, in early MS, some but not all MRI lesions show Gd-enhancement that persists in an individual lesion for 4 to 8 weeks and exhibits a diffuse or open-ring pattern.

> Gd-enhancement with other characteristics should prompt consideration of other diagnoses.

Spinal cord MRI is a useful but frequently underutilized diagnostic tool. Intramedullary T2 hyperintensities in the spinal cord are much more specific for MS than brain lesions and help to point toward the diagnosis of MS if the brain lesions appear nonspecific. MS lesions typically involve 1 to 2 spinal levels, are more frequent in the cervical spine, and often have a patchy distribution. Longitudinally extensive (more than 3 cord segment) lesions are atypical for MS and are more likely to indicate neuromyelitis optica or a metabolic etiology such as B_{12} or copper deficiency. Lesions that are predominantly in the posterior columns are generally seen in tertiary syphilis or B_{12} deficiency. Another red flag on spine imaging is persistent Gd-enhancement which is generally is more concerning for neurosarcoidosis, malignancy, or vascular malformations.

CSF Red Flags

"Classic" CSF findings are outlined earlier in the chapter and include signs of intrathecal antibody production. These can be absent in patients with otherwise typical MS, but in the setting of a marked pleocytosis, particularly if there is a significant proportion of cells other than lymphocytes and macrophages, or markedly elevated protein levels, other diagnoses should be considered, particularly infection, other inflammatory disorders, or malignancy. Conversely, CSF oligoclonal bands and IgG index elevation are often viewed as pathognomonic for MS, but also may be present in other inflammatory or infectious conditions.

> CSF oligoclonal bands and IgG index elevation may be present in other inflammatory or infectious conditions.

MIMICS BY DISEASE CATEGORY

A comprehensive description of all potential MS mimics is outside the scope of this text, but selected key points are outlined here. Other demyelinating etiologies are addressed in detail in separate chapters. The importance of distinguishing neuromyelitis optica from MS is noteworthy because it is often overlooked and the therapeutic approach is different than that for MS.

Infectious etiologies are frequently considered when red flags arise. For example, PML is more likely to cause visual field abnormalities than typical MS vision changes, which most often are due to optic neuropathy. Additional history or exam findings may also point toward an infectious cause, eg, classic erythema migrans raises the possibility of CNS manifestations of Lyme disease. However, it is important to note that evidence of systemic Lyme disease does not prove it as the cause of the MS-like illness; in endemic areas, the infection and MS may be coincident and not causally linked. A broader scope of infectious possibilities should be considered in immunocompromised patients, those with risk factors for HIV infection, or with a history of travel to areas with higher incidences of certain infectious diseases.

Inflammatory and autoimmune diseases can be most difficult to distinguish from MS because the MRI and CSF findings can be similar. In these cases, clinical symptoms may be very helpful in guiding additional diagnostic testing. Classic sicca symptoms are suggestive of Sjogren's syndrome, while a malar rash may suggest systemic lupus erythematosus (SLE). Dry skin and brittle hair/nails suggest thyroid disease (another frequently concomitant rather than causal disease process). Prominent gastrointestinal symptoms warrant additional evaluation for celiac disease. Oral or genital ulcers are concerning for Behçet's disease. Hearing loss warrants consideration of Susac's syndrome. Although cranial nerve nuclei can be affected in MS, extensive cranial nerve involvement is more typical of neurosarcoidosis. Bloodwork may be helpful in confirming inflammatory etiologies, but certain tests—antinuclear antibody (ANA) and angiotensin converting enzyme (ACE) levels—may be modestly elevated in MS and lead to further testing (eg, chest imaging for an elevated ACE level). High ANA titers and the presence of other autoantibodies are more specific for SLE.

Metabolic etiologies should be considered in patients with gastrointestinal malabsorption (eg, history of gastric bypass surgery). In patients with borderline B_{12} (cobalamin) deficiency, blood tests for methylmalonic acid and homocysteine levels should also be checked. Nitrous oxide abuse also leads to functional B_{12} deficiency as it irreversibly binds to the cobalt ion of methylcobalamin and prevents further metabolism. Concurrent myelopathy and sensory neuropathy is characteristic of both B_{12} and copper deficiency. The latter is uncommon but should be considered in patients taking zinc supplements as zinc inhibits the absorption of copper.

The most common malignancy mistaken for MS is primary CNS lymphoma. CSF examination may demonstrate cytologically abnormal lymphocytes but usually is normal or demonstrates only nonspecific abnormalities of protein or pleocytosis. However, spinal tap may still be useful because a finding of oligoclonal bands and an elevated IgG index would argue more strongly in favor of a demyelinating etiology. CNS lymphoma often is steroid responsive, but the response usually is self-limited. Persistent Gd-enhancement or gradual enlargement of MRI lesions should raise the question of malignancy. Ultimately, brain biopsy may be needed for diagnostic confirmation.

> CNS lymphoma often is steroid responsive, but the response usually is self-limited.

DIAGNOSTIC ALGORITHM

If the history, exam, and MRI findings are characteristic of MS, CSF studies and evoked potentials usually are not necessary. Limited additional bloodwork is suggested to look for more common MS mimics as they can often occur concomitantly and may be easily treated (eg, thyroid disease, B_{12} deficiency). Thus, the evaluation of such patients may be limited to:

- Comprehensive medical and neurological history and examination
- Cranial MRI including axial and sagittal FLAIR images, axial proton density or T2-weighted images (better visualization of posterior fossa), and T1-weighted images pre- and post-Gd administration
- Limited blood studies including complete blood count, thyroid stimulating hormone, ANA, syphilis screen (FTA-ABS), vitamin B_{12} level, Lyme titer (in endemic areas).

The utility of more extensive bloodwork is often debated. In patients with manifestations characteristic of MS, the yield is low and false positive results can be misleading.

> Additional testing, such as CSF studies, spinal imaging, and/or VEPs should be considered in less typical cases.

Additional testing, such as CSF studies, spinal imaging, and/or visual evoked potentials (VEPs) should be considered in less typical cases. The specific testing should be guided by the features of the patient, including the presence of red flags.

Patients with abnormal brain MRI in the absence of characteristic clinical manifestations of MS require careful consideration. In patients with atypical histories and nonspecific symptoms, MRI of the brain and spinal cord may be sufficient to rule out MS, but additional tests should be considered as needed. It is important, however, not to assign the diagnosis of MS merely on the basis of exclusion of other diagnoses.

CONCLUSIONS

MS often presents in a typical or straightforward fashion. In such patients, the additional work-up can be limited to MRI studies and modest bloodwork. Clinicians must remain vigilant to ensure that the evolution of manifestations and response to therapy continue to indicate MS. However, many patients referred to MS clinics do not actually have MS. A high proportion of these patients have abnormal brain MRIs and/or nonspecific symptoms and require additional evaluation. It is reasonable to monitor patients periodically in whom testing is equivocal rather than prematurely assigning an MS diagnosis. Careful attention must also be given to identification of red flags because they can indicate the need to search for a potentially uncommon but treatable alternative diagnosis.

KEY POINTS FOR PATIENTS AND FAMILIES

- MS may sometimes be easy to diagnose but there are also times where the diagnosis is unclear and may take time to make.

- MS diagnosis is not based on the number of symptoms, but on the pattern of symptoms, neurological findings on exam, MRI features, and sometimes other diagnostic test results. It requires expertise to make a firm diagnosis of MS.

- Many other conditions may at times look like MS and should be considered when the history, exam, imaging, or other results suggest other diagnoses.

- Many people with nonspecific white matter lesions are evaluated for the diagnosis of MS, but often they do not actually have this disease.

REFERENCES

1. Solomon AJ, Klein EP, Bourdette, D. "Undiagnosing" multiple sclerosis: The challenge of misdiagnosis in MS. *Neurology*. 2012;78:1986–1991.

2. Brettschneider J, Jaskowski TD, Tumani H, et al. Serum anti-GAGA4 IgM antibodies differentiate relapsing remitting and secondary progressive multiple sclerosis from primary progressive multiple sclerosis and other neurological diseases. *J Neuroimmunol*. 2009;217:95–101.

3. Polman CH, Reingold SC, Banwell B, et al. Diagnostic criteria for multiple sclerosis: 2010 revisions to the McDonald Criteria. *Ann Neurol*. 2011;69(2):292–302.

4. Miller DH, Weinshenker BG, Filippi M, et al. Differential diagnosis of suspected multiple sclerosis: A consensus approach. *Mult Scler*. 2008;14:1157–1174.

5. Carminoso MJ, Brousseau KM, Arciniegas DB, et al. Initial evaluations for multiple sclerosis in a university multiple sclerosis center: Outcomes and role of magnetic resonance imaging in referral. *Arch Neurol*. 2005;62:585–590.

6. Boissy AR, Ford, PJ. A touch of MS: Therapeutic mislabeling. *Neurology*. 2012;78:1981–1985.

ADDITIONAL READING

Barned S, Goodman AD, Mattson DH. Frequency of anti-nuclear antibodies in multiple sclerosis. *Neurology*. 1995;45:384–385.

Greco CM, Tassone F, Garcia-Aroncena D, et al. Clinical and neuropathologic findings in a woman with the *FMR1* premutation and multiple sclerosis. *Arch Neurol*. 2008;65(8):1114–1116.

Halperin JJ, Logigian EL, Finkel MF, Pearl RA. Practice parameters for the diagnosis of patients with nervous system Lyme borreliosis (Lyme disease). *Neurology*. 1996;46:619–627.

Kumar N, Gross JB Jr, Ahlskog JE. Copper deficiency myelopathy presents a clinical picture like subacute combined degeneration. *Neurology*. 2004;63(1):33–39.

LaMantia L, Erbetta A. Headache and inflammatory disorders of the central nervous system. *Neurol Sci*. 2004;25(Suppl 3):148–153.

Logigian EL, Kaplan RF, Steere AC. Chronic neurologic manifestations of Lyme disease. *N Engl J Med*. 1990;323:1438–1444.

McDermott C, White K, Bushby K, Shaw P. Hereditary spastic paraparesis: A review of new developments. *J Neurol Neurosurg Psychiatry*. 2000;69(2):150–160.

Natowicz MR, Benjjani B. Genetic disorders that masquerade as multiple sclerosis. *Am J Med Genet*. 1994;49(2):149–169.

O'Riordan JI. Central nervous system white matter diseases other than multiple sclerosis. *Curr Opin Neurol*. 1997;10:211–214.

Rudick RA, Miller AE. Multiple sclerosis or multiple possibilities: The continuing problem of misdiagnosis. *Neurology*. 2012;78: 1904–1906.

Singhal S, Rich P, Markus HS. The spatial distribution of MR imaging abnormalities in cerebral autosomal dominant arteriopathy with subcortical infarcts and leukoencephalopathy and their relationship to age and clinical features. *AJNR*. 2005;26(10): 2481–2487.

Stern BJ. Neurological complications of sarcoidosis. *Curr Opin Neurol*. 2004;17(3):311–316.

Theodoridou A, Settas L. Demyelination in rheumatic diseases. *J Neurol Neurosurg Psychiatry*. 2006;77(3):290–295.

Thompson AJ, Polman CH, Miller DH, et al. Primary progressive multiple sclerosis. *Brain*. 1997;210:1085–1096.

Younger DS. Vasculitis of the nervous system. *Curr Opin Neurol*. 2004;17(3):317–336.

Part III. Treatment

11

Overview of Present Treatment for Relapsing Forms of Multiple Sclerosis

MARY ALISSA WILLIS
RICHARD RUDICK

KEY POINTS FOR CLINICIANS

- Comprehensive management of relapsing forms of multiple sclerosis (MS) involves the treatment of relapses, disease-modifying therapy (DMT), and symptom management.

- The goal of DMT is disease-activity free—no relapses, no MRI activity.

- Although selection of initial therapy is more individualized now than it has been in the past, there are no biomarkers that predict individual response to therapy.

- Monitoring should include routine clinical follow-up at 3 to 6 month intervals and imaging at 6 to 12 months after starting therapy.

- Treatments are only partially effective; breakthrough disease is expected.

Approximately 80% to 85% of patients with multiple sclerosis (MS) initially follow a clinical course characterized by periodic relapses. These are manifest as new or worsened neurological symptoms and deficits with a subsequent period of neurological recovery [1]. In most cases, relapses occur infrequently—1 per year or less. However, relapses do not occur at the same rate for all patients and vary over time for individual patients. Relapses manifest varying clinical patterns, variable severity, and result in varying degrees of permanent disability. When recovery from a relapse is incomplete, neurological impairment and disability can accumulate. Management of MS requires multiple therapeutic approaches. The current management of relapsing-remitting multiple sclerosis (RRMS) involves a triad: treatment of acute relapses, prevention of new disease activity, and management of symptoms affecting the quality of life.

Although the pathogenesis of MS remains poorly understood, remarkable progress in development of new therapies that inhibit disease activity (Figure 11.1) has been witnessed. Using available options, including more effective drugs, there is potential to achieve a new goal—a disease-activity free state that is characterized not only by prevention of relapses but also by the absence of radiological change and disability progression.

RATIONALE FOR EARLY TREATMENT

In longitudinal MRI studies, the frequency of new MRI lesions exceeds the frequency of clinical relapses by a factor of 10 to 20 [2,3]. While short-term recovery may be excellent, clinical relapses and new lesions on imaging represent active tissue destruction. It is known that widespread tissue damage is present at the earliest clinical stages of the disease [4,5]. This ongoing destruction is difficult to reverse and likely sets the stage for progressive disability. The ability to predict disability progression in individual patients is limited, however.

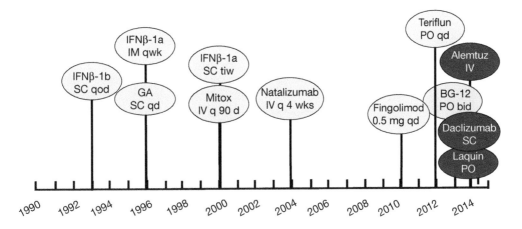

FIGURE 11.1

The changing landscape of MS disease modifying treatment including approved agents (light gray) and a projected timeline for emerging therapies (in dark gray).

IFNβ = interferon beta; GA = glatiramer acetate; Mitox = mitoxantrone; Laquin = laquinimod; BG12 = dimethyl fumarate; Teriflun = teriflunomide; Alemtuz = alemtuzumab

> While short-term recovery may be excellent, clinical relapses and new lesions on imaging represent active tissue destruction.

We now have a variety of DMTs that effectively reduce disease activity and expanded disability status scale (EDSS)-measured disability progression in RRMS. As seen throughout medicine, strategies to prevent tissue injury are more effective than attempts to reverse the injury. A consensus statement of the National Multiple Sclerosis Society endorsed a proactive approach to MS treatment by recommending that these DMTs be started "as soon as possible following a definite diagnosis of MS with active, relapsing disease" [6]. The consensus statement further recommended that therapy should be considered for patients who have had a first episode of demyelination and who are at high risk for developing MS.

> Therapy should be considered for patients who have had a first episode of demyelination who are at a high risk for developing MS.

OVERVIEW OF APPROVED THERAPIES

There are currently 8 medications approved in the United States for treatment of RRMS. A brief summary of these medications is presented in Table 11.1. More detailed descriptions are provided in Chapter 13.

Glatiramer acetate (GA) and the interferon beta preparations are often called *platform agents* or ABCR *drugs*. GA is a mixture of random polymers that are developed to mimic a myelin basic protein. The exact mechanism of action is unclear. Likewise, the immunomodulating effects of interferon (IFN) beta that relate to clinical benefit are incompletely understood. All the platform agents are generally well or moderately tolerated and data accumulated over the past 15 to 20 years suggest strong long-term safety. Each medication has demonstrated reductions in relapse rate and MRI activity compared to placebo. In separate pivotal trials, efficacy on relapse rate was similar between the different injectable therapies, although cross-study comparisons are difficult to interpret. There have been randomized, head-to-head comparison studies that demonstrated comparable clinical benefits of GA and IFN beta-1a SC (Rebif) [7], IFN beta-1b (Betaseron) [8], and IFN beta-1a IM (Avonex) [9]. A randomized head-to-head comparison study indicated a more rapid onset of MRI benefit when using IFN beta-1a SC (Rebif) compared with IFN beta-1b IM (Avonex) [10] although the clinical relevance of that finding is unclear, as benefits beyond 3 months were similar between the 2 treatments. In our opinion, the platform agents are similar in efficacy; selection is generally based on physician and patient preferences and side-effect profile.

> All the platform agents are generally well or moderately tolerated and data suggest strong long-term safety.

Two oral therapies, teriflunomide and dimethyl fumarate, have recently been approved for use as first line agents. The efficacy, safety, and tolerability of these agents are discussed further in Chapter 16.

Natalizumab, fingolimod, and mitoxantrone are more potent medications that are often reserved for patients who have aggressive disease or who have suboptimal response to the platform agents. Natalizumab inhibits the migration of leukocytes into the central nervous system (CNS) by blocking the binding of alpha4beta1 integrin on the leukocytes with

TABLE 11.1
Overview of Currently Approved DMTs for Relapsing MS

AGENT	YEAR APPROVED IN THE UNITED STATES	ROUTE	DOSING FREQUENCY	SPECIFIC CONSIDERATIONS
IFN beta-1b (Betaseron/Extavia)	1993/2009	SC	Every other day	Flu-like side effects; May worsen headaches, depression, spasticity; May cause hepatotoxicity, particularly at higher doses; Avoid IM route for patients on anticoagulants.
IFN beta-1a (Avonex)	1996	IM	Weekly	
Glatiramer acetate (Copaxone)	1996	SC	Daily	Daily injections; Potential for more bothersome site reactions in thin patients.
IFN beta-1a (Rebif)	2000	SC	3 times per week	Same as other interferons.
Mitoxantrone (Novantrone)	2000	IV	Every 3 months (Limited lifetime dose)	Dose-dependent cardiotoxicity; Potential for secondary lymphoid malignancies.
Natalizumab (Tysabri)	2004*	IV	Every 4 weeks	Risk for PML (very low if JCV antibody negative).
Fingolimod (Gilenya)	2010	PO	Daily	Potential for symptomatic bradycardia with first dose; Potential for macular edema; Use with caution in patients with asthma or other lung disease.
Teriflunomide (Aubagio)	2012	PO	Daily	Preganancy category X May cause decreased hair density May cause elevations in liver enzymes
Dimethyl fumarate (Tecfidera)	2013	PO	Twice daily	May cause flushing and gastrointestinal upset

*Withdrawn from the U.S. market in 2005; reapproved in 2006.
IFN beta, interferon beta; IM, intramuscular; IV, intravenous; JCV, JC virus; PML, progressive multifocal encephalopathy; PO, per os (by mouth); SC, subcutaneous.

vascular cell adhesion molecule on vascular endothelial cells [11]. Patients who receive natalizumab require close monitoring for progressive multifocal encephalopathy (PML). Serological testing for antibodies to the JC virus (JCV) helps stratify patients into high- and low-risk categories for PML [12].

Fingolimod is an oral sphingosine 1-phosphate receptor modulator that blocks lymphocyte egress from the lymph nodes and may have direct CNS effects [13]. The use of fingolimod in clinical practice has been limited by concerns for cardiac effects, infection, and macular edema. In response to postmarketing reports of adverse cardiac effects, the U.S. Food and Drug Administration revised first-dose monitoring requirements to increase cardiac monitoring and relative contraindications to fingolimod treatment [14].

> Patients who receive natalizumab require close monitoring for PML.

Mitoxantrone is a chemotherapeutic agent that produces cytotoxicity by interfering with nucleic acid repair and synthesis. Although effective and generally well tolerated, its use has been largely abandoned because of concerns for decreased cardiac function and treatment-related leukemia [15].

CHOOSING INITIAL THERAPY

The DMTs listed in Table 11.1 have all been reported to reduce relapse rate, decrease MRI lesion activity, and most have been reported to slow accumulation of disability. All of the medications have potential tolerability and/or safety concerns. Because there are currently no biomarkers or other objective methods to predict the efficacy of a specific DMT for an individual patient, initial selection of DMTs for patients with MS is largely based on experience and clinical judgement.

Prior to choosing therapy, the rationale and goals of therapy should be thoroughly discussed with the patient. A patient who expects the DMT to restore function or reduce symptoms will usually be disappointed. Such a mismatch between patient and care team expectations may lead to reduced compliance and poorer outcomes.

Any of the IFN beta preparations or GA would be reasonable initial therapy for most patients with MS. Despite modest efficacy and less convenient administration, both IFN beta and GA have the advantage of good long-term safety. As no injectable therapy has shown long-term superiority over another, the selection of DMT is often guided by side-effect profile and patient preference for frequency/route.

> A patient who expects the DMT to restore function or reduce symptoms will usually be disappointed.

In general, GA may be preferable to the IFNs in patients with severe depression, headaches, or spasticity. The less-frequently dosed IFNs may be preferable for patients who are averse to injections. The intramuscular route should be avoided in patients who are chronically anticoagulated. Thin patients may be prone to more bother-some site reactions with GA.

The use of natalizumab and fingolimod as first-line therapy is limited by the risk for more serious side effects and the relative lack of long-term safety data. Use of these medications as first-line agents is appropriate when patients have aggressive disease defined by frequent relapses at initial presentation, poor recovery from relapses, and/or high MRI lesion burden. Evidence suggests that the risk of natalizumab-associated PML is predominantly in patients seropositive for the JCV antibody. Therefore, natalizumab for patients with more aggressive disease who are JCV antibody-negative is favored.

The placement of teriflunomide and dimethyl fuma-rate in the treatment algorithm will become clearer as experience with these medications grows. Both medications are approved for first line use in the United States. As outlined in Chapter 16, risk mitigation strategies seem to be well defined. Protocol for switching between agents (ie, "wash-out periods") has not been established.

TABLE 11.2
Suggested Monitoring

- Baseline MRI of the brain
- Interval history and targeted neurological exam every 3 to 6 months
- Quantitative measures (EDSS, timed 25 foot walk, 9-hole peg test) when feasible
- Repeat MRI brain 6 months after starting therapy (12 months for GA)
- Medication-specific paraclinical testing*:
  - IFN beta—CBC, AST, ALT at months 1, 3, and 6, then every 12 months; Nabs at 12 to 24 months
  - Natalizumab—AST, ALT at months 3 and 6 months, then every 6 months; Nabs at 6 months; JCV serology every 6 to 12 months
  - Fingolimod—CBC, AST, ALT every 6 months; OCT at 3 to 4 months
  - Teriflunomide—TB skin test, CBC, AST, ALT, pregnancy test at baseline; AST, ALT every 6 months
  - Dimethyl fumarate—CBC at baseline and annually

*author opinion.
ALT, alanine transaminase; AST, aspartate transaminase; CBC, complete blood count; JCV, JC virus; OCT, optical coherence tomography.

MONITORING PATIENTS ON THERAPY

Prior to initiating therapy, patients should be fully edu-cated about expected benefits, anticipated and possible side effects, follow-up schedule, and required monitoring and blood testing. After starting therapy, patients should be monitored for compliance, tolerability, safety, and efficacy (Table 11.2). Patients should be seen within a few months of starting a DMT to discuss site reactions or other side effects. Periodic lab work, usually a complete blood count and liver function tests, is recommended for all currently avail-able medications except GA. Clinical assessments includ-ing interval history and targeted neurological exam at 3 to 6 month intervals initially is recommended. Quantitative functional testing (EDSS, timed 25 foot walk, 9-hole peg test) may be helpful in longitudinal assessments. The brain MRI is repeated after 6 months on IFN beta, natalizumab, or fingolimod. Imaging is repeated 1 year after initiation of GA because of a delayed time of onset of efficacy.

DEFINING BREAKTHROUGH DISEASE

All current treatments are only partially effective across a population of MS patients, thus, breakthrough disease is com-mon. About two-thirds of patients with RRMS have a relapse or new MRI lesions within 2 years of starting on IFN beta [16] or GA [17]. Clinical, MRI, and biological measures are used to identify patients with breakthrough disease (Table 11.3).

> Clinical, MRI, and biological measures are used to identify patients with breakthrough disease.

The number of relapses while on treatment is com-monly used to determine efficacy. Sustained worsening in the disability measure EDSS is frequently reported in clini-cal trials to demonstrate worsening. This approach is often not practical in the clinical setting when the EDSS is not con-sistently performed owing to time constraints or when the involvement of multiple examiners increases the variability of the data. On the other hand, patient-reported symptom

TABLE 11.3
Measures of Breakthrough Disease

Clinical measures
Compliance
Patient-reported symptoms
Number of relapses
Disability progression (ie, EDSS)

MRI measures
New or enlarging T2 lesions
Gadolinium-enhancing lesions

Biological measures
IFN beta neutralizing antibodies
Natalizumab neutralizing antibodies

burden often guides treatment decisions although there is no evidence in the literature to support this approach [18].

Longitudinal studies that evaluate predictors of disability progression suggest that MRI is a more sensitive predictor of future disability than clinical relapses [19]. The presence of new or enlarging T2 hyperintense lesions or the presence of gadolinium-enhancing lesions during the course of the DMT suggests future clinical and radiological worsening.

The search continues for biomarkers to guide MS therapy. Neutralizing antibodies (Nabs) to IFN beta and natalizumab may explain poor therapeutic response to those therapies. Nabs to IFN occur in up to 35% of patients and usually appear between 6 and 24 months [20]. Nab frequency is highest with IFN beta-1b (Betaseron), intermediate with IFN beta-1a SC (Rebif), and lowest with IFN beta-1a IM (Avonex). Because occurrence of Nab to IFN beta cannot be predicted in the individual patient, and because persistence of Nabs in high titers blunts the clinical effectiveness of IFN beta, some neurologists choose the least immunogenic IFN beta preparation. Persistence of Nabs to natalizumab also blocks clinical effectiveness, but antibodies only occur in about 6% of patients [21].These antibodies typically appear early—between 3 and 6 months after starting therapy [22].

Other factors that can contribute to suboptimal response to DMT include medication noncompliance; inability to tolerate therapy leading to noncompliance; intercurrent medical illness; comorbidities such as depression, anxiety, diabetes, or obesity; or independent neurological conditions such as cervical cord compression. Addressing compliance issues, comorbidities, and coexisting non-MS conditions is paramount.

CHANGING THERAPY

There is no consensus on the definition of an unacceptable level of disease activity, although new options for disease treatment and monitoring have raised the standards for treatment success. Recently, the concept of freedom from disease activity has emerged as a treatment goal. As currently defined, a patient has achieved freedom from disease activity if there are no new MRI lesions, no relapse activity, and no disability worsening. For patients who have not achieved this therapeutic goal—eg, patients with a clinical relapse, a worsening disability, a new or enlarging T2 lesions on MRI, gadolinium-enhancing lesions on MRI after 6 to 12 months on therapy—change in therapy should be considered.

> Recently, the concept of freedom from disease activity has emerged as a treatment goal.

There is little data to guide therapy changes. Two common approaches to changing DMT are by changing to another platform agent or by escalating therapy to a second-line drug. A third, less common, approach is by using combination therapy. Factors to consider include severity of disease while on the current therapy, degree of recovery from relapses, ongoing disease activity that is visible on MRI, expected tolerance to side effects, patient commitment to disease-free status, and the patient's risk tolerance.

Changing from one injectable to another is reasonable for patients with mild MS disease activity and poor tolerance of the current therapy. In this case, it makes most sense to switch between GA and one of the IFN beta products. Switching from frequent IFN beta to weekly IFN beta-1a may be considered for patients who have troubling IFN beta side effects, as these are dose dependent. As the approved doses of the IFN beta preparations are near the plateau of the dose–clinical response curve, exceeding the recommended dose is more likely to increase side effects than improve efficacy. Likewise, there is no evidence that switching from less-frequent to more-frequent IFN beta increases efficacy. Switching the patient who has breakthrough disease between different platform agents has some rationale (mechanisms of action for IFN beta and GA are almost certainly different), but is not supported by data, and head-to-head studies have failed to demonstrate superiority of any of the platform drugs.

Escalating therapy to natalizumab or fingolimod is a logical approach for patients who have breakthrough disease despite a first-line DMT. This approach is most justified in patients who have frequent relapses, substantial progression of MRI lesion burden, or repeatedly active imaging studies. Factors influencing risk–benefit ratio in individual patients (such as JCV seropositivity when considering natalizumab) should be considered.

DIFFICULT TREATMENT DECISIONS

Treatment dilemmas are common. These include deciding whether to observe the patient with mild disease or start therapy with a disease modifying drug; how much disease activity to tolerate before changing therapy; whether to use a DMT in patients with progressive disease; and when to stop DMT.

The general recommendation for early initiation of DMT does not apply to all patients. DMT should only be used when there is certainty about the diagnosis of MS or in patients who have typical clinically isolated syndromes (CIS) and multiple MRI lesions in locations characteristic to MS. For example, DMT would not be recommended for a patient with only optic neuritis and a few nonspecific brain lesions. Monitoring off-therapy would be appropriate. Observation without DMT is also an appropriate strategy for a subset of patients with a relatively benign course. For patients with mild, intermittent, nonspecific symptoms (ie, headache, fatigue, sensory disturbances) despite MRI findings compatible with MS, initiation of DMT may result in side effects, cost, and risk with little effect on the course of disease [19]. These patients should be followed clinically and radiologically.

As previously mentioned, disease-activity free status is the goal of MS treatment. While there is no consensus on the definition of a tolerable level of active disease, changing to a potentially more effective agent should be considered when a patient has ongoing clinical or sub-clinical disease activity. There are some patients, however, whose ongoing disease activity does not always herald a DMT change. Reduction, but not elimination, of disease activity is an acceptable treatment goal for some patients with very active MS. Other patients may be maintained on a DMT despite breakthrough disease when the risks associated with more potent medications are too great. For example, a JCV seropositive patient with more than 24 months of natalizumab treatment may not be advised to restart natalizumab if subclinical disease activity was detected after 6 months on fingolimod. These difficult decisions must be made on a case-by-case basis.

Deciding when to initiate or continue DMT in patients with secondary progressive MS (SPMS) can be challenging. The inflammatory processes targeted by current DMTs are less prominent in progressive MS. Thus, the medications are less effective at later stages of the disease. The interface between RRMS and SPMS is often nebulous; there is no abrupt transition to a purely progressive mechanism. Patients who have SPMS with a recent onset of progression, superimposed relapses, or ongoing MRI activity are most likely to benefit from DMT [20].

> Deciding when to initiate or continue DMT in patients with secondary progressive MS can be challenging.

There are also no criteria for determining when DMT is no longer needed for patients with either mild disease or with gradual progression. Some patients may elect for monitoring off-therapy when relapses are very infrequent or when side effects, cost, or inconvenience of DMT are more concerning than the possibility of MS disease activity. Other patients with very advanced MS may choose to remain on DMT when this seems futile to the provider. Ultimately, the decision to stop DMT should follow a thoughtful discussion between the patient and the care team.

NEAR-TERM FUTURE

The MS therapeutics field is rapidly developing and evolving. In the next 2–3 years, we expect to see additional treatment options (eg, alemtuzumab; daclizumab; and others). It seems likely that the use of injectables will decline, as oral options become available as first-line agents. As the field grapples with the opportunities and challenges of targeting treatment to achieve disease-activity free status, optimal monitoring and sequencing of first-line and second-line drugs will become central. Finally, information on the effectiveness of more potent drugs very early in the disease, and in patients transitioning to SPMS will guide therapeutic decisions. In the longer term, effective development of pharmacogenomics and pharmacogenetics will guide personalized medicine in the MS field, and result in much improved outcomes.

PATIENT CASE

A 29-year-old woman with recently diagnosed MS presents to establish care 6 months after an episode of partial myelitis with incomplete recovery. She started on GA 6 weeks ago. Her leg weakness and urinary incontinence has worsened during the last 4 weeks. She thinks it may be related to the new medication.

Question: Does this worsening constitute breakthrough disease? What management do you recommend?

Answer: GA is not immediately effective; at least 6 to 12 months is needed to assess its efficacy. Some patients with very active disease may benefit from pulse steroids while waiting for the DMT to take effect. In this case, other causes of worsening symptoms should be investigated. A urinalysis and culture are indicated. Additional studies, such as complete blood count, comprehensive metabolic panel, thyroid stimulating hormone, vitamin B_{12}, and MRI brain/cervical spine, would be reasonable.

She felt better after treatment of her urinary tract infection and vitamin B_{12} deficiency. MRI showed no new or enhancing lesions. Four weeks later she called to report blurry vision and pain with movement of the right eye for 3 days. She reports no missed doses of her GA.

Question: What do you do now?

Answer: This patient describes a relapse after taking GA for 10 weeks. This is still too early to declare a breakthrough disease. A course of high-dose corticosteroids would be appropriate. It would also be reasonable to schedule a clinical follow-up in 3 months.

The patient recovered completely from her optic neuritis. She reported no side effects and no new symptoms at her 3 month follow-up. Her neurological exam results were stable. She called 4 weeks later to say that she has been admitted to a nearby hospital with bilateral lower extremity numbness, weakness, and inability to walk. Her new MRI brain reveals 3 enhancing lesions.

Question: What do you do now?

Answer: The patient has now had 2 clinical relapses and MRI evidence of disease activity after 26 weeks on GA. She reports compliance with her medication. Changing therapy would be indicated. Due to the disease activity and incomplete recovery from the myelitis, escalation of therapy is favored. Either fingolimod or natalizumab would be appropriate. The patient elected to start natalizumab after JCV serology returned with a negative result.

KEY POINTS FOR PATIENTS AND FAMILIES

- Management of MS involves 3 parts:
  1. Treatment of relapses
  2. Prevention of MS disease activity (relapse or MRI change)
  3. Management of symptoms (includes overall wellness, medications, and sometimes rehabilitation services)
- Disease modifying therapy (DMT) to prevent MS disease activity should be started early. For patients with apparently benign disease, or who are being observed for MS, DMT may not be needed.
- DMT does not typically restore function or improve symptoms.
- The care team should be informed of site reactions, side effects, or frequent missed doses.
- Expect to have a follow-up visit and repeat MRI after 6 months of treatment with a DMT.
- The DMT medications are not effective immediately. It often takes 6 to 12 months to assess how well the medication works.
- Other factors that could contribute to worsening symptoms but not necessarily worsening MS are:
  - Infections
  - Thyroid disease, diabetes
  - Vitamin deficiency, anemia
  - Depression, anxiety, poor sleep
  - Arthritis
- A change in therapy does not necessarily indicate aggressive MS or poor prognosis.

REFERENCES

1. Compston A, Coles A. Multiple sclerosis. *Lancet.* 2008; 372(9648):1502–1517.

2. Paty DW, Li DK, UBC MS/MRI study group, The IFNB Multiple Sclerosis Study Group. Interferon beta-1b is effective in relapsing-remitting multiple sclerosis. II. MRI analysis results of a multicenter, randomized, double-blind, placebo-controlled trial. *Neurology.* 1993;43:662–667.

3. McFarland HF, Frank JA, Albert PS, et al. Using gadolinium-enhanced magnetic resonance imaging lesions to monitor disease activity in multiple sclerosis. *Ann Neurol.* 1992;32(6):758–766.

4. Gallo A, Rovaris M, Riva R, et al. Diffusion-tensor magnetic resonance imaging detects normal-appearing white matter damage unrelated to short-term disease activity in patients at the earliest clinical stage of multiple sclerosis. *Arch Neurol.* 2005;62(5):803–808.

5. Rovaris M, Gambini A, Gallo A, et al. Axonal injury in early multiple sclerosis is irreversible and independent of short-term disease evolution. *Neurology.* 2005;65(10): 1626–1630.

6. National Clinical Advisory Board of the National Multiple Sclerosis Society. Disease management consensus statement. 2008; http://www.nationalmssociety.org/PRC

7. Mikol DD, Barkhof F, Chang P, et al. Comparison of subcutaneous interferon beta-1a with glatiramer acetate in patients with relapsing multiple sclerosis (the REbif vs Glatiramer Acetate in Relapsing MS Disease [REGARD] study): A multicentre, randomised, parallel, open-label trial. *Lancet Neurol.* 2008;7(10):903–914.

8. O'Connor P, Filippi M, Arnason B, et al. 250 mcg or 500 mcg interferon beta-1b versus 20mg glatiramer acetate in relapsing-remitting multiple sclerosis: A prospective, randomized multicentre study. *Lancet Neurol.* 2009;8:889–897.

9. Lublin FD, Cofield S, Cutter G, et al. The CombiRx trial: A multi-center, double-blind, randomized study comparing the combined use of interferon beta-1a and glatiramer acetate to either agent alone in participants with relapsing-remitting multiple sclerosis. Presented at the American Academy of Neurology Annual Meeting; April 27, 2012; New Orleans, LA.

10. Panitch HS, Goodin DS, Francis G, et al. Randomized, comparative study of interferon beta 1-a treatment regimens in MS: The EVIDENCE trial. *Neurology.* 2002;59:1496–1506.

11. Ransohoff RM. Natalizumab for multiple sclerosis. *NEJM.* 2007;356(25):2622–2629.

12. Fox RJ, Rudick RA. Risk stratification and patient counseling for natalizumab in multiple sclerosis. *Neurology.* 2012;78(6):436–437.

13. Brinkmann V. FTY720 (fingolimod) in multiple sclerosis: Therapeutic effects in the immune and the central nervous system. *Br J Pharmacol.* 2009;158(5):1173–1182.

14. NDA 22-257. FDA-Approved labeling text for Gilenya (fingolimod) capsules. Updated April 2012.

15. US Food and Drug Administration. Mitoxantrone hydrochloride (marketed as Novantrone and generics). www.fda.gov/Drugs/DrugSafety/PostmarketDrugSafetyInformationfor PatientsandProvides/ucm126445.htm. Published July 29, 2008.

16. Jacobs LD, Cookfair DL, Rudick RA, et al. Intramuscular interferon beta-1a for disease progression in relapsing multiple sclerosis. The Multiple Sclerosis Collaborative Research Group (MSCRG). *Ann Neurol.* 1996;39(3):285–294.

17. Johnson KP, Brooks BR, Cohen JA, et al. Copolymer 1 reduces relapse rate and improves disability in relapsing-remitting multiple sclerosis: Results of a phase III multicenter, double-blind placebo-controlled trial. The Copolymer 1 Multiple Sclerosis Study Group. *Neurology.* 1995;45(7):1268–1276.

18. Rudick RA, Polman CH. Current approaches to the identification and management of breakthrough disease in patients with multiple sclerosis. *Lancet Neurol.* 2009;8(6):545–559.

19. Rudick RA, Lee JC, Simon J, et al. Defining interferon beta response status in multiple sclerosis patients. *Ann Neurol.* 2004;56(4):548–555.

20. Farrell RA, Giovannoni G. Measuring and management of anti-interferon beta antibodies in subjects with multiple sclerosis. *Mult Scler.* 2007;13(5):567–577.

21. Calabresi PA, Giovannoni G, Confavreux C, et al. The incidence and significance of anti-natalizumab antibodies: Results from AFFIRM and SENTINEL. *Neurology.* 2007;69:1391–1403.

22. Polman CH, O'Connor PW, Havrdova E, et al. A randomized, placebo-controlled trial of natalizumab for relapsing multiple sclerosis. *NEJM.* 2006;354(9):899–910.

12

Relapse Management in Multiple Sclerosis

ROBERT J. FOX

KEY POINTS FOR CLINICIANS

- A hallmark of multiple sclerosis (MS) is the clinical relapse, an episode of new or worsening MS symptoms not due to fever or infection lasting more than 1 day.

- In a patient with an established diagnosis of MS, a typical clinical relapse needs little further evaluation besides consideration of infection and alternative diagnoses.

- Relapse management commonly involves high-dose corticosteroids—typically 1,000 mg daily for 3 to 5 days, followed by short oral prednisone taper.

- Symptomatic management of MS symptoms is sometimes helpful.

- Clinical recovery takes several weeks or months, although residual symptoms can persist indefinitely.

In 70% to 80% of patients, multiple sclerosis (MS) begins with a relapsing-remitting course in which neurological manifestations develop in the context of acute relapses. An MS relapse is defined as new or worsening neurological symptoms which persist for more than 24 hours. In clinical trials, the definition of a relapse usually requires objective neurological findings on examination, although in clinical practice, the overall clinical picture is more important than objective findings. Typical symptoms of an MS relapse include blurred vision, diplopia, numbness in an extremity or the trunk, motor weakness, vertigo, or ataxia, but vary from case to case. Symptoms typically come on and worsen over several days or weeks, although occasionally symptoms can be sudden and maximal at onset, mimicking a stroke. Sensory symptoms in the extremity will often start in the toes or fingers and gradually progress proximally up the limb. Sensory symptoms involving the trunk can be described as a tightness sensation, informally called the "MS hug." Weakness can be seen, but usually numbness is more prominent than weakness. Urinary and bowel symptoms can include urgency and frequency, although incontinence is rare during an acute MS relapse.

Neurological findings on examination depend on the affected system. Optic neuritis can present with visual field cut, visual distortion (ie, "looking through glass soda block"), papillitis, and mild retro-orbital pain with eye movement. Diplopia from internuclear ophthalmoplegia is common in MS and manifests with adduction weakness in 1 or both eyes. Sensory symptoms can include numbness, paresthesias, and less commonly pain. Objective sensory loss is often absent despite the patient reporting sensory changes.

Most MS relapses will recover spontaneously over several weeks or months and leave only minor residual symptoms, regardless of treatment. However, not all relapses recovery completely. Early in the disease, most disability accrual is the result of incomplete relapse recovery [1].

Several arguments suggest benefit from active relapse treatment with corticosteroids. First, clinical trials found corticosteroids to accelerate clinical recovery from a relapse. Second, pathological studies have found greater than 10,000 transected axons/mm^3 in MS lesions with active inflammation [2]. This irreversible axonal injury argues for aggressive reduction of inflammation to minimize permanent tissue damage.

> Most MS relapses improve regardless of treatment.

EVALUATION

In a patient without the diagnosis of MS, evaluation of an MS relapse focuses on making an accurate diagnosis of MS and excluding other potential diagnoses (see Chapters 7 and 10). In a patient with an established diagnosis of MS, evaluation is more limited. Since an MS relapse is a clinical diagnosis, imaging studies such as MRI are neither necessary nor indicated during the initial evaluation and management of a typical MS relapse. Infections may precipitate clinical relapses and can probably slow or prevent recovery from relapses. Bladder infections are common in MS patients and should be considered in a patient reporting symptoms suggestive of a relapse. Table 12.1 lists red flags to consider when evaluating patients for relapse. Uncomplicated relapses in a patient with known MS can often be evaluated by telephone.

Pseudorelapse is a worsening of previous MS symptoms during a period of illness, particularly a febrile illness or metabolic derangement. Bladder infections, respiratory infections, and skin infections (eg, decubitus ulcers) are common culprits. Becoming overheated may precipitate a worsening of symptoms. Emotional distress and sleep deprivation can also worsen previous neurological symptoms and mimic an MS relapse through worsened fatigue, sensory symptoms, gait, and overall reduced level of function. Clinical relapses need to be differentiated from transient day-to-day fluctuations in neurological symptoms, which is common in MS patients.

TABLE 12.1
Red Flags of MS Relapse

- Fever: suggests possible infection
- Urinary symptoms: suggests possible urinary infection
- Relapses more than once every 2 to 3 months: suggests pseudorelapses or alternative diagnosis
- Patients receiving highly active anti-inflammatory therapy such as natalizumab: consider opportunistic infection such as PML
- Incomplete response to corticosteroids: although incomplete response to corticosteroids is not rare, it should raise the consideration of alternative diagnosis, including NMO

In a patient currently treated with highly active anti-inflammatory therapy, such as natalizumab, clinical relapses are uncommon. Relapse symptoms early in the course of treatment (ie, less than 6 months) may suggest the presence of neutralizing antibodies against the therapy. Relapse symptoms later in the course of treatment (ie, more than 6 months of therapy) should raise concerns of treatment-related complications. In a patient on natalizumab for over 6 months, progressive multifocal leukoencephalopathy (PML) should always be considered when relapse symptoms develop.

> PML should be considered with relapse symptoms more than 6 months after starting natalizumab.

Superimposed medical conditions need to be differentiated from an MS relapse, particularly when the presentation is atypical for an MS relapse. For example, sudden-onset symptoms should raise a concern for stroke, particularly in patients with vascular risk factors. Cardiac ischemia should be considered in a patient with left arm sensory symptoms, such as pain and heaviness. Paroxysmal events may suggest seizures or tonic spasms. Some patients with MS describe their tonic spasms as "relapses," stating they have multiple "relapses" in a given day. Patients rarely have more than a handful of true relapses in a year, so it is sometimes helpful for a clinician to clarify with patients on their concept of relapses.

> Relapse = Exacerbation = Attack = Bout of MS

Most relapses respond to a single course of corticosteroids. When symptoms do not improve within 1 to 2 weeks, alternative or contributing diagnoses should be considered. Potential conditions include infection (particularly urinary tract infections, which can be asymptomatic), emotional distress, depression, and anxiety. Gradually, progressive neurological symptoms from progressive MS can sometimes be confused with an MS relapse. MRI studies of the affected area (eg, spinal cord for partial transverse myelitis relapse) can help evaluate for persistent inflammation, which manifests as gadolinium-enhancement and edema, as well as a mechanical etiology such as disc disease. On the other hand, imaging at the time of relapse is not usually helpful with either diagnosing the relapse, treating the relapse, or planning changes in therapy. Waiting for an MRI to be performed may slow the beginning of therapy unnecessarily.

MANAGEMENT

The overall goal of relapse management is to stop active inflammation, limit damage secondary to active inflammation,

TABLE 12.2
Typical Management for an MS Relapse

- In a patient with known MS, confirm typical symptoms of MS relapse

- Screen for infection—bladder, respiratory, skin

- Treat with a 3-day course of 1 g/day IVMP, followed by 15-day prednisone taper: 60 mg daily for 3 days, 40 mg daily for 3 days, 20 mg daily for 3 days

- Clinical follow-up in about 6 to 8 weeks to confirm good recovery of symptoms and consider need to change long-term MS therapy

- In a patient with incomplete recovery, consider alternative/contributing conditions, then re-treat with 3 to 5 days of IVMP and prednisone taper

- If still incomplete recovery, consider imaging affected area to help differentiate active inflammation from established injury

IVMP, intravenous methylprednisolone.

TABLE 12.3
Placebo-Controlled Trials of High-Dose Corticosteroids for MS Relapses

STUDY	TREATMENT REGIMENS	N	RESULT
Durelli et al. [15]	15 days of IV MP, tapering from 15 mg/kg per day down to 1 mg/kg per day versus placebo	20	MP better than placebo
Milligan et al. [16]	IV MP 500 mg/day for 5 days versus placebo	22	MP better than placebo
Sellebjerg et al. [12]	Oral MP 500 mg/day for 5 days versus placebo	51	Higher proportion of patients with improvement in oral MP group

IV, intravenous; MP, methylprednisolone; N, total number of subjects.

accelerate and improve clinical recovery, and (ideally) delay the next clinical relapse. Table 12.2 outlines the typical management for MS relapse.

Corticosteroids. The mainstay of MS relapse management is corticosteroids. First reported in 1951 [3], it was not until 1970 that an influential controlled trial showed that adrenocorticotropic hormone (ACTH) improves recovery from a clinical relapse [4]. Reports of benefit from high-dose intravenous methylprednisolone (IVMP) in several autoimmune disorders led to single-arm studies of IVMP in MS [5,6]. Three randomized trials compared the efficacy of ACTH and IVMP [7–9]. The most influential of these trials was a randomized, placebo-controlled, double-blind comparison of IVMP for 3 days verses intramuscular ACTH for 14 days [9]. Both treatment groups improved significantly but there were no significant differences between the groups up to 90 days after treatment. The investigators concluded that IVMP was an effective alternative to ACTH, required shorter treatment durations, and was better tolerated. Most clinicians then abandoned ACTH for treatment of clinical relapses and instead utilized IVMP. ACTH is still available for clinical use, although its prohibitive cost (approximately US$23,000 for a single treatment course), similar efficacy to IVMP, and easy availability of oral MP and other corticosteroid preparations (for patients without IV access) make the use of ACTH in MS predominantly obsolete.

Corticosteroids are the mainstay of MS relapse treatment.

Additional placebo-controlled studies of IVMP provided consistent evidence that high-dose corticosteroids were beneficial compared to placebo (Table 12.3). A meta-analysis and a *Cochrane Review* found convincing evidence to support

the use of IVMP to treat acute relapses [10,11]. Several small studies have followed patients over 1 year after a course of IVMP and reported improved outcomes in the patients treated with IVMP compared to either placebo or low-dose corticosteroids [12–14].

The optimal dose and route of administration for corticosteroids are not clearly defined. Doses ranging from 500 to 2,000 mg/day (IV or oral) for 3 to 5 days have been found to hasten recovery from MS relapses, whereas a single infusion of high-dose corticosteroid was found to be minimally effective (Table 12.4). Doses of 500 to 2,000 mg/day (IV or oral) for 3 to 5 days are appropriate for the treatment of MS relapses. Low or moderate doses of oral corticosteroids are used by some clinicians, particularly for mild relapses. The Optic Neuritis Treatment Trial suggested that low-dose corticosteroids were associated with an increased rate of recurrent optic neuritis, compared with placebo [14]. However, this was not a primary end point for the study and has not been confirmed in other trials. Conventional doses of oral corticosteroids, such as the regimen studied by Barnes et al. [17], cannot be currently recommended, although further studies of oral corticosteroids would help clarify the issue. Accordingly, high-dose corticosteroids are generally preferred wherever possible. Oral administration of high doses of corticosteroids is a reasonable administration option for patients in whom intravenous administration is not possible.

IV corticosteroids can speed up recovery from MS relapses.

Side effects from corticosteroids are common, but typically mild (Table 12.5). Many of the common side effects of corticosteroids can be managed with proper education and over-the-counter medications, when needed (Table 12.6). A common side effect is a feeling of well-being or mild

TABLE 12.4
Clinical Trials Comparing Different Types or Doses of Corticosteroids for MS Relapses

STUDY	TREATMENT REGIMENS	N	OUTCOME
Bindoff et al. [18]	IV MP 1,000 mg/day for 1 day IV MP 1,000 mg/day for 5 days	32	Improved disability in the 5-day-treated group
Alam et al. [19]	IV MP 500 mg/day for 5 days Oral MP 500 mg/day for 5 days	35	No difference between groups over 1 month
La Mantia et al. [13]	IV MP 100 mg/day, tapering off over 14 days versus IV MP 40 mg/day, tapering over 14 days versus IV dexamethasone 8 mg/day, tapering over 14 days	31	High rate of worsening in low-dose MP group after treatment
Barnes et al. [17]	IV MP 1,000 mg/day for 3 days, versus Oral MP 48 mg/day, tapering over 21 days	80	No significant difference in disability over 24 weeks
Oliveri et al. [20]	IV MP 2,000 mg/day for 5 days, versus IV MP 500 mg/day for 5 days	29	No significant difference in disability over 2 months, but lower MRI activity in high-dose group
Martinelli et al. [21]	IV MP 1,000 mg/day for 5 days, versus Oral MP 1,000 mg/day for 5 days	40	No significant difference in reduction in gadolinium-enhancing lesions

IV, intravenous; MP, methylprednisolone.

TABLE 12.5
Side Effects of Corticosteroids

Common side effects associated with a course of corticosteroids

Metallic taste
Insomnia
Dysphoria
Anxiety
Increased appetite
Edema
Headache
Myalgia
Easy bruising
Acne
Gastrointestinal distress/heartburn
Flushing
Palpitations

Uncommon but important adverse effects associated with a course of corticosteroids include:

Anaphylaxis
Osteonecrosis/aseptic necrosis
Psychosis
Euphoria or depression
Exacerbation of preexisting peptic ulcer disease, diabetes mellitus, hypertension, affective disorders
Cataract formation

TABLE 12.6
Key Information for Patients and Families for Clinical Relapse Management

− Clinical relapses are new or worsening neurological symptoms that persist for more than a day or two, and that are not due to infection or fever.

− It is not always easy to differentiate symptoms of an MS relapse from other symptoms. Communicating with your care provider can help recognize what is an MS relapse and what is not.

− Clinical relapses usually are treated with corticosteroids to shorten symptom duration and help improve recovery of inflamed tissue.

− Corticosteroids are typically well tolerated, but can cause some side effects, including:

 − metallic taste
 − irritability
 − insomnia
 − weight gain.

− Rarely, corticosteroids can cause more significant psychiatric symptoms.

− Repeated or long-term corticosteroid use can cause thinning of the bones (osteoporosis), but a short-term course like that used for an MS relapse is not thought to have significant impact on bone health. Rarely, corticosteroids will cause permanent injury to the hip or shoulder joint (aseptic necrosis).

− Most relapse symptoms recover over several weeks to months, but some symptoms can persist long term. Long-term symptoms can often be managed with targeted treatments.

euphoria, which typically is welcomed by patients. Anxiety and irritability, especially in newly diagnosed MS patients, is common and should be treated with reassurance and a short-acting anxiolytic medication, if needed. Insomnia is frequent and can be managed with a short-acting sedative-hypnotic. Patients should be warned about increased appetite. It is often useful for patients to receive their first dose of IVMP under outpatient medical supervision. This supervision helps with medication education, as well as monitoring and management of side effects. Mania and psychosis are rare and, when seen, can be managed with phenothiazines, antipsychotics, or lithium carbonate [22]. Allergic reactions are typically against the preservative, and using preservative-free IVMP preparations can reduce this reaction. Anaphylactoid reactions are rare and thought to be related to IgE response to the succinate portion of methylprednisolone [23]. Sensitization protocols are available for those with severe allergic reactions to preservative-free IVMP but require admission to an intensive care monitoring unit for each treatment.

Symptomatic Therapy. Occasionally, targeted management of relapse symptoms is needed (Table 12.7). This management can include physical or occupational therapy for gait or arm dysfunction, urinary catheter for acute urinary retention, short-term analgesics for pain, antiemetics and phenothiazines for vertigo, antiepileptics for tonic spasms, and eye patch for diplopia. Patient education is an important component of MS relapse management, both regarding MS relapses in general (Table 12.6) as well as management of corticosteroid side effects. Admission for relapses is usually limited to those patients unable to recover at home because of mobility or other functional issues.

Recovery from a clinical relapse usually starts within a couple days of corticosteroid initiation and continues for many months. When relapses do not respond sufficiently to corticosteroid treatment, plasma exchange or immune globulin can be considered, although neither of these are FDA-approved treatments.

A clinical relapse indicates ongoing MS inflammation, which in turn indicates that the current long-term disease-modifying therapy may be insufficient to control the disease. Early in the treatment course of a disease-modifying therapy (ie, less than 6 months), a clinical relapse may be tolerated as the therapy is becoming effective. If a clinical relapse occurs after 6 months on a long-term disease modifying therapy (and perhaps earlier with a highly-effective therapy, such as natalizumab), it may be appropriate to consider changing long-term disease-modifying therapy.

SPECIAL CONSIDERATIONS

Neuromyelitis optica. Neuromyelitis optica (NMO) is a related neuroinflammatory disorder secondary to a specific

TABLE 12.7

Symptomatic Therapy to Consider as Adjunctive Treatment With Corticosteroids

SYMPTOM	TREATMENT
Gait or arm dysfunction	Physical and/or occupational therapy
Urinary retention	Urinary catheter, urology evaluation
Pain	Short-term analgesic
Vertigo	Antiemetic, phenothiazine
Tonic spasm	Antiepileptic medications
Diplopia	Eye patch

autoantibody with the same name NMO. Pathology shows marked tissue injury and necrosis. Patients with NMO often have an incomplete response to corticosteroids and recurrent relapse as early as several weeks or months later. Initial treatment for an NMO relapse is similar to that of MS, but with a longer corticosteroid taper (typically several months) and different long-term treatments (see Chapter 37). Incomplete recovery from an NMO relapse is common. When corticosteroids are not sufficiently effective, plasmapheresis is sometimes used to improve recovery. Treatment for NMO relapses should probably begin as soon as possible after onset given the amount of tissue injury and necrosis associated with NMO relapses. There is therefore a higher urgency to begin treatments for relapses in NMO than in MS.

> NMO relapses are managed somewhat differently and more urgently than MS relapses.

MRI Relapse. By definition, clinical relapses are clinical manifestations of acute MS inflammation. However, active inflammation is sometimes observed as multiple gadolinium-enhancing lesions on MRI in patients without any symptoms. The severe tissue injury observed in pathological studies of active inflammation suggest that this MRI relapse may benefit from a course of corticosteroids, although no studies have formally evaluated this potential benefit.

ACKNOWLEDGMENT

Supported by RG 4103A4/2 from the National Multiple Sclerosis Society (USA).

PATIENT CASE

A 36-year-old woman with a 3 year history of known MS calls reporting 5 days of gradually progressive paresthesia in her left leg—starting first in her toes, and now up to her waist. She has never had these symptoms before.

Question: What evaluation is needed? What management do you recommend?

Answer: The clinical picture is most consistent with a partial myelitis secondary to an MS relapse. After asking her about potential infections, no further evaluation is typically needed. It is reasonable to treat her at this point with a course of high-dose corticosteroids (eg, 3 days of 1 g/day IVMP, followed by a 12 day prednisone taper). Information about the side effects of corticosteroids and expectation of treatment response should be reviewed with her.

She calls during the last few days of the prednisone taper and reports that although sensory symptoms improved for a few days immediately after IV corticosteroids, they now have returned and have progressed to involve her left hand and arm to the shoulder.

Question: What do you do now?

Answer: This still appears most consistent with an MS relapse, despite not responding to a course of high-dose corticosteroids. At this point, it is important to exclude infection, so a urinalysis would be appropriate, even without urinary symptoms. A repeat course of high-dose corticosteroids is indicated (eg, 5 days of 1 g/day IVMP, followed by a 12 day prednisone taper). It would also be appropriate to schedule a follow-up in about 2 to 3 weeks with MRI of the cervical spine (likely location of the symptomatic lesion), and imaging here will evaluate both for active inflammation and alternative etiologies, such as compressive disc disease. Brain MRI would also be helpful as a broad-based assessment of ongoing inflammation. At the follow-up visit, consideration should include whether her current disease-modifying therapy is sufficiently effective in controlling active inflammation.

KEY POINTS FOR PATIENTS AND FAMILIES FOR CORTICOSTEROID TREATMENT

- Limit concentrated sugars (to lessen the risk of hyperglycemia), limit salt (to decrease fluid retention), and encourage foods rich in potassium (to avoid hypokalemia).
- To help prevent gastritis, an acid blocker (eg, ranitidine) may be helpful.
- Insomnia typically responds to short-acting hypnotic at bedtime.
- In patients with known hypertension, blood pressure should be monitored by the infusion nurse.
- In patients with known diabetes mellitus or past history of corticosteroid-associated hyperglycemia, blood sugar should be monitored closely. Involvement of the patient's primary care provider can be helpful.
- Irritability is common, although typically only needs patient counseling.
- Severe affective side effects (eg, psychosis) are rare, but may respond to antipsychotic medication such as lithium.

REFERENCES

1. Lublin FD, Baier M, Cutter G. Effect of relapses on development of residual deficit in multiple sclerosis. *Neurology.* 2003;61:1528–1532.

2. Trapp BD, Peterson J, Ransohoff RM, et al. Axonal transection in the lesions of multiple sclerosis. *N Eng J Med.* 1998;338:278–285.

3. Glaser GH, Merritt HH. Effects of ACTH and cortisone in multiple sclerosis. *Trans Am Neurol Assoc.* 1951;56:130–133.

4. Rose AS, Namerow NS, Kuzma JW, et al. Cooperative study in the evaluation of therapy in multiple sclerosis. ACTH vs. placebo-final report. *Neurology.* 1970;20:1–59.

5. Dowling PC, Bosch VV, Cook SD. Possible beneficial effect of high-dose intravenous steroid therapy in acute demyelinating disease and transverse myelitis. *Neurology.* 1980;30(7 Pt 2):33–36.

6. Buckley C, Kennard C, Swash M. Treatment of acute exacerbations of multiple sclerosis with intravenous methylprednisolone. *J Neurol Neurosurg Psychiatry.* 1982;45(2):179–180.

7. Abbruzzese G, Gandolfo C, Loeb C. "Bolus" methylprednisolone versus ACTH in the treatment of multiple sclerosis. *Ital J Neurol Sci.* 1983;4:169–172.

8. Barnes MP, Bateman DE, Cleland PG, et al. Intravenous methylprednisolone for multiple sclerosis in relapse. *J Neurol Neurosurg Psychiatry.* 1985;48:157–159.

9. Thompson AJ, Kennard C, Swash M, et al. Relative efficacy of intravenous methylprednisolone and ACTH in the treatment of acute relapse in MS. *Neurology.* 1989;39:969–971.

10. Miller DM, Weinstock-Guttman B, Bâethoux F, et al. A meta-analysis of methylprednisolone in recovery from multiple sclerosis exacerbations. *Mult Scler.* 2000;6(4):267–273.

11. Filippini G, Brusaferri F, Sibley W, et al. Corticosteroids or ACTH for acute exacerbations in multiple sclerosis. *Cochrane Database Syst Rev.* 2000;(4):CD001331.

12. Sellebjerg F, Frederiksen JL, Nielsen PM, Olesen J. Double-blind, randomized, placebo-controlled study of oral, high-dose methylprednisolone in attacks of MS. *Neurology.* 1998;51: 529–534.

13. La Mantia L, Eoli M, Milanese C, et al. Double-blind trial of dexamethasone versus methylprednisolone in multiple sclerosis acute relapses. *Eur Neurol.* 1994;34(4):199–203.

14. Beck RW, Cleary PA, Anderson MM, et al. A randomized, controlled trial of corticosteroids in the treatment of acute optic neuritis. *N Engl J Med.* 1992;326:581–588.

15. Durelli L, Cocito D, Riccio A, et al. High-dose intravenous methylprednisolone in the treatment of multiple sclerosis: Clinical-immunologic correlations. *Neurology.* 1986;36:238–243.

16. Milligan NM, Newcombe R, Compston DAS. A double-blind controlled trial of high dose methylprednisolone in patients with multiple sclerosis: 1. clinical effects. *J Neurol Neurosurg Psychiatry.* 1987;50:511–516.

17. Barnes D, Hughes RA, Morris RW, et al. Randomised trial of oral and intravenous methylprednisolone in acute relapses of multiple sclerosis. *Lancet.* 1997;349(9056):902–906.

18. Bindoff L, Lyons PR, Newman PK, Saunders M. Methylprednisolone in multiple sclerosis: A comparative dose study. *J Neurol Neurosurg Psychiatry.* 1988;51(8):1108–1109.

19. Alam SM, Kyriakides T, Lawden M, Newman PK. Methylprednisolone in multiple sclerosis: A comparison of oral with intravenous therapy at equivalent high dose. *J Neurol Neurosurg Psychiatry.* 1993;56:1219–1220.

20. Oliveri RL, Valentino P, Russo C, et al. Randomized trial comparing two different doses of methylprednisolone in MS. A clinical and MRI study. *Neurology.* 1998;50:1833–1836.

21. Martinelli V, Rocca MA, Annovazzi P, et al. A short-term randomized MRI study of high-dose oral vs intravenous methylprednisolone in MS. *Neurology.* 2009;73:1842–1848.

22. Falk WE, Mahnke MW, Poskanzer DC. Lithium prophylaxis of corticotropin-induced psychosis. *JAMA.* 1979;241:1011–1012.

23. Burgdorff T, Venemalm L, Vogt T, et al. IgE-mediated anaphylactic reaction induced by succinate ester of methylprednisolone. *Ann Allergy Asthma Immunol.* 2002;89(4):425–428.

13

Disease-Modifying Therapies in Relapsing Multiple Sclerosis

JIWON OH
PETER A. CALABRESI

KEY POINTS FOR CLINICIANS

- There are currently 9 FDA-approved disease-modifying treatments for relapsing-remitting multiple sclerosis: interferon beta-1a (Avonex and Rebif), interferon beta-1b (Betaseron and Extavia), glatiramer acetate (Copaxone), natalizumab (Tysabri), fingolimod (Gilenya), teriflunomide (Aubagio), and mitoxantrone (Novantrone).

- Glatiramer acetate and the interferon beta class of drugs are considered first-line agents for the treatment of relapsing multiple sclerosis, largely based on their benign side-effect profiles. Natalizumab, fingolimod, and mitoxantrone are efficacious agents in reducing disease activity in multiple sclerosis, but carry the risk of rare but potentially serious adverse effects.

- Patients considering treatment with natalizumab can be stratified for their risk of developing progressive multifocal leukoencephalopathy based on the presence or absence of known risk factors which include: serum JC virus antibody status, prior history of immunosuppression, and duration of treatment with natalizumab.

- The adverse-effect profile of fingolimod is evolving with postmarketing surveillance. The most concerning adverse effects associated with fingolimod are cardiac events, severe or fatal infections, and macular edema. Patients considering fingolimod need to be screened for the presence of factors that put them at an increased risk for adverse cardiac events, and should be counseled and monitored appropriately.

- The use of mitoxantrone is limited by concerns of serious adverse effects, including cardiac ventricular dysfunction and therapy-related acute leukemia.

Over the past 2 decades, the available treatment armamentarium for relapsing-remitting multiple sclerosis (RRMS) has been continuously expanding. Choosing a specific disease-modifying therapy (DMT) can be challenging for both patients and clinicians, and it is a decision that requires consideration of a variety of factors, including disease characteristics, personal preference, and tolerability.

At present, there are 9 FDA-approved treatments for RRMS. This chapter summarizes the currently available treatment options for RRMS, with a brief description of each agent and its proposed mechanism of action, indications for use, adverse effects, patient selection, pretesting/interval monitoring recommendations, and a brief discussion of when to discontinue or change

At present, there are 9 FDA-approved treatments for RRMS.

DMTs. A few patient cases are presented at the end of this chapter for illustrative purposes.

Dimethyl fumarate (otherwise known as BG-12, trade name TECFIDERA) and teriflunomide (Aubagio) received FDA approval after the preparation of this chapter. Please see Chapter 16 on emerging therapies for a full discussion of this medication.

DESCRIPTION OF AVAILABLE DMTs IN RRMS

Glatiramer Acetate

Glatiramer acetate (Copaxone) (GA) was originally developed to simulate the encephalitogenic properties of myelin basic protein. Surprisingly, when used in the laboratory, GA was found to demonstrate beneficial effects in animal models of MS, thus was further developed for clinical trial testing in humans. GA is comprised of a mixture of synthetic polypeptides derived from 4 amino acids, including L-alanine, L-glutamic acid, L-lysine, and L-tyrosine [1]. The precise mechanism of action of this drug is unclear, but is likely multifactorial. Experimental evidence suggests that GA induces CD4+ T cells to preferentially differentiate into Th2 cells, which promotes an anti-inflammatory state. In addition, GA is known to interact with both regulatory T cells, CD8+ T cells, and antigen presenting cells (including dendritic cells and monocytes). These interactions produce an overall shift in the immune cytokine profile from a Th1 state, which is thought to be more proinflammatory, to a Th2 state, which is thought to be more anti-inflammatory, resulting in its observed beneficial effects. Finally, there is evidence that suggests that GA may have direct neuroprotective effects through an upregulation of neurotrophic factors [2].

GA is typically administered at a dose of 20 mg subcutaneously daily.

Interferon Beta

Four formulations of the interferon beta (IFN beta) class of drugs have been FDA-approved for use in the treatment of RRMS: IFN beta-1a (Avonex and Rebif) and IFN beta-1b (Betaseron and Extavia). IFN beta-1a is a recombinant peptide produced in Chinese hamster ovary cells, while IFN beta-1b is a recombinant peptide produced in E. coli bacteria. Of note, Betaseron and Extavia are identical medications that are even produced in the same facility, but branded differently by 2 independent pharmaceutical companies.

The mechanism by which the IFN beta class of drugs acts to reduce MS-related disease activity is incompletely understood, but likely acts on multiple cellular functional levels. IFN beta agents bind to the type I IFN receptor, modifying the expression of a spectrum of proteins, including: increases in the expression and concentration of anti-inflammatory (Th2) cytokines (IL-10 and IL-4, among others) and decreases in the expression of proinflammatory (Th1 and Th17) cytokines (IFN gamma, osteopontin, IL-17, and tumor necrosis factor [TNF] alpha, among others). In addition, the IFN beta drugs reduce cellular trafficking of inflammatory cells across the blood–brain barrier by modulating very late antigen (VLA)-4, soluble vascular cell adhesion molecule (sVCAM), and matrix metalloproteases [3,4].

The dosing and route of administration of the IFN beta drugs depends on the specific formulation. One formulation of IFN beta-1a (Avonex) is administered at 30 mcg intramuscularly once weekly, while another formulation (Rebif) is administered at either 22 mcg or 44 mcg subcutaneously, 3 times weekly. Of note, of the 2 doses of Rebif, only the higher dose (44 mcg 3 times weekly) is approved for use in RRMS by the FDA. Avonex is typically titrated over 3 weeks, while Rebif is titrated over 4 weeks to reach the target dose. IFN beta-1b (Betaseron and Extavia) is administered at 0.25 mg (8 million international units) every other day, subcutaneously. Both Betaseron and Extavia are also titrated to achieve the target dose, typically over 6 weeks. All forms are now available using an autoinjection system.

Natalizumab

Natalizumab (Tysabri) is a humanized monoclonal antibody (Ab) that is classified as a selective adhesion molecule inhibitor, developed for use in Crohn's disease and MS. Natalizumab is directed against the alpha4 subunit of the alpha4beta1 integrin dimer, which is a cell surface adhesion molecule present on most leukocytes. Integrins play an important role in immune cell adhesion and migration across endothelial surfaces [5]. In MS, natalizumab is thought to exert its beneficial effects by blocking the alpha4 integrin, thereby preventing autoreactive T cells from crossing the blood–brain barrier, inhibiting one of the primary steps in MS pathogenesis. In addition, natalizumab plays a role in regulating immune cell activation in inflammatory tissue, which may also contribute to its beneficial clinical effects [6,7].

Natalizumab is administered at a dose of 300 mg intravenously every 4 weeks.

Fingolimod

Fingolimod (FTY720, Gilenya) is an oral medication that was developed for use in MS and organ transplant. Fingolimod acts in MS by binding with the sphingosine-1-phosphate (S1P) receptor on lymphocytes causing downregulation of the S1P receptor, thereby preventing egress of lymphocytes from lymph nodes. This results in a diminution of peripherally circulating lymphocytes. This ultimately prevents autoaggressive lymphocytes from crossing the blood–brain barrier, thus inhibiting one of the primary steps in MS pathogenesis. There is also evidence that fingolimod may have neuroprotective effects by modulating S1P receptors on glial and neural cells [8–13].

Fingolimod is typically administered at a dose of 0.5 mg orally daily.

Mitoxantrone

Mitoxantrone (Novantrone) is a cytotoxic drug, originally developed for use as an antineoplastic agent. Classified as an anthracenedione compound, mitoxantrone acts by inhibiting DNA topoisomerase and causing DNA intercalation, which results in disruptions in DNA synthesis and repair. In MS, mitoxantrone's clinical effects are thought to be mediated by T-cell modulation and suppression of humoral immunity [14].

Mitoxantrone is typically administered at 12 mg/m² intravenously every 3 months. The maximum lifetime dose is 140 mg/m² because of the risk of lymphoproliferative disorders (including therapy-related acute leukemia [TRAL]) and cardiac toxicity. A "black box" warning regarding cardiotoxicity in the U.S. package insert recommends assessment of left ventricular ejection fraction before each dose.

Table 13.1 provides a summary of clinically relevant information of each of the DMTs discussed.

INDICATIONS FOR USE

At present, GA and the IFN beta class of drugs are considered "first-line" agents for the treatment of patients with RRMS, largely based on their benign adverse-effect profiles. In regard to treatment efficacy, these agents have fairly similar effects on diminishing relapse rate (approximately 30%), reducing MRI evidence of disease activity (percentage reduction varies depending on MRI measure), and on disability progression (12%–37% diminished risk of sustained disability progression over 2–3 years) [15–23]. Evidence from unblinded or single-blinded head-to-head clinical trials suggest that the high-dose formulations of the IFN beta agents (Rebif and Betaseron) are more efficacious than the low-dose formulation (Avonex) with respect to clinical and MRI evidence of disease activity [24,25]. On the other hand, unblinded head-to-head clinical trials comparing GA to the high-dose formulations of IFN beta agents (Rebif and Betaseron) have demonstrated that the clinical efficacy of GA is similar to these agents [26,27]. The Therapeutics and Technology Assessment Subcommittee of the American Academy of Neurology (TTA-AAN) has concluded that IFN beta demonstrates established evidence (Level A) of diminishing relapse rate in RRMS, and probable evidence (Level B) of producing a beneficial effect on MRI measures of disease severity, and

on disease progression [28]. Similarly, the AAN has concluded that GA shows established evidence (Level A) of diminishing relapse rate in RRMS, and possible evidence (Level C) of a beneficial effect on MRI measures of disease severity, and slowing disability progression [28]. The *Cochrane Review* concluded that the IFN beta drugs had modest efficacy in reducing relapse rate and disease progression in RRMS [29]. With GA, however, the *Cochrane Review* concluded partial efficacy in RRMS in terms of relapse-related clinical outcomes, without any significant effect on sustained disability [30].

Overall, although the efficacy of these agents in reducing MS-related disease activity is moderate, they are considered first-line agents because of their superior adverse-effect profiles in comparison to the other available agents. Common adverse effects associated with these agents (subsequently outlined in more detail) are mild in severity, and they require only infrequent laboratory monitoring. The choice between first-line agents is often a matter of personal preference with regard to dosing frequency, route of administration, side-effect profile, and requirements for laboratory monitoring, which are outlined in detail in other sections of this chapter.

Other agents used in the treatment of RRMS have shown efficacy in reducing MS-related disease activity, with some agents showing evidence of greater efficacy in reducing MS-related disease activity in comparison to first-line agents. Natalizumab has been shown to reduce relapse rate by 68%, markedly reduce MRI evidence of disease activity (percentage reduction varies by specific MRI measure), and decrease disability progression at 2 years by 42% in comparison to placebo [31]. The TTA-AAN has concluded that natalizumab shows established evidence (Level A) in reducing clinical and radiographic evidence of disease activity in MS [32], and the *Cochrane Review* similarly concludes that natalizumab shows robust evidence in decreasing relapse rate and disability [33]. Natalizumab likely has greater efficacy in reducing MS-related disease activity in comparison to first-line agents. However, at present, in the absence of a head-to-head clinical trial, it is difficult to definitively conclude if this is the case.

More recently, fingolimod has been shown to reduce relapse rate by 54% and disability progression by 30% in comparison to placebo, with MRI measures of disease activity supporting these clinical findings [8]. In a head-to-head trial against IFN beta-1a weekly therapy, fingolimod showed a greater reduction in relapse rate (approximately 30%) and a concomitant reduction of MRI measures of disease activity, but no difference in disease progression [34].

> Natalizumab, fingolimod, and mitoxantrone are efficacious agents in the treatment of RRMS, but are considered second-line primarily owing to the potential for rare, but serious side effects.

> GA and the IFN beta class of drugs are considered "first-line" agents for treatment of patients with RRMS, based on their benign adverse-effect profiles.

Finally, mitoxantrone has been shown to diminish a composite of relapse rate and disability progression in

TABLE 13.1
Summary of Current FDA-Approved DMTs in RRMS*

GENERIC DRUG (TRADE NAME)	DOSING	MECHANISM OF ACTION	ADVERSE EFFECTS	LABORATORY MONITORING	PREGNANCY RISK CATEGORY
Glatiramer acetate (Copaxone)	20 mg SC daily	Promotes Th2 cell differentiation Interacts with T cells and APCs to promote Th2 state Upregulation of neurotrophic factors	Injection site reactions Postinjection reaction	None required	B
Interferon beta-1a (Avonex) (Rebif)	30 mcg IM weekly 44 mcg SC 3 times weekly	Promotes shift from Th1 to Th2 state Reduces cellular trafficking of inflammatory cells across BBB	Injection site reactions Flu-like reactions Hematological abnormalities Elevated liver enzymes Exacerbation in preexisting thyroid disease	Baseline CBC, LFTs CBC, LFTs at 1, 3, and 6 months after treatment initiation Periodic CBC, LFTs thereafter (typically twice annually) Baseline thyroid function in patients with preexisting thyroid disease, then periodically with clinical symptoms	C
Interferon beta-1b (Betaseron) (Extavia)	0.25 mg SC every other day 0.25 mg SC every other day				
Natalizumab (Tysabri)	300 mg IV monthly	Blocks alpha4 integrin on leukocytes, preventing migration of inflammatory T cells across BBB	Hypersensitivity reactions PML (overall risk of about 1:500)	Prior to initiation: Serum JCV-Ab, MRI-brain with contrast, baseline CBC, LFTs In all patients: Annual (or more frequent) MRI-brain with contrast Clinical assessment every 6 months Periodic CBC, LFTs as needed Consider anti-natalizumab antibody assessment if evidence of diminished clinical efficacy of natalizumab or hypersensitivity reaction In JCV-Ab negative patients: serum JCV-Ab annually In JCV-Ab positive patients: CSF JCV PCR with new MRI lesions	C
Fingolimod (Gilenya)	0.5 mg po daily	Binds S1P receptor on autoaggressive lymphocytes preventing egress from lymph nodes	Bradycardia, atrioventricular conduction slowing (prolonged QT$_c$) Macular edema Herpes virus infections Hypertension Elevated liver enzymes	Baseline LFTs, renal function, VZV serology (consider immunization if no evidence of prior immunity) Baseline ECG, further cardiac assessment if necessary Baseline ophthalmological assessment, and reassessment at 3 to 4 months, then with clinical symptoms Periodic CBC, LFTs as needed	C
Mitoxantrone (Novantrone)	12 mg/m² IV every 3 months, maximum cumulative lifetime dose of 140 mg/m²	Inhibits topoisomerase, causes DNA intercalation resulting in disruptions in DNA synthesis and repair	Cardiac ventricular dysfunction, congestive heart failure Leukemia	Baseline CBC, LFTs, LVEF CBC, LFTs, and LVEF prior to each dose Assess LVEF pre/post dose when more than 100 mg/m² Assess LVEF annually even after mitoxantrone discontinuation	D

*In women of child-bearing age, a pregnancy test is suggested prior to initiation of any of these treatments.
APC, antigen presenting cells; BBB, blood–brain barrier; CBC, complete blood count; CSF, cerebrospinal fluid; IM, intramuscular; IV, intravenous; JCV Ab, JC virus antibody; LFT, liver function tests; LVEF, left ventricular ejection fraction; PCR, polymerase chain reaction; po, by mouth; QT$_c$, corrected QT; S1P, sphingosine-1-phosphate; SC, subcutaneous; VZV, varicella zoster virus.

comparison to placebo [35]. The TTA-AAN concluded that there is probable evidence (Level B) that mitoxantrone reduces relapse rate in RRMS [36]. Similarly, the *Cochrane Review* has concluded that there is moderate evidence that mitoxantrone reduces relapse rate and disease progression in MS, but advises that this agent should be reserved for treatment-refractory patients because of the concern for long-term side effects [37].

Natalizumab, fingolimod, and mitoxantrone are considered second-line agents in the treatment of RRMS, primarily owing to the potential for rare, but serious side effects. In general, if a patient has demonstrated significant breakthrough disease on first-line therapies, or alternatively, is unable to tolerate adverse effects related to first-line therapy, these second-line agents should be considered for use. In some exceptional circumstances where patients have extremely aggressive disease, or in circumstances precluding the use of a first-line agent (needle phobia), second-line agents could be considered prior to the use of a first-line agent. However, this practice should be undertaken only after a frank discussion of risks and benefits with the patient.

Table 13.2 summarizes the pivotal placebo-controlled clinical trials for FDA-approved DMTs in RRMS.

Common and Uncommon Side Effects

Glatiramer Acetate
Adverse effects attributable to GA are generally mild in severity. Injection site skin reactions are common and typically manifest with erythema, pain, and can be seen in 60% to 80% of patients. These skin reactions are usually mild and transient, and rarely result in skin necrosis. With chronic use, lipodystrophy can occur at injection sites [3].

> Adverse effects attributable to GA are generally mild in severity and consist of injection site reactions and an immediate postinjection systemic reaction.

In approximately 10% to 15% of patients, an immediate postinjection systemic reaction can occur, with onset typically within seconds to minutes of injection with GA. Symptoms can include tachycardia, palpitations, chest tightness, shortness of breath, anxiety, and flushing. These symptoms usually last for a total duration of 10 to 20 minutes. This reaction is self-limited, and does not result in any permanent adverse effects, nor does it portend any adverse consequences from a cardiovascular standpoint [3,39].

No adverse effects with GA have been reported with other organ systems, making one of the greatest benefits of GA therapy the lack of a need for periodic monitoring of laboratory markers. There are no known drug interactions with GA therapy, and no evidence of neutralizing antibodies with this medication [40].

IFN Beta
Adverse effects associated with the IFN beta class of drugs are generally mild. The most common adverse effects include injection-site skin reactions (with subcutaneous preparations mostly), flu-like symptoms, and transient laboratory evidence of hepatic or hematological abnormalities [3].

TABLE 13.2
Summary of Results of Pivotal Placebo-Controlled Clinical Trials for FDA-Approved DMTs in RRMS

DRUG	RELATIVE EFFECT ON RELAPSE RATE	RELATIVE EFFECT ON DISABILITY	RELATIVE EFFECT ON MRI MEASURES (NEW T2 LESIONS, GD+ LESIONS, BURDEN OF DISEASE)
IFN beta-1a 30 mcg IM qweekly [15,16]	18% decrease	37% decrease	4% to 42% decrease*
IFN beta-1a 44 mcg SC TIW [17,23]	32% decrease	30% decrease	15% to 88% decrease*
IFN beta-1b 0.25 mg SC qOD [18–20]	34% decrease	29% NS decrease	17–83% decrease*
GA 20 mg SC qdaily [21,22]	29% decrease	12% (NS) decrease	8% to 38% decrease*
MITO 12 mg/m² IV q3monthly [35,38]	42% decrease	75% decrease	79% decrease*
Natalizumab 300 mg IV qmonthly [31]	68% decrease	42% decrease	18% to 92% decrease*
Fingolimod 0.5 mg po qdaily [8]	54% decrease	30% decrease	23% to 40% decrease**

Adapted from [32].
*Calculated using difference in median % change between treated and placebo group.
**Calculated using difference in mean % change between treated, placebo group.
GA, glatiramer acetate; IM, intramuscular; NS, non-significant; po, by mouth; qOD, every other day; SC, subcutaneous; TIW, three times weekly.

Skin reactions are common with the IFN beta drugs, and occur in over 60% of patients [18,20,41]. These reactions are typically mild to moderate in severity, but somewhat more severe than that seen with GA, with up to 5% of cases resulting in skin necrosis [18,20,41]. Symptoms of injection-site skin reactions can include erythema, pain, bruising, infection, atrophy, and necrosis. Skin reactions that are mild to moderate in severity do not necessitate discontinuation of IFN beta; however, with more severe reactions such as skin necrosis or infections, the medication may need to be discontinued. Route of administration and injection site can affect the severity of skin reactions, with intramuscular dosing and buttock injections typically causing milder skin reactions. In addition, assistive devices or methods such as autoinjectors or changing needles after the drug has been drawn into the syringe can also improve the severity and frequency of skin reactions [42–44].

Flu-like symptoms, which include fever, myalgias, arthralgias, headache, fatigue, and malaise, occur in up to 75% of patients on IFN beta agents. These symptoms typically begin within hours of injection, and resolve within 24 hours. Most patients experience flu-like symptoms immediately upon initiating IFN beta therapy, with subsequent resolution over the next 3 months. To minimize the effect of flu-like symptoms, strategies such as a gradual dose escalation with treatment initiation and dosing at bedtime can be utilized. Administration of medications such as acetaminophen or nonsteroidal anti-inflammatory drugs, especially naproxen sodium, before and after medication injection can substantially alleviate the flu-like symptoms. For those that do not respond to over-the-counter medications, low-dose prednisone may be considered, but this should only be used within the first 3 months of medication initiation.

> Adverse effects of the IFN beta class of drugs are generally mild and include injection-site skin reactions, flu-like symptoms, and transient laboratory evidence of hepatic or hematological abnormalities.

Pentoxyfilline has also been used during the first 6 months of medication initiation. Where flu-like reactions persist, regular dosing with acetaminophen or nonsteroidal anti-inflammatory drugs (NSAIDs) with IFN beta injections may be necessary [44].

Hematological laboratory abnormalities can transiently be seen in patients on IFN beta therapy, and most commonly consist of leukopenia, although anemia and thrombocytopenia have also been reported. Typically, these abnormalities are asymptomatic and resolve within 6 months of medication initiation. Table 13.1 outlines a recommended laboratory monitoring schedule. Should hematological toxicity exist (leukocytes less than $3.0 \times 10^9/L$, granulocytes less than $1.5 \times 10^9/L$, lymphocytes less than $1.0 \times 10^9/L$, hemoglobin less than 10 g/dL, platelets less than $75 \times 10^9/L$), the dose of IFN beta should be reduced and laboratory values reassessed. If hematological toxicity

persists, IFN beta should be discontinued. Experience from the pivotal IFN beta clinical trials and postmarketing surveillance show that only 0.3% of patients on IFN beta therapy require medication discontinuation because of severe hematological toxicity [44–46].

An asymptomatic elevation in hepatic laboratory markers can also be seen in patients, typically within the first year of IFN beta therapy. Most commonly, hepatic transaminases are elevated. These abnormalities are usually asymptomatic and resolve within 6 months of medication initiation. Table 13.1 outlines a recommended laboratory monitoring schedule. Should severe hepatic toxicity persist (elevations that exceed 3 times the upper limit of normal), a dose reduction or medication discontinuation should be pursued. Postmarketing surveillance shows that only 0.4% of patients on IFN beta agents experience serious liver toxicity [44,45,47,48].

An exacerbation in thyroid function in patients with preexisting thyroid disease has been described with IFN beta therapy. The current recommendation is to assess thyroid function prior to initiation of IFN beta therapy, and with any clinical evidence of thyroid dysfunction thereafter [49,50].

The link between depression and IFN beta therapy is unclear, thus the presence of depression is not a contraindication for initiation of IFN beta therapy. However, both clinician and patient awareness of this issue is important, and should depressive symptoms become intractable or severe, another DMT should be considered [51–54].

Natalizumab

In general, natalizumab is a well-tolerated agent. Uncommon adverse effects associated with natalizumab include infusion reactions, hypersensitivity reactions, headache, infections, anxiety, sinus congestion, peripheral edema, among others [31,55].

> Natalizumab is generally a well-tolerated agent, but the most concerning serious adverse effect is PML, which occurs at an overall incidence of 2.1 per 1,000.

Infusion reactions typically manifest with symptoms of headache, dizziness, and nausea, and are not a reason to discontinue natalizumab. They are treated conservatively by a combination of measures, including decreasing the infusion rate, or preinfusion treatment with antihistamines, acetaminophen, NSAIDs, or steroids.

Immediate and delayed hypersensitivity reactions can occur in approximately 2% to 9% of patients, with 1% experiencing anaphylactoid reactions [32]. Hypersensitivity reactions occur most commonly during the second infusion [56,57]. Should a hypersensitivity reaction develop, the current recommendation is to discontinue treatment with natalizumab and not to re-treat. However, this recommendation needs further assessment, as selecting those that do not have persistent neutralizing antibodies and pretreating with antihistamines and corticosteroids prior to infusion may allow for the continued safe administration of natalizumab [58].

Treatment with natalizumab also results in a reversible elevation in lymphocytes, monocytes, eosinophils, and basophils, which is in keeping with its known mechanism of action [55].

The most concerning serious adverse effect of natalizumab is progressive multifocal leukoencephalopathy (PML), which occurs at an overall incidence of 2.1 per 1,000. The risk can change substantially from 1:11,000 or less to 1:90 based on the presence of various risk factors. Three identified factors that substantially alter an individual's risk of PML include duration of natalizumab treatment, prior history of immunosuppression, and serum anti-JC virus (JCV) Ab status. Natalizumab treatment duration exceeding 24 months, a prior history of immunosuppressant use, and anti-JCV Ab positivity results in the greatest risk of PML at 1:90 (Figure 13.1) [59–61].

Prior to initiating natalizumab, patients should be tested for the presence of JCV Ab to more accurately understand their risk of PML. In addition, patients should undergo a baseline MRI-brain with gadolinium contrast. Patients on natalizumab who develop any clinical features concerning for PML should immediately undergo an MRI-brain. Cerebrospinal fluid (CSF) studies assessing for the presence of JCV should be pursued if the MRI-brain shows evidence of lesions that raise concern for PML. Current guidelines regarding clinical and MRI surveillance, and JCV Ab testing are further outlined in a subsequent section in this chapter, and in Table 13.1 [59,62].

The availability of postmarketing surveillance safety data and a commercial JCV Ab test allows for improved risk stratification of patients, which will enable more informed clinical decision making with regard to natalizumab use. It is important to keep in mind, however, that decisions regarding treatment should always be made on a case-by-case basis, because a patient's risk tolerance and disease severity are factors that need to be taken into consideration in a discussion of risks and benefits [59,60].

Fingolimod

The adverse-effect profile of fingolimod has been evolving with postmarketing surveillance. In the pivotal clinical trials, the majority of reported adverse effects were mild to moderate (77%–90%), with upper respiratory tract infections, headache, back pain, and diarrhea being among the most commonly reported effects. Serious adverse effects associated with fingolimod include bradycardia and atrioventricular conduction block with treatment initiation, elevated liver enzymes, macular edema, hypertension, and herpes virus infections (including 2 fatal cases), and skin cancer [8,34].

> The adverse effect profile of fingolimod has been evolving with postmarketing surveillance. The most concerning adverse effects include cardiac events, fatal infections, and macular edema.

Specifically, the cardiovascular adverse effects seen seem to reach a nadir within 4 to 5 hours of onset, with symptom resolution in affected patients within 24 hours [8]. Thus, patients receiving their first dose of fingolimod are required to be monitored for 6 hours in an infusion center, and for a total of 24 hours if bradycardia or QT prolongation exists.

However, postmarketing surveillance suggests that the observed cardiovascular effects may manifest for a considerably longer duration (more than 24 hours) after fingolimod initiation. Recently, a variety of risk factors that may put individuals at greater risk for cardiovascular adverse effects with fingolimod have been identified, including concomitant use of medications that affect the heart rate and/or QT interval (including beta-blockers, calcium channel blockers, digoxin, and any drug associated with prolongation of the corrected QT [QT_c]) and preexisting cardiac dysfunction. Contraindications to treatment with fingolimod, and patient factors associated with higher cardiac risk are summarized in Figures 13.2 and 13.3. In

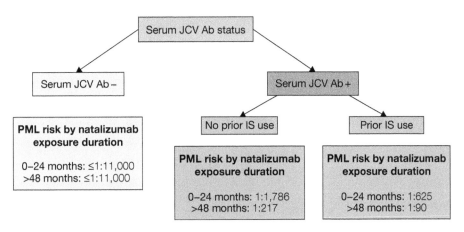

FIGURE 13.1
Incidence of PML stratified by known risk factors. *Source: Modified from [60].*

- Recent history (<6 months) of myocardial infarction (MI), unstable angina, stroke, transient ischemic attack (TIA), decompensated heart failure
- Mobitz type II second degree atrio-ventricular (AV) block, third degree AV block, or sick sinus syndrome if no pacemaker
- QT_c interval >500 msec
- Use of class Ia anti-arrythmic (quinidine, procainamide) or class III (amiodarone, sotalol, dofetilide, ibutilide)

FIGURE 13.2
Contraindications to fingolimod use.

- Prior history of: ischemic heart disease, congestive heart failure, cerebrovascular disease, symptomatic bradycardia, recurrent syncope, severe untreated sleep apnea, atrio-ventricular block, sino-atrial heart block
- Prolonged QT interval
- Risk factors for prolonged QT interval (hypokalemia, hypomagnesemia, congential long QT syndrome, drugs known to prolong QT interval [citalopram, chlorpromazine, haloperidol (and other antipsychotics), methadone, erythromycin]
- Use of beta blockers, digoxin, some calcium-channel blockers (verapamil, diltiazem)

FIGURE 13.3
Patients at higher risk for cardiac adverse events with fingolimod use.

individuals at higher risk for cardiovascular adverse effects, overnight monitoring is required with the first dose of fingolimod [63].

In keeping with the known mechanism of action of fingolimod, an average decrease in peripheral blood lymphocyte count of approximately 70% was observed in clinical trials. As this decrease is an expected effect of fingolimod, a drop in lymphocyte count does not warrant medication discontinuation unless levels fall to below 0.2×10^9/L, at which point the risk of infection may be higher. In clinical trial settings, patients with lymphocyte counts less than 0.2×10^9/L discontinued fingolimod, thus the exact risk of infection with significant lymphopenia is unclear [64].

Baseline and interval monitoring recommendations for fingolimod are summarized in a subsequent section and in Table 13.1.

Further experience with fingolimod will enable a more accurate characterization of its full adverse-effect profile. Currently, given the lack of long-term experience with fingolimod, this agent should be used with careful monitoring, and particularly in those with additional risk factors for cardiovascular adverse effects.

Mitoxantrone

In MS clinical trials, mitoxantrone has generally been a well-tolerated agent. Reported mild to moderate adverse effects associated with mitoxantrone include nausea, alopecia, menstrual disorders, urinary tract infections, leukopenia, and elevated gamma-glutamyl transpeptidase [35].

> The use of mitoxantrone is limited by concerns of serious adverse effects, including cardiac ventricular dysfunction, and therapy-related acute leukemia.

The use of mitoxantrone is limited, however, by concerns of serious adverse effects, including cardiac ventricular dysfunction, which is directly related to the cumulative lifetime dose, as well as TRAL. Postmarketing surveillance has revealed that the incidence of these serious complications is higher than initially reported, with the incidence of significant ventricular dysfunction estimated to be as high as 12%, congestive heart failure 0.8%, and TRAL as high as 0.3%, based on a consolidation of the available current literature on mitoxantrone toxicity [65]. Baseline and interval monitoring of cardiac function and hematological markers are required in patients on mitoxantrone are summarized in a subsequent section and in Table 13.1 [66].

Patient Selection

As a general rule of thumb, newly diagnosed RRMS patients should be initiated on one of the first-line DMTs. Choice of first-line agent is generally influenced by patient preference of dosing frequency and route, and tolerability of side effects.

> As a general rule of thumb, newly diagnosed RRMS patients should be initiated on one of the first-line DMTs, although there may be exceptional circumstances in which a second-line agent may be considered in treatment-naïve RRMS patients.

There may be special circumstances in which one of the second-line agents may be considered in a treatment-naïve RRMS patient. In a newly diagnosed individual with very active, polysymptomatic disease with MRI evidence of tissue destruction (T1 black holes and atrophy), initiating with a second-line therapy may be indicated. Also, in refractory needle-phobia, natalizumab or fingolimod may be the only feasible option, and may be considered after a discussion in which the patient demonstrates a clear comprehension of the risks and benefits of such an approach.

Individuals who are unable to tolerate side effects of one of the first-line agents may need to be switched to a second-line agent if side effects (flu-like reactions, skin reactions) cannot be managed adequately with conservative measures.

Finally, in female patients of child-bearing age, family planning may factor into the discussion of when to initiate treatment. With respect to FDA pregnancy risk categories, GA is classified as category B, and is thus the safest FDA-approved DMT for use in RRMS [40]. The remaining DMTs, including the IFN beta class of drugs, natalizumab, fingolimod, and mitoxantrone, are classified as pregnancy risk category D.

In the setting of an unplanned pregnancy, there are existing studies suggesting that GA may be relatively safe in pregnancy [67,68]. On the other hand, retrospective analyses of data from clinical trials involving IFN-beta drugs demonstrated an increased rate of spontaneous abortion with in utero exposure to IFN beta. In addition, lower birth weights, higher rates of miscarriages and still-births, and incidence of major malformations have been reported on the basis of data obtained from drug safety services [69]. Despite these retrospective analyses, however, the specific effects of IFN beta drugs in pregnancy are inconclusive.

In light of the fact that there are no existing controlled human studies demonstrating the safety of existing MS DMTs in pregnancy, and taking into account the evidence from animal studies as well as retrospective data, these issues should be addressed in female MS patients of child-bearing age when discussing DMT initiation and continuation. The general practice is to either discontinue IFN beta for 2 menstrual cycles, or delay initiation of DMTs in a patient actively attempting to conceive, and during pregnancy. Fortunately, MS relapse rates have been shown to be lower in the second and third trimesters of pregnancy [70]. Breastfeeding is also not recommended with resumption of DMT postpartum, as it is unknown whether DMTs are secreted in breast milk [40,45].

Pretesting and Interval Monitoring

GA

GA is not known to cause adverse effects on any internal organs [40]. It is therefore not necessary to check any baseline laboratory markers or to periodically monitor laboratory markers in patients on GA.

IFN Beta Drugs

Prior to initiation of any of the IFN beta class of drugs, a complete blood count (CBC) with differential, and liver function tests (LFTs) including aspartate aminotransferase (AST), alanine aminotransferase (ALT), alkaline phosphatase (ALP), and bilirubin should be obtained. After

initiation of treatment, CBC and LFTs should be checked at 1, 3, 6, and 12 months, and periodically thereafter. Of note, FDA guidelines suggest the aforementioned laboratory monitoring schedule for Rebif, Betaseron, and Extavia. For Avonex, FDA guidelines recommend monitoring CBC and LFTs every 6 months. However, in practice, most clinicians utilize the former, more frequent laboratory monitoring schedule for all patients on the IFN beta class of drugs. In patients with preexisting thyroid dysfunction, baseline thyroid function should be assessed, and thereafter as clinically indicated [3,44,45] (Table 13.1).

Natalizumab

Prior to initiation of natalizumab, patients should be screened for the presence of serum JCV Ab and a prior history of immunosuppression. Those who are positive for JCV Ab (approximately 50%–60% of MS patients) [60,71] and those with prior immunosuppression are at an increased risk category for PML, thus the risk and benefits of initiating natalizumab should be discussed in light of these factors. In all patients initiating natalizumab, a baseline brain MRI with contrast should be obtained, which will serve as a comparative scan should concern arise for PML. In addition, a baseline MRI-brain will enable a more accurate assessment of treatment response.

All patients on natalizumab should be reassessed clinically every 6 months at a minimum, and an annual MRI-brain with contrast should be performed to monitor for the presence of PML, as well as evidence of MS disease activity. In patients who are JCV Ab negative, JCV Ab should be tested for every 6 to 12 months to assess for seroconversion or an initial false negative test, as this substantially changes an individual's PML risk longitudinally. Furthermore, once a patient has been on natalizumab treatment for about 24 months, another discussion regarding PML risk should be undertaken before continuing treatment, as treatment duration for over 24 months is also a known risk factor for PML [59,60].

In a patient with new symptoms or signs that raise the concern for PML, a repeat MRI-brain with contrast should be obtained urgently, and CSF studies should be obtained to assess for the presence of JCV by polymerase chain reaction (PCR).

In regard to routine serum laboratory monitoring, there are no consensus guidelines. However, periodic CBC and LFTs are performed in some centers [62]. The presence of anti-natalizumab antibodies may be useful to assess in individuals with evidence of diminished clinical efficacy of natalizumab, or hypersensitivity reactions [72] (Table 13.1).

Fingolimod

Prior to initiation of fingolimod, CBC, LFTS, and renal laboratory markers should be obtained. In addition, immunity for varicella zoster virus should be assessed by serological tests, and immunization considered if there is no evidence of prior immunity. A baseline ECG should be obtained, and patients should be screened for any preexisting cardiovascular history or medication use that are either contraindications or put them at an increased risk for an adverse cardiovascular event with fingolimod (Figures 13.2 and 13.3). In individuals at a higher risk for cardiovascular events, overnight monitoring with the first dose of fingolimod is recommended [8,34,63].

An ophthalmological assessment should be performed to assess for preexisting macular damage and to obtain a baseline assessment given the risk of macular edema with fingolimod. Another ophthalmological assessment should be performed 3 to 4 months after initiation and if clinically indicated thereafter [73].

There are no consensus recommendations for monitoring of routine laboratory markers with fingolimod; however, periodical CBC, LFTs, and renal markers are typically performed [73] (Table 13.1).

Mitoxantrone

Prior to initiation of mitoxantrone, patients should have their cardiac function evaluated by echocardiography, specifically to assess the left ventricular ejection fraction (LVEF). In individuals with LVEF of less than 50% of normal, mitoxantrone is not recommended. Individuals who develop a clinically significant decrease in LVEF or congestive heart failure while on mitoxantrone should discontinue the drug [35,66].

Previous guidelines recommended assessing cardiac function before and after each individual dose when a cumulative lifetime dose of more than 100 mg/m² is reached [66]. However, more recent guidelines recommend assessing cardiac function before each dose of mitoxantrone, regardless of cumulative dose, and on an annual basis even after discontinuation, given the potential for delayed development of cardiotoxicity [65].

With respect to serum laboratory markers, a CBC with differential and LFTs should be assessed prior to initiation and before each subsequent dose of mitoxantrone. In individuals with neutrophils less than $1.5 \times 10^9/L$ and in those with laboratory evidence of hepatic dysfunction, mitoxantrone is not recommended. Given the potential teratogenicity in women of child-bearing potential, a pregnancy test is recommended prior to initiation [66] (Table 13.1).

Change or Discontinuation of DMTs

There is no consensus on the optimal approach to breakthrough disease; however, it is a commonly encountered situation in clinical practice. In this section, we present a practical approach to this commonly encountered dilemma.

Broadly speaking, breakthrough disease is defined as ongoing clinical or radiographic evidence of MS-related disease activity despite being on an accepted DMT for RRMS. Definitions of breakthrough disease have been proposed by various groups, and include: an increase in clinical relapse rate in comparison to the baseline relapse rate of 6 to 12 months after being on a first-line DMT, no decrease in relapse rate while on a first-line DMT, clinical

progression (which is typically defined as an increase in the Expanded Disability Status Scale [EDSS] score $f > 1$ sustained over 6 months), or MRI disease activity (which can refer to the presence of new enhancing lesions, new T1 black holes, or new T2 hyperintense lesions) although the precise number of lesions necessary to constitute "breakthrough disease" is difficult to define [74–79]. Thus, true "breakthrough disease" needs to be considered on an individual basis.

> Although there is no consensus definition, breakthrough disease is generally thought to be ongoing clinical or radiographic evidence of disease despite being on a DMT.

In individuals with breakthrough disease, 2 different approaches are reasonable. If the patient has not tried one of the alternate classes of first-line DMTs, this may be pursued. However, if the patient has evidence of severe breakthrough disease, then a more potent second-line agent may be considered immediately, which can include natalizumab, fingolimod, or mitoxantrone, but an extensive discussion of the risks and benefits of these agents must be undertaken with the patient.

> In individuals with breakthrough disease, one of the alternate classes of first-line injectable medications, this may be pursued, or a more potent second-line agent may be considered.

Situations other than breakthrough disease may also necessitate a change in DMT. These can include change from a relapsing to a progressive course of disease, as well as intolerable side effects. In the situation where a patient transitions to the progressive phase of MS, the decision can be challenging. If the patient continues to experience relapses superimposed on progression, then the continued use of a DMT may be justifiable. If, however, there are no superimposed relapses, then DMT discontinuation could be discussed with the patient, although it remains possible that the reason there are no superimposed relapses is because the DMT is successfully treating this aspect of the disease.

With respect to adverse effects, every attempt should be made to manage them symptomatically. However, if the patient remains intolerant of these adverse effects, change to another first-line class of drugs or second-line agent should be considered.

ACKNOWLEDGMENT

Supported by Multiple Sclerosis Society of Canada Postdoctoral Fellowship (to JO), National Multiple Sclerosis Society (NS041435 (PAC) and NMSS CA to PAC).

PATIENT CASE 1

A previously healthy 27-year-old woman presents with symptoms of eye pain and blurred vision in the left eye. She is seen by her neurologist and diagnosed with optic neuritis. She is given a 5 day course of intravenous steroids and undergoes an MRI-brain with gadolinium contrast administration. She has MRI lesions meeting the criteria set forth in the International Panel Criteria for RRMS, with 1 lesion in each of the periventricular, infratentorial, and juxtacortical regions of the brain, as well as the simultaneous presence of 1 enhancing lesion and 2 nonenhancing lesions.

Her neurologist recommends starting treatment with a first-line DMT to decrease the chance of future relapses and to diminish the chance of accumulating disability on a long-term basis. The patient is presented with the option of starting GA or one of the available IFN beta class of drugs. She is given information on each of these agents in the form of pamphlets and online resources, and is instructed to contact her neurologist's office to commence treatment when she had decided on a DMT. Of note, she denies having any plans to conceive in the near future, and is currently regularly taking an oral contraceptive medication.

The patient leads a very active lifestyle, and works long hours as a marketing executive. Owing to her unpredictable work schedule, she finds it difficult to schedule regular visits to a medical laboratory for laboratory monitoring, thus, would prefer being on a medication with minimal monitoring requirements. She also values having a routine to follow on a daily basis. Based on her personal preferences, she chooses to start GA, which is a daily injectable medication with no requirements for laboratory monitoring.

PATIENT CASE 2

A 32-year-old woman presents with symptoms of right-sided arm and leg numbness and paresthesia that evolved over a few days, and that have persisted for the past 1½ weeks. When questioned further, she recalls having had bilateral lower limb numbness and paresthesia 3 years earlier, which resolved completely. She undergoes an MRI-brain and cervical spine, which show evidence of lesions in the brain and spine that are characteristic of MS. She is given a diagnosis of RRMS, and presented with first-line DMT options.

Prior to initiating treatment, her neurologist inquires whether she has immediate plans to start a family. She reveals that she and her husband are intending to conceive within the next 6 months to 1 year, and asks about the risk of DMTs in pregnancy.

Her neurologist discusses with her that there is only limited information regarding pregnancy risk and the first-line DMTs. GA is in pregnancy risk category B, while the IFN beta drugs are in pregnancy risk category C. However, given the lack of definitive evidence, the current practice is to avoid DMT use during both the preconception period and pregnancy. Furthermore, the use of DMTs is not recommended with breast-feeding either.

Since this patient has immediate plans to conceive, the patient decides to delay starting treatment until she delivers her first child, at which point, she can discuss with her neurologist the optimal time to start a DMT. Should she have difficulty conceiving, the discussion of initiating a DMT can be resumed with her neurologist at that time.

PATIENT CASE 3

A 42-year-old man presented with bilateral lower limb weakness and urinary symptoms 3 years previously. He underwent multiple investigations at that time, including an MRI-brain and spine, and was given a diagnosis of RRMS. He initially started treatment with GA, but had 2 additional relapses and MRI evidence of active disease after 1 year of treatment.

He discontinued GA at that time, and started Rebif. On Rebif, he has had 3 relapses over 2 years, and his most recent MRI-brain shows evidence of a new enhancing lesion, as well as new nonenhancing lesions in comparison to his MRI from 6 months previously. From a clinical perspective, although he has recovered for the most part from most of his relapses, he notices that he is no longer able to run, and needs to sit and rest when he walks for more than a few hundred meters. He also has persistent numbness in his feet bilaterally.

Given both the clinical and radiographic evidence of breakthrough disease, his neurologist has a discussion with him about approved second-line agents for breakthrough MS disease. They discuss the risks and benefits of natalizumab and fingolimod. The patient is interested in trying natalizumab. He has no prior history of immunosuppression. The patient has his serum JCV Ab checked, which is negative, putting him at a significantly reduced risk for PML. He initiates treatment with natalizumab, and his follow-up MRI at 3 months shows no gadolinium enhancement, and he remains stable clinically with no new symptoms or signs suggestive of a relapse.

KEY POINTS FOR PATIENTS AND FAMILIES

- MS DMTs are intended to prevent new areas of inflammation, which is measured both by clinical relapses and new lesions on MRI.

- Since these MS therapies are intended to prevent inflammation, they generally do not improve symptoms of MS.

- There are several different first-line DMTs for MS.

- The choice of first-line therapy is often guided by patient preference, dosing frequency, route of administration, and tolerability of side effects.

- There may be special circumstances in which one of the second-line agents may be considered in a treatment-naïve RRMS patient.

- Patients who do not tolerate or respond sufficiently to a first-line agent may be changed to a second-line therapy.

- Female patients who intend to get pregnant should discuss this with their care team so that appropriate plans can be made for their MS treatment.

REFERENCES

1. Wolinsky JS. Glatiramer acetate for the treatment of multiple sclerosis. *Expert Opin Pharmacother.* 2004;5:875–891.

2. Farina C, Weber MS, Meinl E, et al. Glatiramer acetate in multiple sclerosis: Update on potential mechanisms of action. *Lancet Neurol.* 2005;4:567–575.

3. Mehta LRG, Andrew D. Multiple sclerosis. *Continuum: Lifelong Learning in Neurology.* 2007;13:144–180.

4. Kieseier BC. The mechanism of action of interferon-beta in relapsing multiple sclerosis. *CNS Drugs.* 2011;25:491–502.

5. Hynes RO. Integrins: A family of cell surface receptors. *Cell.* 1987;48:549–554.

6. Frenette PS, Wagner DD. Adhesion molecules—Part 1. *N Engl J Med.* 1996;334:1526–1529.

7. Frenette PS, Wagner DD. Adhesion molecules—Part II: Blood vessels and blood cells. *N Engl J Med.* 1996;335:43–45.

8. Kappos L, Radue EW, O'Connor P, et al. A placebo-controlled trial of oral fingolimod in relapsing multiple sclerosis. *N Engl J Med.* 2010;362:387–401.

9. Matloubian M, Lo CG, Cinamon G, et al. Lymphocyte egress from thymus and peripheral lymphoid organs is dependent on S1P receptor 1. *Nature.* 2004;427:355–360.

10. Mandala S, Hajdu R, Bergstrom J, et al. Alteration of lymphocyte trafficking by sphingosine-1-phosphate receptor agonists. *Science (NY).* 2002;296:346–349.

11. Bartholomaus I, Kawakami N, Odoardi F, et al. Effector T cell interactions with meningeal vascular structures in nascent autoimmune CNS lesions. *Nature.* 2009;462:94–98.

12. Brinkmann V. Sphingosine 1-phosphate receptors in health and disease: Mechanistic insights from gene deletion studies and reverse pharmacology. *Pharmacol Ther.* 2007;115:84–105.

13. Miron VE, Jung CG, Kim HJ, et al. FTY720 modulates human oligodendrocyte progenitor process extension and survival. *Ann Neurol.* 2008;63:61–71.

14. Crespi MD, Ivanier SE, Genovese J, Baldi A. Mitoxantrone affects topoisomerase activities in human breast cancer cells. *Biochem Biophys Res Commun.* 1986;136:521–528.

15. Jacobs LD, Cookfair DL, Rudick RA, et al. Intramuscular interferon beta-1a for disease progression in relapsing multiple sclerosis. The Multiple Sclerosis Collaborative Research Group (MSCRG). *Ann Neurol.* 1996;39:285–294.

16. Simon JH, Jacobs LD, Campion M, et al. Magnetic resonance studies of intramuscular interferon beta-1a for relapsing multiple sclerosis. The Multiple Sclerosis Collaborative Research Group. *Ann Neurol.* 1998;43:79–87.

17. Randomised double-blind placebo-controlled study of interferon beta-1a in relapsing/remitting multiple sclerosis. PRISMS (Prevention of Relapses and Disability by Interferon beta-1a Subcutaneously in Multiple Sclerosis) Study Group. *Lancet.* 1998;352:1498–1504.

18. Interferon beta-1b is effective in relapsing-remitting multiple sclerosis. I. Clinical results of a multicenter, randomized, double-blind, placebo-controlled trial. The IFNB Multiple Sclerosis Study Group. *Neurology.* 1993;43:655–661.

19. Paty DW, Li DK. Interferon beta-1b is effective in relapsing-remitting multiple sclerosis. II. MRI analysis results of a multicenter, randomized, double-blind, placebo-controlled trial. UBC MS/MRI Study Group and the IFNB Multiple Sclerosis Study Group. *Neurology.* 1993;43:662–667.

20. Interferon beta-1b in the treatment of multiple sclerosis: Final outcome of the randomized controlled trial. The IFNB Multiple Sclerosis Study Group and The University of British Columbia MS/MRI Analysis Group. *Neurology.* 1995;45:1277–1285.

21. Johnson KP, Brooks BR, Cohen JA, et al. Copolymer 1 reduces relapse rate and improves disability in relapsing-remitting multiple sclerosis: Results of a phase III multicenter, double-blind placebo-controlled trial. The Copolymer 1 Multiple Sclerosis Study Group. *Neurology.* 1995;45:1268–1276.

22. Comi G, Filippi M, Wolinsky JS. European/Canadian multicenter, double-blind, randomized, placebo-controlled study of the effects of glatiramer acetate on magnetic resonance imaging—measured disease activity and burden in patients with relapsing multiple sclerosis. European/Canadian Glatiramer Acetate Study Group. *Ann Neurol.* 2001;49: 290–297.

23. Li DK, Paty DW. Magnetic resonance imaging results of the PRISMS trial: A randomized, double-blind, placebo-controlled study of interferon-beta1a in relapsing-remitting multiple sclerosis. Prevention of relapses and disability by interferon-beta1a subcutaneously in multiple sclerosis. *Ann Neurol.* 1999;46: 197–206.

24. Durelli L, Verdun E, Barbero P, et al. Every-other-day interferon beta-1b versus once-weekly interferon beta-1a for multiple sclerosis: Results of a 2-year prospective randomised multicentre study (INCOMIN). *Lancet.* 2002;359:1453–1460.

25. Panitch H, Goodin DS, Francis G, et al. Randomized, comparative study of interferon beta-1a treatment regimens in MS: The EVIDENCE Trial. *Neurology.* 2002;59:1496–1506.

26. O'Connor P, Filippi M, Arnason B, et al. 250 microg or 500 microg interferon beta-1b versus 20 mg glatiramer acetate in relapsing-remitting multiple sclerosis: A prospective, randomised, multicentre study. *Lancet Neurol.* 2009;8:889–897.

27. Mikol DD, Barkhof F, Chang P, et al. Comparison of subcutaneous interferon beta-1a with glatiramer acetate in patients with relapsing multiple sclerosis (the REbif vs Glatiramer Acetate in Relapsing MS Disease [REGARD] study): A multicentre, randomised, parallel, open-label trial. *Lancet Neurol.* 2008;7: 903–914.

28. Goodin DS, Frohman EM, Garmany GP Jr, et al. Disease modifying therapies in multiple sclerosis: Report of the Therapeutics and Technology Assessment Subcommittee of the American Academy of Neurology and the MS Council for Clinical Practice Guidelines. *Neurology.* 2002;58:169–178.

29. Rice GP, Incorvaia B, Munari L, et al. Interferon in relapsing-remitting multiple sclerosis. *Cochrane Database Syst Rev.* (Online) 2001;(4):CD002002.

30. La Mantia L, Munari LM, Lovati R. Glatiramer acetate for multiple sclerosis. *Cochrane Database Syst Rev.* (Online) 2010;(5):CD004678.

31. Polman CH, O'Connor PW, Havrdova E, et al. A randomized, placebo-controlled trial of natalizumab for relapsing multiple sclerosis. *N Engl J Med.* 2006;354:899–910.

32. Goodin DS, Cohen BA, O'Connor P, et al. Assessment: The use of natalizumab (Tysabri) for the treatment of multiple sclerosis (an evidence-based review): Report of the Therapeutics and Technology Assessment Subcommittee of the American Academy of Neurology. *Neurology.* 2008;71:766–773.

33. Pucci E, Giuliani G, Solari A, et al. Natalizumab for relapsing remitting multiple sclerosis. *Cochrane Database of Syst Rev.* (Online) 2011;(10):CD007621.

34. Cohen JA, Barkhof F, Comi G, et al. Oral fingolimod or intramuscular interferon for relapsing multiple sclerosis. *N Engl J Med.* 2010;362:402–415.

35. Hartung HP, Gonsette R, Konig N, et al. Mitoxantrone in progressive multiple sclerosis: A placebo-controlled, double-blind, randomised, multicentre trial. *Lancet.* 2002;360:2018–2025.

36. Goodin DS, Arnason BG, Coyle PK, et al. The use of mitoxantrone (Novantrone) for the treatment of multiple sclerosis: Report of the Therapeutics and Technology Assessment Subcommittee of the American Academy of Neurology. *Neurology.* 2003;61:1332–1338.

37. Martinelli Boneschi F, Rovaris M, Capra R, Comi G. Mitoxantrone for multiple sclerosis. *Cochrane Database Syst Rev.* (Online) 2005;(4):CD002127.

38. Krapf H, Morrissey SP, Zenker O, et al. Effect of mitoxantrone on MRI in progressive MS: Results of the MIMS trial. *Neurology.* 2005;65:690–695.

39. *Physician Desk Reference.* Montvale, NJ: Thomson PDR; 2005.

40. Perumal J, Filippi M, Ford C, et al. Glatiramer acetate therapy for multiple sclerosis: A review. *Expert Opin Drug Metab Toxicol.* 2006;2:1019–1029.

41. Placebo-controlled multicentre randomised trial of interferon beta-1b in treatment of secondary progressive multiple sclerosis. European Study Group on interferon beta-1b in secondary progressive MS. *Lancet.* 1998;352:1491–1497.

42. Frohman EM, Brannon K, Alexander S, et al. Disease modifying agent related skin reactions in multiple sclerosis: Prevention, assessment, and management. *Mult Scler (England).* 2004;10:302–307.

43. Elgart GW, Sheremata W, Ahn YS. Cutaneous reactions to recombinant human interferon beta-1b: The clinical and histologic spectrum. *J Am Acad Dermatol.* 1997;37:553–558.

44. Walther EU, Hohlfeld R. Multiple sclerosis: Side effects of interferon beta therapy and their management. *Neurology.* 1999;53:1622–1627.

45. Kremenchutzky M, Morrow S, Rush C. The safety and efficacy of IFN-beta products for the treatment of multiple sclerosis. *Expert Opin Drug Saf.* 2007;6:279–288.

46. Rieckmann P, O'Connor P, Francis GS, et al. Haematological effects of interferon-beta-1a (Rebif) therapy in multiple sclerosis. *Drug Saf.* 2004;27:745–756.

47. Francis GS, Grumser Y, Alteri E, et al. Hepatic reactions during treatment of multiple sclerosis with interferon-beta-1a: Incidence and clinical significance. *Drug Saf.* 2003;26:815–827.

48. Tremlett HL, Yoshida EM, Oger J. Liver injury associated with the beta-interferons for MS: A comparison between the three products. *Neurology.* 2004;62:628-631.

49. Monzani F, Caraccio N, Casolaro A, et al. Long-term interferon beta-1b therapy for MS: Is routine thyroid assessment always useful? *Neurology.* 2000;55:549–552.

50. Monzani F, Caraccio N, Dardano A, Ferrannini E. Thyroid autoimmunity and dysfunction associated with type I interferon therapy. *Clin Exp Med.* 2004;3:199–210.

51. Feinstein A, O'Connor P, Feinstein K. Multiple sclerosis, interferon beta-1b and depression A prospective investigation. *J Neurol.* 2002;249:815–820.

52. Goeb JL, Even C, Nicolas G, et al. Psychiatric side effects of interferon-beta in multiple sclerosis. *Eur Psychiatry.* 2006;21:186–193.

53. Mohr DC, Goodkin DE, Likosky W, et al. Treatment of depression improves adherence to interferon beta-1b therapy for multiple sclerosis. *Arch Neurol.* 1997;54:531–533.

54. Mohr DC, Likosky W, Dwyer P, et al. Course of depression during the initiation of interferon beta-1a treatment for multiple sclerosis. *Arch Neurol.* 1999;56:1263–1265.

55. Rudick RA, Stuart WH, Calabresi PA, et al. Natalizumab plus interferon beta-1a for relapsing multiple sclerosis. *N Engl J Med.* 2006;354:911–923.

56. Phillips JT, O'Connor PW, Havrdova E, et al. Infusion-related hypersensitivity reactions during natalizumab treatment. *Neurology.* 2006;67:1717–1718.

57. Hellwig K, Schimrigk S, Fischer M, et al. Allergic and nonallergic delayed infusion reactions during natalizumab therapy. *Arch Neurol.* 2008;65:656–658.

58. Kappos L, Bates D, Edan G, et al. Natalizumab treatment for multiple sclerosis: Updated recommendations for patient selection and monitoring. *Lancet Neurol.* 2011;10:745–758.

59. O'Connor P. The use of JC viral antibody status to assist in PML risk determination in natalizumab-treated patients. In: ACTRIMS. San Diego, CA; 2012.

60. Bloomgren G, Richman S, Hotermans C, et al. Risk of natalizumab-associated progressive multifocal leukoencephalopathy. *N Engl J Med.* 2012;366:1870–1880.

61. Sorensen PS, Bertolotto A, Edan G, et al. Risk stratification for progressive multifocal leukoencephalopathy in patients treated with natalizumab. *Mult Scler (England).* 2012;18:143–152.

62. Rudick RA, Panzara MA. Natalizumab for the treatment of relapsing multiple sclerosis. *Biologics.* 2008;2:189–199.

63. *Gilenya Full Prescribing Information.* East Hanover, NJ: Novartis Pharmaceuticals Corporation; 2012.

64. Saidha S, Eckstein C, Calabresi PA. New and emerging disease modifying therapies for multiple sclerosis. *Ann NY Acad Sci.* 2012;1247:117–137.

65. Marriott JJ, Miyasaki JM, Gronseth G, O'Connor PW. Evidence Report: The efficacy and safety of mitoxantrone (Novantrone) in the treatment of multiple sclerosis: Report of the Therapeutics and Technology Assessment Subcommittee of the American Academy of Neurology. *Neurology.* 2010;74:1463–1470.

66. Scott LJ, Figgitt DP. Mitoxantrone: A review of its use in multiple sclerosis. *CNS Drugs.* 2004;18:379–396.

67. Fragoso YD, Finkelsztejn A, Kaimen-Maciel DR, et al. Long-term use of glatiramer acetate by 11 pregnant women with multiple sclerosis: A retrospective, multicentre case series. *CNS Drugs.* 2010;24:969–976.

68. Salminen HJ, Leggett H, Boggild M. Glatiramer acetate exposure in pregnancy: Preliminary safety and birth outcomes. *J Neurol.* 2010;257:2020–2023.

69. Sandberg-Wollheim M, Frank D, Goodwin TM, et al. Pregnancy outcomes during treatment with interferon beta-1a in patients with multiple sclerosis. *Neurology.* 2005;65:802–806.

70. Confavreux C, Hutchinson M, Hours MM, et al. Rate of pregnancy-related relapse in multiple sclerosis. Pregnancy in Multiple Sclerosis Group. *N Engl J Med.* 1998;339:285–291.

71. Trampe AK, Hemmelmann C, Stroet A, et al. Anti-JC virus antibodies in a large German natalizumab-treated multiple sclerosis cohort. *Neurology.* 2012;78:1736–1742.

72. Calabresi PA, Giovannoni G, Confavreux C, et al. The incidence and significance of anti-natalizumab antibodies: Results from AFFIRM and SENTINEL. *Neurology.* 2007;69:1391–1403.

73. Hyland MH, Cohen JA. Fingolimod. *Neurol Clin Pract.* 2011;1:61–65.

74. Rudick RA, Polman CH. Current approaches to the identification and management of breakthrough disease in patients with multiple sclerosis. *Lancet Neurol.* 2009;8:545–559.

75. Marriott JJ, O'Connor PW. Definitions of breakthrough disease and second-line agents. *Neurol Clin.* 2011;29:411–422.

76. O'Connor PW. Use of natalizumab in multiple sclerosis patients. *Can J Neurol Sci.* 2010;37:98–104.

77. Freedman MS, Forrestal FG. Canadian treatment optimization recommendations (TOR) as a predictor of disease breakthrough in patients with multiple sclerosis treated with interferon beta-1a: Analysis of the PRISMS study. *Mult Scler (England).* 2008;14:1234–1241.

78. Cohen BA, Khan O, Jeffery DR, et al. Identifying and treating patients with suboptimal responses. *Neurology.* 2004;63:S33–S40.

79. Greenberg BK, Kramer JF. Current and emerging multiple sclerosis therapeutics. *Continuum: Lifelong Learning in Neurology.* 2010;16:19.

14

Primary Progressive Multiple Sclerosis

KATHLEEN HAWKER

KEY POINTS FOR CLINICIANS

- Primary progressive multiple sclerosis (PPMS) is defined by a progressive accrual of disability in the absence of relapses.

- Unlike relapsing-remitting multiple sclerosis, the incidence of PPMS is equal in males and females and patients tend to be older at the time of diagnosis.

- Diagnosis may be difficult because of the insidious onset of the disease.

- Lesions on the MRI of the brain are identical to other forms of multiple sclerosis but typically show a paucity of lesions as compared to the relapsing forms of the disease.

- There is currently no approved treatments for slowing disability in patients with PPMS, although a subset of patients may respond to disease-modifying treatments.

In contradistinction to relapsing multiple sclerosis (MS), approximately 10% to 15% of MS patients present with a slow, insidious onset of symptoms. This is known as primary progressive MS (PPMS). PPMS most commonly presents with a myelopathy [1]. Owing to the slow onset over a period of months and occasionally years, patients may delay seeking medical advice and even when seen by a doctor, the diagnosis is delayed as compared to relapsing-remitting MS (RRMS). Other features of PPMS that differ from the more common RR form include an older age at onset (40 to 50 years). Most studies show that patients with PPMS are approximately 10 years older on average than RRMS patients. Despite the typically older age at presentation, younger patients in their 20s and 30s may present with PPMS [1,2].

PPMS affects males and females in equal numbers in distinction to the 1:3 ratio seen in relapsing forms [1,2]. Although a hormonal basis may be postulated as a reason,

the 1:1 sex ratio is similar in pre and postmenopausal cohorts of females with PPMS [1,2].

> Misdiagnosis or delay in diagnosis is common in PPMS.

A relatively rare subtype of MS, progressive-relapsing multiple sclerosis (PRMS), accounts for approximately 1% of all cases of MS [1]. Patients may present with the typically insidious course of PPMS but have very infrequent superimposed relapses. Occasionally, patients experience

> A small subset of patients present with rare relapses superimposed upon progression.

an initial relapse followed by the progressive course. Of interest, this subgroup of patients tends to have a more aggressive course than PPMS overall and MRI of the brain tends to show more lesions on average than those seen on MRIs of PPMS patients [3].

GENETICS AND EPIDEMIOLOGY

It had been argued that PPMS is a distinct disease from RRMS and many have questioned whether PPMS is autoimmune mediated [1]. Several genetic and environmental risk factors are similar to those for RRMS, however, suggesting a common link between the 2 phenotypes. Similar to RRMS, patients with PPMS have an increased incidence of the same human leukocyte antigen (HLA) loci and if positive for *HLA-DRB1*1501* tend to have a poorer prognosis [4,5]. Patients with PPMS and their families have an increased risk of developing other autoimmune diseases, such as Graves' disease, systemic lupus erythematous, and type 1 diabetes, likely due to common susceptibility genes [5]. Finally, family and twin studies have shown that there is an increase in the incidence of both PPMS and RRMS in siblings [5]. Thus, the evidence suggests a strong link between the 2 subtypes of MS although it is presently unclear as to what factors determine the ultimate phenotype.

> PPMS patients have a higher risk of developing other autoimmune diseases.

Similar to RRMS, there is a higher incidence in northern Europeans, being uncommon in African Americans (6%), and rare in other ethnic groups [5].

It is presently unclear why some patients develop PPMS as opposed to RRMS and whether certain factors, such as age, hormonal influences, and environmental triggers, may modify the immune response and thus the clinical phenotype.

CLINICAL PRESENTATION

The initial symptoms of PPMS vary. By far, the most common symptom at onset is a gradually progressive myelopathy, primarily affecting walking. Typically, patients develop a spastic paraparesis, with upper limb difficulties occurring later in the course [1,2]. Initial patient symptoms include catching their toe, tripping and stumbling, and difficulty walking and running (exertional fatigue). Given the insidious onset, the symptoms are commonly ascribed to fatigue, shoe issues, or orthopedic problems. The symptoms are often aggravated by fatigue, heat, infection, and overexertion. Stiffness, pain, and cramps in the legs and low thoracic and lumbar spine may occur because of the spasticity,

causing poor exercise endurance and occasionally sleep disturbances. It is common for the weakness and spasticity to be asymmetric, beginning on one side and then slowly progressing. Initially, the myelopathy predominantly affects the legs although a minority of patients may complain of symptoms in their hands, such as difficulty doing buttons or fastening necklaces.

> A progressive myelopathy is by far the most common presenting feature.

Symptoms of a neurogenic bladder (urgency, frequency, and double voiding) tend to coexist with the walking difficulties. Owing to detrusor sphincteric dysynergy, urinary post void residuals may be elevated, leading to an increased risk for urinary tract infections and some patients with PPMS may present to their family doctors with multiple urinary tract infections requiring antibiotic use. Initial symptoms of bowel dysfunction are less common; however, constipation, difficulty evacuating the rectum, and rarely diarrhea may accompany bladder complaints. Sexual difficulties can manifest as erectile dysfunction, problems with ejaculation, and poor sensation with difficulty achieving orgasm.

> Bladder, bowel, and sexual difficulties tend to coexist with the myelopathy.

Although myelopathic complaints are by far the most common initial symptoms, a minority of patients may present with a constellation of symptoms consistent with brain stem dysfunction. Patients may report progressive diplopia, blurred vision, imbalance and incoordination although typically myelopathic features are present either on the clinical exam or ensue shortly after the initial brain stem presentation [1,2]. Other less common complaints include visual blurring or visual loss consistent with a unilateral or bilateral optic neuritis, albeit at a lesser rate than RRMS [1,2].

> A progressive onset of brain stem or optic neuritis symptoms can be seen.

It had previously been thought that cognition was relatively spared in PPMS though recent studies have shown

> Cognition, depression, and fatigue are common effects in PPMS.

evidence of dysfunction similar to, but less severe, than RRMS [6]. Depression and generalized fatigue are common but again, less so than experienced in RRMS [7].

Symptom management is identical to that of other forms of MS and is tailored toward specific patient concerns. Physical therapy and exercise as well as treatment of spasticity are paramount to prevent disuse atrophy and further deterioration of limb weakness.

PROGNOSIS

There is marked heterogeneity in the rate of progression among patients, with 25% needing a cane within 7 years of diagnosis, 50% by 13 years, and 15% needing a wheelchair by 20 years. Yet, up to 30% are still partially ambulatory by 30 years [8]. Although there is heterogeneity among patients, the rate of progression for an individual patient is typically steady. A relatively sudden acceleration in the rate of progression should trigger a search for other causes (for example, infection, medication side effect, superimposed stroke, spinal cord compression, etc.). Since the incidence of other autoimmune diseases is increased in PPMS, B_{12} and thyroid testing, in addition to other tests dependent on patient symptoms, should be considered.

Typically, disability has been assessed using the Expanded Disability Status Scale (EDSS). However, the 25 foot timed walk has been correlated with progression and is a simpler method to use for clinicians and patients.

Factors that indicate a poorer prognosis include initial involvement of the brain stem or cerebellum, or significant spinal cord lesions [1,2]. Younger ages (of less than 51 years), increased lesions on the brain MRI, a rapid increase

> Younger age, more than 3 systems involved, a rapid increase in EDSS in the first 2 years, large lesion load on brain and spine MRIs, and a positive CSF are negative prognostic factors.

in EDSS in the first 2 years, more than 3 systems' involvement at the time of diagnosis, and a positive cerebrospinal fluid (CSF) may negatively affect the outcome (see Table 14.1).

There are 3 very rare presentations of PPMS: progressive visual loss consistent with optic neuritis, progressive cognitive dysfunction, and progressive cerebellar dysfunction (dysarthria, imbalance, and incoordination). The absence of other symptoms (although there may be other signs on the clinical exam) may confound clinicians and the diagnosis may be delayed in many cases [1,2].

DIAGNOSIS

The diagnosis is established by using a combination of the clinical presentation, MRI findings, and exclusion of other diseases. The revised International Diagnostic Criteria for PPMS includes 1 year of disease progression, and 2 of 3 of the following criteria: a classic T2 lesion in the brain, 2 or more T2 lesions in the spinal cord, or positive CSF (oligoclonal bands or an elevated IgG index) [9] (see Table 14.2).

> Diagnosis requires typical lesions on the brain and/or spine plus a year of progression.

The mandate for a year of disease progression, as well as the typical insidious onset of the disease, can make an early diagnosis of MS difficult. Indeed, several studies have suggested that PPMS may take 2 to 3 years longer to diagnose than RRMS and 50% of patients have a moderate amount of weakness in their legs at the time of diagnosis [8]. It is not uncommon for a misdiagnosis of another disorder to be made prior to the true diagnosis of PPMS.

TABLE 14.1
Indicators of Poor Prognosis in PPMS

Younger age

Possibly male gender

Shorter time to reach EDSS score of 3.0

Increase in EDSS score in the first 2 years of disease

Poor 25 foot (7.6 m) timed walk at onset of the disease

More than 3 systems involved at the time of diagnosis

Increased number of T2 lesions

Gd lesions on the brain MRI

More severe brain and/or spinal atrophy

Positive CSF testing

TABLE 14.2
Revised McDonald Criteria for the Diagnosis of PPMS

One-year disease progression plus at least 3 of the following:

One Gd-positive lesion[a] or 9 T2 hyperintense lesions if no Gd lesion is present

Four T2 lesions and a positive visual-evoked potential

At least 1 infratentorial lesion

At least 1 juxtacortical lesion

At least 3 periventricular lesions

Two spinal cord lesions[b]

Positive CSF (oligoclonal band or IgG index)

[a]A Gd-positive spinal cord lesion = a brain Gd-positive lesion.
[b]Spinal cord lesion = infratentorial lesion.

Many other diseases, including cervical spondylopathy (the most common), vitamin deficiencies, leukodystrophies, arteriovenous malformations (including dural arteriovenous fistulas of the cord), spinal cord tumors, hereditary spastic paraparesis, infectious etiologies, and paraneoplastic syndromes may mimic PPMS, thus further complicating the diagnosis (see Table 14.3; Figure 14.1). It is important to remember that other conditions may coexist with PPMS, particularly spinal stenosis, vitamin B_{12} deficiency (pernicious anemia), and hypothyroidism (Graves' disease), and aggravate the symptoms of PPMS.

> Many other diseases can mimic PPMS and a complete work-up should be performed.

There may be several factors to be considered that may aid in the correct diagnosis, including the age of the patient, concomitant symptoms, and family history. Other tests to rule out other mimics should be performed (see Table 14.4). Although reports of MRI scans of the brain may describe "white matter lesions," nonspecific lesions thought to represent microvascular changes, are common in older individuals. It is important to review the MRI of the brain personally to determine whether the lesions are truly classical (periventricular and juxtacortical) for MS before a diagnosis is made. Requesting a sagittal fluid attenuation and inversion recovery (FLAIR) image as part of the MRI study to see whether Dawson's fingers exist may help differentiate MS from microvascular disease [10]. Age-related lesions on T2-weighted MRI spinal cord scans would be very rare; thus, imaging of the cervical and thoracic cord may help elucidate the diagnosis. Spinal cord lesion extending over more than 2 spinal cord segments, persistently enhancing lesions despite the use of steroids or expansile lesions, suggest an alternative diagnosis.

> A sagittal FLAIR brain MRI can clarify whether the MRI lesions represent PPMS or microvascular disease.

If MRI findings are equivocal, spinal fluid analysis (oligoclonal bands and IgG index) used in conjunction with the history may help elucidate the diagnosis although up to 10% of patients may have a negative CSF study [11]. It

TABLE 14.3
Differential Diagnosis of PPMS

Structural Causes
Cervical stenosis
Arteriovenous malformation or dural venous fistula
Syrinx
Tumor

Infections
Human T lymphotropic virus, type 1
HIV
Progressive multifocal leukoencephalopathy
Lyme disease

Nutritional Deficiencies
Vitamin B_{12} deficiency
Copper deficiency
Vitamin E deficiency
Wernicke's syndrome

Metabolic Disorders
Adrenomyeloneuropathy

Genetic
Hereditary spastic paraparesis
Spinal cerebellar ataxias

Other
Primary lateral sclerosis
Cerebral autosomal dominant arteriopathy with subcortical infarcts and leukoencephalopathy
Sarcoidosis
Lupus cerebritis

TABLE 14.4
Testing for Alternative Diagnoses

Vitamin B_{12}	CBC, MCV, B_{12} level, homocysteine, methylmalonic acid
Copper deficiency	Blood and urinary copper, ceruloplasm
Vitamin E deficiency	Vitamin E levels
HTLV	HTLV-1 antibodies in serum and CSF, PCR, 50% elevated lymphocytes and protein in CSF, oligoclonal bands, IgG index
ADL	VLCFA, elevated CSF protein, corticotrophin stimulation test, elevated protein in CSF, genetic blood test
PML	JC virus DNA PCR serum and CSF, brain biopsy
Sarcoidosis	ACE level, CXR, gallium scan lungs, bronchial lavage, PFT's, serum and urinary calcium, serum gamma globulin, endocrine study, biopsy lymph nodes
SLE	CBC, renal function, anti ds DNA Ab, anti Sm, anti Ro, anti RNP, anti cardiolipin Ab, CSF-decrease glucose, mild increase lymphocytes and protein
CADASIL	Serum for CADASIL
SCA	Specific genetic testing for various SCA
HSP	Specific genetic testing for various HSP
PLS	Nerve conduction and EMG

Ab, antibodies; ACE, angiotensin converting enzyme; CXR, chest x-ray; ds, double stranded; EMG, electromyography; MCV, mean corpuscular volume; PFT, pulmonary function test; VLCFA, very long chain fatty acids.

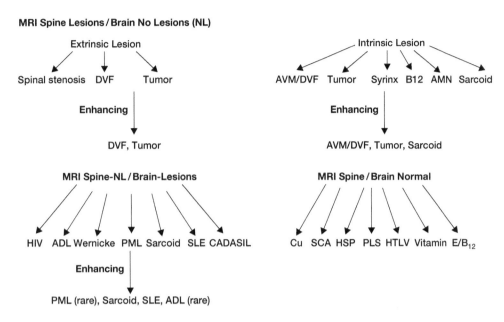

FIGURE 14.1

Differential diagnosis for PPMS. *ADL, adrenoleukodystrophy; AMN, adrenomyeloneuropathy; AVM, arteriovenous malformation; CADASIL, cerebral autosomal dominant arteriopathy and subcortical infarcts and leukoencephalopathy; cu, copper deficiency; DVF, dural venous fistula; B$_{12}$, vitamin B$_{12}$; HSP, spastic paraparesis; HTLV, human trophic lymphocytic virus; PLS, primary lateral sclerosis; PML, progressive multifocal leukodystrophy; SCA, spinocerebellar atrophy; SLE, systemic lupus erythematous; vitamin E/B$_{12}$, vitamin E or vitamin B$_{12}$ deficiency.*

is important to note that oligoclonal bands and an elevated IgG index are nonspecific and can occur in other inflammatory and infectious disorders; thus, a positive result has to be considered in conjunction with the MRI and other diagnostic serology (see Table 14.3).

> CSF can be negative in up to 10% of patients and a positive CSF can be seen in other diseases.

IMAGING OF PPMS

It was previously thought that neurodegeneration was the hallmark of PPMS; however, more recent MRI and autopsy studies revealed evidence of both inflammation and degeneration.

Patients with PPMS display the same classic periventricular, juxtacortical, and spinal cord lesions in the white matter, identical to those seen in RRMS (see Table 14.5). Despite the qualitative similarities, early studies found that PPMS was associated with fewer T2 brain lesions than either secondary progressive MS (SPMS) or RRMS [12]. This observation has since been replicated and extended to gadolinium (Gd)-enhancing lesions in many other studies [13–16]. Despite the quantitative differences between the groups, there is evidence of an early, clinically silent inflammatory component in PPMS. Several studies using double-dose Gd found enhancing lesions in approximately

40% to 50% of early stage PPMS patients as compared to 80% of RRMS patients [13]. Other studies have reported a lower proportion of patients with Gd enhancing lesions, possibly reflecting disease duration [14].

> MRI lesions are identical to those seen in RRMS.

> Gd positive lesions are seen in 50% of patients with early stage PPMS. Double-dose Gd may reveal more lesions.

Spinal cord lesions are common in PPMS, occurring in greater than 75% of patients as reported in several MRI studies. The lesions are indistinguishable to lesions seen in RRMS, being more common in the cervical and upper thoracic cord and spanning less than 2 spinal cord segments [16].

> Spinal cord lesions are common and scans of the cervical and thoracic cord may help with diagnosis and prognosis.

Both gray and white matter atrophy, as measured by conventional MRI, have been shown in PPMS and some studies have suggested that white matter atrophy

TABLE 14.5
MRI and CSF Characteristics in Patients with PPMS at the Time of Diagnosis

MRI/TEST	NUMBER OF LESIONS	PERCENTAGE OF PATIENTS (%)
Brain MRI	9 or more	65
	4 to 8	15
	Less than 4	20
Spinal cord MRI	2 or more	40
	1	20
	Normal	40
Abnormal CSF		82
Abnormal visual-evoked potential		65

occurs earlier in this disease than in RRMS. The atrophy described in PPMS has a much higher correlation with long-term disability, although several studies have also shown a weaker correlation between T2 lesions and disability [17–22]. Cord atrophy occurs in progressive disease in addition to brain atrophy, and in different studies the degree of atrophy, a lower EDSS at baseline and gray matter mean diffusivity (a measure of diffusion of water), predicts disability [20,23,24]. The small size of the spinal cord limits the precision of atrophy measures using cord imaging.

Advances in MRI technology are also changing our understanding of the pathogenesis of MS subtypes. The nonconventional MRI techniques, magnetization transfer MRI, diffusion tensor MRI, and magnetic resonance spectroscopy, have shown that compared with healthy controls, patients with PPMS have widespread changes to the normal-appearing tissues of the brain and spinal cord in both normal-appearing white matter (NAWM) and especially normal-appearing gray matter (NAGM) [18,25,26]. Measurement of NAWM and NAGM seem to have a higher correlation to disability outcomes and may become useful in the future.

> Newer MRI methods (NAWM, NAGM) have a higher correlation to disability.

TREATMENT

There are currently no FDA-approved treatments to alter the course of PPMS. Although overall results from drug trials have been negative, results have suggested that a subset of PPMS may benefit from disease-modifying therapies. Several factors predict a response to treatment.

> There are no FDA-approved drugs for PPMS.

There have been 2 particularly well-designed trials providing class 1 evidence in PPMS. The PROMIsE trial randomized 943 PPMS patients to treatment with either subcutaneous glatiramer acetate (Copaxone) or placebo and measured sustained progression over 3 years. The study was terminated after only 2 years when a futility analysis demonstrated no difference between glatiramer acetate and placebo. Further subanalysis revealed a trend favoring treatment in more rapidly progressing males. Of interest, patients with a positive spinal fluid tended to have a higher burden of disease on MRI (T2 and Gd lesions) and a faster rate of progression occurred in patients with Gd lesions at baseline [11].

The OLYMPUS study used rituximab (Rituxan), a monoclonal antibody that depletes B cells, in 439 patients in a randomized, double-blind, placebo-controlled trial. Confirmed disability progression was measured over a 2 year period and overall showed no difference between the treated and placebo groups. A preplanned secondary analysis showed that rituximab treated patients who were younger (less than 51 years old), those with 1 or more Gd lesion on a baseline MRI, or a combination of both (less than 54 years old and at least 1 Gd lesion) on a brain MRI at baseline had slowing of disability as compared to placebo, irrespective of disease duration. Further analysis noted that younger patients had a proportionally higher percentage of Gd-positive scans and the slowing of disability in these patients was likely driven by inflammation rather than their younger age. These subgroups, like the male cohort in the PROMIsE trial, had a more rapid rate of progression [27]. A robust beneficial effect of rituximab on T2 lesion volume was noted in the overall treatment group. All patients had positive spinal fluid at baseline, so assessment of the impact of CSF could not be ascertained.

> Studies suggest that younger patients and positive Gd on MRI can predict a response to treatment.

Many other controlled trials have been conducted in PPMS. Proper interpretation of their results is difficult for a variety of reasons, including small sample size, open label design, a lack of a placebo, nonreporting of baseline and study MRI data, inclusion of both PPMS and secondary progressive MS patients, and heterogeneity in baseline patient characteristics entered into the studies. The trials tended to be divided into 2 groups on the basis of patient characteristics; those studies that included only patients with a diagnosis of PPMS and others that selected patients with clinically rapidly progression. Therapies

PPMS Trial Characteristics

	RANDOMIZED	DOUBLE-BLIND	PLACEBO-CONTROLLED	POWERED FOR SIZE	ENTRY CRITERIA PUBLISHED	BASELINE CRITERIA PUBLISHED	MIXED (PPMS/SPMS)	OUTCOME ON DISABILITY
Glatiramer	Yes	Yes	Yes	Yes	Yes	Yes	No	Negative[a]
Rituximab	Yes	Yes	Yes	Yes	Yes	Yes	No	Negative overall; Positive if Gd lesions at baseline
IFN B-1b	Yes	Yes	Yes	No	No	No	No	Negative
IFN B-1a (30 or 60 mcg)	Yes	Yes	Yes	No	Yes	Yes	No	Negative
Mito xantrone	Yes	Yes	Yes	No	Yes	No	No	Negative
Cladribine	Yes	Yes	Yes	No	Yes	Yes	Yes	Negative
IVIG	Yes	Yes	Yes	No	Yes	Yes	Yes	Positive
CYC	Yes	Yes	Yes	No	Yes	Yes	Yes	Negative (Open label trial was positive)
MTX	Yes	Yes	Yes	No	Yes	Yes	Yes	Positive
IV Steroids	No	No	No	No	Yes	Yes	Yes	Positive

CYC, cyclophosphamide; EDSS, Expanded Disability Status Scale; IFN B-1b, interferon beta-1b; IFN B-1a, interferon beta-1a; IVIG, intravenous gamma globulin; MTX, methotrexate.
All trials were planned for a 2 year duration except glatiramer. Glatiramer data is from 2 year interim analysis; study was stopped after this interim analysis.
[a]Data from 2-year interim analysis; study was stopped after this interim analysis.

studied included intravenous and intrathecal steroids, methotrexate, intravenous gamma globulin (IVIG), cladribine, azathioprine, mitoxantrone, cyclophosphamide, and beta interferons (IFN) [1,28–36].

Outcomes were generally mixed, although a slowing of disability was seen with intravenous methylprednisolone [35], methotrexate [32], IVIG [31], and an open label trial of cyclophosphamide [33]. The beta-IFNs and methotrexate trials observed a decrease in Gd-enhancing and T2 lesions on MRI [28,29]. One factor was consistent among all the trials with a positive effect on disability: the enrolled patients had been rapidly progressing prior to entry into the study.

> Treatment tends to have an effect in patients who have been progressing rapidly.

Therefore, several conclusions can be drawn from previous treatment trials; patients with a rapid clinical course

from the onset and certain MRI characteristics (Gd lesion on MRI of the brain) may predict a poorer prognosis but also a greater likelihood of response to therapy. Thus, MRI findings (or early rapid progression) early in the course of the disease may help differentiate those patients that may benefit from treatment. It is not clear whether a certain drug has advantages over others and the risk and benefit to the patient must be considered.

SUMMARY

Although PPMS is a clinically distinct phenotype of MS, it shares many characteristics of RRMS, including genetic determinants, epidemiological similarities, and MRI evidence of inflammation and degeneration. Although a paucity of data exists as compared to RRMS, the evidence suggests that predictive factors including MRI findings and the initial clinical course may identify a group of patients amenable to effective treatment. Further studies to determine appropriate treatments for these patients are needed in the future.

PATIENT CASE 1

A 42-year-old female presented with difficulty running and catching her right toe and tripping. Within 6 months she had progressed, having difficulty walking and she had problems getting on her horse. She was seen by a neurologist, diagnosed with PPMS, and started on IFN beta-1a. She had no slowing of her progression and temporary worsening of her spasticity in her legs due to side effects of the interferon. She was changed to mitoxantrone but continued to progress at a faster rate than before. She then was seen at a university center for a second consultation.

Clinical exam revealed a spastic paraparesis with grade 3+ strength proximally as well as weakness in her hands. Bladder ultrasound showed a post void residual of 250 mL of urine. Her MRI of the head was unremarkable. MRI of the cervical spine was normal. The thoracic MRI showed an intramedullary enhancing lesion from T5 to T8.

A spinal angiogram was done which revealed an arteriovenous fistula (AVM) in the thoracic cord, which was ablated.

Discussion. The initial very rapid progression, followed by a change in the rate of progression is atypical for PPMS. The lack of lesions elsewhere, combined with a long, persistently enhancing lesion in the spinal cord should raise the possibility of another diagnosis, such as an AVM or spinal cord tumor. Sarcoidosis may also have persistently enhancing lesions but the lack of other symptoms after a year of neurological disease makes sarcoidosis a less likely diagnosis.

PATIENT CASE 2

A 32-year-old male presented with a 1 year history of problems with visual blurring, walking difficulties, intermittent hand tremor, and short-term memory problems. He had to take disability from his job 6 months after the onset of symptoms. On exam, he had a bilateral INO and had a tremor in both hands with incoordination and past pointing. Gait was ataxic and wide-based, and mini-mental exam showed impaired short-term memory. He had been started on IFN beta-1a 8 months ago with little effect.

Brain MRI showed multiple deep white matter, juxtacortical, and periventricular lesions, some of which were enhancing, mainly seen throughout the cerebellum and brain stem. MRIs of the cord were normal.

Blood tests were performed and were normal. The CSF showed 3 oligoclonal bands with a minimally elevated IgG index. Gallium scan showed no other evidence of inflammation. Owing to the rapid progression, a brain biopsy was performed that showed demyelination with no evidence of tumor, PML, or vasculitis.

He was started on an immunomodulating therapy.

Discussion. The patient presents with the rare subtype of PPMS that mainly affects the posterior fossa. Owing to the very fast progression, a biopsy was done to rule out infections or a vasculitis. Immunomodulating therapy was used (off label) as the patient was young, had enhancements and was rapidly progressing.

PATIENT CASE 3

A 56-year-old female had a 7 year history of slowly progressive weakness and pain in her legs and thoracolumbar area. Clinically she had a mild bilateral spastic paraparesis, a right afferent papillary defect and a left intranuclear opthalmoplegia. Brain MRI showed bilateral periventricular and juxtacortical lesions, and spine MRI showed nonenhancing lesions at C3, C5, and T2.

She was diagnosed with PPMS and treated with antispasticity medications to reduce the pain in her spine and legs.

She had very mild progression over the next 3 years, and then presented with a 4 month history of rapid progression. Pain had worsened and she had developed increasing bladder problems. MRI of the brain showed 2 new nonenhancing lesions. MRI of the cervical spine was unchanged. MRI of the thoracic cord showed a herniated disc with cord compression at T8.

She underwent neurosurgery for removal of the disc and her neurological exam improved to the point where she was prior to her deterioration.

Discussion. The change in the rate of progression should trigger a search for other causes. Disc disease is common and new MRIs may help aid in the diagnosis.

KEY POINTS FOR PATIENTS AND FAMILIES

- PPMS can be misdiagnosed as other conditions, including foot or spine problems, and a delay in diagnosis is common.

- An MRI of the upper or mid spine (cervical or thoracic) is more useful than the lower spine (lumbar).

- The most common symptom is weakness and stiffness in the legs and exercise, including stretching, is very important to maintain mobility.

- Other conditions can coexist with PPMS and abrupt changes in the rate of progression are unusual. Checking with your doctor for other causes is important.

- An MRI of the brain performed intermittently can be important to assess whether therapy may be helpful.

- Certain therapies may be helpful to slow progression in some patients; however, therapeutics may have risks and a specific discussion of the benefit and risks of each drug is important.

REFERENCES

1. Miller DH, Leary SM. Primary-progressive multiple sclerosis. *Lancet Neurol.* 2007;6(10):903–912.

2. Leary S, Thompson A. Primary progressive multiple sclerosis. *CNS Drugs.* 2005;19(6):369–376.

3. Stevenson VL, Miller DH, Rovaris M, et al. Primary and transitional progressive MS: A clinical and MRI cross-sectional study. *Neurology.* 1999;52:839–845.

4. Vasconcelos CC, Fernández O, Leyva L, et al. Does the DRB1*1501 allele confer more severe and faster progression in primary progressive multiple sclerosis patients? *J Neuroimmunol.* 2009;214:101–103.

5. Hauser SL, Oksenberg JR. The neurobiology of multiple sclerosis: Genes, inflammation, and neurodegeneration. *Neuron.* 2006;52(1):61–76.

6. Camp SJ, Stevenson VL, Thompson AJ, et al. A longitudinal study of cognition in primary progressive multiple sclerosis. *Brain.* 2005;128(Pt 12):2891–2898.

7. Boissy A, Cohen J. Multiple sclerosis symptom management. *Expert Rev Neurother.* 2007;9:1213–1222.

8. Tremlett H, Paty D, Devonshire V. The natural history of primary progressive MS in British Columbia, Canada. *Neurology.* 2005;65(12):1919–1923.

9. Polman CH, Reingold SC, Edan G, et al. Diagnostic criteria for multiple sclerosis: 2005 revisions to the "McDonald criteria." *Ann Neurol.* 2005;58(6):840–846.

10. Sahraian M, Eshaghi O. Role of MRI in diagnosis and treatment of multiple sclerosis. *Clin Neurol Neurosurg.* 2010;112(7):609–615.

11. Wolinsky JS, Narayana PA, O'Connor P, et al. Glatiramer acetate in primary progressive multiple sclerosis: Results of a multinational, multicenter, double-blind, placebo-controlled trial. *Ann Neurol.* 2007;61(1):14–24.

12. Thompson AJ, Kermode AG, MacManus DG, et al. Patterns of disease activity in multiple sclerosis: Clinical and magnetic resonance imaging study. *BMJ.* 1990;300:631–634.

13. Ingle GT, Sastre-Garriga J, Miller DH, Thompson AJ. Is inflammation important in early PPMS?: A longitudinal MRI study. *J Neurol Neurosurg Psychiatry.* 2005;76(9):1255–1258.

14. Ingle GT, Stevenson VL, Miller DH, et al. Two-year follow-up study of primary and transitional progressive multiple sclerosis. *Mult Scler.* 2002;8(2):108–114.

15. Lycklama à Nijeholt GJ, Van Wlderveen MA, Castelijins JA, et al. Brain and spinal cord abnormalities in multiple sclerosis. Correlation between MRI parameters, clinical subtypes and symptoms. *Brain.* 1998;121:687–697.

16. Kidd D, Thorpe JW, Thompson AJ, et al. Spinal cord MRI using multi-array coils and fast spin echo. II. Findings in multiple sclerosis. *Neurology.* 1993;43(12):2632–2637.

17. Ramio-Torrenta L, Sastre-Garriga J, Ingle GT, et al. Abnormalities in normal appearing tissues in early primary progressive multiple sclerosis and their relation to disability: A tissue specific magnetisation transfer study. *J Neurol Neurosurg Psychiatry.* 2006;77(1):40–45.

18. Filippi M, Rovaris M, Rocca MA. Imaging primary progressive multiple sclerosis: The contribution of structural, metabolic, and functional MRI techniques. *Mult Scler.* 2004;10(Suppl 1):S36–S44.

19. Sastre-Garriga J, Ingle GT, Chard DT, et al. Grey and white matter volume changes in early primary progressive multiple sclerosis: A longitudinal study. *Brain.* 2005;128(Pt 6):1454–1460.

20. Khaleeli Z, Ciccarelli O, Manfredonia F, et al. Predicting progression in primary progressive multiple sclerosis: A ten year multicenter study. *Ann Neurol.* 2008;63(6):790–793.

21. Confavreux C, Vukusic S. Accumulation of irreversible disability in multiple sclerosis: From epidemiology to treatment. *Clin Neurol Neurosurg.* 2006;108(3):327–332.

22. Filippi M, Rocca MA. MR Imaging of gray matter involvement in multiple sclerosis: Implications for understanding disease pathophysiology and monitoring treatment efficacy. *AJNR.* 2010;31(7):1171–1177.

23. Losseff NA, Webb SL, O'Riordan JI, et al. Spinal cord atrophy and disability in multiple sclerosis. A new reproducible and sensitive MRI method with potential to monitor disease progression. *Brain.* 1996;119(Pt 3):701–708.

24. Rovaris M, Judica E, Gallo A, et al. Grey matter damage predicts the evolution of primary progressive multiple sclerosis at 5 years. *Brain.* 2006;129(Pt 10):2628–2634.

25. Rovaris M, Judica E, Sastre-Garriga J, et al. Large-scale, multicentre, quantitative MRI study of brain and cord damage in primary progressive multiple sclerosis. *Mult Scler.* 2008;14:455–464.

26. Filippi M, Agosta F. Magnetization transfer MRI in multiple sclerosis. *J Neuroimaging.* 2007;17(Suppl 1):22S–26S.

27. Hawker K, O'Connor P, Freedman MS, et al. Efficacy and safety of rituximab in patients with primary progressive multiple sclerosis: Results of a randomized, double-blind, placebo-controlled, multicenter trial. *Ann Neurol.* 2009;66(4):460–471.

28. Leary SM, Miller DH, Stevenson VL, et al. Interferon beta-1a in primary progressive MS: An exploratory, randomized, controlled trial. *Neurology.* 2003;60(1):44–51.

29. Montalban X. Overview of European pilot study of interferon beta-Ib in primary progressive multiple sclerosis. *Mult Scler.* 2004;10(Suppl 1):S62–S64.

30. Stüve O, Kita M, Pelletier D, et al. Mitoxantrone as a potential therapy for primary progressive multiple sclerosis. *Mult Scler.* 2004;10(Suppl 1):S58–S61.

31. Pohlau D, Przuntek H, Sailer M, et al. Intravenous immunoglobulin in primary and secondary progressive multiple sclerosis: A randomized, controlled multicenter study. *Mult Scler.* 2007;13(9):1007–1017.

32. Goodkin DE, Rudick RA, VanderBrug MS, et al. Low-dose (7.5 mg) oral methotrexate is effective in reducing the rate of progression of neurological impairment in patients with chronic progressive multiple sclerosis. *Ann Neurol.* 1995;37:30–40.

33. Zephir H, de Seze J, Duhamel A, et al. Treatment of progressive forms of multiple sclerosis by cyclophosphamide: A cohort study of 490 patients. *J Neurol Sci.* 2004;218:73–77.

34. Rice G, Filippi M, Comi G, et al. The Cladribine Clinical Study Group and for the Cladribine MRI Study Group. Cladribine and progressive MS: Clinical and MRI outcomes of a multicenter controlled trial. *Neurology.* 2000;54:1145–1155.

35. Pirko I, Rodriguez M. Pulsed intravenous methylprednisolone therapy in progressive multiple sclerosis: Need for a Controlled Trial. *Arch Neurol.* 2004;61:1148–1149.

36. Hoffmann V, Kuhn W, Schimrigk S, et al. Repeat intrathecal triamcinolone acetonide application is beneficial in progressive MS patients. *Eur J Neurol.* 2006;13(1):72–76.

15

Secondary Progressive Multiple Sclerosis

ALESSANDRO SERRA
ROBERT J. FOX

KEY POINTS FOR CLINICIANS

- Secondary progressive multiple sclerosis (SPMS) is defined as an initial relapsing-remitting disease followed by gradual clinical progression with or without relapses.

- About 50% of patients with relapsing-remitting MS (RRMS) develop SPMS within 10 years from onset of the disease.

- Increasing evidence support the theory that degenerative changes are more predominant in progressive forms of MS whereas focal infiltrative inflammation is more typical of relapsing forms.

- As overt inflammation plays a minor role in SPMS, disease-modifying therapies (DMT) are generally less effective, while health maintenance and rehabilitation are particularly important for patients in this stage.

- Future therapy developments should aim at slowing degeneration and promoting neuroaxonal repair and remyelination.

Secondary progressive multiple sclerosis (SPMS) was defined by a panel of experts as "an initial relapsing-remitting disease followed by progression with or without relapses, minor remissions and plateaus" [1]. Several epidemiological studies have shown that up to 50% of initial relapsing MS cases evolve into a progressive phase within 10 years of onset [2]. However, when also including patients presenting with a distinct clinically isolated syndrome (CIS) [3], a more realistic estimate of the median time between relapsing disease onset and secondary progression phase in the general MS population is about 19 years [4].

The secondary progressive phase of MS is characterized by worsening of neurological impairment both with superimposed relapses or, more typically, without. This is in contrast to the relapsing phase of the disease, where (by definition) patients do not get worse gradually between relapses although they might recover only partially from an exacerbation.

One problem posed in clinical practice, which in turn limits the development of effective therapeutic strategies, is the difficulty of precisely identifying the date of transition to disease progression, which is typically defined as a period of about 6 to 12 months of continuous worsening following the relapsing phase. Thus, such change in the disease course can be estimated only retrospectively and perhaps when the pathogenetic process leading to accumulation of fixed disability is already at an advanced stage. Furthermore, reliable clinical and laboratory predictors of time to transition to the secondary progressive phase of MS have not been clearly identified, which again creates difficulties when designing clinical trials. However, a few factors have been shown in most studies to be associated with a shorter time interval to progression: advanced age at onset of disease; initial presentation with sensory, visual, and brain stem-related symptoms; an incomplete recovery from the initial exacerbations; a higher number of relapses during the first 2 to 5 years; and a higher disability score early in the disease [3,5–8]. More controversial seems to be the notion that men with RRMS develop secondary progression faster than women, as many but not all studies have shown such a trend [3,5–7].

> SPMS = 6 to 12 months of continuous clinical worsening.

UNDERLYING PATHOGENESIS

While clearly distinct pathogenetic hallmarks of progression in MS have not been identified, there is growing evidence that focal infiltrative inflammation, predominant in the relapsing-remitting phase, eventually subsides leaving neuroaxonal degeneration and often diffuse inflammation as the most predominant aspects of secondary (as well as primary) progression. In this respect, a few pathological studies have shown reduced inflammatory activity in and around lesions in SPMS, although this activity seems to be still more prominent than in primary progressive MS lesions. In SPMS, diffuse axonal loss and diffuse inflammation are also evident [9,10]. What immunological phenomena and molecular and cellular mechanisms actually drive the shift from a predominantly infiltrative "inflammatory" relapsing-remitting course to a mostly "degenerative" secondary progressive stage is unknown. An alternative explanation comes from a whole different concept of MS as a disease [11]. According to this view, the "inside-out" hypothesis, the underlying *primum movens* of the disease in MS would be a "cytodegeneration" involving the olygodendrocytes and myelin, beginning years before any clinical manifestation. According to this hypothesis, it would then be the level of the host's imunocompetency and intensity of response to highly autoantigenic components, released as a consequence of degeneration, to determine the episodes of inflammation that correspond to clinical relapses. Thus, at one end of the spectrum people with an immune system particularly predisposed to react to antigens would present with aggressive tumefactive MS (the so called Marburg variant) [12], while at the other end of the spectrum those with a weaker immune system would exhibit a classic primary progressive course with few or no relapses. The majority of MS patients who present with the typical relapsing-remitting course would be those within these 2 extremes of immunological response. When these patients exhaust the immune responsiveness, a secondary

progressive course takes place where the initial underlying neurodegeneration is again the main protagonist [11]. The authors who propose this hypothesis also argue that the most-used animal model for MS, the experimental autoimmune encephalomyelitis (EAE) [13], which reproduces mostly inflammatory changes, may not be an accurate representation of the underlying disease mechanisms, whereas other models of neurodegeneration, such as the cuprizone model of copper deficiency-related central nervous system (CNS) demyelination [14], would be a better representation of the MS degenerative stage and an ideal ground for testing drugs' efficacy in SPMS.

> Immunopathology of transition from RRMS to SPMS is unknown.

Finally, this view is in accordance with recent evidence that chronic oxidative axonal damage and chronic demyelination in progressive MS might accelerate and amplify neurodegeneration because of exhausted brain functional reserve capacity due to accumulation of tissue damage despite decreased tissue inflammation [15].

> MS might be originally a neurodegenerative disease with later superimposed inflammation.

EVALUATION AND TREATMENT

In clinical practice, identification of the exact time when MS transitions from the relapsing-remitting to the progressive phase is not easy and usually a retrospective estimation is the only possible way. This clearly represents a management challenge, especially when deciding on further management (which may include stopping a certain DMT), for example in cases where secondary progression is still accompanied by occasional relapses. As a general guide, a patient is considered to have entered a progressive phase if disability progresses continuously for 6 to 12 months. Thus, in evaluating a patient in this stage of the disease, it is essential to focus on new onset symptoms and gradual worsening of preexisting ones that can negatively affect daily functioning, along with relying on objective scales to quantify disability and quality of life.

While MRI is paramount in driving evaluation and therapeutic decisions in RRMS, its utility in SPMS is not as obvious and markers of disease progression are less defined. However, a few MRI findings may help guide the clinician's assessment in distinguishing between relapsing phase and progression: (a) In general, the average burden of brain T2 hyperintense lesions in SPMS compared to RRMS tends to be higher, as well as the load of focal spinal cord lesions; (b) The number of gadolinium-enhancing lesions tends to be less in SPMS than in RRMS; (c) The number of T1 hypointense lesions tend to be more in SPMS than in RRMS [16].

Because of the lack of reliable discriminants between RRMS and SPMS, the challenge of how to predict onset and time to onset of progression in a patient with typical RRMS remains. In this regard, evidence suggest that the distribution pattern of cerebral atrophy, rather than the rate of atrophy accumulation, and the frequency of large and ring-enhancing lesions are possibly predictive of subsequent Expanded Disability Status Scale (EDSS) worsening [16].

As a consequence of focal inflammation and corresponding clinical relapses being less prominent in progressive MS, the overall goal of SPMS management lies in promoting rehabilitation and health maintenance to allow acceptable daily functioning. In fact, DMTs have shown to be only marginally effective in this stage of the disease. Here, we briefly review the most important clinical trials to date in SPMS.

Interferon Beta

There have been four large-scale, double-blind, randomized, placebo-controlled studies to assess the effectiveness of IFN-beta in SPMS (see Table 15.1): (a) The European multicenter trial on IFN beta-1b in SPMS (EUSPMS) [17] studied 718 patients treated with either IFN beta-1b or placebo for up to 3 years with the primary outcome being the time to confirmed progression of disability (ie, sustained increase in EDSS for at least 3 months). While this study showed that disability progression was significantly delayed in treated patients, subgroup analysis suggested that the patients who benefited the most from treatment and had associated better health-related quality of life were those who had a high prestudy relapse rate; (b) The SP Efficacy Trial of Rebif

(IFN beta-1a) in MS (SPECTRIMS) [18] studied 618 patients who received IFN beta-1a or placebo for 3 years with the primary outcome being time to confirmed progression in disability. While this study showed no significant benefit from active treatment, a trend of greater benefit in women and in patients who had reported more than one relapse in the 2 years before the study was suggested; (c) The North American Study of IFN beta-1b in SPMS (NASPMS) [19] studied 939 patients who were randomly assigned placebo or IFN beta-1b with the primary end point being time to confirmed progression of disability (ie, EDSS increase sustained for 6 months or more). This study was stopped early because of a lack of efficacy; (d) The International MS SP Avonex Clinical Trial (IMPACT) [20] study included 436 patients who were randomized to receive IFN beta-1a or placebo with the primary outcome measure being "baseline to month 24" change in the MS functional composite (MSFC). Active treatment had no significant effect on EDSS, but did show a benefit on MSFC.

> Only the European trial has shown efficacy of IFN-beta on slowing disability in SPMS.

Among these studies, the EUSPMS was the only trial to show a significant positive effect of treatment on the accumulation of sustained disability, which characterizes the secondary progressive phase of MS, as measured by EDSS. This led to approval of IFN beta-1b in Europe as a DMT in SPMS. On the other hand, not surprisingly, all these studies showed significant positive effects of treatment on relapse rate in SPMS, increase in T2 lesion load, and MRI measures of MS activity. It has been suggested that the differences among these studies could have been due, at least in part, to the different patient populations included.

TABLE 15.1
Placebo-Controlled Trials of IFN-Beta in SPMS

STUDY	TREATMENT REGIMENS	N	OUTCOME	RESULT
European multicenter trial on IFN beta-1b in SPMS (EUSPMS) [17]	Either IFN beta-1b or placebo for up to 3 years	718	Sustained increase in EDSS for at least 3 months	Disability progression was significantly delayed in treated patients
The SP Efficacy Trial of Rebif (IFN beta-1a) in MS (SPECTRIMS) [18]	IFN beta-1a (22 mcg or 44 mcg) or placebo subcutaneously 3 times per week for 3 years	618	Time to confirmed progression in disability	No significant benefit from active treatment
The North American Study of IFN beta-1b in SPMS (NASPMS) [19]	Placebo, an IFN beta-1b dose of 8 million IU, or an IFN beta-1b dose adjusted for bodyweight and size (5 million IU/mL)	939	EDSS increase sustained for 6 months or more	Study stopped early because of lack of efficacy
The International MS SP Avonex Clinical Trial (IMPACT) [20]	IFN beta-1a (60 mcg) or placebo by weekly intramuscular injections for 2 years	436	"Baseline to month 24 change" in the MSFC	Active treatment had no significant effect on EDSS

EDSS, Expanded Disability Status Scale; MSFC, MS functional composite; N, number.

Intravenous Immunoglobulins

Intravenous immunoglobulin efficacy (1 g/kg administered every 4 weeks for 26 months) was assessed in 318 patients who exhibited clinically active SPMS during the preceding 2 years. The results of this study showed no significant effect of treatment on time to EDSS sustained increase, relapse rates, or T2 lesion load on MRI [21,22].

Immunosuppressants

Several agents, such as methotrexate, cladribine, cyclophosphamide, methylprednisolone, azathioprine, cyclosporine, and mitoxantrone have been used in patients with SPMS: (a) Methylprednisolone was administered every other month for up to 2 years to 108 patients with SPMS [23]. This study showed that treatment with high-dose methylprednisolone might have a modest benefit in delaying time to onset of sustained progression of disability; (b) Controlled and uncontrolled trials of cyclophosphamide have reported a strong effect in patients with SPMS with poor response to other disease-modifying treatments, while other studies did not confirm these benefits [24,25]; (c) Intravenous cladribine, an antineoplastic drug approved for the treatment of hairy-cell leukemia, did not show any clinical benefit in a phase 3 trial of progressive MS [26]; (d) Mitoxantrone, a synthetic anthracenedione chemotherapeutic agent with broad immunosuppressive and cytotoxic activity, was used in the "Mitoxantrone in MS Study" (MIMS) [27,28] which included 194 patients with worsening RRMS or SPMS. While patients treated with mitoxantrone had significant benefit at 24 months, this effect was reported in the total group and not specifically in those patients with SPMS. Mitoxantrone is the only FDA-approved treatment for SPMS, but its use is limited by rare but potentially serious adverse effects such as bone-marrow suppression, dose-related cardiotoxicity, and lymphoproliferative disorders including leukemia; (e) Alemtuzumab, a humanized antileukocyte monoclonal antibody, which causes prolonged T-lymphocyte depletion, was shown to reduce the relapse rate and conventional MRI activity in 36 patients with SPMS who were followed for more than 8 years [29,30]. However, sustained accumulation of disability was unaffected as demonstrated by progressive cerebral atrophy on follow-up MRI scans.

> Immunosuppressive therapies are used with caution in progressive MS because of the potentially serious side effects.

Finally, a number of trials are underway to test efficacy of other medications such as fingolimod and laquinimod in slowing neurodegeneration in progressive MS.

CONCLUSIONS

The majority of patients with MS present with a typical relapsing-remitting course followed in 10 years or more by a secondary phase where progression of disability occurs steadily over 6 to 12 months with or without associated clinical relapses. This phase is characterized by accumulation of T2 lesion burden on MRI and progressive cerebral atrophy. Although the immunopathology of this transition is not understood, it seems that recurring focal inflammation typical of RRMS plays only a marginal role in SPMS, which is reflected by the limited efficacy of DMT shown by several international trials. This poses problems in clinical practice when the neurologist is faced with the decision of whether to continue a DMT in a patient who is worsening or to try a stronger agent, and deal with its potential side effects, in an attempt to slow down the progression. This is further complicated by the difficulty of determining when a patient with RRMS has entered the secondary progressive phase, as explained earlier.

In general, particular attention by the clinician to the disability score and its progression, especially in the 6 to 12 months period, should be the main aspect of the clinical assessment. As the relapsing-remitting phase subsides and the patient enters the progressive phase, typically without relapses, the challenge is whether to discontinue DMTs previously employed. Although no guidelines are available on when exactly to stop the treatment, population studies conducted in the United States have shown that DMTs are unlikely to be cost effective in progressive forms of the disease, and that their cost-effectiveness is maximized if started early in the relapsing phase and stopped when the patient requires nursing home care [31]. In SPMS, it is reasonable to stop the DMT if the burden of treatment (eg, costs, side effects) outweighs perceived potential benefits (eg, relapse rate reduction, stability of MRI disease burden). Immunosuppressive therapies, such as mitoxantrone, should be used with caution in selected cases because of possible serious side effects. Thus, the focus of management in SPMS should be switched to health maintenance, physical rehabilitation, and treatment of chronic disabling symptoms such as fatigue, including energy conservation strategies [32], spasticity, and bladder, bowel, and sexual dysfunction. The efforts of a multidisciplinary rehabilitation approach in this phase should be directed at maximizing functional independence and safety, minimizing complications due to decreased mobility, restoring and maintaining function, and improving quality of life.

The future of SPMS management is to develop effective therapeutic strategies that target neuroaxonal loss and cerebral atrophy promoting axonal repair and remyelination, based on models of disease that more accurately reflect the underlying immunopathology of the progressive phase.

PATIENT CASE

A 44-year-old woman with a 20-year history of initially RRMS, who has not seen a neurologist for the past 2 years, presents to the clinic complaining of increasing fatigue and spasticity. You learn from the history that she had her last relapse, treated with IV methylprednisolone, 10 years ago and that afterward her functioning, in particular her gait, got slowly worse without further relapses. In fact, she started using a cane to walk at age 35, a rollator at age 37, and she is wheelchair-bound since age 41. She was on Copaxone before, which was stopped 8 years ago. Her last brain MRI 2 years ago was stable.

Question: What evaluation is needed? What management do you recommend?

Answer: The clinical picture is mostly consistent with SPMS and the focus of the evaluation should be on assessing and quantifying disability and quality of life with standard scales. A major portion of the treatment plan should be directed at maximizing independent functioning through a MS-specific physical therapy program. Management of disabling symptoms such as fatigue and spasticity is imperative. While spasticity can be managed by a specialized MS team that might include Botox use along with physical therapy and stretching exercises, fatigue is more challenging to manage. First, causes for secondary fatigue such as poor sleep and depression should be assessed and treated. Then, medications such as amantadine, modafinil, or amphetamine/dextroamphetamine should be tried although their effectiveness might be limited. Finally, energy conservation strategies might be beneficial in improving interference of fatigue with daily functioning. Education and monitoring for complications arising from decreased mobility, such as infections, is also crucial in this phase.

KEY POINTS FOR PATIENTS AND FAMILIES

- SPMS is a form of MS that follows relapsing MS. In this stage, patients may still get relapses but in between relapses gradually worsen over time.

- Patients with SPMS who continue to have either relapses or new MRI lesions may benefit from DMTs.

- There is no MRI or clinical sign that diagnoses SPMS; it is based on the course of the disease.

REFERENCES

1. Lublin FD, Reingold SC, for the National Multiple Sclerosis Society (USA) Advisory Committee on Clinical Trials of New Agents in Multiple Sclerosis. Defining the clinical course of multiple sclerosis: Results of an international survey. *Neurology*. 1996;46:907–911.

2. Weinshenker BG, Bass B, Rice GP, et al. The natural history of multiple sclerosis: A geographically based study I: Clinical course and disability. *Brain*. 1989;112:133–146.

3. Eriksson M, Andersen O, Runmarker B. Long-term follow-up of patients with clinically isolated syndromes, relapsing-remitting and secondary progressive multiple sclerosis. *Mult Scler*. 2003;9:260–274.

4. Confavreux C, Compston DAS. The natural history of multiple sclerosis. In: Compston DAS, ed. *McAlpine's Multiple Sclerosis*, 4th ed. London: Churchill-Livingstone; 2005.

5. Confavreux C, Aimard G, Devic M. Course and prognosis of multiple sclerosis assessed by the computerized data processing of 349 patients. *Brain*. 1980;103:281–300.

6. Vukusic S, Confavreux C. Prognostic factors for progression of disability in the secondary progressive phase of multiple sclerosis. *J Neurol Sci*. 2003;206:135–137.

7. Amato MP, Ponziani G. A prospective study on the prognosis of multiple sclerosis. *Neurol Sci*. 2000;21(Suppl 2):831–838.

8. Müller R. Studies on disseminated sclerosis: With special reference to symptomatology, course and prognosis. *Acta Med Scand*. 1949;133(Suppl 222):1–214.

9. Prineas JW, Kwon EE, Cho ES, et al. Immunopathology of secondary-progressive multiple sclerosis. *Ann Neurol*. 2001;50:646–657.

10. Kutzelnigg A, Lucchinetti CF, Stadelmann C, et al. Cortical demyelination and diffuse white matter injury in multiple sclerosis. *Brain*. 2005;128:2705–2712.

11. Stys PK, Zamponi GW, van Minnen J, Geurts JJ. Will the real multiple sclerosis please stand up? *Nat Rev Neurosci.* 2012 Jun 20;13(7):507–514.

12. Capello E, Mancardi GL. Marburg type and Balò's concentric sclerosis: Rare and acute variants of multiple sclerosis. *Neurol Sci.* 2004 Nov;25(Suppl 4):S361–S363.

13. Pachner AR. Experimental models of multiple sclerosis. *Curr Opin Neurol.* 2011 Jun;24(3):291–299.

14. Kipp M, Clarner T, Dang J, et al. The cuprizone animal model: New insights into an old story. *Acta Neuropathol.* 2009 Dec;118(6):723–736.

15. Lassmann H, van Horssen J, Mahad D. Progressive multiple sclerosis: Pathology and pathogenesis. *Nat Rev Neurol.* 2012 Sep 25;168. [Epub ahead of print]

16. Rovaris M, Confavreux C, Furlan R, et al. Secondary progressive multiple sclerosis: Current knowledge and future challenges. *Lancet Neurol.* 2006 Apr;5(4):343–354.

17. European Study Group on interferon β-1b in secondary progressive MS. Placebo-controlled multicentre randomised trial of interferon beta-1b in treatment of secondary progressive multiple sclerosis. *Lancet.* 1998;352:1491–1497.

18. Secondary Progressive Efficacy Clinical Trial of Recombinant Interferon-beta-1a in MS (SPECTRIMS) Study Group. Randomized controlled trial of interferon-beta-1a in secondary progressive MS: Clinical results. *Neurology.* 2001;56:1496–1504.

19. Panitch H, Miller A, Paty D, et al. Interferon beta-1b in secondary progressive MS: Results from a 3-year controlled study. *Neurology.* 2004;63:1788–1795.

20. Cohen JA, Cutter GR, Fischer JS, et al. Benefit of interferon beta-1a on MSFC progression in secondary progressive MS. *Neurology.* 2002;59:679–687.

21. Hommes OR, Sorensen PS, Fazekas F, et al. Intravenous immunoglobulin in secondary progressive multiple sclerosis: Randomised placebo-controlled trial. *Lancet.* 2004;364:1149–1156.

22. Fazekas F, Sorensen PS, Filippi M, et al. MRI results from the European study on intravenous immunoglobulin in secondary progressive multiple sclerosis (ESIMS). *Mult Scler.* 2005;11: 433–440.

23. Goodkin DE, Kinkel RP, Weinstock-Guttman B, et al. A phase II study of i.v. methylprednisolone in secondary-progressive multiple sclerosis. *Neurology.* 1998;51:239–245.

24. La Mantia L, Eoli M, Salmaggi A, et al. Cyclophosphamide in chronic progressive multiple sclerosis: A comparative study. *Ital J Neurol Sci.* 1998;19:32–36.

25. The Canadian Cooperative Multiple Sclerosis Study Group. The Canadian cooperative trial of cyclophosphamide and plasma exchange in progressive multiple sclerosis. *Lancet.* 1991;337:441–446.

26. Rice GP, Filippi M, Comi G. Cladribine and progressive MS: Clinical and MRI outcomes of a multicenter controlled trial. *Neurology.* 2000;54:1145–1155.

27. Hartung HP, Gonsette R, Konig N, et al. Mitoxantrone in progressive multiple sclerosis: A placebo-controlled, double-blind, randomised, multicentre trial. *Lancet.* 2002;360: 2018–2025.

28. Krapf H, Morrissey SP, Zenker O, et al. Effect of mitoxantrone on MRI in progressive MS: Results of the MIMS trial. *Neurology.* 2005;65:690–695.

29. Coles AJ, Wing MG, Molyneux P, et al. Monoclonal antibody treatment exposes three mechanisms underlying the clinical course of multiple sclerosis. *Ann Neurol.* 1999;46:296–304.

30. Paolillo A, Coles AJ, Molyneux P, et al. Quantitative MRI in patients with secondary progressive MS treated with monoclonal antibody Campath 1H. *Neurology.* 1999;53: 751–757.

31. Noyes K, Bajorska A, Chappel A, et al. Cost-effectiveness of disease-modifying therapy for multiple sclerosis: A population-based study. *Neurology.* 2011 Jul 26;77(4):355–363.

32. Mathiowetz VG, Finlayson ML, Matuska KM, et al. Randomized controlled trial of an energy conservation course for persons with multiple sclerosis. *Mult Scler.* 2005 Oct;11(5): 592–601.

16

Emerging Therapies for Relapsing Multiple Sclerosis

DANIEL ONTANEDA
ROBERT J. FOX

There have been significant improvements in the treatment of multiple sclerosis (MS) over the last 20 years. The FDA approved 8 disease-modifying agents for use in relapsing forms of the disease [1]. A combination of incomplete effectiveness, inconvenient routes of administration, and safety concerns with currently approved agents have stimulated the search for better therapies. This chapter provides a brief overview of the overall process through which MS therapies are developed (see Table 16.1), followed by a description of therapies in the late stages of development (see Table 16.2).

DEVELOPMENT OF MS THERAPEUTICS

Animal Models

The first step in the development of successful therapeutics is a basic understanding of the physiology and biology of the underlying disease. Experimental animal models of human disease serve both to understand disease processes and also to test potential therapeutic compounds with targets along the pathogenic pathway of the disease. Experimental autoimmune encephalomyelitis (EAE) is the principal animal model used to emulate MS. EAE is induced through either the inoculation of myelin and other brain proteins or through adoptive transfer of lymphocytes reactive to the same proteins. Models have been developed for relapsing MS and optic neuritis, with more limited models of progressive MS [2]. The possibility of screening a large variety of compounds in animal models has led to the development of several approved medications for MS, including mitoxantrone, glatiramer acetate, fingolimod, and natalizumab [3]. Despite these successes, EAE is still an imperfect model of MS and the majority of agents which show promise in EAE have not shown beneficial effects in humans—and some have even shown paradoxical proinflammatory responses in

humans [4]. Standardized scoring systems, dosing regimens, medication delivery, and careful selection of EAE models are all important features in order to identify compounds at a high success rate. More recently, several other animal models including autoimmune demyelination (as opposed to induced demyelination) in zebrafish and neurodegeneration also in zebrafish have shown promise [5].

> Experimental animal models of human disease serve both to understand disease processes and also to test potential therapeutic compounds with targets along the pathogenic pathway of the disease.

Phase 1 Trials

Once potential therapeutics have been identified, through animal models or through repositioning (compounds derived from experience in other conditions that carry some shared feature with MS), agents enter a clinical trial stage during which human safety is evaluated in patients or healthy controls. Phase 1 trials involve establishing a dose at which adverse effects are tolerable and also assessing the pharmacodynamic properties of the compound. Typical outcomes for these types of trials include the presence of dose-limiting toxicity and side effects. The study is typically carried out in a small group of subjects and involves a dose escalation regimen. A "3 + 3" design is commonly used where an initial group of 3 patients receives a dose, and this dose is increased in subsequent participants only if all participants do not experience toxicity. If toxicity is observed, an additional 3 patients are treated and the dose is escalated only if 1 (or none) of the subjects experience toxicity. Otherwise, the maximum tolerated dose is considered to be that level. Several accelerated titration designs are now being

TABLE 16.1
Phases of Drug Developments in MS

	PRIMARY PURPOSE	PARTICIPANTS/ARMS	PRIMARY OUTCOMES	DURATION	ESTIMATED SAMPLE SIZE
Preclinical	Identify compounds and effectiveness along certain pathways; screen for animal toxicity	Animal Models, EAE	EAE clinical scoring	25–40 days	10–20
Phase 1	Dose finding (for toxicity)	Treatment arm only	Dose limiting toxicity Maximum tolerated dose Minimum tolerated dose	1–6 months	20–80
Phase 2	Dose finding (for efficacy)	Treatment arm Placebo arm Active comparator arm	GAD lesions T2 lesion volume Enlarging lesions Brain atrophy measures	12–24 months	100–300
Phase 3	Definitive efficacy and safety	Treatment arm Placebo arm Active comparator arm	ARR Proportion of relapse free Confirmed EDSS disability progression	24–36 months	500–1500
Phase 4	Postmarketing studies	Open label treatments	Relapse rate EDSS progression Safety measures	1–10+ years	Variable

ARR, annualized relapse rate; EAE, experimental autoimmune encephalomyelitis; EDSS, Expanded Disability Status Score; GAD, gadolinium enhancing.

used which minimize participant exposure to lower tolerable doses without clinical effects using stochastic simulations [6].

> Phase 1 trials involve establishing a dose at which adverse effects are tolerable and also assessing the pharmacodynamic properties of the compound.

Phase 2 Trials

The principal objective of phase 2 trials is to establish the activity of investigational compounds at several doses. Typically, the trials are powered to detect differences in biological markers of disease, in part to limit the size and expense of the study. An investigational compound is compared against either placebo or a standard therapy (active comparator). Treatment assignment is randomized, and typically allocation is concealed (ie, patients and investigators are not able to tell what arm the patient would be randomized to). MS phase 2 trials typically involve repeated MRI as the primary outcome [7]. When studying immunomodulating agents, inflammatory measures of disease activity are used, such as new gadolinium enhancing (GAD) lesions, new combined unique lesions (GAD and T2), and T2 lesions volume. Scans are typically acquired every 4 to 6 weeks to ensure enhancing lesions are captured, and the duration of these studies is typically 6 to 12 months. Measures related to disease progression in phase 2 trials sometimes include brain atrophy metrics. Potential

measures of neuroprotection such as T1 black hole conversion have also been proposed and used. Safety and tolerability is also assessed during phase 2 studies and in many occasions toxicities are first identified at this stage.

> MS phase 2 trials involve a repeated MRI as the primary outcome.

Phase 3 Trials

Phase 3 studies determine the clinical efficacy and safety of investigational compounds in a broad population and serve as the definitive evidence for submission to regulatory agencies for approval and marketing. In phase 3 trials, participants are randomized to the investigational drug and either placebo or an active comparator. Wherever possible, treatment assignment is also blinded. The primary outcomes of phase 3 trials are typically clinical measures with significant relevance to patient's function. Phase 3 trials are powered to detect changes in these clinical end points which are typically less sensitive to change than MRI markers. Consequently, phase 3 studies typically involve over 1,000 patients, which require multiple study sites in various countries and continents. Study duration is normally 24 months or more, and the study may involve different stages where participants are crossed over from placebo to active medication. These studies also commonly have extension phases where the longer-term safety and tolerability of

TABLE 16.2
Emerging Therapies in MS

	MECHANISM OF ACTION	ROUTE OF ADMINISTRATION/DOSE	EVIDENCE OF EFFICACY/ONGOING TRIALS	SAFETY CONCERNS/ADVERSE EFFECTS
Dimethyl fumarate (BG-12)	Activates nuclear factor E2 related factor 2. Anti-inflammatory, antioxidant, neuroprotectant effects	PO 240 mg BID or 240 mg TID	Phase 3: DECIDE (vs. placebo) ARR reduction (48%–53%) Disability reduction (34%–38%) Phase 3: CONFIRM (vs. placebo) ARR reduction (44%–51%) Disability reduction (21%–24%)	Flushing, gastrointestinal intolerance Risk mitigation strategies: • Baseline and annual CBC
Teriflunomide	Inhibition of dihydroorotate dehydrogenase Inhibits de novo pyrimidine synthesis	PO 7 mg daily or 14 mg daily	Phase 3: TEMSO (vs. placebo) ARR reduction 31% Disability reduction 29.8% (14 mg dose) Phase 3: TOWERS (vs. placebo) ARR reduction 36% Disability reduction 31.5% Phase 3: TENERE Did not show noninferiority over IFN beta-1a Ongoing phase 3 studies: TOPIC (clinically isolated syndrome)	Gastrointestinal intolerance, elevation of liver function enzymes, hair thinning Leflunomide: pregnancy category X Risk mitigation strategies: • LFTs at baseline and every 6 months • CBC at baseline • Baseline testing for latent tuberculosis • Baseline pregnancy test • Confirm contraception • BP at baseline and monitoring
Laquinimod	Modulates expression of cytokines and has an effect on antigen presentation, T cells, B cells, and microglia	PO 0.6 mg	Phase 3: ALLEGRO (vs. placebo) ARR reduction 23% Disability reduction 36% Phase 3: BRAVO (vs. placebo) ARR reduction: Did not reach significance	Elevation in liver function enzymes Proinflammatory effects Increased CRP, ESR
Alemtuzumab	Humanized monoclonal antibody directed at CD52	IV 12 mg daily for 5 days followed by 12 mg daily for 3 days after 1 year	Phase 3: CARE MS I (vs. subcutaneous IFN beta-1a in the treatment-naive) ARR reduction 55% Disability reduction did not reach significance Phase 3: CARE MS II (vs. subcutaneous IFN beta-1a in treatment failure) ARR reduction 49% Disability reduction 42%	Infusion-related reactions, mild/moderate respiratory infections. Autoimmune reactions including hyperthyroidism, immune thrombocytopenic purpura, and Goodpasture's syndrome. Increased rate of infections
Ocrelizumab	Humanized/chimeric monoclonal antibody directed at CD20	IV 300 mg for 2, 2 weeks apart or 1000 mg for 2, 2 weeks apart	Phase 2: Ocrelizumab vs. placebo reduction in GAD lesions and relapse rate Ongoing phase 3 in RRMS and PPMS	Infusion related reactions, sinus and urinary tract infections. Phase 2 ocrelizumab: 1 death reported due to disseminated intravascular coagulation
Daclizumab	Humanized monoclonal antibody directed at interleukin-2 receptor	SC 150 mg every 4 weeks	Phase 2: Daclizumab showed decrease in GAD lesions Ongoing phase 3: DECIDE daclizumab vs. IM IFN beta-1a	Skin reactions, rash increase infection rate. Two malignancies in phase 2 trial

ARR, annualized relapse rate; BP, blood pressure; CBC, complete blood count; CRP, C-reactive protein; ESR, erythrocyte sedimentation rate; GAD, gadolinium enhancing; IM, intramuscular; IV, intravenous; LFT, liver function tests; PO, orally; SC, subcutaneous.

investigational drugs are tested. MS phase 3 trials typically include a measure of relapse activity—most commonly the annualized relapse rate (ARR) or the proportion of participants who are relapse-free at the completion of the study. Progression of neurological disability is usually measured as a worsening in the Kurtzke Expanded Disability Status Scale (EDSS) [8] which remains sustained for a certain period of time (usually 3–12 months) [9]. More sensitive and quantitative measures of disability have been used in clinical trials such as the Multiple Sclerosis Functional Composite, which is comprised of the timed 25 foot walk, the 9-hole peg test, and the paced auditory serial addition test [10]. MRI measures are also employed as secondary and tertiary outcomes, but typically scans are acquired only every 6 to 12 months and include a variety of lesional and atrophy measures [7].

> Phase 3 studies determine the clinical efficacy and safety of investigational compounds in a broad population and serve as the definitive evidence for submission to regulatory agencies for approval and marketing.

THERAPIES IN LATE STAGE OF DEVELOPMENT

Dimethyl Fumarate

Dimethyl fumarate, otherwise known as BG-12, is a fumaric acid ester with immunomodulatory and potential neuroprotective effects. The mechanism of action of BG-12 in MS is thought to be related to its effect on nuclear factor-E2-related factor (Nrf) 2 [11]. Fumaric acid esters have been used to treat psoriasis in German-speaking countries under the trade name Fumaderm, where it has been shown to have a favorable safety profile [12]. In a phase 2 trial, BG-12 at a dose of 240 mg 3 times daily demonstrated a 69% reduction in GAD lesions [13]. BG-12 has been tested in 2 phase 3 trials. The DEFINE trial studied 2 regimens of BG-12 (240 mg twice daily and 240 mg thrice daily) against placebo [14]. The study showed a 48% to 53% reduction in ARR compared to placebo, and a 34% to 38% reduction in risk of disability progression. MRI measures of disease activity were also reduced in the BG-12 arms when compared to placebo. A second phase 3 trial examined the same dosing regimens of BG-12 compared with placebo, but also included glatiramer acetate as an active comparator (CONFIRM Trial) [15]. A significant benefit was observed in both BG-12 groups compared to placebo, with a 44% to 51% reduction in ARR. A slowing of disability progression was not significant in this study. Although the preplanned did not include a comparison of BG-12 to glatiramer acetate, post hoc analyses found BG-12 superior on several clinical and imaging outcomes.

The most frequent adverse effects encountered in phase 3 trials were gastrointestinal upset and flushing [16]. These symptoms were most prominent during the first 2 months of treatment and improved significantly thereafter. Concomitant use of aspirin reduces flushing associated with BG-12 [17]. No increased rate of serious adverse events was seen in the BG-12 arms in the phase 3 trials, and infections were similar between BG-12 and placebo arms. Lymphopenia was observed in approximately 2% of patients on BG-12 in clinical trials but there was no increase in infections among those patients. The data from both phase 2 and phase 3 trials in MS confirms the overall favorable safety profile observed with fumarates in psoriasis.

BG-12 was approved for use in relapsing forms of MS in April of 2013 by the FDA. A starting dose of 120 mg twice daily for seven days followed by a maintenance dose of 240 mg twice daily was approved. A baseline complete blood count prior to initiation and annually on the medication are recommended given lymphopenia associated with BG-12.

Teriflunomide

Teriflunomide (2-hydroxyethylidene-cyanoacetic acid-4-trifluoromethyl anilide) is the active metabolite of leflunomide and is an oral therapy which inhibits the de novo synthesis of pyrimidine nucleotides through the inhibition of dihydroorotate dehydrogenase [18]. Teriflunomide inhibits T-cell activation and cytokine production along with cytostatic effects on proliferating B and T cells [19].

A phase 2 study of teriflunomide showed beneficial effects over placebo on combined unique brain MRI lesions and also on clinical measures of disease activity [20]. Teriflunomide has also shown efficacy on GAD lesions in a phase 2 add on study to interferon beta (IFN beta) [21]. The Teriflunomide Multiple Sclerosis Oral Trial (TEMSO) was a phase 3 trial that compared doses of 7 mg and 14 mg once daily against placebo [22]. A 31% reduction in ARR was observed for both doses, with a 29.8% reduction in disability progression for the 14 mg dose. Teriflunomide also had beneficial effects on total lesion volume, GAD lesions, and unique active lesions. Measures of brain atrophy were not significantly different between placebo and teriflunomide. A phase 3 trial comparing teriflunomide against subcutaneous IFN beta-1a (TENERE) failed to show superiority [23]. A second placebo-controlled phase 3 trial in relapsing-remitting MS (RRMS) (TOWER) showed that teriflunomide decreased ARR by 36.3% compared to placebo, with a 31.5% reduction in 12 week sustained progression of disability [24]. A third placebo-controlled trial (TOPIC) will study patients with clinically isolated syndrome (or a first attack of MS).

In phase 2 and phase 3 trials, teriflunomide was safe and relatively well tolerated. No increase in opportunistic infections was observed and most adverse effects related to the medication were transitory. The most frequent adverse effects include gastrointestinal symptoms, decrease in hair density, and mild elevations in liver function enzymes. Rash and fatigue were also commonly encountered with teriflunomide. A single long-term safety study showed that teriflunomide was safe over 8.5 years of follow-up [25]. Leflunomide is a pregnancy category X medication and it is likely that teriflunomide carries similar embryonic/fetal risks in both male and female MS patients. The removal of teriflunomide from the body can be accelerated with cholestyramine [22]. The beneficial effects on clinical and imaging outcomes along with a favorable safety profile suggests that teriflunomide will be a useful treatment option for relapsing MS, although it is likely that teratogenicity will limit its use in patients of child-bearing potential.

Teriflunomide was approved for use in relapsing forms of MS in September of 2012. Both the 7 mg and 14 mg daily doses were approved. Warnings regarding serious hepatotoxicty and risk of teratogencity were included in the label. Liver function tests are recommended at baseline and every 6 months while on the medication. A baseline and 6 month complete blood count is recommended. Testing for latent tuberculosis prior to initiation should also be conducted with a tuberculin skin test or with interferon release assays. Terfilunomide is a category X medication for pregnancy. Pregnancy must be excluded in all women of child bearing potential and reliable contraception should be confirmed for both women and men. Rapid elimination with cholestyramine or charcoal are recommended in cases of suspected pregnancies or serious infections on the medication.

Laquinimod

Laquinimod is an oral quinoline 3-carboxamide derivative which is closely related to roquinimex and has wide immune effects on antigen presentation, T cells, B cells, and microglia [26]. Roquinimex had shown promise in EAE and phase 2 trials, but a phase 3 trial in MS was halted because of rare systemic proinflammatory adverse events, including vasculitis [27]. Laquinimod has shown efficacy in EAE as monotherapy [28] as well as synergistic effect when used with IFN beta [29]. Phase 2 clinical trials showed a beneficial effect of laquinimod on GAD lesions, new T2 lesions, and cerebral volume loss [30,31]. The Assessment of Oral Laquinimod in Preventing Progression in Multiple Sclerosis (ALLEGRO) trial was a phase 3 randomized study which compared 0.6 mg of oral laquinimod daily with placebo [32]. A 23% reduction in ARR was observed along with a 36% reduction in disability progression. Brain atrophy was also reduced by 33% in patients receiving laquinimod. A second phase 3 trial (BRAVO) failed to meet the primary end point in ARR and did not show statistically significant differences in disability progression.

The overall safety profile of laquinimod appears favorable. Phase 2 and phase 3 studies did not show the serious adverse events observed with linomide, although 5 cases of appendicitis occurred in the active arm of the ALLEGRO trial, while only 1 occurred in the placebo arm. Elevated liver enzymes were observed in the laquinimod groups but were usually transient. Risk of infection was similar in placebo and active medication groups. A third, 2 year trial in relapsing MS was started in 2012, with the primary end point of sustained progression of disability.

Alemtuzumab

Alemtuzumab is a humanized monoclonal antibody directed at CD52, a molecule which plays a role in T-cell activation and proliferation [33]. It is administered by intravenous injection at a dose of 12 mg daily for 5 days followed by a 3 day repeat treatment course at 12 months. Alemtuzumab causes a rapid depletion of lymphocytes and was approved for use in B-cell chronic lymphocytic leukemia until the company voluntarily withdrew it from the market in 2012. Following preliminary studies in the 1990s, alemtuzumab was studied in relapsing MS in a randomized rater-blinded phase 2 study against subcutaneous IFN beta-1a [34]. Alemtuzumab showed a reduction in T2 lesion load and had beneficial effects on brain atrophy. A long-term follow-up of the phase 2 trials showed a 69% reduction in ARR and a 72% reduction of disability progression over IFN beta-1a [35]. Two phase 3 trials have been completed. CARE-MS I showed a relapse reduction of 55% when compared with subcutaneous IFN beta-1a in treatment-naïve patients, but did not show a benefit on disability progression [36]. CARE MS II also showed a significant reduction in relapses (49%) and disability progression (42%) when compared with subcutaneous IFN beta-1a in patients who relapsed on prior MS treatments [37].

Alemtuzumab has been linked to episodes of humoral autoimmunity which are felt to be related to faulty reconstitution of B lymphocytes. Autoimmune thyroid disease is the most common humoral autoimmunity and appears to affect 16% to 30% of individuals treated with alemtuzumab [38]. Autoimmune thrombocytopenic purpura has been identified at a rate of about 1%, and in one case resulted in fatality due to a cerebral hemorrhage [34,36,37]. Several cases of antiglomerular basement disease (Goodpasture's syndrome) have also occurred. It appears autoimmune events may occur even years after initial treatment. An ongoing screening strategy (thyroid, liver, and renal tests) will likely be recommended for long-term monitoring. The incidence of infections was approximately 2-fold higher with alemtuzumab than IFN beta-1a. Alemtuzumab is also associated with infusion reactions likely due to release of cytokines.

MORE DISTANT THERAPIES

Daclizumab

Daclizumab is a monoclonal antibody directed at the interlukin-2 (IL-2) receptor and was initially designed for treatment of T-cell leukemia. Daclizumab results in both a decrease in CD4+ T cells and an increase in natural killer regulatory cells [39]. Subcutaneous daclizumab was studied in a phase 2 trial against placebo and IFN beta where it showed significant benefit on new or enlarging GAD lesions. Infections and rash were more common with daclizumab treatment. Two cases of malignancy were detected in daclizumab-treated patients (breast cancer, pseudomyxoma peritonei). Daclizumab is currently being studied in a phase 3 active comparator trial against subcutaneous IFN beta-1a. The study is expected to enroll 1,500 participants and daclizumab will be administered at a dose of 150 mg every 4 weeks. A large phase 2 study (SELECT) will also examine 2 different doses of daclizumab (150 mg and 300 mg) and is expected to enroll 600 participants.

Ocrelizumab

Ocrelizumab is a humanized monoclonal antibody directed at CD20 currently being studied in relapsing MS after positive phase 2 results of rituximab (a chimeric monoclonal antibody directed against CD20) [40]. Similar to rituximab, ocrelizumab depletes circulating B cells and is felt to be less immunogenic than rituximab (ie, induces less anti-ocrelizumab antibodies), although the presence of anti-rituximab antibodies has not been shown to diminish the effect of rituximab [41]. In a phase 2 study, 600 and 2,000 mg of ocrelizumab were compared against placebo and intramuscular IFN beta-1a. Ocrelizumab reduced enhancing or enlarging lesions by over 90%, and approximately two-thirds of the ocrelizumab patients had no MRI disease activity (relapses or new lesions) at 96 weeks. Serious infections were similar across treatment arms; however one death related to disseminated intravascular coagulation has been reported. Two phase 3 studies in relapsing MS and 1 in primary progressive MS were underway in 2012.

CONCLUSION

Over the next several years, many new agents to treat RRMS are expected to be introduced into the market. Several will have superior efficacy over current injectable first-line therapies, but may also have significant risks, too. The treatment of MS and the balance between treatment-related risk and efficacy will become progressively more complex for patients and health care providers. An understanding of the drug development process along with up-to-date information about new therapies at different stages of testing will allow clinicians to critically appraise new medications as they become available.

REFERENCES

1. Miller AE, Rhoades RW. Treatment of relapsing-remitting multiple sclerosis: Current approaches and unmet needs. *Curr Opin Neurol.* 2012;25(Suppl):S4–S10.

2. Steinman L, Zamvil SS. How to successfully apply animal studies in experimental allergic encephalomyelitis to research on multiple sclerosis. *Ann Neurol.* 2006;60:12–21.

3. Bolton C. The translation of drug efficacy from in vivo models to human disease with special reference to experimental autoimmune encephalomyelitis and multiple sclerosis. *Inflammopharmacology.* 2007;15:183–187.

4. Friese MA, Montalban X, Willcox N, et al. The value of animal models for drug development in multiple sclerosis. *Brain.* 2006;129:1940–1952.

5. Warford J, Robertson GS. New methods for multiple sclerosis drug discovery. *Expert Opin Drug Discov.* 2011;6:689–699.

6. Penel N, Isambert N, Leblond P, et al. "Classical 3 + 3 design" versus "accelerated titration designs": Analysis of 270 phase 1 trials investigating anti-cancer agents. *Invest New Drugs.* 2009;27(6):552–556.

7. Barkhof F, Simon JH, Fazekas F, et al. MRI monitoring of immunomodulation in relapse-onset multiple sclerosis trials. *Nat Rev Neurol.* 2011;8:13–21.

8. Kurtzke JF. Rating neurologic impairment in multiple sclerosis: An expanded disability status scale (EDSS). *Neurology.* 1983;33:1444–1452.

9. Healy B, Chitnis T, Engler D. Improving power to detect disease progression in multiple sclerosis through alternative analysis strategies. *J Neurol.* 2011;258:1812–1819.

10. Rudick R, Antel J, Confavreux C, et al. Recommendations from the national multiple sclerosis society clinical outcomes assessment task force. *Ann Neurol.* 1997;42:379–382.

11. Linker RA, Lee DH, Ryan S, et al. Fumaric acid esters exert neuroprotective effects in neuroinflammation via activation of the Nrf2 antioxidant pathway. *Brain.* 2011;134:678–692.

12. Reich K, Thaci D, Mrowietz U, et al. Efficacy and safety of fumaric acid esters in the long-term treatment of psoriasis—a retrospective study (FUTURE). *J Dtsch Dermatol Ges.* 2009;7:603–611.

13. Kappos L, Gold R, Miller DH, et al. Efficacy and safety of oral fumarate in patients with relapsing-remitting multiple sclerosis: A multicentre, randomised, double-blind, placebo-controlled phase IIb study. *Lancet.* 2008;372:1463–1472.

14. Gold R, Kappos L, Bar-Or A. Clinical efficacy of BG-12, an oral therapy, in relapsing-remitting multiple sclerosis: Data from the phase 3 DEFINE trial. *Program and abstracts of the 5th Joint Triennial Congress of the European and Americas Committees for Treatment and Research in Multiple Sclerosis (ECTRIMS/ACTRIMS);* 19–22 October 2011; Amsterdam, The Netherlands; 2011.

15. Fox R, Miller D, Phillips JT, et al. Clinical efficacy of BG-12 in relapsing-remitting multiple sclerosis (RRMS): Data from the phase 3 CONFIRM study (S01.003). *Neurology.* 2012;78:S01.003.

16. Phillips JT, Fox R, Miller D, et al. Safety and tolerability of BG-12 in patients with relapsing-remitting multiple sclerosis (RRMS): Analyses from the CONFIRM study (S41.005). *Neurology.* 2012;78:S41.005.

17. Sheikh S, Nestorov I, Russell H, et al. Safety, tolerability, and pharmacokinetics of BG-12 administered with and without aspirin: Key findings from a randomized, double-blind, placebo-controlled trial in healthy volunteers (P04.136). *Neurology.* 2012;78:P04.136.

18. Greene S, Watanabe K, Braatz-Trulson J, et al. Inhibition of dihydroorotate dehydrogenase by the immunosuppressive agent leflunomide. *Biochem Pharmacol.* 1995;50:861–867.

19. Xu X, Blinder L, Shen J, et al. In vivo mechanism by which leflunomide controls lymphoproliferative and autoimmune disease in MRL/MpJ-lpr/lpr mice. *J Immunol.* 1997;159:167–174.

20. O'Connor PW, Li D, Freedman MS, et al. A phase II study of the safety and efficacy of teriflunomide in multiple sclerosis with relapses. *Neurology.* 2006;66:894–900.

21. Freedman MS, Wolinsky JS, Wamil B, et al. Teriflunomide added to interferon-beta in relapsing multiple sclerosis: A randomized phase II trial. *Neurology.* 2012;78:1877–1885.

22. O'Connor P, Wolinsky JS, Confavreux C, et al. Randomized trial of oral teriflunomide for relapsing multiple sclerosis. *N Engl J Med.* 2011;365:1293–1303.

23. Genzyme Corporation. Genzyme reports top-line results for TENERE study of oral teriflunomide in relapsing multiple sclerosis; 2012.

24. Genzyme Corporation. Genzyme reports positive top-line results of TOWER, a pivotal phase III trial for AUBAGIOTM* (teriflunomide) in relapsing multiple sclerosis; 2012.

25. Confavreux C, Li DK, Freedman MS, et al. Long-term follow-up of a phase 2 study of oral teriflunomide in relapsing multiple sclerosis: Safety and efficacy results up to 8.5 years. *Mult Scler.* 2012;18(9):1278–1289.

26. Jonsson S, Andersson G, Fex T, et al. Synthesis and biological evaluation of new 1,2-dihydro-4-hydroxy-2-oxo-3-quinolinecarboxamides for treatment of autoimmune disorders: Structure-activity relationship. *J Med Chem.* 2004;47:2075–2088.

27. Noseworthy JH, Wolinsky JS, Lublin FD, et al. Linomide in relapsing and secondary progressive MS: Part I: Trial design and clinical results. North American Linomide Investigators. *Neurology.* 2000;54:1726–1733.

28. Yang JS, Xu LY, Xiao BG, et al. Laquinimod (ABR-215062) suppresses the development of experimental autoimmune encephalomyelitis, modulates the Th1/Th2 balance and induces the Th3 cytokine TGF-beta in lewis rats. *J Neuroimmunol.* 2004;156:3–9.

29. Runstrom A, Leanderson T, Ohlsson L, et al. Inhibition of the development of chronic experimental autoimmune encephalomyelitis by laquinimod (ABR-215062) in IFN-beta k.o. and wild type mice. *J Neuroimmunol.* 2006;173:69–78.

30. Polman C, Barkhof F, Sandberg-Wollheim M, et al. Treatment with laquinimod reduces development of active MRI lesions in relapsing MS. *Neurology.* 2005;64:987–991.

31. Comi G, Pulizzi A, Rovaris M, et al. Effect of laquinimod on MRI-monitored disease activity in patients with relapsing-remitting multiple sclerosis: A multicentre, randomised, double-blind, placebo-controlled phase IIb study. *Lancet.* 2008;371:2085–2092.

32. Comi G, Jeffery D, Kappos L, et al. Placebo-controlled trial of oral laquinimod for multiple sclerosis. *N Engl J Med.* 2012;366: 1000–1009.

33. Hu Y, Turner MJ, Shields J, et al. Investigation of the mechanism of action of alemtuzumab in a human CD52 transgenic mouse model. *Immunology.* 2009;128:260–270.

34. CAMMS223 Trial Investigators, Coles AJ, Compston DA, et al. Alemtuzumab vs. interferon beta-1a in early multiple sclerosis. *N Engl J Med.* 2008;359:1786–1801.

35. Coles AJ, Fox E, Vladic A, et al. Alemtuzumab more effective than interferon beta-1a at 5-year follow-up of CAMMS223 clinical trial. *Neurology.* 2012;78:1069–1078.

36. Coles A, Brinar V, Arnold D, et al. Efficacy and safety results from comparison of alemtuzumab and rebif(R) efficacy in multiple sclerosis I (CARE-MS I): A phase 3 study in relapsing-remitting treatment-naive patients (S01.006). *Neurology.* 2012;78:S01.006.

37. Cohen J, Twyman C, Arnold D, et al. Efficacy and safety results from comparison of alemtuzumab and rebif(R) efficacy in multiple sclerosis II (CARE-MS II): A phase 3 study in relapsing-remitting multiple sclerosis patients who relapsed on prior therapy (S01.004). *Neurology.* 2012;78:S01.004.

38. Costelloe L, Jones J, Coles A. Secondary autoimmune diseases following alemtuzumab therapy for multiple sclerosis. *Expert Rev Neurother.* 2012;12:335–341.

39. Bielekova B, Catalfamo M, Reichert-Scrivner S, et al. Regulatory CD56(bright) natural killer cells mediate immunomodulatory effects of IL-2Ralpha-targeted therapy (daclizumab) in multiple sclerosis. *Proc Natl Acad Sci USA.* 2006;103:5941–5946.

40. Hauser SL, Waubant E, Arnold DL, et al. B-cell depletion with rituximab in relapsing-remitting multiple sclerosis. *N Engl J Med.* 2008;358:676–688.

41. van Meerten T, Hagenbeek A. CD20-targeted therapy: The next generation of antibodies. *Semin Hematol.* 2010;47:199–210.

Part IV. Rehabilitation and Symptom Management

17

Overview of Rehabilitation in Multiple Sclerosis

FRANCOIS BETHOUX

KEY POINTS FOR CLINICIANS

- Rehabilitation refers to a variety of interventions that aim at preserving or improving function and quality of life.

- In multiple sclerosis (MS), rehabilitation is a component of the comprehensive care approach and is a useful complement to disease-modifying and symptomatic therapies.

- The International Classification of Functioning, Disability, and Health (ICF) is increasingly used as a conceptual framework to describe the consequences of MS, and to assess the results of rehabilitation.

- The nature, intensity, and setting of rehabilitation interventions are determined on the basis of the patient's needs and on mutually agreed upon goals.

Rehabilitation refers to an array of skilled interventions which aim at optimizing function in patients with a variety of health conditions. The World Health Organization (WHO) defines rehabilitation as "a proactive and goal-oriented activity to restore function and/or to maximize remaining function to bring about the highest possible level of independence, physically, psychologically, socially and economically" [1]. Traditionally, rehabilitation is indicated after an acute injury (eg, brain or spinal cord injury) or health event (eg, stroke, surgery). The expectation is that the patient will achieve functional gains during the rehabilitation period, then will be returned to his or her usual environment, or to the appropriate setting (assisted living, nursing home), depending on the patient's ultimate functional status, personal characteristics, and environmental factors (such as socioeconomic conditions).

Applying this traditional rehabilitation framework to multiple sclerosis (MS) requires a change in paradigm, as disability is expected to increase over time in a majority of patients. Therefore, delaying or slowing functional loss becomes a valuable goal of MS rehabilitation. In a consensus statement on rehabilitation in MS, a task force convened by the National Multiple Sclerosis Society defined rehabilitation as, "a process that helps a person achieve and maintain maximal physical, psychological, social and vocational potential, and quality of life consistent with physiologic impairment, environment, and life goals. Achievement and maintenance of optimal function are essential in a progressive disease such as MS" [2].

Even though rehabilitation is integrated to be an important component of the comprehensive care of MS [3], obstacles to its implementation remain, and evidence to guide decision making remains insufficient. In this chapter, we introduce the rehabilitation process, instruments used to measure the results of rehabilitation, and practical applications of rehabilitation in MS. Additional details are found in many other chapters in this book.

THE REHABILITATION PROCESS

Referral

A patient's access to rehabilitation services is most often contingent upon a referral from the neurology treating team. Tables 17.1 and 17.2 describe the main goals for referring a patient to specific rehabilitation professionals and specialized rehabilitation services. To maximize the chances of a positive outcome, the main elements of the referral must be kept in mind:

1. To *which rehabilitation professional(s) should the patient be referred?* Rehabilitation is by nature a multidisciplinary specialty, but all professionals do not always need to be involved in the care of a particular patient at all times. Even though there is a partial overlap in the expertise and problems addressed, it is important to refer the patient to the appropriate professional. The list provided in Table 17.1 is extensive, but not exhaustive. For example, psychologists, social workers, recreation therapists, and music or art therapists also can be involved in the rehabilitation process. Another important component is the professional's knowledge and expertise in MS. Some MS centers offer rehabilitation services on site, but in many instances the patient needs to be referred to a therapist in the community. It is therefore important to establish a referral network, seeking therapists with neurorehabilitation training and expertise.

2. *What is the purpose/goal of the referral to rehabilitation services?* It is essential that the reason for the referral and the expected outcome be discussed with the patient (and family when appropriate) as precisely as possible. This promotes an understanding of how rehabilitation "fits" within the individualized MS management plan, gives patients an opportunity to talk about their own goals, increases their motivation, and helps set realistic expectations regarding the results of rehabilitation.

TABLE 17.1
Professionals Involved in MS Rehabilitation

REHABILITATION PROFESSIONALS	EXAMPLES OF INDICATIONS
Physiatrist [4] Rehabilitation nurse, advanced practice nurse, physician assistant	Complex symptom management and functional issues requiring the coordination of multiple rehabilitation interventions (eg, spasticity management)
Physical therapist [5]	Lower extremity impairments Teaching of home exercise program Gait/balance training Mobility aides fitting/training
Occupational therapist [6]	Upper extremity impairments Limitation of self-care activities Fatigue management Upper extremity splinting Use of assistive devices for ADLs Home/work modifications
Speech language pathologist	Language and speech impairment Dysphagia
Orthotist	Fabrication and fitting of orthotics

ADLs, activities of daily living.

TABLE 17.2
Specialized Rehabilitation Services

SERVICE	MAIN GOALS
Driver rehabilitation	To assess driving performance (in the office and on the road, sometimes with a driving simulator) To provide on-the-road training To determine the need for vehicle adaptations (eg, hand controls) and train patients to their use
Vocational rehabilitation	To help gain or maintain employment despite functional limitations
Wheelchair/seating clinic	To determine the most appropriate wheeled mobility device and seating arrangement for the patient, provide the information needed for reimbursement, train the patient, and assess the need for wheelchair/seating adjustments over time
Functional capacity evaluation	To assess the need for work accommodations To document physical performance for disability application
Cognitive rehabilitation	To perform exercises that aim at enhancing cognitive performance in daily activities To teach compensatory strategies

This information should also be shared with the rehabilitation professional. Goals and expectations may be adjusted over time on the basis of feedback from the therapist and from the patient. Specialized rehabilitation services may be sought to address specific needs, such as driving.

3. *What is the best rehabilitation setting to address the patient's needs?* In most cases, MS rehabilitation interventions are provided in an outpatient setting where space, setup, and equipment are often optimized. However, for patients who cannot drive or have adequate transportation, or when the goal is specifically to assess performance and work on functional tasks within the home environment, home rehabilitation services should be considered. Inpatient rehabilitation is indicated when patients have more complex needs and require more intensive rehabilitation involving several types of therapies. In most cases, patients are transferred to inpatient rehabilitation from a medical or surgical acute inpatient unit after a major health event (eg, severe MS exacerbation, sepsis, surgery). Less commonly, admission to inpatient rehabilitation may also occur directly from home; for example, when patients experience a rapid functional decline within a relatively short time frame, compromising their ability to function at home, but have a good potential to regain function. Telerehabilitation potentially offers the ability to monitor the patient's functional status and provide rehabilitation interventions from a distance, but is not yet widely used.

Assessment

Rehabilitation professionals share common concepts in order to describe a patient's current functional status and rehabilitation goals. The most accepted framework for rehabilitation worldwide is the International Classification of Functioning, Disability, and Health (ICF), published by the WHO [7]. The ICF classifies the consequences of medical conditions (eg, disease, injury, malformation) in terms of body function and structure, activities, and participation. In addition, the ICF takes into account personal and environmental factors. The ICF is useful in identifying problems and goals relevant to rehabilitation. For example, a patient in the early stages of MS after an exacerbation with partial transverse myelitis, who works on an assembly line in a factory, may experience chronic weakness and spasticity in 1 leg (alteration of body function), resulting in difficulty walking and standing for long periods (activity limitation), and consequent inability to perform work duties full time (participation restriction). After rehabilitation, the patient's ability to work may be preserved by improving spasticity via stretching and symptomatic medication, by improving walking through physical therapy and the use of an ankle-foot orthosis, and by recommending modifications to the work environment.

Examples of assessment tools that can be used for rehabilitation are listed in Table 17.3. This list is not exhaustive,

and more comprehensive information can be found in specific chapters (eg, spasticity, fatigue). The same instruments are used to measure individual patient performance and to set quantitative goals in the course of a series of rehabilitation sessions, and to assess changes at the group level in clinical trials of rehabilitation.

OBSTACLES TO REHABILITATION IN MS

As the awareness of the role of rehabilitation grows among patients and health care providers, it is important to acknowledge limitations and obstacles and to take them into account when planning a referral. Some limitations stem from the disease itself. Fatigue and depression may decrease the patient's motivation to engage in a rehabilitation program. MS symptoms often worsen transiently with exertion, making it necessary to determine the right "dose" and type of exercises for each patient. Fluctuations in symptoms and functional performance over time require adjustments to the goals and contents of rehabilitation. Access to rehabilitation services may be compromised by the absence of neurorehabilitation specialists in the patient's area, by difficulty getting transportation, and by limits imposed by third-party payors (many patients have a limited number of physical therapy [PT] and occupational therapy [OT] sessions covered per year, and maintenance of functional performance is generally not accepted as a valid indication to start or continue rehabilitation). Patient education, communication between providers, and assistance with access problems all help overcome these obstacles.

FOR WHAT PURPOSE SHOULD REHABILITATION BE USED IN MS?

Education and Teaching of a Home Exercise Program

The development of an exercise program, to be performed by the patient at home or in a gym, independently or with a helper, is one of the goals of most rehabilitation programs. Randomized studies have demonstrated the benefits of exercise in MS on fitness, fatigue, muscle strength, mood, quality of life, and function. A meta-analysis based on results from 22 publications showed a small but significant improvement of walking performance after exercise training [8]. Both aerobic (endurance) exercise and resistance training were shown to be effective [9].

In practice, it is often difficult for patients with MS to initiate a physical exercise routine on their own, owing to the obstacles discussed. This limitation further exposes them to physical deconditioning, and increases the risk of comorbidities such as osteoporosis and cardiovascular conditions. Therefore, a referral to a PT or OT is strongly recommended to optimize patients' exercise routines. At the early stages of MS, one visit may be sufficient to teach an individualized program. Later in the course of the disease, a series of sessions is often needed to initiate an adapted exercise routine.

TABLE 17.3
Examples of Assessment Tools for MS Rehabilitation

ASSESSMENT TOOL	RATED BY	ICF LEVEL	COMMENTS
Global assessment			
Expanded Disability Status Scale	Clinician	Body function Activity	Scores based on neurological examination and ambulation status
Environmental Status Scale	Clinician	Participation	Scores based on the ability to perform complex activities (eg, work, use of transportation, social life)
Functional Independence Measure	Clinician	Activity	Scores based on the level of assistance needed to perform daily activities
Incapacity Status Scale	Clinician	Body function Activity	Scores based on the need for assistive devices or physical assistance to perform activities and the functional impact of symptoms
MS Impact Profile	Patient	Body function Activity Participation	Assesses the perception of disability related to MS
MS Impact Scale-29	Patient	Body function Activity Participation	Asks how much problems related to MS bothered the patient during the past 2 weeks
NeuroQOL	Patient	Body function Activity Participation	Assesses the health-related quality of life of individuals with neurological disorders
Community Integration Questionnaire	Patient	Participation	Assesses limitations in the ability to perform social roles (home integration, social integration, productive activity)
Targeted Assessment			
Manual Muscle Testing, Dynamometry	Clinician	Body function	Measures strength
Ashworth Scale, Tardieu scale	Clinician	Body function	Measures spasticity
MS Spasticity Scale-88	Patient	Body function Activity Participation	Asks how much spasticity bothered the patient in the past 2 weeks
Goniometry	Clinician	Body function	Measures range of motion
Timed walking tests (eg, Timed 25 foot walk, 2- or 6-minute walk, Timed up and go)	Clinician	Activity	These tests are frequently used in clinical practice and clinical trials of rehabilitation interventions
MS Walking Scale-12	Patient	Activity	Asks the patient how much MS has limited various aspects of walking in the past 2 weeks
Balance scales (eg, Berg Balance Scale, BESTest, Dynamic Gait Index, Functional Reach Test)	Clinician	Activity	Most of these scales consist of a series of tests assessing static and dynamic balance
Activities-specific Balance Confidence scale	Patient	Activity	Asks about the level of self-confidence about performing activities without losing balance
Timed upper extremity function tests (eg, 9-hole peg test, Box and Block Test)	Clinician	Activity	These tests are easy and quick to administer
Modified Fatigue Impact Scale	Patient	Body function Activity Participation	Assesses the impact of fatigue in terms of effects of fatigue in terms of physical, cognitive, and psychosocial functioning

ICF: International Classification of Functioning, Disability, and Health.

The general rule for exercise in MS is to begin with a short duration and low intensity, and to increase very gradually ("start low, go slow"). If overheating causes a transient worsening of symptoms, it can be avoided by using a fan or cooling garments, or by exercising in water. Although clinicians used to discourage patients from exercising because of fears of overheating, this is now recognized to only cause transient symptoms in a subset of patients and does not cause permanent neurologic injury.

Comprehensive Symptom Management

Rehabilitation can be integrated into the management of MS symptoms, particularly fatigue and spasticity. In fact, rehabilitation may at times be the first line of treatment, before medications or other interventions.

Fatigue is one of the most frequently reported symptoms by MS patients, and has a profound impact on functional performance and quality of life. The comprehensive management of MS fatigue includes behavioral changes aimed at improving and preserving energy, often initiated by OTs or PTs, and encompasses exercise, modification of daily activities, and the use of assistive devices. Detailed recommendations for the management of fatigue can be found in Chapter 18.

Spasticity is another frequent indication for referral to PT and OT, often in conjunction with other treatment modalities (see Chapter 27) [10]. All patients with spasticity should initiate a stretching routine under the supervision of a rehabilitation professional, to ensure that the stretches will be performed with an effective and safe technique. In patients with severe disability, family members and home health aides need to be trained to perform stretching. Other rehabilitation modalities relevant to spasticity management are splinting, serial casting, brace fitting, and functional training. In addition, botulinum toxin therapy and intrathecal baclofen therapy are often managed by physiatrists [11].

Even though there is evidence suggesting that a rehabilitation approach is helpful in chronic pain management, specific evidence related to MS is lacking.

Task-Specific Rehabilitation

Task-specific rehabilitation is focused on training the patient to a specific function or activity, and can play an essential role in helping to maintain a patient's independence. The function that has been the most studied is walking, with treatment modalities including conventional gait training and the use of advanced technology such as body weight supported treadmill training and the use of robotics (see Chapter 28). Other examples include balance and a variety of activities of daily living (ADLs; basic ADLs mostly represent self-care tasks, while instrumented ADLs [IADLs] refer to more complex activities such as cooking a meal and managing bills). Assessment and rehabilitation for dysphagia and dysphonia, performed by speech language pathologists, also fall into this category. Cognitive rehabilitation involves task-specific training, and aims at improving specific impairments (eg, attention/concentration deficit) and teaching compensatory strategies (eg, use of memory aids) [12]. Driving is an essential activity for community mobility, and as a consequence a patient's ability to drive safely is a sensitive discussion topic. Driver rehabilitation specialists (often OTs) perform in-office and on-the-road (or via a driving simulator) assessments [13], and can help preserve a patient's ability to drive when indicated by providing training, and by recommending vehicle adaptations and modifications, such as hand controls. Another important goal of MS management is to preserve the patients' ability to work, as the disease affects them at the peak of their productive years. A functional capacity evaluation (FCE), usually performed by a PT or an OT, helps quantify a patient's physical ability in relation to employment (eg, sedentary versus more physically demanding work). FCEs are often used to support an application for disability, but may also help formulate recommendations for workplace accommodations. Vocational rehabilitation services (discussed in Chapter 34) can provide further assistance in maintaining a patient's ability to work.

Evaluation and Training for Assistive Devices and Orthotics

Even though a prescription from a physician, a physician assistant, clinical nurse specialist, or nurse practitioner is required to obtain assistive devices and orthotics, rehabilitation professionals play a key role in determining which type of equipment is most appropriate for the patient, in providing supporting information to obtain reimbursement (particularly for wheeled mobility devices), in helping with fitting and adjustments, and in training patients to use their devices efficiently and safely. A comprehensive description of orthoses and assistive devices that can be prescribed to patients with MS are discussed in Chapter 28. Extensive information about assistive technology, including suppliers, can be found at www.abledata.com. More specific information related to MS is available on the National MS Society website (www.nationalmssociety.org/living-with-multiple-sclerosis/mobility-and-accessibility/assistive-technology/index.aspx).

Rehabilitation After MS Exacerbations

MS exacerbations resulting in new onset of functional limitations, or worsening of preexisting disability (particularly those resulting from lesions involving the spinal cord and brain stem) constitute a valid indication for rehabilitation. The loss of function typically occurs over a short time period, and even though some recovery is expected in the following weeks and months, residual disability from exacerbations is common [14,15]. A randomized controlled trial of inpatient rehabilitation in 40 MS patients treated with intravenous steroids for an MS exacerbation showed improvement in neurological disability and functional performance at 3 months, compared to routine care [16]. Another study of inpatient rehabilitation after treatment with corticosteroids for MS exacerbation, using an uncontrolled pre–post intervention design, showed improvement of Expanded Disability Status Scale scores and functional performance scores (Barthel Index, Functional Independence Measure) at the time of discharge [17]. Contrasting with these findings, a randomized single-blind clinical trial of outpatient rehabilitation twice per week for 6 weeks, starting 4 weeks after IV methylprednisolone treatment for an exacerbation of MS, showed no significant between-group differences in Incapacity Status Scale and SF-36 scores at 3 months or 1 year [18]. These observations suggest that the intensity of rehabilitation plays a role in the efficacy of the intervention. In practice, the onset of rehabilitation may need to be delayed until the peak of the relapse has passed, to ensure that the patient is able to tolerate the therapies.

Rehabilitation for Progressive MS

An emphasis has been placed recently on finding treatments for progressive forms of MS [19], which do not usually respond to currently available disease-modifying therapies. There is evidence showing that rehabilitation is effective in this patient population. A randomized single-blind controlled trial of inpatient rehabilitation showed improvement of activity performance (FIM) and self-reported health status (SF-36) after 3 weeks in the treatment group, compared to a no-intervention group (approximately 80% of the subjects in each group had progressive MS) [20]. Another study of inpatient rehabilitation in patients with progressive MS showed improvement of disability, handicap, psychological status, and perceived physical health status, which was sustained for at least 6 months [21]. Di Fabio et al. observed a significant decrease in symptom frequency and fatigue at 1 year, and a slower progression of disability in MS patients receiving outpatient rehabilitation, compared to no intervention [22]. A more recent randomized controlled trial compared a 12 month comprehensive rehabilitation intervention (inpatient followed by outpatient) to usual care (wait list), and found a significant improvement of FIM-motor scores in the treatment group. A significantly greater proportion of patients in the control group exhibited a worsening of functional performance on the FIM (58.7% versus 16.7%; $P < .001$). No significant benefit was observed on self-report measures (MS Impact Scale and General Health Questionnaire) [23]. Altogether, these studies suggest that both inpatient and outpatient multidisciplinary rehabilitation improves or stabilizes functional status in some patients with progressive MS, although the carryover of the benefit after the end of rehabilitation needs to be determined.

CONCLUSION

Rehabilitation should be considered in the management of MS at all stages of the disease. The nature, intensity, and setting of rehabilitation interventions are determined on the basis of the patient's needs and on mutually agreed upon goals. As the success of rehabilitation relies on long-term behavioral modifications, it is important to initiate these interventions early, and to explain to the patient how they fit within the overall management plan for their disease. As the patient will often be referred to 1 or several professionals outside of the neurology practice, ongoing communication is essential in ensuring that outcomes are optimized.

KEY POINTS FOR PATIENTS AND FAMILIES

- Rehabilitation is an important part of the comprehensive management of MS. Rehabilitation can be performed at home, in an outpatient office or clinic, or in a hospital as an inpatient, depending on your needs.

- Examples of rehabilitation professionals include physiatrists (physicians specialized in rehabilitation), physical therapists, occupational therapists, speech therapists, and many other professionals and services.

- The main goal of rehabilitation is to optimize a person's ability to function in daily life. Rehabilitation can be helpful all along the course of the disease, both to the persons with MS and to loved ones that are involved in their care.

- It is important to mention to your neurology team symptoms that prevent you from carrying out daily activities, so you can be referred to the appropriate rehabilitation professional or service when indicated.

- Specific goals need to be agreed upon with the person with MS before starting rehabilitation, so the effects of rehabilitation can be assessed.

REFERENCES

1. *A Glossary of Terms for Community Health Care and Services for Older Persons. World Health Organization Centre for Development, Ageing and Health Technical Report*, Vol. 5. Geneva: World Health Organization; 2004.

2. Medical Advisory Board of the National Multiple Sclerosis Society. *Rehabilitation: Recommendations for Persons with Multiple Sclerosis.* National Multiple Sclerosis Society; 2005:10 pp.

3. *European-wide Recommendations on Rehabilitation for people affected by Multiple Sclerosis.* European Multiple Sclerosis Platform; 2008:63 pp.

4. McKee K, Bethoux F. Team focus: Physiatrist. *Int J MS Care.* 2009;11:144–147.

5. Sutliff M. Team focus: Physical therapist. *Int J MS Care.* 2008;10:127–132.

6. Forwell SJ, Zackowski KM. Team focus: Occupational therapist. *Int J MS Care.* 2008;10:94–98.

7. *International Classification of Functioning, Disability and Health.* Geneva: World Health Organization; 2001.

8. Snook EM, Motl RW. Effect of exercise training on walking mobility in multiple sclerosis: A meta-analysis. *Neurorehabil Neural Repair.* 2009;23:108–116.

9. Dalgas U, Stenager E, Ingemann-Hansen T. Multiple sclerosis and physical exercise: Recommendations for the application of resistance-, endurance- and combined training. *Mult Scler.* 2008;14(1):35–53.

10. Brar SP, Smith MB, Nelson LM, et al. Evaluation of treatment protocols on minimal to moderate spasticity in multiple sclerosis. *Arch Phys Med Rehabil.* 1991;72(3):186–189.

11. Rizzo M, Hadjimichael O, Preiningerova J, Vollmer T. Prevalence and treatment of spasticity reported by multiple sclerosis patients. *Mult Scler.* 2004;10:589–595.

12. O'Brien AR, Chiaravalloti N, Goverover Y, Deluca J. Evidenced-based cognitive rehabilitation for persons with multiple sclerosis: A review of the literature. *Arch Phys Med Rehabil.* 2008;89(4):761–769.

13. Schultheis MT, Weisser V, Ang J, et al. Examining the relationship between cognition and driving performance in multiple sclerosis. *Arch Phys Med Rehabil.* 2010;91(3):465–473.

14. Bethoux F, Miller D, Kinkel R. Recovery following acute exacerbations of multiple sclerosis: From impairment to quality of life. *Mult Scler.* 2000;7:137–142.

15. Lublin FD, Baier M, Cutter G. Effect of relapses on development of residual deficit in multiple sclerosis. *Neurology.* 2003;61:1528–1532.

16. Craig J, Young CA, Ennis M, et al. A randomised controlled trial comparing rehabilitation against standard therapy in multiple sclerosis patients receiving steroid treatment. *J Neurol Neurosurg Psychiatry.* 2003;74:1225–1230.

17. Liu C, Playfird ED, Thompson AJ. Does neurorehabilitation have a role in relapsing remitting multiple sclerosis? *J Neurol.* 2003;250(10):1214–1218.

18. Bethoux F, Miller DM, Stough D. Efficacy of outpatient rehabilitation after exacerbations of multiple sclerosis. *Arch Phys Med Rehabil.* 2005;84:A10.

19. Fox RJ, Thompson A, Baaker D, et al. Setting a research agenda for progressive multiple sclerosis: The International Collaborative on Progressive MS. *Mult Scler.* 2012;18:1534–1540.

20. Solari A, Filippini G, Gasco P, et al. Physical rehabilitation has a positive effect on disability in multiple sclerosis patients. *Neurology.* 1999;52:57–62.

21. Freeman J, Langdon D, Hobart J, Thompson A. Inpatient rehabilitation in multiple sclerosis: Do the benefits carry over in the community? *Neurology.* 1999;52:50–56.

22. Di Fabio R, Soderberg J, Choi T, et al. Extended outpatient rehabilitation: Its influence on symptom frequency, fatigue, and functional status for persons with progressive multiple sclerosis. *Arch Phys Med Rehabil.* 1998;79:141–146.

23. Khan F, Pallant JF, Brand C, Kilpatrick TJ. Effectiveness of rehabilitation intervention in persons with multiple sclerosis: A randomised controlled trial. *J Neurol Neurosurg Psychiatry.* 2008;79(11):1230–1235.

18

Fatigue in Multiple Sclerosis

SUSAN FORWELL

KEY POINTS FOR CLINICIANS

- Fatigue is experienced by 75% to 90% of persons with multiple sclerosis (MS), of which 50% indicate it is one of their worst problems.

- The pathogenesis of fatigue continues to be unclear.

- Factors that contribute to fatigue include depression, sleep problems, medication side effects, deconditioning, chronic stressors, and comorbid conditions.

- Primary MS fatigue refers to the fatigue experience that is directly related to the MS disease process, while nonprimary MS fatigue refers to fatigue that is related to other factors.

- The approach to fatigue management should be individual-centered, comprehensive, systematic, and sensitive to the individual's experience and priorities.

- It is helpful to use a 4-phase iterative process (identifying the presence of fatigue, screening, comprehensively assessing, and implementing an appropriate program of intervention) when managing fatigue.

- Fatigue management should target nonprimary and primary fatigue.

Fatigue in multiple sclerosis (MS) is real, disabling, and pervasive.

All human beings experience fatigue after hours of being awake or following activity. For this normal fatigue, rest or sleep restores the body's energy. Like the rest of us, those with MS experience this normal fatigue. In addition, persons with MS experience fatigue that is beyond normal fatigue and is related to the MS disease process and other contributing factors.

"Fatigue gets in the way of living my life" is a shared sentiment among persons with MS, as it has been shown to influence the ability to participate in paid work, domestic roles and responsibilities, and for some it creates challenges in taking care of oneself. Like that of pain and depression, the invisibility of fatigue brings a host of issues. Because it is difficult to objectively measure [1],

understanding the fatigue experience primarily rests with patient report. In a society where behaviors and attitudes that are represented by statements like "no pain no gain" or "beating it against all odds" are valued and rewarded, reporting fatigue may feel like complaining or not trying. A person with MS who experiences overwhelming fatigue may feel that there are times when they are not believed or that those around them do not understand the magnitude of the problem. It is on the functional, personal, social, and

> A person with MS who experiences fatigue may have concerns about not being believed or not being understood by others.

economic impact of fatigue on daily life, and its ubiquitous experience for persons with MS, that the premise of this chapter rests.

This chapter provides an overview of the issues related to fatigue in MS, of the factors that may contribute to or augment the fatigue experience, and of the process to address fatigue. This process is described in a 4-phase iterative framework that includes identifying the presence of fatigue, screening, comprehensive assessment, and intervention.

FATIGUE IN MS

Fatigue is experienced by 75% to 90% of persons with MS, of which 50% indicate it is one of their worst problems [1,2]. It negatively affects quality of life and employment, the latter of which may result in dire economic consequences [3–5]. Consistently, studies have demonstrated that there are physical, cognitive, and emotional aspects related to the fatigue experience in MS. Contradictory findings were reported regarding the correlation between fatigue and aspects of cognitive function, with some studies showing a correlation with action control (attention, motivation) and effortful wordlist learning with immediate verbal recall, while other studies found no significant correlation [6–8]. Cognitive difficulties, however, have been shown to influence fatigue as well as social function [9]. The demographic characteristics of age and sex are not associated with fatigue, nor is MS disease duration [10].

> Fatigue negatively affects quality of life and employment.

Pathogenesis

The pathogenesis of fatigue continues to be unclear. Studies using neuroimaging to understand potential anatomical correlates of MS fatigue show no correlation with T2 lesion load, but otherwise lack consensus in their findings [10,11]. With functional neuroimaging, preliminary evidence suggests that individuals with MS and fatigue have decreased glucose metabolism in the frontal cortex and basal ganglia [12]. While there has been some evidence related to neurotransmitter function, the role of the hypothalamus, and the contribution of amino acids, these remain preliminary findings [13,14].

> The pathogenesis of fatigue remains unclear.

Definition of Fatigue in MS

There are numerous definitions offered to capture the construct of fatigue in MS. Some address the duration and

impact, others the chronic nature of fatigue [15,16] while further definitions focus on the causes of fatigue [16] or the complexity of the entity [17]. For the purpose of this chapter, the definition of fatigue in MS is "a subjective lack of physical and/or mental energy that is perceived by the individual or caregiver to interfere with usual and desired activities" [15].

Factors That May Contribute to Fatigue in MS

Several factors appear to contribute to fatigue, including depression, sleep problems, side effects of medications, deconditioning, chronic stressors, comorbid medical conditions, and mobility impairment [18,19].

> Factors that may contribute to fatigue in MS are depression, sleep problems, side effects of medications, deconditioning, chronic stressors, comorbid medical conditions, and mobility impairment.

Depression plays a significant role in MS fatigue [20,21], and when depression is effectively treated the reported experience of fatigue is reduced [22]. The link, however, between depression and primary MS fatigue is considered by some to be an artifact that is, in part, because of fatigue being a symptom of depression as well as MS [6,7].

Sleep problems affect up to 58% of individuals with MS, the most common being sleep apnea–hypopnea [18,23]. Poor sleep quality is associated with fatigue, and when sleep disorders are treated there is a significant improvement in fatigue [24,25].

Medication side effects of fatigue are common for persons with MS. This includes disease-modifying therapies [26] as well as drugs used for symptomatic management, such as those prescribed for neuropathic pain and spasticity.

Deconditioning has been shown to be a contributor to fatigue in MS. Persons with MS are less active and the presence of muscle weakness and decreased endurance requires more energy to engage in activity [27,28]. Exercise programs reduce the impact of fatigue in MS [29].

Chronic stressors have been linked to fatigue in MS, such that if one feels they have control over their physical and social environment, they experience reduced fatigue and stress [30].

Comorbid medical conditions present a host of complications for persons with MS, among them fatigue. Treating comorbid conditions (eg, thyroid disease, infections, arthritis, anemia, cardiovascular disease) will have an impact on the fatigue experience in MS [31].

A relationship between *mobility impairment* and fatigue has been recently established [32], suggesting that maximizing efficient ambulation may have an impact on reducing fatigue.

Types of Fatigue in MS

While there have been many different labels for the various experiences and factors contributing to fatigue in MS, 6 types of fatigue are described here. Some of these are overlapping, some discrete, and all are relevant in the overall picture of MS fatigue.

Central fatigue (also called generalized fatigue) refers to the overall exhausted feeling that is a full body experience and has both a physical and mental component [33]. Simple resting does not remediate central fatigue.

Peripheral fatigue (also called motor fatigue) is the depletion, fatiguing, or progressive weakening of a muscle group with prolonged use [33]. For example, after walking a distance, one may experience increasing weakness of the ankle dorsiflexors such that the foot begins to slap or drag. Sufficient rest is typically therapeutic for this type of peripheral fatigue [33].

Primary MS fatigue refers to the fatigue experience that is directly related to the MS disease process such as demyelination, autoimmune phenomenon, or axonal loss [11].

Nonprimary MS fatigue refers to fatigue that is not directly related to the MS disease process and is considered to represent additional factors that contribute to fatigue in MS. Subtypes of nonprimary MS fatigue are secondary, acute, and chronic fatigue.

Secondary fatigue, a subset of nonprimary fatigue, refers to the fatigue resulting from or secondary to other symptoms of MS. For example, with increased walking challenges due to weakness or spasticity, more energy is required to move around.

Acute fatigue, another subset of nonprimary MS fatigue, refers to fatigue that occurs for a short period. It emerges as a result of a short-term condition or circumstance such as acute infection (eg, the common cold) or stressful events (eg, moving residence) [15].

Chronic fatigue, the final subset of nonprimary MS fatigue, refers to fatigue that lasts more than 6 months and emerges with long-term issues [15] such as depression and comorbid conditions.

Approach to Addressing Fatigue in MS

The diverse impact and factors related to fatigue clearly underscore the complex nature of the problem and the need for a targeted yet comprehensive approach. The principles of this approach are 4-fold: individual-centered, comprehensive, systematic, and sensitive.

> The principles for addressing fatigue in MS are individual-centered, comprehensive, systematic, and sensitive.

Individual-centered refers to ensuring the individual with MS identifies their priorities, preferences, and constraints related to fatigue, and its impact on their life. Their priorities may be as diverse as maintaining employment to attending a child's soccer game, while preferences may be related to valuing physical exercise or an interest in social activities. Constraints will also differ. For example, economic issues may present a barrier for some, while time to integrate suggestions is a concern for others.

Comprehensiveness refers to identifying and addressing not only the primary fatigue related to MS, but also factors that contribute to the fatigue experience. As the number of contributing factors increases, the severity of fatigue is enhanced [11].

Systematic refers to using a process that sequences assessment and intervention and allows for reevaluation and monitoring of all aspects and factors of the fatigue experience. Using the 4-phase process described here follows this principle.

The principle of *sensitivity* refers to addressing the area of fatigue in MS thoughtfully, recognizing that psychosocial attitudes, values, and experiences have shaped the individual's perception of normalcy, acceptability, stigma, and usefulness of reporting and addressing the issues of fatigue.

Process for Addressing Fatigue in MS

Mindful of these principles, a 4-phase iterative process is provided that includes identifying the presence of fatigue, screening, comprehensively assessing, and implementing an appropriate program of intervention. Figure 18.1 provides a graphic representation of this process.

> A 4-phase process to address fatigue in MS is: (a) Identifying the problem, (b) screening, (c) comprehensively assessing, and (d) implementing an appropriate program of intervention.

1. **Identify the presence of fatigue.** This phase establishes whether the person with MS has fatigue that interrupts or impacts everyday life. Questions to ask might include: "Is fatigue a problem for you?" or "Does fatigue get in the way of doing the things you need and want to do?"

   It is also critical to establish whether addressing the issue of fatigue is a priority or something the patient would like to deal with. While fatigue may be considerable and have a profound impact, other aspects of life or symptoms of MS may be a priority. In this situation, it will be important to account for fatigue in other interventions (for example, during a mobility program, vocational assessment, or when recommending home modifications).

2. **Screen for severity of fatigue.** If fatigue is an issue and priority for the individual, then moving onto screening for the severity of fatigue is recommended. The reason for screening is to

   - determine the level or severity of fatigue;
   - ensure fatigue is targeted for treatment, if appropriate;

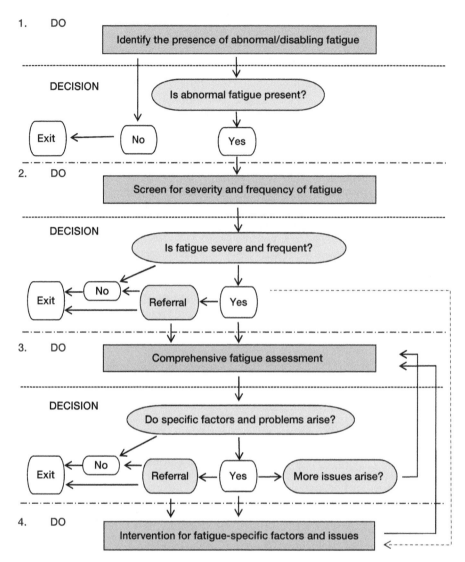

FIGURE 18.1
Evaluation and intervention process for fatigue in MS. *Adapted from Figure 14.1 in [34].*

- account for fatigue when treating other issues of MS or other chronic conditions;
- identify an outcome measure to establish a baseline and attest to the efficacy of intervention for fatigue.

There are no clinical laboratory tests or imaging techniques for fatigue. Rather, the measures that screen for the presence and severity of fatigue in MS are usually self-report tools completed using paper and pencil, smart technology (eg, electronic tablets) or computers. These measures are usually valid and reliable, include between 1 and 40 items, and are typically statements evaluated on Likert scales (for example, from 0–4) or visual analog scales (for example, marking a point on a line from least to most fatigue).

There are a number of measures to screen for fatigue in the general population (eg, the Occupational Fatigue Exhaustion Recovery, the Fatigue Symptom Checklist) as well as for specific groups with chronic conditions,

including MS. It is recommended that when screening for fatigue in MS, measures developed for or tested with the MS population be used. Table 18.1 provides examples of such measures. It is useful to select one of these measures and have it readily available, to be used as needed, during clinical visits.

> Use screening measures developed for or tested with the MS population.

In a consensus conference [43] with a multidisciplinary group of clinicians and researchers in MS, the following characteristics were deemed important for selecting an outcome measure of fatigue in MS:

- Measures the impact of fatigue on *activities* and *participation* as defined in the International Classification of Function (ICF) framework

TABLE 18.1
Measures to Screen for Fatigue in MS

MEASURE	NUMBER OF ITEMS	FORMAT	SCORING	DESCRIPTION	SOURCE
Short measures (5–7 minutes to complete)					
Fatigue Severity Scale (FSS)	9	Likert Scale; 1–7 for each item	Sum values and divide by 9. Score is out of 7. Higher score = worse fatigue	Items are phrases related to severity and impact on activities	[35]
Daily Fatigue Impact Scale (D-FIS)	8	Likert Scale; 0–4 for each item	Sum score. Score is out of 32. Higher score = worse fatigue	Items are phrases related to current daily changes in life attributable to fatigue	[36]
PROMIS v1.0 Fatigue Short Form	7	Likert Scale; 1–5	Sum score. Score is out of 35 with higher score = worse fatigue	Items are phrases related to feelings of tiredness and sense of exhaustion that decrease the ability to execute daily activities and family/social roles	[37] www.nihpromis.org/assessment
Visual Analog Scale for fatigue	1	100 mm line	Divide the line into one-thirds—mild, moderate, and severe fatigue	Ends of line are "Not fatigued at all" and "Extremely fatigued"	[35]
Categorical					
Fatigue Impact Scale (FIS)	36	Likert Scale; 0–4 for each item	Summed scores. Score is out of 144 with higher scores = worse fatigue	3 Three dimensions: cognitive (10 items), physical (10 items), social (16 items)	[1]
Modified Fatigue Impact Scale (MFIS)	21	Likert Scale; 0–4 for each item	Summed scores; Score is out of 84 with higher scores = worse fatigue	3 Three subscales: cognitive (10 items), physical (9 items), psycho-social (2 items)	[1]
Multicomponent Fatigue Scale (MFS)	15	Likert Scale; 0–4 for each item	Summed scores. Score is out of 60 with higher scores = worse fatigue	3 Two subscales: cognitive (7 items), physical (8 items)	[38]
Fatigue Scale for Motor & Cognitive Functions (FSMC)	20	Likert Scale; 0–4 for each item	Summed scores. Score is out of 80 with higher scores = worse fatigue	3 Two subscales: cognitive (10 items), physical (10 items)	[39]
Noncategorical					
Fatigue Assessment Instrument (FAI)	29	Likert Scale; 1–7 for each item	Sum values. Score ranges from 29 to 203. Higher score = worse fatigue	Items are phrases capturing quantitative and qualitative components of fatigue	[40]
Würzburg Fatigue Inventory for MS (WEIMuS)	17	Likert Scale; 0–4 for each item	Sum values. Score is out of 68 with higher score = worse fatigue	Items are phrases related severity and impact on activities and cognition	[41]
Rochester Fatigue Diary (RFD)	24	24 lines (one for each hour of the day). Ends are "Energetic, no fatigue" to "Exhausted, severe fatigue"	Divide the line into one-thirds—mild, moderate, and severe fatigue	Place a mark on the line rating average energy for each hour. If asleep, the line is not marked for that hour.	[42]

- Time efficient, easy, quick
- Has established psychometric properties for validity and reliability for MS
- Applicable over the MS disease course
- Could be self-report or administered by a health professional

- Includes features of self efficacy
- Includes content related to managing fatigue and contributing factors

Each of the measures described in Table 18.1 were evaluated to ascertain their fit with these characteristics [43].

It was shown that most measures address issues of impact on activities and participation, are time efficient, have established psychometrics for MS, and are self-administered. The majority of these measures, however, do not address issues of self-efficacy in the face of fatigue, methods used to manage fatigue, or other factors that contribute to fatigue [43]. It is, however, unrealistic to expect outcome measures or tools used to screen for the level of fatigue to also provide indepth information related to these elements. Rather, once the screening measure has identified the severity of fatigue, a comprehensive assessment that can provide information on these areas and guide intervention decisions is recommended. Completing phases 1 and 2 can be done efficiently, and in most cases does not take more than 15 minutes.

Even at this screening phase, however, as shown in Figure 18.1, there may be an opportunity to provide targeted interventions. For example, if heat is identified as impacting fatigue tolerance, there might be consideration for trying a cooling garment.

3. **In-depth assessment of fatigue in MS.** After screening for the level of fatigue in MS, completing an indepth assessment is essential. The comprehensive assessment provides information to

- identify and ascertain the scope of potential factors contributing to fatigue;
- ensure factors contributing to fatigue are addressed;
- guide intervention decisions.

Studies have shown that factors that may contribute to nonprimary MS fatigue are present for 72% to 74% of persons with MS who experience fatigue [18,19] (see Table 18.2) and that this subgroup experiences a higher level of fatigue [18]. Furthermore, some of these factors can be treated, or at least partially alleviated, such as depression, sleep problems, mobility challenges, and medication side effects.

A comprehensive assessment of fatigue in MS can begin with a series of self-report questionnaires that assess factors which may contribute to the fatigue experience. Because these questionnaires cover a broad spectrum of issues, they take time to complete. These questionnaires can be forwarded to the individual to be completed in advance of the appointment with the health care provider (HCP). In an unhurried setting, the questionnaires can then be completed more thoughtfully, with less stress, and may allow for input from others who know them well, all of which increase the ecological validity of responses. The completed questionnaires are then reviewed at the next visit by the HCP, typically the occupational therapist, who can quickly see the issues and target discussion and intervention priorities.

> Comprehensive assessments can be completed in advance of the appointment with the HCP.

TABLE 18.2
Frequency of Coexisting Factors for Persons With Fatigue and MS

	n (%) [18]	n (%) [19]
Non-MS fatigue-CHRONIC	**36 (72%)**	**945 (74%)**
Acute	4 (8%)	—
Chronic		
• Sleep problems	29 (58%)	313 (25%)
• Depression	20 (40%)	567 (44%)
• Medications	10 (20%)	105 (8%)
• Deconditioning	10 (20%)	—
• Significant chronic stressors	3 (6%)	255 (20%)
• Concomitant medical problems	2 (4%)	181 (14%)
Secondary MS fatigue		
• Unmanaged mobility impairment	26 (52%)	282 (22%)
• Respiratory problems	2 (4%)	—
Primary MS fatigue	**14 (28%)**	**335 (26%)**

Preliminary work has been completed on a Comprehensive Fatigue Assessment Battery for MS [44] that assesses the presence of comorbid conditions, fatigue and self-efficacy, pain, sleep, stress, depression, anxiety, mobility, environment, nutrition, and fatigue management history. To review the completed questionnaires, the HCP and patient will take, on average, 10 to 30 minutes depending on the number of issues identified and the clarifying discussion that follows.

Along with this information, it may be necessary to complete performance-based assessments related to mobility or methods of fatigue management. It is important to remember that clinically observed performance does not necessarily correlate with the experience of fatigue.

4. **Intervention.** In the fourth phase, intervention begins with treating the factors that contribute to fatigue, and followed by or concurrently treating the primary MS fatigue.

   a. Treating factors that may contribute to fatigue in MS. Most often, several factors contribute to the fatigue experience in MS, and fortunately many of these factors have intervention pathways, either through referral or directly attending to the issue. For example,

   - depression can be treated with counseling, psychotherapy, medication, or group interventions;
   - fatiguing side effects of medications can be identified through a review of the medications, and adjustments might then be made to the administration schedule, type, or dosage of drug;
   - sleep problems, depending on the nature, may be addressed through educating on sleep hygiene principles, providing strategies to manage the social

environment that interrupts sleep, medications, and in some cases referral to a sleep specialist to assess and treat possible sleep disorders; and

• inefficient mobility or deconditioning is typically managed through an appropriate exercise or activity program.

> Typically many factors contribute to fatigue. Fortunately, many are treatable either through referral or directly attending to the issue.

b. Treating primary MS fatigue. The intervention plan for primary MS fatigue usual follows a multipronged approach. There are 3 types of interventions for primary MS fatigue: (i) Pharmacotherapy, (ii) psychoeducation and behavioral programs, and (iii) complementary and alternative strategies.

i. **Pharmacotherapy**. For primary MS fatigue has had a modest effect. Table 18.3 lists the agents that have been tested, their dosage, and the results. Of these, amantadine and modafinil have shown the greatest promise.

ii. **Psychoeducation and behavioral programs** have also been tested with favorable results. There are 2 energy management programs that utilize a self-management approach and are efficacious as an intervention for addressing fatigue in MS.

a. An *Energy conservation program* that is offered in 6 weekly 2 hour group sessions [53,54]. The content of the program includes the importance of rest, communicating about fatigue, body mechanics, energy efficiency devices, ergonomics and modifying the environment, goal setting, activity analysis, and life style review. The efficacy of this program has been established for different formats including face-to-face format, teleconference, and online [54–56].

b. A video series, *Fatigue: Take Control*, consists of 5 15 to 25 minute videos and has shown a positive effect on reducing the fatigue experience [57]. The content of these videos include medical management of fatigue, cognitive fatigue, heat sensitivity, diet, goal setting, exercise, changes at home/work, mobility, energy conservation, ergonomics, and analyzing and modifying activities.

TABLE 18.3
Evidence for Pharmacotherapy for Treating Fatigue in MS

AUTHOR	DOSAGE	MEASURE	METHOD	RESULT
Amantadine				
[45] (n = 32)	100 mg twice a day	Fatigue Assessment Scale	Double-blind, controlled study	Moderate—marked improvement
[46] (n = 115)	100 mg twice daily	VAS and ADLs	Cross-over design	Small but significant improvement
[47] (n = 22)	100 mg twice daily	5-point scales for energy, strength, cognition, and well-being	Double-blind, controlled study	Higher self-report ratings
[48] (n = 93)	100 mg twice daily	MS-specific FSS; FSS	Randomized, double-blind, placebo-controlled study	Significant improvement
Pemoline				
[48] (n = 93)	18.75 mg daily in wk 1 37.5 mg daily in wk 2 56.25 mg daily wks 3–6	FSS	Randomized, double-blind, placebo-controlled study	No significant improvement at 56.25 mg/day
[49] (n = 41)	75 mg daily for 2 4-wk periods	VAS	Double-blind, placebo-controlled, crossover trial	Good—excellent improvement
3,4 diaminopyridine				
[50] (n = 8)	50–60 mg/according to body size, taken for 3 wks	FSS	Open label clinical trial	Improvement observed
Modafinil				
[51] (n = 72)	200 mg/day for 2 wks followed by 400 mg/day for 2 wks	FSS, MFIS, fatigue VAS	Single blind, pilot study	Significant Improvement
[52] (n = 115)	200 mg/day for 1 wk based on tolerance, increased to: 300 mg/day in wk 2 400 mg/day in wk 3	MFIS	5 week randomized, double-blind, placebo-controlled	No difference

ADLs, activities of daily living; FSS, fatigue severity scale; MFIS, modified fatigue impact scale; VAS, visual analog scale.

c. Exercise programs have also been shown to have a mitigating effect on fatigue. These include vestibular training [58], treadmill training [59], elliptical exercise [60], and progressive resistance training [29].

iii. **Complementary and alternative strategies.** The use of complementary and alternative methods (CAM) is widely accepted among persons with MS, with 65% to 90% using at least 1 kind of CAM [61,62]. CAM strategies demonstrating some modest impact on reducing the effects of fatigue in MS include yoga, cooling therapy, ginko, hydrotherapy (Ai Chi aqua therapy), and mindfulness training [63–66]. CAM that showed no effect were hyperbaric oxygen, polyunsaturated fatty acid diets, dental amalgam removal, and bee venom therapy [19]. In general, while the benefit derived from CAM may have a modest impact on reducing fatigue, there may be significant benefit relative to feelings of well-being, along with the fact that most of these strategies pose no added risk.

CONCLUSION

The understanding of fatigue in MS has significantly progressed in the last 20 years. There are now numerous screening measures available and diverse, though still limited number of, treatment strategies. The systematic, thorough approach offered here facilitates the comprehensive management of this complex and common problem among those with MS. Gaps, however, remain. A further understanding of the pathogenesis of fatigue in MS is required to better hone assessment and intervention tools. Adding to the repertoire of interventions that can be easily incorporated by the individual with MS is the key to successfully managing this pervasive problem.

KEY POINTS FOR PATIENTS AND FAMILIES

- Fatigue is very frequent with MS, and has a significant impact on activities and quality of life.

- Fatigue has been named one of the "invisible symptoms of MS," because it is primarily a subjective symptom.

- While it is sometimes difficult to communicate the experience of fatigue to others, questionnaires have been developed to reliably measure MS fatigue.

- Although the cause of MS fatigue remains unclear, effective interventions have been identified.

- It is important to identify and address factors that contribute to fatigue, such as mood and sleep problems, medication side effects, lack of physical activity, and other health problems.

- Interventions that may help with MS fatigue include educational programs, exercise programs, medications, as well as complementary and alternative strategies.

- Prioritizing activities and planning rest periods are important steps in managing energy throughout the day.

- It is essential to communicate with your HCP about your fatigue; for example, how fatigue affects you, if your fatigue has worsened, and whether treatments for fatigue were effective or not.

REFERENCES

1. Fisk JD, Pantefract A, Ritvo PG, et al. The impact of fatigue on patients with multiple sclerosis. *Can J Neurol Sci.* 1994;21:9–14.

2. Freal JE, Kraft G, Coryell J. Symptomatic fatigue in multiple sclerosis. *Arch of Phys Med Rehabil.* 1984;65:135–138.

3. Julian LJ, Vella L, Vollmer T, et al. Employment in multiple sclerosis. Exiting and re-entering the work force. *J Neurol.* 2008;255(9):1354–1360.

4. Janardhan V, Bakshi R. Quality of life in patients with multiple sclerosis: The impact of fatigue and depression. *J Neurol Sci.* 2002;205:51–58.

5. Edgley K, Sullivan MJL, Deboux E. A survey of multiple sclerosis. Part 2: Determinants of employment status. *Can J Rehabil.* 1991;4(3):127–132.

6. Penner IK, Bechtel N, Raselli C, et al. Fatigue in multiple sclerosis: Relation to depression, physical impairment, personality and action control. *Mult Scler.* 2007;13(9):1161–1167.

7. Morrow SA, Weinstock-Guttman B, Munschauer FE, et al. Subjective fatigue is not associated with cognitive impairment in multiple sclerosis: Cross-sectional and longitudinal analysis. *Mult Scler.* 2009;15(8):998–1005.

8. Diamond BJ, Johnson SK, Kaufman M, Graves L. Relationships between information processing, depression, fatigue and cognition in multiple sclerosis. *Arch Clin Neuropsychol.* 2008;23(2):189–199.

9. Patti F. Cognitive impairment in multiple sclerosis. *Mult Scler.* 2009;15(1):2–8.

10. Mainero C, Faroni J, Gasperini C, et al. Fatigue and magnetic resonance imaging activity in multiple sclerosis. *J Neurol.* 1999;246:454–458.

11. Kos D, Kerckhofs E, Nagels G, et al. Origin of fatigue in multiple sclerosis: Review of the literature. *Neurorehabil Neural Repair.* 2008 Jan–Feb;22(1):91–100.

12. Roelcke U, Kappos L, Lechner-Scott J, et al. Reduced glucose metabolism in the frontal cortex and basal ganglia of multiple sclerosis patients with fatigue: A 18F-fluorodeoxyglucose positron emission tomography study. *Neurology.* 1997;48:1566–1571.

13. Heilman K, Watson R. Fatigue. *Neurol Network Communication.* 1997;1:283–287.

14. Newsholme EA, Blomstrand E. The plasma level of some amino acids and physical and mental fatigue. *Experientia.* 1996;52:413–415.

15. Multiple Sclerosis Council for Clinical Practice Guidelines. *Fatigue and Multiple Sclerosis: Evidence-Based Management Strategies for Fatigue in Multiple Sclerosis.* Washington DC: Paralyzed Veterans of America; 1998.

16. Induruwa I, Constantinescu CS, Gran B. Fatigue in multiple sclerosis-A brief review. *J Neurol Sci.* 2012;323:9–15.

17. Braley TJ, Chervin RD. Fatigue in multiple sclerosis: Mechanisms, evaluation, and treatment. *Sleep.* 2010;33(8):1061–1067.

18. Forwell S, Brunham S, Tremlett H, et al. Primary and non primary fatigue in multiple sclerosis. *Int J MS Care.* 2008;10:14–20.

19. Stewart TM, Tran ZV, Bowling AC. Factors related to fatigue in multiple sclerosis. *Int J MS Care.* 2007;9:29–34.

20. Bol Y, Duits AA, Hupperts RMM, et al. The impact of fatigue on cognitive functioning in patients with multiple sclerosis. *Clin Rehabil.* 2010;24:854–862.

21. Patrick E, Christodoulou C, Krupp LB. Longitudinal correlates of fatigue in multiple sclerosis. *Mult Scler.* 2009;15(2):258–261.

22. Mohr DC, Hart SL, Goldberg A. Effects of treatment for depression on fatigue in multiple sclerosis. *Psychosom Med.* 2003;65(4):542–547.

23. Trojan DA, Da Costa D, Bar-Or A, et al. Sleep abnormalities in multiple sclerosis patients (Abstract). *Mult Scler.* 2008;14(Suppl 1):S160.

24. Trojan DA, Arnold D, Collet JP, et al. Fatigue in multiple sclerosis: Association with disease-related, behavioural and psychosocial factors. *Mult Scler.* 2007;13(8):985–995.

25. Lobentanz IS, Asenbaum S, Vass K, et al. Factors influencing quality of life in multiple sclerosis patients: Disability, depressive mood, fatigue and sleep quality. *Acta Neurol Scand.* 2004;110(1):6–13.

26. Neilley LK, Goodin DS, Goodkin DE, Hauser SL. Side effect profile of interferon beta-1b in MS Results of an open label trial. *Neurology.* 1996;46(2):552–553.

27. Motl RW, Gosney JL. Effect of exercise training on quality of life in multiple sclerosis: A meta-analysis. *Mult Scler.* 2008;14(1):129–135.

28. Motl WR, Goldman M. Physical inactivity, neurological disability, and cardiorespiratory fitness in multiple sclerosis. *Acta Neurol Scand.* 2011;123(2):98–104.

29. Dalgus U, Stenager E, Jakobsen J, et al. Fatigue, mood and quality of life improve in MS patients after progressive resistance training. *Mult Scler.* 2010;16(4):480–490.

30. Schwartz CE, Coulthard Morris L, Zeng Q. Psychosocial correlates of fatigue in multiple sclerosis. *Arch Phys Med Rehabil.* 1996;77:165–170.

31. Marrie RA, Horwitz RI. Emerging effects of comorbidities on multiple sclerosis. *Lancet Neurol.* 2010;9(8):820–828.

32. Motl RW, Sandroff BM, Suh Y, Sosnoff JJ. Energy cost of walking and its association with gait parameters, daily activity, and fatigue in persons with mild multiple sclerosis. *Neurorehabil Neural Repair.* 2012;26(8):1015–1021.

33. Chaudhuri A, Behan PO. Fatigue in neurological disorders. *Lancet.* 2004 Mar 20;363(9413):978–988.

34. Forwell SJ, Perrin Ross A. Self Care. In: Finlayson M, ed. *Multiple Sclerosis Rehabilitation: From Impairment to Participation.* Taylor & Francis LLC; 2012:327–354.

35. Krupp L, LaRocca N, Muir-Nash J, Steinberg AD. The fatigue severity scale: Application to patients with multiple sclerosis and systemic lupus erythematosus. *Ach Neurol.* 1989;46:1121–1123.

36. Benito-León J, Martínez-Martín P, Frades B, et al. Impact of fatigue in multiple sclerosis: The fatigue impact scale for daily use (D-FIS). *Mult Scler.* 2007;13(5):645–651.

37. Patient Reported Outcome Measurement Information System. 2011. PROMIS Scoring Guide.

38. Paul R, Beatty W, Schneider R, et al. Cognitive and physical fatigue in multiple sclerosis: relations between self-report and objective performance. *Appl Neuropsychol.* 1998;5:143–148.

39. Penner IK, Raselli C, Stöcklin M, et al. The Fatigue Scale for Motor and Cognitive Functions (FSMC): Validation of a new instrument to assess multiple sclerosis-related fatigue. *Mult Scler.* 2009;15(12):1509–1517.

40. Schwartz JE, Jandorf L, Krupp LB. The measurement of fatigue: A new instrument. *J Psychosom Res.* 1993;37(7):753–762.

41. Flachenecker P, Meissner H. Fatigue in multiple sclerosis presenting as acute relapse: subjective and objective assessment. *Mult Scler.* 2008;14(2):274–277.

42. Schwid SR, Covington M, Segal BM, Goodman AD. Fatigue in multiple sclerosis: Current understanding and future directions. *J Rehabil Res Dev.* 2002;39(2):211–224.

43. Hutchinson B, Forwell SJ, Bennett S, et al. Towards a consensus on rehabilitation outcomes in MS: Gait and fatigue CSMC consensus conference. *Int J MS Care.* 2009;11:67–78.

44. Forwell SJ, Ghahari S. Comprehensive Fatigue Assessment Battery for Multiple Sclerosis: Clinico-metric Properties. Council of Occupational Therapists from the European Countries (COTEC), Stockholm, Sweden; May 2012.

45. Murray TJ. Amantadine therapy for fatigue in multiple sclerosis. *Can J Neurol Sci.* 1985;12:251–254.

46. Canadian MS Research Group. A randomized controlled trial of amantadine in fatigue associated with multiple sclerosis. *Can J Neurosci.* 1987;14:273–278.

47. Cohen RA, Fisher M. Amantadine treatment of fatigue associated with multiple sclerosis. *Arch Neurol.* 1989;46:676–680.

48. Krupp LB, Coyle PK, Doscher C, et al. Fatigue therapy in multiple sclerosis: Results of a double-blind, randomized, parallel trial of amantadine, pemoline, and placebo. *Neurology.* 1995;45:1956–1961.

49. Weinshenker BG, Penman M, Bass B, et al. A double-blind, randomized, crossover trial of pemoline in fatigue associated with multiple sclerosis. *Neurology.* 1992;42:1468–1471.

50. Sheean GL, Murray NM, Rothwell JC, et al. An open-labelled clinical and electrophysiological study of 3,4-diaminopyridine in the treatment of fatigue in multiple sclerosis. *Brain.* 1998;121:967–975.

51. Rammohan KW, Rosenberg JH, Lynn DJ, et al. Efficacy and safety of modafinil (Provigil) for the treatment of fatigue in multiple sclerosis: A two centre phase 2 study. *J Neurol Neurosurg Psychiatry.* 2002;72(2):179–183.

52. Stankoff B, Waubant E, Confavreux C, et al. Modafinil for fatigue in MS: A randomized placebo-controlled double-blind study. *Neurology.* 2005;64(7):1139–1143.

53. Packer TL, Sauriol A, Brouwer B. Fatigue secondary to chronic illness: Postpolio syndrome, chronic fatigue syndrome and multiple sclerosis. *Arch Phys Med Rehabil.* 1995;75:1122–1126.

54. Mathiowetz V, Finlayson ML, Matuska KM, et al. Randomized controlled trial of an energy conservation course for persons with multiple sclerosis. *Mult Scler.* 2005;11:592–601.

55. Finlayson M, Holberg C. Evaluation of a teleconference-delivered energy conservation education program for people with multiple sclerosis. *Can J Occup Ther.* 2007;74(4):337–347.

56. Ghahari S, Packer TL, Passmore AE. Effectiveness of an online fatigue self-management program for people with chronic neurological conditions: A randomized controlled trial. *Clin Rehabil.* 2010;24(8):727–744.

57. Hugos CL, Copperman LF, Fuller BE, et al. Clinical trial of a formal group fatigue program in multiple sclerosis. *Mult Scler.* 2010;16(6):724–732.

58. Hebert JR, Corboy JR, Manago MM, Schenkman M. Effects of vestibular rehabilitation on multiple sclerosis-related fatigue and upright postural control: A randomized controlled trial. *Phys Ther.* 2011;91(8):1166–1183.

59. Pilutti LA, Lelli DA, Paulseth JE, et al. Effects of 12 weeks of supported treadmill training on functional ability and quality of life in progressive multiple sclerosis: A pilot study. *Arch Phys Med Rehabil.* 2011;92(1):31–36.

60. Huisinga JM, Filipi ML, Stergiou N. Elliptical exercise improves fatigue ratings and quality of life in patients with multiple sclerosis. *J Rehabil Res Dev.* 2011;48(7):881–890.

61. Bowling AC. Complimentary and alternative medicine in multiple sclerosis: Dispelling common myths about CAM. *Int J MS Care.* 2005;7(2):42–44.

62. Olsen SA. A review of complementary and alternative medicine (CAM) by people with multiple sclerosis. *Occup Ther Int.* 2009;16(1):57–70.

63. Bowling AC. Complementary and alternative medicine and multiple sclerosis. *Neurol Clin.* 2011;29(2):465–480.

64. Johnson SK, Diamond BJ, Rausch S, et al. The effect of Ginkgo biloba on functional measures in multiple sclerosis: A pilot randomized controlled trial. *Explore (NY).* 2006;2(1):19–24.

65. Castro-Sánchez AM, Matarán-Peñarrocha GA, Lara-Palomo I, et al. Hydrotherapy for the treatment of pain in people with multiple sclerosis: A randomized controlled trial. *Evid Based Complement Alternat Med.* 2012;2012:473963.

66. Grossman P, Kappos L, Gensicke H, et al. MS quality of life, depression, and fatigue improve after mindfulness training: A randomized trial. *Neurology.* 2010 Sep 28;75(13):1141–1149.

19

Emotional Disorders in Multiple Sclerosis

ELIAS A. KHAWAM

KEY POINTS FOR CLINICIANS

- Emotional disorders are common in multiple sclerosis (MS) and cause significant disturbances in patients' quality of life and compliance with treatment.

- Depression is the most common psychiatric comorbidity encountered in MS and can affect up to 54% of patients. The etiology of major depression in MS is multifactorial and includes both biological and psychological factors. Early recognition and treatment is essential to decrease morbidity and mortality.

- Screening tools are available to identify depressed patients. The Hospital Anxiety and Depression Scale and the Beck Depression Inventory-Fast Screen have been validated for MS patients.

- Treatment for psychiatric disorders in MS should be individualized and involve psychopharmacology, psychotherapy, or combined treatment.

- The suicide rate in MS is elevated compared to the general population. Patients' suicidal ideations should be taken seriously. If the patient appears at high risk, a psychiatric evaluation should be immediately requested.

- Pseudobulbar affect (PBA) causes significant distress and has a negative impact on patients and caregivers. Center for Neurologic Study-Lability Scale (CNS-LS) is a useful tool for the assessment of PBA. Medications are available to effectively treat this condition.

Multiple sclerosis (MS) is a chronic and disabling demyelinating disorder of the central nervous system. It causes multiple neuropsychiatric disturbances including mood, affect, behavior, and cognitive abnormalities. Psychiatric conditions cause significant disturbances in patients' social life, occupation, and family structure, in addition to affecting compliance with treatment.

Despite their higher prevalence in MS compared to the general population [1,2] and their negative effect on quality of life [3], psychiatric disorders remain underdiagnosed and undertreated.

While depression has been the most studied, other psychiatric disorders, such as anxiety disorders, bipolar disorder, euphoria, pseudobulbar affect, and psychotic disorders, received less attention. We review in this chapter the most common psychiatric disorders in MS. Cognitive disorders are discussed in Chapter 20.

MAJOR DEPRESSION IN MS

Depression disorder is the most common psychiatric comorbidity encountered in MS. Its prevalence in MS is 2-folds that of the general population (Table 19.1). Depression causes significant personal suffering and adversely affects physical activity, fatigue, pain, and quality of life.

Diagnosis of Depression

Physicians should be able to differentiate between depressed mood as a symptom and major depressive disorder (MDD), which represents a cluster of symptoms and necessitates treatment.

Depressed mood could be a symptom of other psychiatric disorders. Patients with adjustment disorder, for example, develop a group of symptoms involving emotions, such as depressed mood or anxiety, or behavior. These symptoms occur within 3 months of the onset of an identifiable stress. The prevalence of adjustment disorder with depressed mood was 22% in patients who were examined within 2 months of an MS diagnosis [10]. Adjustment disorder does not necessarily require psychopharmacological therapy except in severe cases. Psychotherapy is usually the primary treatment modality.

The Diagnostic and Statistical Manual DSM-IV-R criteria for major depressive episode require the presence of 5 or more of the following symptoms within a 2 week period with at least 1 symptom being either depressed mood or loss of interest or pleasure:

- Depressed mood
- Loss of interest or pleasure in all or almost all activities
- Weight loss or weight gain
- Insomnia or hypersomnia

- Psychomotor retardation or agitation
- Fatigue or loss of energy nearly every day
- Feelings of worthlessness, or excessive inappropriate guilt
- Diminished ability to think or concentrate
- Recurrent thoughts of death

Symptoms are present most of the day, nearly every day and cause significant functioning impairment.

Diagnosing major depression in MS based on DSM-IV-R criteria could be challenging because of an overlap between neurological impairments and the vegetative symptoms of MDD. Symptoms such as fatigue, insomnia, and decreased concentration and appetite occur in many MS patients in the absence of depression. The presence of inappropriate guilt, self-blaming, and passive thoughts of death or active suicidal ideations should not be considered a normal reaction to a chronic illness. Symptoms such as anger, irritability, worry, and discouragement have been associated with depression in MS. Isolation, hopelessness, helplessness, and worthlessness are often associated with MDD.

Some features that may help physicians differentiate between somatic symptoms related to depression versus MS symptoms are:

- Persistent low mood and loss of interest or pleasure beyond what is expected as a normal reaction to stress, even after the resolution of such stress
- Worsening mood despite neurological improvement
- Initial or middle insomnia are more prevalent in MS than in depression
- Fatigue tends to get worse as the day progresses in MS compared to some improvement or fluctuation of energy level in depressed patients
- Dramatic worsening of fatigue and concentration, compared to baseline level, in association with depressed mood.

Early recognition and treatment of MDD in MS patients is essential to decrease morbidity and mortality

TABLE 19.1
Prevalence and Common Psychopharmacological Treatment for Emotional Disorders in MS

EMOTIONAL DISORDERS	PREVALENCE	PSYCHOPHARMACOLOGICAL TREATMENT
Major depressive disorder	12 months: 15.7% [1]	SSRIs, SNRIs, bupropion, mirtazapine, TCAs
	Life time: 27%–54% [1,4,5]	
Bipolar disorder	2.4%–13% [6,7]	Lithium, Depakote, carbamazepine, atypical antipsychotics
Euphoria	Up to 13% [8]	None
Anxiety disorders	35.7% [2]	SSRIs, SNRIs, buspirone
Psychotic disorders	2%–3% [9]	Atypical antipsychotics, typical antipsychotics

SNRI, serotonin norepinephrine reuptake inhibitors; SSRI, selective serotonin reuptake inhibitors; TCA, tricyclic antidepressant.

TABLE 19.2
Screening Tools for Depression in MS

Hospital Anxiety and Depression Scale (HADS) [11]	14-item scale self-report questionnaire split equally between anxiety and depression questions. A threshold score of 8 or greater has 90% sensitivity and 87.3% specificity for the depression subscale.
Beck Depression Inventory-Fast Screen (BDI-FS) [12]	Self-report questionnaire that consists of 7 items: dysphoria, anhedonia, suicide, and 4 items that measure nonsomatic criteria for major depressive disorder.
Beck Depression Inventory (BDI) [10]	21-item self-report inventory that has been used widely for depression screening in MS. A cut-off score of 13 has 71% sensitivity and 79% specificity for depression.
Patient Health Questionnaire-9 (PHQ-9) [13]	The PHQ-9 uses the DSM-IV criteria for depression and asks the patient to rate them from "0" (not at all) to "3" (nearly every day). A score equal to or greater than 10 had 88% sensitivity and 88% specificity for major depression. Scores of 5, 10, 15, and 20 correlate respectively with mild, moderate, moderately severe, and severe depression.
Center for Epidemiologic Studies-Depression Scale (CES-D) [14]	Depression screening tool that has been used in epidemiological studies.
Chicago Multiscale Depression Inventory (CMDI) [15]	This inventory is divided into 3 depression scales which help differentiating mood, vegetative, and depressive cognitive symptoms.
Inventory for Depressive Symptomatology (IDC) [16]	Combines a clinician-Rated (IDS-C) and a self-report (IDS-SR) scale.

and to improve quality of life. Physicians are encouraged to use screening tools (Table 19.2) to identify depressed patients, keeping in mind that the clinical interview remains the golden standard to diagnose major depression. The Hospital Anxiety and Depression Scale [11] and the Beck Depression Inventory-Fast Screen [12] have been validated for MS patients. We have found that the Patient Health Questionnaire-9 (PHQ-9) items are a useful screening tool for depression in our center.

The Goldman Algorithm [17,18] recommends a regular screening for depression for all MS patients by either the 2-question screen (2QS), the Beck Depression Inventory (BDI), or the PHQ-9. In case of positive screening, a diagnostic interview for depression is recommended, including an assessment for suicidality. Referral to psychiatry is warranted if severe depression is identified. Otherwise, the neurologist should discuss the treatment options, including pharmacotherapy, psychotherapy (supportive, interpersonal, or cognitive behavioral therapy), or both, in addition to setting up a follow-up assessment.

Etiology of Depression in MS

The etiology of major depression in MS is multifactorial and includes both biological and psychological factors (Table 19.3). Structural neuroimaging studies highlighted the association between depression in MS and an increase in lesion load in the left suprainsular region, the right temporal lobe [19], and the superior frontal and parietal white matter, as well as frontal atrophy [20].

A growing body of evidence suggests an association between brain inflammation, autoimmune dysregulation, and endocrine dysfunction in MS-related depression. Lower CD8+ cell numbers and higher CD4/CD8 ratio were

TABLE 19.3
Factors Associated With Depression in MS

- Brain lesion location
- Autoimmune dysregulation
- Endocrine abnormalities
- MS somatic symptoms (pain, fatigue, etc.)
- Cognitive impairment
- Unpredictability of disease progression
- Psychosocial stressors
- MS effects on social life, occupation, and family
- Poor coping strategies
- Limited support system
- History of mood disorder

linked to increased depression in chronic progressive MS patients. The production of the cytokine interferon (IFN) gamma in relapsing-remitting MS is related to depression, and its production was reduced in association with depression treatment. Several other studies confirmed the association between elevated cytokine levels and depression [21].

Fassbender et al. [22] studied the relationship between depressive symptoms and Hypothalamic-Pituitary-Adrenal (HPA) axis function in MS patients. When compared to a control group, MS patients failed to suppress corticotropin releasing hormone (CRH)-induced corticotrophin and cortisol response after dexamethasone administration. A higher level of depression and anxiety is associated with increased serum cortisol level following a dexamethasone CRH Suppression Test.

Treatment for Major Depression

Treatment for depression in MS should be individualized and involve psychopharmacology, psychotherapy, or combined treatment [17]. Despite the common use of antidepressants among depressed MS patients and empirical evidence of its clinical effectiveness, rigorous evidence is lacking.

There are only 2 published randomized controlled trials (RCTs) so far studying the effectiveness of antidepressants on major depression in MS. In a 5 week small RCT (N = 28), desipramine was found to be more effective when compared to control group [23]. Side effects including postural hypotension, constipation, and dry mouth, limited desipramine dose increase. Paroxetine was compared to placebo in a double-blind 12 week RCT (N = 42) [24]. Patients who were treated with paroxetine showed improvement of depressive symptoms. However, patients in both trials did not achieve full remission of depression. The effectiveness of antidepressants was also documented in open label trials (sertraline and moclobemide) and case reports (fluoxetine).

The effectiveness of psychotherapy for the treatment of depression in MS has been assessed in a number of studies. Individual cognitive behavior therapy (CBT) has been compared to supportive expressive group psychotherapy (SET) and to sertraline. CBT and sertraline were found to be equally effective, and superior to SET, in the treatment of major depression [25]. CBT delivered by telephone was found to be valuable and more beneficial compared to telephone-delivered SET [26].

The combination of psychopharmacology and psychotherapy was found to be superior to either one delivered alone. Patients receiving combined treatments of desipramine and individual psychotherapy showed more improvement than psychotherapy and placebo [23]. A meta-analysis from the general psychiatry literature also supports the advantage of combining psychotherapy and psychopharmacology versus medication alone [27].

When choosing an antidepressant, 4 principles should be taken into consideration. The optimum choice is an antidepressant that

- has minimum potential side effects;
- has low potential for drug–drug interactions;
- targets multiple depressive symptoms (insomnia, decreased appetite and energy);
- targets other MS symptoms (pain, fatigue, etc.).

Selective serotonin reuptake inhibitors (SSRIs) are often the first choice of treatment for major depression in MS given their favorable side-effect profile, low number of contraindications, and lower chance of drug–drug interaction. However, other antidepressants could be used as first-line therapy on the basis of the need to target other MS symptoms (Table 19.4).

What if the first medication fails to achieve full remission despite a good therapeutic trial? Evidence on how to proceed is generated from the general psychiatry literature. The 2 most commonly used strategies are augmentation with another antidepressant, or switching to a different medication. Results from the STAR-D trial suggest that patients who did not achieve complete response after 12 weeks or more of therapy might benefit more from augmentation therapy compared to switching medication [28].

SUICIDE

Epidemiological studies report various rates of suicide, but all show an elevated suicidal rate in MS patients when compared to the general population. Suicidal risk in MS was at least twice as great than the general population rate [29]. Feinstein et al. reported that the lifetime prevalence of suicidal intent in MS is 28.6% [30]. Suicide was identified as the cause of 15% of deaths in an MS clinic in a Canadian

TABLE 19.4

Medication for Depression That Is Associated With Other Comorbid Conditions

ANTIDEPRESSANTS	COMMON ADDITIONAL USES AND BENEFITS	CAUTIONS AND COMMON SIDE EFFECTS
SNRIs (Venlafaxine, duloxetine)	Neuropathic pain Comorbid anxiety	Increased risk of serotonin syndrome if combined with SSRI Discontinuation syndrome
Bupropion	No sexual side effects No weight gain Improved energy Smoking cessation Could alleviate sexual side effects caused by SSRIs	Lowers seizure threshold
Mirtazapine	Loss of appetite Sleep disturbance	Sedation Worsening fatigue
TCAs	Sleep disturbance Neuropathic pain Nocturia	Sedation Cardiovascular side effects Anticholinergic side effects including urinary retention Avoid abrupt discontinuation

SNRI, serotonin norepinephrine reuptake inhibitors; SSRI, selective serotonin reuptake inhibitors; TCA, tricyclic antidepressants.

study [31] and the suicidal rate was 7.5 times greater compared to age-matched controls from the general population in a Danish study [32]. Suicide risk factors include male gender, young age of onset of MS symptoms [29], severity of depression, social isolation, recent functional deterioration, and alcohol abuse [30]. Even though only a minority of patients complete suicide, patients' suicidal ideations should be taken seriously. If the patient appears at high risk, a psychiatric evaluation should be immediately requested.

BIPOLAR DISORDER

The association between MS and bipolar disorder has been documented in multiple case reports. The prevalence of bipolar disorder in MS is higher than in the general population [6,7] (Table 19.1). Mania has been reported as an initial presentation of MS. There are no data linking bipolar disorder to specific brain lesions.

There have been no studies on the treatment of bipolar disorder in MS. Anecdotal reports suggest successful management of mania with mood stabilizers, antipsychotics, and benzodiazepines. Lithium has been used to treat acute mania. Patients who are treated with lithium for bipolar disorder should maintain adequate hydration, which might be a problem in MS patients, as they sometimes restrict their fluid intake owing to bladder dysfunction. Carbamazepine and valproate sodium are effective but they should be monitored closely because of potential side effects such as tremor, weight gain, and drug–drug interactions. Lamotrigine is approved for maintenance therapy of bipolar depression and does not prevent manic episodes. All atypical antipsychotics are used for the treatment of bipolar mania. They also should be monitored closely because of risks of extrapyramidal symptoms (EPS), metabolic syndrome, and worsening of fatigue. The use of antidepressants alone should be avoided in bipolar depression as they might precipitate a manic or mixed episode.

EUPHORIA

Euphoria is defined as a fixed mental state of well-being and optimism despite the presence of severe physical disability. It is similar to mania in that euphoric patients have elevated mood, but other manic symptoms are lacking. Patients with euphoria usually have significant neurological disability, severe cognitive impairment, enlarged ventricles, cerebral atrophy, and a high lesion load, often with an extensive frontal lobe involvement [33]. There is no treatment for this condition that does not cause suffering to patients but might cause caregiver distress.

ANXIETY DISORDERS

Although anxiety disorders are common in MS, they have received less attention in the literature and often have been overlooked in clinical practice. The lifetime prevalence of any anxiety disorder in MS is higher compared to the general population (Table 19.1). Generalized anxiety disorder was identified as the most common among anxiety disorders with a prevalence of 18.6%. Panic disorder and obsessive compulsive disorder prevalence rates were 10% and 8.6%, respectively.

Patients with anxiety disorders are more likely to be female [2,34], and to have a history of major depression and alcohol abuse. They are also more likely to report greater social stress, a limited support system, and a higher rate of suicidal intent and self-harm attempts [2]. It was noted that a psychiatric diagnosis has been previously given to one-third of these patients, but none were previously diagnosed with anxiety disorder. Moreover, more than one-half of anxiety disorder patients did not receive any type of treatment. Anxiety has not been linked to specific brain lesions [35].

Treatment for anxiety disorders has not been studied in the MS population. Most of the body of knowledge is obtained from studies conducted in general psychiatry. Multiple medications have been approved for the treatment of anxiety disorders. SSRIs are safe and reliable; however, they do not have a rapid onset of action. Serotonin norepinephrine reuptake inhibitors (SNRIs) and buspirone are other effective options for the treatment of generalized anxiety disorder. Short-term treatment with benzodiazepines in combination with SSRIs or SNRIs might be considered for quick relief of anxiety symptoms. However, clinicians should be aware of the potential side-effect profile of benzodiazepines. Side effects include sedation, cognitive decline, worsening of fatigue, and increased risk of falls. Psychotherapy is also effective in anxiety disorders, with or without medication. Patients should be educated on all options and encouraged to participate in both types of treatment in cases of moderate to severe anxiety disorders.

PSYCHOTIC DISORDERS

An elevated rate of psychosis was reported in MS compared to the general population [9] (Table 19.1). However, the majority of the data is derived from case reports. Multiple types of psychotic symptoms have been reported in MS, including hallucinations, paranoid delusion, Capgras syndrome, erotomanic delusion, and delusion of mercury poisoning.

Antipsychotic medications should be considered, starting initially with small doses, to target psychotic symptoms. Close monitoring is advised because of potential side effects such as EPS, metabolic syndrome, and worsening fatigue.

PSEUDOBULBAR AFFECT

Pseudobulbar affect (PBA) describes a disconnection between the patient's affect and mood. Patients may laugh or cry spontaneously, out of proportion to, or in the absence of, specific feelings. PBA causes significant distress and has a negative impact on patients and caregivers. It is often overlooked or underdiagnosed.

PBA has been also referred to as pathological laughing and crying, emotional incontinence, and involuntary emotional expressive disorder (IEED). It has been recognized in MS for many years and affects approximately 10% of MS patients [36]. The etiology is unclear and PBA has been considered as a disconnection syndrome resulting from the loss of brain stem inhibition of the putative center for laughing and crying. PBA has been recently linked to lesions in the frontal, parietal, and brain stem regions [37]. PBA is associated with cognitive impairment, particularly on tasks that are mediated by the frontal lobe, increased physical disability, and chronic progressive forms of MS.

The Center for Neurologic Study-Lability Scale (CNS-LS) is a useful tool for the assessment of PBA. It is short (7 questions) and should be completed by patients. The CNS-LS has been validated for the screening of PSA in MS [38], and has been used in clinical and research settings.

SSRIs are recommended as first-line therapy for PBA and patients usually respond quickly within a few days (1 to 3 days). Other treatment options include tricyclic antidepressants (TCAs) and levodopa. Dextromethorphan/Quinidine (DM/Q) was shown to be effective in the treatment of PBA in a randomized control trial [39], with improved quality of life, quality of relationship, and pain intensity scores. Dizziness was the only side effect that occurred more often in the DM/Q group. Headache and nausea were also reported, but the difference between the DM/Q and the placebo group was not significant.

PSYCHIATRIC EFFECTS OF MS TREATMENTS

There have been concerns that disease-modifying agents cause depression. This concern was initially raised after reports of increased suicidal risk during the IFN beta-1b trial. However, data from the same study showed a decrease in the rate of depression in the treatment group [40]. An increase in depression has been reported in clinical trials during the first 2 to 6 months of treatment with IFN beta-1a and IFN beta-1b. However, this increase in depression symptoms appears to be related to a prior history of depression disorder rather than to the treatment itself [41]. Several studies showed no difference in depression rates [42], while other studies showed improvement of mood with IFN treatment [43].

History of depression prior to initiation of IFN is the main risk factor for worsening depression during IFN therapy. Therefore, in the presence of severe depression, the use of another agent should be considered. If a patient develops depression after IFN therapy initiation, it is not necessarily an indication to discontinue IFN, but rather to initiate treatment for depression.

Corticosteroids can be associated with mood instability. Mania and depression represent 75% of cases. Other side effects include insomnia, irritability, anxiety, psychosis, and delirium. Treatment of neuropsychiatric symptoms includes tapering corticosteroids and administering an antidepressant, lithium, or an antipsychotic in case of mania or psychosis.

CONCLUSION

Multiple sclerosis has a high association with a wide spectrum of emotional disorders which can profoundly affect the quality of life and overall well-being of patients and their family. While depression has been widely studied in MS, other psychiatric disturbances cause significant suffering and deserve more attention. Screening and recognition of emotional disturbances is essential, and effective treatment is available for almost all emotional issues. Our knowledge of the psychiatric disorders in MS has improved over the years; however, further research is still needed, particularly regarding their pathophysiology and the effectiveness of various treatment strategies.

REFERENCES

1. Schubert DS, Foliart RH. Increased depression in multiple sclerosis patients: A meta analysis. *Psychosomatics.* 1993;34: 124–130.

2. Korostil M, Feinstein A. Anxiety disorders and their clinical correlates in multiple sclerosis patients. *Mult Scler.* 2007;13: 67–72.

3. Amato MP, Ponziani G, Rossi F, et al. Quality of life in multiple sclerosis: The impact of depression, fatigue and disability. *Mult Scler.* 2001;7:340–344.

4. Patten SB, Beck CA, Williams JV, et al. Major depression in multiple sclerosis: A population based perspective. *Neurology.* 2003;61:1524–1527.

5. Minden SL, Orav J, Reich P. Depression in multiple sclerosis. *Gen Hosp Psychiatry.* 1987;9:426–434.

6. Marrie RA, Horwitz R, Cutter G, et al. The burden of mental comorbidity in multiple sclerosis: Frequent, underdiagnosed, and undertreated. *Mult Scler.* 2009;15(3):385–392.

7. Joffe RT, Lippert GP, Gray TA, et al. Mood disorder and multiple sclerosis. *Arch Neurol.* 1987;44:376–378.

8. Diaz-Olavarrieta C, Cummings JL, Velazquez J, et al. Neuropsychiatric manifestations of multiple sclerosis. *J Neuropsychiatry Clin Neurosci.* 1999;11:51–57.

9. Patten SB, Svenson LW, Metz LM. Psychotic disorders in MS: Population-based evidence of an association. *Neurology.* 2005;65:1123–1125.

10. Sullivan MJ, Weinshenker B, Mikail S, Bishop SR. Screening for major depression in the early stages of multiple sclerosis. *Can J Neurol Sci.* 1995;22(3):228–231.

11. Honarmand K, Feinstein A. validation of the Hospital Anxiety and Depression Scale for use with multiple sclerosis patients. *Mult Scler.* 2009;15:1518–1524.

12. Benedict RH, Fishman I, McClellan MM, et al. Validity of the beck depression inventory-fast screen in multiple sclerosis. *Mult Scler.* 2003;9:393–396.

13. Kroenke K, Spitzer RL, Williams JB. The PHQ-9: Validity of a brief depression severity measure. *J Gen Intern Med.* 2001; 16(9):606–613.

14. Verdier-Taillefer MH, Gourlet V, Fuhrer R, et al. Psychometric properties of the center for epidemiologic studies-depression scale in multiple sclerosis. *Neuroepidemiology.* 2001;20(4): 262–267.

15. Nyenhuis DL, Rao SM, Zajecka JM, et al. Mood disturbance versus other symptoms of depression in multiple sclerosis. *J Int Neuropsychol Soc.* 1995;1(3):291–296.

16. Rush AJ, Gullion CM, Basco MR, et al. The Inventory of Depressive Symptomatology (IDS): Psychometric properties. *Psychol Med.* 1996;26(3):477–486.

17. Goldman Consensus Group. The Goldman Consensus Statement on depression in multiple sclerosis. *Mult Scler.* 2005;11: 328–337.

18. Schiffer RB. Depression in neurological practice: Diagnosis, treatment, implications. *Semin Neurol.* 2009;29:220–233.

19. Berg D, Supprian T, Thomae J, et al. Lesion pattern in patients with multiple sclerosis and depression. *Mult Scler.* 2000;6: 156–162.

20. Bakshi R, Czarnecki D, Shaikh ZA, et al. Brain MRI lesions and atrophy are related to depression in multiple sclerosis. *Neuroreport.* 2000;11:1153–1158.

21. Schiepers OJ, Wichers MC, Maes M. Cytokines and major depression. *Prog Neuropsychopharmacol Biol Psychiatry.* 2005;29: 201–217.

22. Fassbender K, Schmidt R, Mossner R, et al. Mood disorders and dysfunction of the hypothalamic-pituitary-adrenal axis in multiple sclerosis. *Arch Neurol.* 1998;55:66–72.

23. Schiffer RB, Wineman NM. Antidepressant pharmacotherapy of depression associated with multiple sclerosis. *Am J Psychiatry.* 1990;147:1493–1497.

24. Ehde DM, Kraft GH, Chwastiak L, et al. Efficacy of paroxetine in treating major depressive disorder in persons with multiple sclerosis. *Gen Hosp Psychiatry.* 2008;30(1):40–48.

25. Mohr DC, Boudewyn AC, Goodkin DE, et al. Comparative outcomes for individual cognitive-behavioral therapy, supportive-expressive group psychotherapy and sertraline for the treatment of depression in multiple sclerosis. *J Consult Clin Psychology.* 2001;69:942–949.

26. Mohr DC, Hart SL, Julian L, et al. Telephone-administered psychotherapy for depression. *Arch Gen Psychiatry.* 2005;62: 1007–1014.

27. Pampallona S, Bollini P, Tibaldi G, et al. Combined pharmacotherapy and psychological treatment for depression: A systematic review. *Arch Gen Psychiatry.* 2004;61:714–719.

28. Gaynes BN, Dusetzina SB, Ellis AR, et al. Treating depression after initial treatment failure: Directly comparing switch and augmenting strategies in STAR*D. *J Clin Psychopharmacol.* 2012;32(1):114–119.

29. Brønnum-Hansen H, Stenager E, Nylev Stenager E, et al. Suicide among Danes with multiple sclerosis. *J Neurol Neurosurg Psychiatry.* 2005;76(10):1457–1459.

30. Feinstein A. An examination of suicidal intent in patients with multiple sclerosis. *Neurology.* 2002;59:674–678.

31. Sadovnik AD, Eisen RN, Ebers GC, et al. Cause of death in patients attending multiple sclerosis clinics. *Neurology.* 1991;41:1193–1196.

32. Stenager EN, Stenager E, Koch-Henrikson N, et al. Suicide and multiple sclerosis: An epidemiological investigation. *J Neurol Neurosurg Psychiatry.* 1992;55:542–545.

33. Rabins PV. Euphoria in multiple sclerosis. In: Rao SM, ed. *Neurobehavioral Aspects of Multiple Sclerosis.* New York: Oxford University Press; 1990:180–185.

34. Feinstein A, O'Connor P, Gray T, Feinstein K. The effects of anxiety on psychiatric morbidity in patients with multiple sclerosis. *Mult Scler.* 1999;5:323–326.

35. Zorzon M, de Masi R, Nasuelli D, et al. Depression and anxiety in multiple sclerosis. A clinical and MRI study in 95 subjects. *J Neurol.* 2001;248:416–421.

36. Feinstein A, Feinstein K, Gray T, et al. Prevalence and neurobehavioral correlates of pathological laughing and crying in multiple sclerosis. *Arch Neurol.* 1997;54:1116–1121.

37. Ghaffar O, Chamelian L, Feinstein A. The neuroanatomy of pseudobulbar affect. *J Neurol.* 2008;255(3):406–412.

38. Smith RA, Berg JE, Pope LE, et al. Validation of the CNS emotional lability scale for pseudobulbar affect (pathological laughing and crying) in multiple sclerosis patients. *Mult Scler.* 2004;10(6):679–685.

39. Panitch HS, Thisted RA, Smith RA, et al. Randomized, controlled trial of dextromethorphan/quinidine for pseudobulbar affect in multiple sclerosis. *Ann Neurol.* 2006;59:780–787.

40. University of British Columbia MS/MRI Analysis Group. IFNB Multiple Sclerosis Study Group, Interferon beta-1b in the treatment of multiple sclerosis: Final outcome of the randomized controlled trial. *Neurology.* 1995;45:1277–1285.

41. Polman CH, Thompson AJ, Murray TJ, McDonald WI, eds. *Multiple Sclerosis: The Guide to Treatment and Management*, 5th ed. New York: Demos Publishing; 2001:7–43.

42. Patten SB, Metz LM. SPECTRIMS Study Group. Interferon beta 1a and depression in secondary progressive MS: Data from the SPECTRIMS trial. *Neurology.* 2002;59:744–746.

43. Feinstein A, O'Connor P, Feinstein K. Multiple sclerosis, interferon beta-1b and depression: A prospective investigation. *J Neurol.* 2002;249:815–820.

20

Cognitive Dysfunction in Multiple Sclerosis

STEPHEN M. RAO

KEY POINTS FOR CLINICIANS

Cognitive dysfunction

- Occurs in 43%–65% of patients with MS.

- Is often under-recognized or misdiagnosed as depression, stress, or personality disorder

- Is assessed with neuropsychological testing. The most common deficits are seen on measures of recent memory and information processing speed.

- Contributes significantly to unemployment, motor vehicle accidents, impairment in activities of daily living, and loss of social contacts.

- Is strongly related to the extent of white matter lesion volume and brain atrophy on MRI.

- May be treated with disease-modifying and symptomatic treatments with modest success.

Cognitive function is often impaired in multiple sclerosis (MS) patients [1]. Nearly 43% to 65% of MS patients exhibit some degree of impairment on standardized neuropsychological (NP) tests [1]. Cognitive impairment can have devastating consequences for the MS patient in the areas of employment [2,3], driving skills and safety [4], social activities [2], personal and community independence [2,3], and the likelihood of benefiting from rehabilitation [5]. Not surprisingly, it is a major source of caregiver strain [6].

Cognitive impairment is the direct result of MS-related cerebral pathology. Brain abnormalities, as visualized by various MRI techniques (for a recent review, see [7]), correlate with NP tests. Cognitive deficits have been shown to correlate with T2- and T1-weighted white matter lesions as well as lesions in gray matter and brain atrophy. They also correlate with microscopic pathology, as visualized by magnetization transfer, diffusion tensor,

and proton spectroscopy, in both lesions and normal-appearing brain tissue. Furthermore, longitudinal studies have shown that deteriorating cognitive function is associated with increased lesion burden and atrophy [8–10].

> Cognitive impairment is the direct result of MS-related cerebral pathology. Brain abnormalities, as visualized by various MRI techniques, correlate with NP tests.

Secondary progressive MS patients typically perform more poorly on NP testing than do patients with relapsing-remitting MS (RRMS) or primary progressive MS [11]. Surprisingly, NP test scores correlate only weakly with disease duration and neurological disability [12]. The weak cross-sectional correlations between cognitive dysfunction and disease duration may be due to the high variability in symptom presentation in MS: some patients exhibit cognitive dysfunction as an early presentation of the disease, whereas other patients may never exhibit problems with cognition.

Neurological disability, as typically assessed by the Expanded Disability Status Scale (EDSS), correlates only modestly with the degree of cognitive dysfunction [13]. The EDSS tends to emphasize disability associated with ambulation. As a consequence, lesions affecting primarily the brain regions associated with higher cognitive functions may not have an impact on the EDSS; likewise, lesions of the spinal cord may impact ambulation and the EDSS score, but have no effect on cognitive functions.

Not all cognitive functions are equally susceptible to disruption by MS. Deficits in learning and recall of new information (episodic memory) and in information processing speed and working memory (ie, the ability to simultaneously buffer and manipulate information) are the most common [14]. Less common, but significant deficits are observed on visuospatial abilities and executive functions (including reasoning, problem solving, and planning/sequencing) [14]. In contrast, very few MS patients exhibit deficits on measures of auditory attention span and language abilities, although recent natural history studies suggest that deficits in these domains become evident when cohorts are followed for longer periods of time [3]. The severity and pattern of cognitive deficits may vary considerably across individual MS patients [15]. This heterogeneity of NP impairment can best be appreciated when large samples of patients are administered a comprehensive NP test battery [16].

> Most common deficits are in the areas of recent memory and information processing speed.

The natural history of MS-related cognitive impairment has been reported from studies [3,17–20] conducted prior to the appearance of disease-modifying drugs (see Table 20.1). Progression rates vary considerably across patients and across cognitive functions, but on average, approximately 5% to 9% of patients will experience deterioration on NP tests annually. In general, cognitive impairment is unlikely to remit to any significant extent, but cognitive deficits may remain stable for long periods of time before worsening. Acute exacerbations and remissions involving cognitive functions can be seen (see Figure 20.1).

EVALUATION

Cognitive dysfunction is typically evaluated by a board-certified clinical neuropsychologist. The purposes of such an evaluation can vary and involve questions of differential diagnosis (depression vs. cognitive dysfunction), disability assessment (eg, Social Security), design of cognitive

TABLE 20.1
Indicators of Cognitive Dysfunction in MS

- Need for help with activities of daily living not attributable to physical disability

- Underemployment or unemployment not attributable to physical disability

- Change in mood or behavior (eg, increased irritability, disinhibition) not attributable to anxiety or depression

- Withdrawal from usual social activities not attributable to anxiety or depression

- MRI showing global atrophy and a high lesion load on T2-weighted imaging

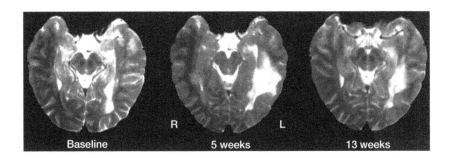

FIGURE 20.1
A female RRMS patient (age 37) had normal cognitive functions at baseline NP testing. At 5 weeks, she developed a selective impairment in verbal episodic memory in association with the development of a large white matter hyperintensity in the left temporal lobe on T2-weighted MRI imaging. The white matter lesion had decreased in size at 13 weeks postbaseline with an improvement in verbal episodic memory, although her test performance did not return to baseline. Her performance in NP tests of visuospatial episodic memory and information processing speed were unchanged during the 3 examinations.

rehabilitation interventions, and clinical management with symptomatic and disease-modifying drugs. Comprehensive assessment will necessarily involve several measures that capture different cognitive domains. An example of a comprehensive battery for monitoring MS patients is the Minimal Assessment of Cognitive Function in MS (MACFIMS) (see Table 20.2) [21]. The MACFIMS takes approximately 90 minutes to administer and was created on the basis of a consensus panel of neuropsychologists. The brief repeatable NP battery (BRB) [22] is an alternative battery that takes approximately 30 minutes to administer.

> NP evaluations are needed to gauge the severity and pattern of cognitive deficits.

A major challenge in clinical practice is the identification of MS patients who would benefit from a comprehensive NP evaluation. Numerous studies have shown that self-report of cognitive dysfunction is frequently inaccurate. Patients with depression may over-report cognitive symptoms but perform normally on NP testing. Conversely, patients with significant cognitive dysfunction on objective NP testing may lose self-awareness and minimize the report of their cognitive deficits. There is some evidence to suggest that the observer ratings of close family members are more likely to predict impairment on NP testing. Because the cognitive deficits in MS typically do not involve language or communication deficits, physicians who specialize in MS do not typically identify cognitive dysfunction from the mental status examination. Furthermore, screening examinations for dementia, such as the Mini Mental State Examination, are insensitive to the cognitive dysfunction in MS. Single test screening examinations using measures of information processing speed, like the Paced Auditory Serial Addition Test (PASAT) or the Symbol Digit Modalities Test (SDMT), are capable of identifying 45% to 74% of patients diagnosed with cognitive dysfunction relative to results derived from a comprehensive NP battery [14,23]. This approach, however, will be insensitive to MS patients with cognitive dysfunction in other domains (eg, episodic memory).

> Self-report of cognitive impairment can be unreliable.

MANAGEMENT

Disease-Modifying Medications

As the prevalence and functional consequences of MS-related cognitive dysfunction were recognized, several randomized, placebo-controlled trials of disease-modifying medications for RRMS and progressive MS incorporated NP outcome measures. Tables 20.3 (RRMS) and 20.4 (progressive MS) provide an overview of these trials. The studies indicate that the beneficial effects of disease-modifying therapies can extend to cognitive function, although these effects may be subtle. Statistically significant NP effects were most often observed on composite NP outcome measures.

> Modest success has been shown in treating cognitive dysfunction with disease-modifying drugs.

TABLE 20.2
Minimal Assessment of Cognitive Function in MS (MACFIMS) [21]

TEST	ESTIMATED ADMINISTRATION TIME
Information processing speed	
Paced Auditory Serial Addition Test (PASAT)	10 minutes
Symbol Digit Modalities Test (SDMT)	5 minutes
Episodic memory	
California Verbal Learning Test-II (CVLT-2)	25 minutes
Brief Visuospatial Memory Test-Revised (BVMT-R)	10 minutes
Executive functions	
California Sorting Test (CST)	25 minutes
Visuospatial perception	
Judgment of Line Orientation Test (JLO)	10 minutes
Language/Other	
Controlled Oral Word Association Test (COWAT)	5 minutes

TABLE 20.3
Randomized Clinical Trials of Disease-Modifying Medications With NP Outcome Assessment: RRMS

TRIAL	INITIAL SAMPLE	NP MEASURES AND DESIGN	NP OUTCOME
Betaseron (IFN beta-1b) [24,25]	372 patients EDSS = 0.0–5.5	Focused battery (WMS Logical Memory and Visual Reproduction, Trails A & B, Stroop) at 2 years and 4 years only (*n* = 30 at a single site)	Treatment effect on Delayed Visual Reproduction, favoring high-dose group, with a similar trend on Trails B
Copaxone (glatiramer acetate) [26,27]	248 patients EDSS = 0.0–5.0	Focused battery (Selective Reminding Test, 10/36 SRT, PASAT, SDMT, and Word List Generation) at baseline, 12 months, and 24 months	No significant treatment effects
Avonex (IFN beta-1a) [28,29]	166 patients EDSS = 0.0–3.5	Broad-spectrum battery at baseline and 2 years, and focused battery every 6 months for 24 months	Significant treatment effects on memory and information processing, with a trend on visuospatial abilities and executive functions
Tysabri (natalizumab) [30–32]	942 patients EDSS = 0.0–5.5	PASAT-3″ (as component of MS Functional Composite) at baseline, then every 3 months for 24 months	Sustained worsening was 7% in natalizumab group and 12% in placebo group

EDSS, Expanded Disability Status Scale; IFN, interferon; PASAT, paced auditory serial addition text; SDMT, symbol digit modalities test; SRT, simple reaction time; WMS, Wechsler Memory Scale.

TABLE 20.4
Randomized Clinical Trials of Disease-Modifying Medications With NP Outcome Assessment: Progressive MS

TRIAL	INITIAL SAMPLE	NP MEASURES AND DESIGN	NP OUTCOME
Methotrexate [33,34]	60 CPMS patients EDSS = 3.0–6.5	Broad-spectrum battery at baseline, 12 months, 24 months (*n* = 40); focused NP battery every 6 weeks for 24 weeks to a subset of patients	Trend toward beneficial overall treatment effect, due primarily to effects on PASAT; effect on PASAT was evident early in treatment
Betaferon (IFN beta-1b) [35,36]	718 SPMS patients EDSS = 3.0–6.5	Broad-spectrum battery (Selective Reminding Test, 10/36 SRT, PASAT, SDMT, Word List Generation) at baseline, 12 months, 24 months, and 36 months	No significant treatment effect; secondary analyses indicated that fewer IFN beta-1b patients met criteria for new or worsened cognitive impairment at 24 months
Avonex (IFN beta-1a) [37]	436 SPMS patients EDSS = 3.5–6.5	PASAT (as component of MS Functional Composite) at 3 baseline visits, then every 3 months for 24 months	Trend toward beneficial treatment effect on PASAT

CPMS, Chronic progressive MS; EDSS, Expanded Disability Status Scale; SPMS, secondary progressive MS; NP, neuropsychological; PASAT, paced auditory serial addition test; SDMT, symbol digit modalities test; SRT, simple reaction time.

Symptomatic Therapy

Table 20.5 summarizes clinical trials designed to assess the efficacy of medications designed to symptomatically treat cognitive impairment. Patients enrolling in these symptomatic trials were required to have documented cognitive deficits or at minimum subjective cognitive complaints. The typical trial involved a relatively small number of patients (*n* < 70) and was conducted at a single site, although larger (*n* > 100), multisite trials have begun to appear in the literature [38,39]. Results of these trials have been mixed. Medications approved for the treatment of Alzheimer's disease (donepezil, rivastigmine, memantine) show either no clinical benefit or a very modest benefit in treating MS-related cognitive dysfunction. Likewise, *Ginkgo biloba* does not appear to be effective for treatment of cognitive dysfunction. Surprisingly, L-amphetamine sulfate, a stimulant, appears to

have a promising effect on verbal and visuospatial episodic memory, but no effect on measures of information processing speed and attention. Also promising is the effect of modafinil on measures of simple attention and working memory.

> Some symptomatic therapies involving drugs and cognitive rehabilitation show improved cognitive function.

Cognitive rehabilitation techniques are designed to either restore functions or develop strategies to compensate for cognitive dysfunction. Recently, rigorous randomized controlled trials [46] have begun to appear in the literature supporting the use of these interventions in MS.

TABLE 20.5
Placebo-Controlled Clinical Trials of Symptomatic Medications for Cognitive Dysfunction in Patients With Documented or Subjective Cognitive Deficits at Entry

STUDY	SAMPLE/STUDY DESIGN	NP MEASURES	OUTCOME
IV physostigmine [40]	4 patients (EDSS 3.0–6.0) with documented memory impairment; 6-week placebo-controlled crossover (no washout)	Focused battery (Buschke SRT and Digit Span Forward) at baseline, then weekly for 6 weeks	Significant treatment effects on selected Buschke SRT variables (LTS, LTR, STR) and consistent trends on others; no effect on Digit Span
Donepezil hydrochloride (10 mg/day for 24 weeks) [41]	N = 69 MS patients with documented cognitive impairment; 24-week randomized, double-blind, parallel group	Broad-spectrum battery (Brief Repeatable Battery, Tower of Hanoi) at baseline and 24 weeks	Significant treatment effect on primary outcome measure, Buschke SRT; nonsignificant trend for PASAT; no effect on 10/36, SDMT, Word List Generation, and Tower of Hanoi
Ginkgo biloba (240 mg/day for 12 weeks) [42]	N = 39 MS patients with documented impairment on PASAT or CVLT-II; 12-week randomized, double-blind, parallel group	Broad-spectrum battery (PASAT, CVLT-II, Stroop, Symbol Digit, Stroop, Useful Field of View Test) at baseline and 12 weeks	No significant treatment effects; a trend for improved function in the drug group on the Stroop test; more impaired patients at baseline demonstrated a stronger treatment effect
Modafinil (200 mg/day for 16 weeks) [43]	N = 49 RRMS patients with documented impairment on attention measures; 6-week randomized, single-blind, parallel group	Broad-spectrum battery (PASAT, CPT, CVLT, Trails, ANAM, Digit Span, Digit Symbol, verbal and visuospatial fluency)	Significant treatment effects on measures of simple attention span, working memory, and verbal fluency; nonsignificant trends on measures of sustained attention and episodic memory
Rivastigmine (6 mg/day for 12 weeks) [44]	N = 60 MS patients (19 RR, 31 SP, 10 PP) with documented impairment on WMS; 12 week, randomized, double-blind, parallel group	Focused Battery (subtests of Wechsler Memory Scales)	No significant treatment effects observed on the WMS General Memory score or subtest scores
Rivastigmine (9 mg/day for 16 weeks) [45]	N = 15 MS patients (12 RR and 3 SP) with subjective complaints of cognitive impairment; 32-week randomized, single-blind, crossover (no washout)	Broad-spectrum battery (Brief Repeatable Battery, Stroop, N-Back) at baseline, 16 and 32 weeks	Nonsignificant trend on BRB for improved cognitive function on versus off rivastigmine; no performance effects of drug on Stroop and N-Back
L-amphetamine sulfate (30 mg/day for 29 days) [24]	N = 151 MS patients with documented impairment on Symbol Digit or CVLT-II or PASAT; 28 day, randomized, double-blind, parallel group (2:1 drug:placebo)	Broad-spectrum battery (Symbol Digit, CVLT-II, Brief Visual Memory Test, PASAT) at baseline and at 29 days	No significant effect on primary NP outcome measure (Symbol Digit); significant treatment effects observed on memory measures
Memantine (20 mg/day for 16 weeks) [38l]	N = 114 MS patients (RR, PP, and SP) with documented impairment on PASAT or CVLT-II; 16-week randomized, double-blind, parallel group	Broad-spectrum battery (PASAT, CVLT-II, Stroop, Symbol Digit, COWAT, DKEFS) at baseline and 16 weeks	No significant treatment effects observed on the primary (PASAT, CVLT-II) and secondary NP outcome measures

BRB, brief repeatable NP battery; EDSS, Expanded Disability Status Scale; IV, intravenous; NP, neuropsychological; PASAT, paced auditory serial addition test; PP, primary progressive; RR, relapsing-remitting; SP, secondary progressive; SRT, simple reaction time; WMS, Wechsler Memory Scale.

PATIENT CASE

A married male with 15 years of education was diagnosed with MS at the age of 45. At age 48, his primary symptoms and signs included spastic paraparesis, ataxic gait (requiring the use of a cane), dysarthria, bilateral upper extremity numbness, back pain, and bladder dysfunction. His clinical course was progressive with an EDSS score of 3.5. The patient was performing most activities of daily living without difficulty and was working full-time as a computer technician. He denied memory or other cognitive symptoms; his wife, however, reported that he was experiencing mild recent memory disturbance.

Question: What evaluation is needed?

Answer: Self-report of cognitive deficits is generally less reliable than those of close relatives and friends. The wife's report of memory disturbance would suggest referral for an NP evaluation and a cranial MRI. NP testing indicated that the patient obtained a verbal IQ of 101, which is in the average range but perhaps lower than expected for his educational background. Cognitive deficits were confined to measures of verbal and nonverbal recent memory. Performance was normal on an executive function task involving conceptual reasoning. MRI showed multiple confluent and focal periventricular areas with high signal intensity on T2-weighted images throughout the cerebral white matter, left cerebellum, and pons. In addition, the corpus callosum was abnormally thin. Lesion volume in the frontal lobes was relatively minimal.

The patient was reevaluated 3 years later. He was wheelchair bound as a result of increased truncal and lower extremity ataxia; EDSS score increased to 8.0. He also demonstrated more pronounced dysarthria and a reduction in fine motor control of the upper extremities. The patient was no longer able to work. His wife expressed concerns over a change in his cognitive and personality functioning, characterized by impaired judgment, anger outbursts, recent memory loss, word-finding difficulties, and decreased self-awareness. The patient nearly drowned in the family pool when he decided to swim without a life vest. He also experienced 2 cases of heat exhaustion when he failed to protect himself from overexposure to the sun.

Question: What do you do now?

Answer: Both NP testing and MRI were repeated. NP testing was relatively unchanged on measures of verbal intelligence, recent memory, and language. In contrast, a prominent decrement in performance was observed on an executive function task, with the patient experiencing a large number of perseverative responses suggesting cognitive inflexibility. MRI demonstrated a marked increase in white matter lesions within the frontal lobes (360% increase in frontal white matter lesion volume; by contrast, only a 29% increase was observed in non-frontal lesion volume). This case illustrates the point that the location and severity of intracranial lesions can have an important influence on the expression of cognitive deficits.

KEY POINTS FOR PATIENTS AND FAMILIES

Disorders of cognition

- (Memory, speed of processing information, naming things) is often affected in MS though is more common later in the course of MS
- May be misdiagnosed as depression, stress, or a personality disorder
- May affect social functions, driving, and employment
- May benefit from treatment to some extent

REFERENCES

1. Bobholz JA, Rao SM. Cognitive dysfunction in multiple sclerosis: A review of recent developments. *Curr Opin Neurol.* 2003 Jun;16(3):283–288.

2. Rao SM, Leo GJ, Ellington L, et al. Cognitive dysfunction in multiple sclerosis. II. Impact on employment and social functioning. *Neurology.* 1991 May;41(5):692–696.

3. Amato MP, Ponziani G, Siracusa G, Sorbi S. Cognitive dysfunction in early-onset multiple sclerosis: A reappraisal after 10 years. *Arch Neurol.* 2001 Oct;58(10):1602–1606.

4. Schultheis MT, Garay E, Millis SR, DeLuca J. Motor vehicle crashes and violations among drivers with multiple sclerosis. *Arch Phys Med Rehabil.* 2002 Aug;83(8):1175–1178.

5. Langdon DW, Thompson AJ. Multiple sclerosis: A preliminary study of selected variables affecting rehabilitation outcome. *Mult Scler.* 1999 Apr;5(2):94–100.

6. Chipchase SY, Lincoln NB. Factors associated with carer strain in carers of people with multiple sclerosis. *Disabil Rehabil.* 2001 Nov 20;23(17):768–776.

7. Filippi M, Rocca MA, Benedict RH, et al. The contribution of MRI in assessing cognitive impairment in multiple sclerosis. *Neurology.* 2010 Dec 7;75(23):2121–2128.

8. Hohol MJ, Guttmann CR, Orav J, et al. Serial neuropsychological assessment and magnetic resonance imaging analysis in multiple sclerosis. *Arch Neurol.* 1997 Aug;54(8):1018–1025.

9. Sperling RA, Guttmann CR, Hohol MJ, et al. Regional magnetic resonance imaging lesion burden and cognitive function in multiple sclerosis: A longitudinal study. *Arch Neurol.* 2001 Jan;58(1):115–121.

10. Zivadinov R, Sepcic J, Nasuelli D, et al. A longitudinal study of brain atrophy and cognitive disturbances in the early phase of relapsing-remitting multiple sclerosis. *J Neurol Neurosurg Psychiatry.* 2001 Jun;70(6):773–780.

11. Fischer JS. Using the Wechsler Memory Scale-Revised to detect and characterize memory deficits in multiple sclerosis. *Clin Neuropsychol.* 1988;2:149–172.

12. Beatty WW, Goodkin DE, Hertsgaard D, Monson N. Clinical and demographic predictors of cognitive performance in multiple sclerosis. Do diagnostic type, disease duration, and disability matter? *Arch Neurol.* 1990 Mar;47(3):305–308.

13. Whitaker JN, McFarland HF, Rudge P, Reingold SC. Outcomes assessment in multiple sclerosis clinical trials: A critical analysis. *Mult Scler.* 1995 Apr;1(1):37–47.

14. Rao SM, Leo GJ, Bernardin L, Unverzagt F. Cognitive dysfunction in multiple sclerosis. I. Frequency, patterns, and prediction. *Neurology.* 1991 May;41(5):685–691.

15. Beatty WW, Wilbanks SL, Blanco CR, et al. Memory disturbance in multiple sclerosis: Reconsideration of patterns of performance on the selective reminding test. *J Clin Exp Neuropsychol.* 1996 Feb;18(1):56–62.

16. Fischer JS, Jacobs LD, Cookfair DL, et al. Heterogeneity of cognitive dysfunction in multiple sclerosis. *Clin Neuropsychol.* 1998;12:286Abs.

17. Amato MP, Ponziani G, Pracucci G, et al. Cognitive impairment in early-onset multiple sclerosis. Pattern, predictors, and impact on everyday life in a 4-year follow-up. *Arch Neurol.* 1995 Feb;52(2):168–172.

18. Jennekens-Schinkel A, Laboyrie PM, Lanser JB, van der Velde EA. Cognition in patients with multiple sclerosis after four years. *J Neurol Sci.* 1990 Nov;99(2-3):229–247.

19. Kujala P, Portin R, Ruutiainen J. The progress of cognitive decline in multiple sclerosis. A controlled 3-year follow-up. *Brain.* 1997 Feb;120(Pt 2):289–297.

20. Bobholz JA, Rao SM, Sweet LH, et al. Cognitive decline in multiple sclerosis: An 8-year longitudinal investigation. *J Int Neuropsychol Soc.* 1998;4:35.

21. Benedict RH, Fischer JS, Archibald CJ, et al. Minimal neuropsychological assessment of MS patients: A consensus approach. *Clin Neuropsychol.* 2002 Aug;16(3):381–397.

22. Rao SM, NMSS Cognitive Function Study Group. *A Manual for the Brief Repeatable Battery of Neuropsychological Tests in Multiple Sclerosis.* New York: National MS Society; 1990.

23. Rosti E, Hamalainen P, Koivisto K, Hokkanen L. PASAT in detecting cognitive impairment in relapsing-remitting MS. *Appl Neuropsychol.* 2007;14(2):101–112.

24. The IFNB Multiple Sclerosis Study Group. Interferon beta-1b is effective in relapsing-remitting multiple sclerosis. I. Clinical results of a multicenter, randomized, double-blind, placebo-controlled trial. *Neurology.* 1993 Apr;43(4):655–661.

25. Pliskin NH, Hamer DP, Goldstein DS, et al. Improved delayed visual reproduction test performance in multiple sclerosis patients receiving interferon beta-1b. *Neurology.* 1996 Dec;47(6):1463–1468.

26. Johnson KP, Brooks BR, Cohen JA, et al. Copolymer 1 reduces relapse rate and improves disability in relapsing-remitting multiple sclerosis: Results of a phase III multicenter, double-blind placebo-controlled trial. The Copolymer 1 Multiple Sclerosis Study Group. *Neurology.* 1995 Jul;45(7):1268–1276.

27. Weinstein A, Schwid SI, Schiffer RB, et al. Neuropsychologic status in multiple sclerosis after treatment with glatiramer acetate (Copaxone). *Arch Neurol.* 1999 Mar;56(3):319–324.

28. Jacobs LD, Cookfair DL, Rudick RA, et al. Intramuscular interferon beta-1a for disease progression in relapsing multiple sclerosis. The Multiple Sclerosis Collaborative Research Group (MSCRG) 35. *Ann Neurol.* 1996 Mar;39(3):285–294.

29. Fischer JS, Priore RL, Jacobs LD, et al. Neuropsychological effects of interferon beta-1a in relapsing multiple sclerosis. Multiple Sclerosis Collaborative Research Group. *Ann Neurol.* 2000 Dec;48(6):885–892.

30. Polman CH, O'Connor PW, Havrdova E, et al. A randomized, placebo-controlled trial of natalizumab for relapsing multiple sclerosis. *N Engl J Med.* 2006 Mar 2;354(9):899–910.

31. Havrdova E. The effects of natalizumab on a test of cognitive function in patients wiuth relapsing multiple sclerosis (MS). *Eur J Neurol.* 2006;13(Suppl 2):307.

32. Polman CH, Rudick RA. The multiple sclerosis functional composite: A clinically meaningful measure of disability. *Neurology.* 2010 Apr 27;74(Suppl 3):S8–S15.

33. Goodkin DE, Rudick RA, VanderBrug MS, et al. Low-dose (7.5 mg) oral methotrexate reduces the rate of progression in chronic progressive multiple sclerosis. *Ann Neurol.* 1995 Jan;37(1):30–40.

34. Goodkin DE, Fischer JS. Treatment of multiple sclerosis with methotrexate. In: Goodkin DE, Rudick RA, eds. *Multiple Sclerosis: Advances in Clinical Trial Design, Treatment and Future Perspectives.* London: Springer; 1996:251–289.

35. European Study Group on interferon beta-1b in secondary progressive MS. Placebo-controlled multicentre randomised trial of interferon beta-1b in treatment of secondary progressive multiple sclerosis. *Lancet.* 1998 Nov 7;352(9139): 1491–1497.

36. Langdon DW, Thompson AJ, Hamalainen P, et al. Effect of IFNB-1b on cognition in secondary progressive multiple sclerosis. 2006. Unpublished Work.

37. Cohen JA, Cutter GR, Fischer JS, et al. Benefit of interferon beta-1a on MSFC progression in secondary progressive MS. *Neurology.* 2002 Sep 10;59(5):679–687.

38. Morrow SA, Kaushik T, Zarevics P, et al. The effects of L-amphetamine sulfate on cognition in MS patients: Results of a randomized controlled trial. *J Neurol.* 2009 Jul;256(7): 1095–1102.

39. Lovera JF, Frohman E, Brown TR, et al. Memantine for cognitive impairment in multiple sclerosis: A randomized placebo-controlled trial. *Mult Scler.* 2010 Jun;16(6):715–723.

40. Leo GJ, Rao SM. Effects of intravenous physostigmine and lecithin on memory loss in multiple sclerosis: Report of a pilot study. *J Neurol Rehabil.* 1988;2:123–129.

41. Krupp LB, Christodoulou C, Melville P, et al. Donepezil improved memory in multiple sclerosis in a randomized clinical trial. *Neurology.* 2004;63:1579–1585.

42. Lovera J, Bagert B, Smoot K, et al. Ginkgo biloba for the improvement of cognitive performance in multiple sclerosis: A randomized, placebo-controlled trial. *Mult Scler.* 2007 Apr;13(3): 376–385.

43. Wilken JA, Sullivan C, Wallin M, et al. Treatment of multiple sclerosis-related cognitive problems with adjunctive modafinil: Rationale and preliminary supportive data. *Int J MS Care.* 2008;10:1–10.

44. Shaygannejad V, Janghorbani M, Ashtari F, et al. Effects of rivastigmine on memory and cognition in multiple sclerosis. *Can J Neurol Sci.* 2008 Sep;35(4):476–481.

45. Cader S, Palace J, Matthews PM. Cholinergic agonism alters cognitive processing and enhances brain functional connectivity in patients with multiple sclerosis. *J Psychopharmacol.* 2009 Aug;23(6):686–696.

46. Chiaravalloti ND, DeLuca J, Moore NB, Ricker JH. Treating learning impairments improves memory performance in multiple sclerosis: A randomized clinical trial. *Mult Scler.* 2005 Feb;11(1):58–68.

21

Epilepsy, Sleep Disorders, and Transient Neurological Events in Multiple Sclerosis

ALEXANDER D. RAE-GRANT

In multiple sclerosis (MS), symptoms vary widely from patient to patient. Relapses in MS are typically well recognized and do not lead to much clinical confusion (for example, optic neuritis, brain stem syndromes, and spinal cord syndromes). However, there are other paroxysmal events that occur in MS which may be less expected. These may lead to an extensive and potentially unnecessary investigation for what is a known problem in MS. In this chapter, we focus on a variety of paroxysmal events in MS which may not receive much attention but which can be disruptive to patients. These include the occurrence of epilepsy or sleep disorders, both of which occur at an increased frequency in the MS population and may have implications for therapy. We discuss the common, sometimes weird, and often under-recognized phenomena of transient neurological events (including tonic spasms) which may be distressing to patients. The hope of this chapter is to help clinicians recognize and treat this fascinating set of issues in MS and perhaps both save patients unneeded investigations and expedite their pathway to effective intervention.

EPILEPSY AND MULTIPLE SCLEROSIS

KEY POINTS FOR CLINICIANS REGARDING EPILEPSY AND MS

- Seizures occur in about 3% of multiple sclerosis patients (MS).
- Seizures of all types have been described.
- Seizures may be refractory in some patients.
- Seizures may resolve as relapses or lesions regress.
- Treatment is as per standard epilepsy protocols.
- Carbamazepine and phenytoin may increase MS symptoms.
- Some medicines used in MS treatment may make seizures more likely.
- Insomnia is best treated with nonpharmacological approaches, including sleep hygiene, avoidance of caffeine and stimulants, and treatment of depression.

Epidemiology

Kelley and Rodriguez in 2009 performed a systematic review of the literature on seizures in the MS population [1]. The best data came from 6 population-based studies. Overall, these studies included 1,843 patients of whom 3.8% had epilepsy. Taken together, they indicated a prevalence rate in the MS population of 3% to 4%, which is approximately 3 times that expected in the general population [1]. Hospital-based series, which would be expected to show a higher risk because of more severely affected patients, actually showed a similar risk, with estimates ranging from 1.8% to 7.5%. Prevalence is highest in electroencephalography (EEG) cohorts, likely because of selection bias [2].

Types of Seizures

Patients with MS and seizures had a variety of seizure types, including simple partial, complex partial, secondary generalized seizures, as well as convulsive status epilepticus [3]. Specific case reports of musicogenic epilepsy [4], aphasic status epilepticus [5], and epilepsia partialis continua [6] attest to the variety of seizure types that can occur in the setting of MS.

Relationship With Clinical and Paraclinical Measures

Seizures have been reported throughout the course of MS, with occasional case reports of MS presenting with seizures [1]. One study using a prospective MS database showed an increased risk of epilepsy among progressive forms of MS [7]. Seizures during a relapse are in the minority in published cases [3]. There is limited prognostic data on the course of epilepsy other than to say that it varies [3]. In some cases, seizures resolve spontaneously or with treatment of an acute relapse, while in others they can persist [8]. Some case series suggested that seizures may continue to occur in many patients with MS [9].

A variety of studies looking at EEG findings in MS patients with seizures have been published. Study design, timing of EEG, and other parameter differences make comparison of this data difficult. The prevalence of EEG changes varied from 60% to 100%, with focal or generalized slowing being the most common finding [10]. Epileptiform discharges (both interictal and ictal) have been reported in such studies. The absence of EEG change does not rule out seizure, a finding similar to that of epilepsy in general.

MRI findings also vary. In 1 case control study, Truyen et al. found a higher cortical-subcortical lesion burden in MS patients with seizures than those without [11]. One study using double inversion recovery (DIR) (which detects cortical plaques) showed an increase in intracortical lesions in those with epilepsy [12]. Confounding this issue is that cortical lesions are common but frequently not visible on standard MRI studies [13]. Newer techniques such as DIR MRI increase the yield for such cortical lesions, although many cortical lesions remain invisible using this technique [14].

Pathogenesis of Seizures in MS

Pathological data has emphasized the early [15] and frequent [16] involvement of cortical regions in MS. This likely underlies some seizures in MS. Of course, some patients may have epilepsy based on genetic factors or other causes similar to the general population. Medicines used in MS may also precipitate seizures. For example, patients suddenly withdrawing from Lioresal can have status epilepticus (usually seen in Lioresal pump patients) [17]. The use of extended-release dalfampridine is associated with an increased risk of seizures [18], likely due to its stimulatory effect on demyelinated axons. Individual case reports of focal cortical epilepsy have shown a lesion/seizure focus correlation [13]. However, most patients with MS have multiple cortical and subcortical lesions making specific lesional diagnosis problematic.

Treatment of Seizures in the MS Population

No randomized controlled trials of antiepileptic medicines have been done in this population [19]. Because seizures may resolve spontaneously, particularly in the setting of acute relapse or acute new MRI lesion formation, many clinicians wait until repeated seizures occur to treat patients. There is no clear data to guide selection of individual antiepileptic medicines. There is some theoretical risk with the use of sodium channel blocking agents based on animal model experience, but it is not clear if this is an issue in humans [20,21]. There is also case report literature of symptomatic worsening with the use of carbamazepine in the MS population. Solaro et al. showed frequent "relapse like" events with carbamazepine with fewer events related to gabapentin and none related to lamotrigine use in MS [22]. A case report showed improvement of refractory tonic clonic seizures after treatment with natalizumab, but there is limited data about the use of immune therapies for MS related seizures [23].

KEY POINTS FOR PATIENTS ABOUT EPILEPSY AND MS

- Seizures occur in some patients with MS.
- They can usually be treated with medications.
- They likely occur because of MS affecting the surface of the brain (cortex).

SLEEP EVENTS AND MS

KEY POINTS FOR CLINICIANS REGARDING SLEEP AND MS

- Sleep disorders are common in MS and should be considered particularly when patients have fatigue, complaints of sleep disruption, or cognitive deficits.

- Consider formal sleep study and consultation where there is sleep disruption or excess fatigue.

- Restless leg syndrome (RLS) and rapid eye movement (REM) sleep behavior disorders can be treated per standard protocol (ropinirole for RLS, clonazepam for REM behavior disorder).

- Rarer sleep disorders include narcolepsy, Kleine–Levin syndrome, and REM behavior disorder.

- Narcolepsy has been correlated with hypothalamic lesions and low cerebrospinal fluid (CSF) hypocretin-1 levels in MS patients in one study.

- Insomnia is best treated with nonpharmacological approaches, including sleep hygiene, avoidance of caffeine and stimulants, and treatment of depression.

Introduction

Traditionally, sleep disorders have not been among the phenomena that MS clinicians recognize in their MS patients. While fatigue is very commonly seen in MS, it has been thought to be part of the MS spectrum and based on mechanisms such as cytokine activation, increased brain activation for a functional task, medication effect, or depression [24]. In fact, recent studies have shown an increase in frequency of sleep disorders in the MS population. Case reports have also highlighted a variety of unusual manifestations of sleep disease in the MS population of which health care practitioners should be aware. Finally, some studies have shown a correlation between daytime fatigue and sleep disorders in MS patients, prompting clinicians to look further for sleep disorders in this population.

Epidemiology

Prevalence of Sleep Disorders in MS Population
Studies of the prevalence of sleep disorders naturally vary depending on the patient population (neurology clinic, MS clinic, sleep lab, population, etc.) and ascertainment methodology (eg, clinical evaluation, sleep questionnaires, sleep studies, etc.). Clark et al. in 1992 studied a selected outpatient MS population using the Minnesota Multiphasic Personality Inventory (MMPI) and found that patients reported sleep problems more frequently than controls on 3 sleep-related items, especially the statement "Is my sleep fitful and disturbed?" [25]. Tachibana et al. studied 28 outpatients with MS from an MS clinic using clinical parameters, all-night oximetry, and polysomnography (PSG) in a small subset [26]. They found sleep disorders in more than one-half, including frequent awakenings due to spasms or leg discomfort, difficulty initiating or maintaining sleep, habitual

snoring, and nocturia. One small PSG study of MS patients found evidence of reduced sleep efficiency and more frequent awakenings compared to controls but otherwise normal sleep latency and sleep architecture [27].

Stanton et al. assessed a convenience sample of patients attending an outpatient MS clinic in London, United Kingdom, using the Fatigue Severity Scale (FSS), Epworth Sleepiness Scale (ESS), and a 7 day sleep diary [28]. They showed a significant association between the FSS score and number of days in which the subjects reported "middle insomnia" (waking at least 2 times per night). More than one-half of the patients reported problems on 2 or more nights a week with falling asleep, waking during the night, or early waking.

A study of outpatient and inpatient MS patients from a Berlin MS clinic assessed mobile outpatient PSG in a subgroup of 66 patients [29]. Seventy-four percent of this group was found to have a "clinically relevant" sleep disorder which could cause daytime sleepiness. Another study compared 15 patients with MS and fatigue with 15 MS patients without fatigue from an MS clinic using actigraphy [30] and showed that in the fatigued patients, 2 had a delayed sleep phase disorder and 10 had disrupted sleep. Twelve of fifteen nonfatigued patients had normal sleep recordings, 1 had an irregular sleep phase, and 2 had disrupted sleep. The authors concluded that sleep disturbance was correlated with fatigue in the MS population.

A large self-report mail survey of individuals recruited through a National MS society chapter (Washington State) compared responses to those of participants in a postmenopausal women's study [31]. MS participants had more sleep-related difficulties than controls. In addition, women with MS were more likely than men to report sleep disorders, and the overall prevalence of moderate to severe sleep disturbances was 51.5%.

Kaminska et al. evaluated MS patients without known sleep disorders and healthy controls with PSG

TABLE 21.1
Narcolepsy and MS Case Reports

SOURCE	AGE/SEX	AGE ONSET MS/ NARCOLEPSY	IMAGING	COMMENT
[38]	M/31	31/23	No imaging	
[38]	F/42	33/31	No imaging	
[39]	M/48	26/28	No imaging	Noted familial clustering of MS
[39]	F/52	38/26	No imaging	
[39]	F/40	20/29	No imaging	
[40]	F/62	31/56	CT atrophy	Monozygotic twin, twin not affected
[41]	M/46	40/17	T2 lesions paraventricular and peduncular	MSLT SOREMP
[41]	F/46	13/45	Right frontal, paraventricular	MSLT SOREMP
[42]	F/45	Not reported	Hypothalamic lesion	Hypocretin less than 40 pg/mL
[42]	F/21	Not reported	Hypothalamic lesion	Hypocretin less than 40 pg/mL
[42]	F/54	Not reported	Hypothalamic lesion	Hypocretin 184 pg/mL
[42]	M/61	Not reported	Hypothalamic lesion	Hypocretin 173 pg/mL

MSLT, multiple sleep latency test; SOREMP, sleep onset rapid eye movement periods.
Hypocretin less than 40 to 110 pg/mL markedly reduced, 110 to 200 pg/mL markedly reduced.

and multiple sleep latency tests (MSLT) [32]. They found obstructive sleep apnea (OSA) in 36 of 62 MS and 15 of 32 controls (no significant difference). They found that fatigue was correlated with OSA in MS but not controls.

Types of Sleep Disorders in MS Population
Insomnia appears to be common in the MS population [33]. In 1 study, 40% of those studied had insomnia with difficulty initiating and maintaining sleep [26]. Factors associated with this insomnia include muscle spasms, pain, periodic limb movements, restless leg syndrome (RLS), nocturia, medication effects, and psychiatric syndromes such as depression. Particularly of note is the occasional use of stimulant medications during the day for fatigue, which may inadvertently compromise night time sleeping.

OSA appears to be similar in frequency to the general population, but may not be immediately apparent on clinical questioning and may be correlated with fatigue in the MS population [32].

Nocturnal movement disorders appear to be more common in the MS population than the general population [27,34]. In 1 study, RLS was seen in 36% of participants versus estimates of 5% to 15% in the general population [27].

Nocturia and pain frequently interrupt sleep in MS patients. Nocturia affects as many as 70% to 80% of MS patients [35]. Pain can disrupt sleep causing daytime somnolence and worsening fatigue, as well as reducing pain threshold [36].

Rarer Sleep Disorders Reported in MS
NARCOLEPSY. A handful of case reports have noted the presence of narcolepsy in a few patients with MS. Whether this is a chance association is unclear. Most reported cases have an older age of onset than sporadic narcolepsy (23.4 and 24.4

years in 2 large population-based studies) [37], suggesting an association with MS and not simply representing sporadic narcolepsy (see Table 21.1).

KLEIN–LEVIN SYNDROME. There is a single case report of Klein–Levin syndrome at onset of MS [43]. A 20-year-old male presented with 2 episodes of daytime hypersomnia, orthostatic hypotension, compulsive masturbation and hyperphagia, with well-defined MS-like brain lesions and CSF oligoclonal bands. Whether cases of hypersomnolence in MS represent part of this spectrum or vice versa is unclear, but such cases probably share hypothalamic involvement.

REM BEHAVIOR DISORDERS. Patients with REM sleep behavioral disorder (RBD) have been described in the MS population in some case reports [44,45]. A large case control study of 135 MS patients and 118 controls assessed by history found 4 patients in the MS group with RBD, and none in the control group [46].

ONDINE'S CURSE. Two case reports in patients with sudden death during sleep showed multiple medulla oblongata lesions [47]. Lesions overlying the ventral nuclear complex of respiratory control were present in both cases.
Practical suggestions for clinicians:

• Inquire about sleep disorders in the MS population.
• Consider formal sleep study and consultation where there is sleep disruption or excess fatigue.
• RLS and RBD can be treated per standard protocol (ropinarole for RLS, clonazepam for RBD).
• Insomnia is best treated with nonpharmacological approaches including sleep hygiene, avoidance of caffeine and stimulants, and treatment of depression.

KEY POINTS FOR PATIENTS ABOUT MS AND SLEEP DISORDERS

- Sleep disorders occur commonly in MS and may require treatment.

- Snoring, frequent awakening at night, and fatigue in the morning may be symptoms of a sleep disorder.

- Insomnia is common in MS and is best treated with nonmedication approaches.

TRANSIENT NEUROLOGICAL EVENTS (PAROXYSMAL EVENTS) IN MS

Case

A 49-year-old male delivery man presents with recurrent events of speech arrest. He notices an odd sensation in his throat, followed a few seconds later by tingling on his right face. For the next 30 to 60 seconds he stutters, and has trouble getting his words out. He may have episodes 2 to 3 times a day, and they occur more frequently when he is working as a volunteer toastmaster. His health has been good other than treated hypertension. MRI with and without contrast shows multiple paraventricular and infratentorial lesions on fluid-attenuated inversion recovery (FLAIR) and T2 imaging without enhancing lesions (Figure 21.1). CSF shows oligoclonal banding and a mild lymphocytic pleocytosis. Over the ensuing year the patient develops some gait spasticity, fatigue, paresthesia of the legs, and new nonenhancing MRI lesions. His episodes spontaneously resolve after 4 months.

Overview

Clinicians caring for patients with MS are well aware of relapses of MS, as well as of the progressive nature of MS in many patients. However, many MS patients describe transient, stereotyped, even bizarre sounding events lasting seconds that do not conform to a typical relapse or epileptic, migranous, or sleep phenomena. Such events have been called various things (tonic spasms, painful tonic spasms, paroxysmal attacks, paroxysmal symptoms). However, none of these terms capture the full group of phenomena that have the following general characteristics which distinguish them from others.

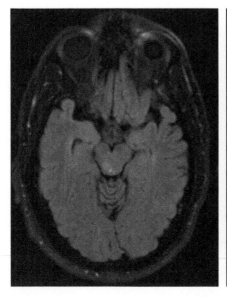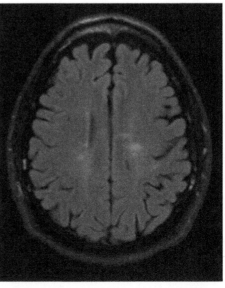

FIGURE 21.1
FLAIR axial views showing callosal, paraventricular, and mesencephalic lesions consistent with demyelination.

KEY POINTS FOR CLINICIANS REGARDING TRANSIENT NEUROLOGICAL EVENTS IN MS

Transient neurological events

- Occur in setting of MS or other demyelinating syndrome.

- Last usually seconds (typically less than 60 seconds) rather than minutes or hours.

- Are stereotyped.

- May have a combination of different types of sensory, motor, or visual activity or sensation (eg, blurred vision due to nystagmus, dysarthria, focal sensory symptoms).

- May occur multiple times a day up to hundreds of times a day.

- Are more common early in MS but may occur any time during the course of the disease.

- Do not conform to more usual descriptions of focal seizures or migrainous events.

- May last for few weeks and resolve spontaneously, sometimes in the setting of acute relapse.

- Typically respond to antiepileptic medicines. Antiepileptic medications are usually effective. We tend to taper these off after a few months if possible.

While clinicians may under-recognize these events, for patients and their families they are very disruptive and a source of concern and anxiety. They may lead to a fruitless search for epilepsy or sleep disorders, and result in extensive testing.

PATHOPHYSIOLOGICAL CONCEPTS

Many MS symptoms are likely related to conduction block, slowed conduction, loss of axons, reduced safety factor, and other disruption of neural transmission. Positive symptoms such as paroxysmal events may have a variety of underlying mechanisms. Positive symptoms such as paresthesias, Lhermitte's phenomenon, and tonic spasms may be caused by spontaneously generated trains of spurious impulses arising in an area of demyelination and propagating along axons in both directions [48]. In experimental models of central demyelination, newly demyelinated axons do not seem to have this property, but develop it after a week or two [49]. Different patterns of spontaneous bursting have been seen in demyelinated fibers, including trains of evenly spaced impulses at frequencies of 10 to 50 Hz for periods of 0.1 to 5 seconds, and bursts of impulses [50]. These patterns may have differing mechanisms based on sodium or potassium channel activity, but the exact correlations in experimental models are unclear. "Spontaneous bursting" patterns can sometimes be provoked by stimulating axons at physiological frequencies, providing a model for the precipitation of Lhermitte's phenomenon with neck movement. In addition, positive phenomena are often enhanced by hyperventilation [51] which increases axonal excitability by reducing membrane surface charge due to reduced extracellular free calcium [52]. Other mechanisms have been proposed for positive phenomena in MS. In a demyelinated fiber, conduction may be slow enough to re-excite backward the normal area which has recovered from the refractory period [53]. Impulse conduction may activate adjacent fibers via ephaptic transmission [54]. Clinically it is unclear which of these mechanisms, if any, are causing positive symptoms but some or all are likely to underlie the phenotypic expression of symptoms.

CLINICAL DESCRIPTION

Events lasting a few seconds that are apparent to patients with MS have been described for years, but often go under-recognized by patients and physicians. The description of these events varies and many neurologists recognize some but not all of the paroxysmal events in MS. Most neurologists separate such paroxysmal events from epilepsy by their brevity, high frequency, absence of change in awareness, and lack of typical seizure aura, but it is unclear whether this separation is artificial as the mechanisms of paroxysmal symptoms in MS are not fully worked out. No prospective study has been done in an MS population to define the frequency of transient neurological events.

Paroxysmal events in MS usually last seconds and can be stereotyped. They may occur hundreds of times a day or only on occasion. Sometimes their time course overall is clustered in a few weeks, similar to the time course of a relapse. The relationship between paroxysmal events and relapse has not been fully elucidated. They appear to occur more frequently early in the disease course, and may be related to the time of a relapse. However, they can occur throughout the disease and independent of an acute relapse.

The phenomenology of paroxysmal events varies as much as other manifestations of MS. Essentially, any part of the central neuraxis can be affected. Sensory symptoms (usually a spreading sensation of some kind), motor symptoms (tonic spasms, transient inhibition of motor function, or ataxia), brain stem symptoms (dysarthria, blurred vision

TABLE 21.2
Types of Transient Neurological Events, System Involved, and Localization

SYMPTOM	SIGN	SYSTEM INVOLVED	LOCALIZATION (IF KNOWN)	COMMENTS
Tonic spasm [55]	Movement with dystonic component lasting seconds	Motor	Posterior internal capsule, cerebral peduncle, spinal cord	May be triggered by movement, hyperventilation
Bilateral tonic spasm [56]	Bilateral tonic movements	Motor	Medulla	
Paroxysmal dysarthria [57]	Transient slurred speech often with ataxia	Cerebellar connections, corticobulbar fibers	Various	
Paroxysmal itching, other paresthesiae [56]	None	Sensory afferents	Unknown	May last minutes to hours
Paroxysmal akinesia [58]	Transient loss of motor function	Unclear		Usually lower limb involved
Kinesogenic choreoathetosis [59]	Complex movement of limb with or without other signs	Unclear	Unclear	
Paroxysmal diplopia [56]		Unclear		Responded to carbamazepine
Ocular convergence spasm [60]	Convergence spasm	Convergence system midbrain	Brainstem lesion MLF	

MLF, medial longitudinal fasciculus.

or diplopia, vertigo) or gustatory symptoms (altered taste, taste hallucination) can all be seen (see Table 21.2).

Tonic Spasms

The original description of tonic spasms in MS was by Matthews in 1958 [61]. Since that time, multiple publications have described this most well defined of paroxysmal events in MS. Tonic spasms can be triggered by movement, hyperventilation, or other stimuli. They may be accompanied or preceded by sensory symptoms such as tingling, burning, or itching, suggesting involvement of nearby sensory fibers during the event. When unilateral, they are often generated by a focal plaque in the contralateral corticospinal pathways, most typically the cerebral peduncle or internal capsule [55,62]. They have also been referred to as tonic seizures; however, this term may imply a cortical localization for their generation, which may not be correct.

Matthews characterized "tonic seizures" as [58,61]

- brief (duration up to 90 seconds);
- frequent (up to hundreds per day);
- usually intensely painful or uncomfortable;
- limbs on one side adopt a tetanic posture;
- often precipitated by movement or sensory stimulation;
- remit completely in weeks.

Matthews and others have noted that such tonic spasms are neither accompanied by surface EEG changes nor by altered consciousness.

TABLE 21.3
Descriptions of Transient Neurological Events

"'cramp' in the left leg followed by sensation heat without pain, lasting 1 minute, up to 15 times per day" [56]

"Sudden sensation of right knee 'locked'...lost tone muscles right leg...seconds...30 times a day...lasted 6 months" [56]

"Attacks in which she felt as if her eyes were turning in. Her head would turn slightly to the right and the left eye would adduct. These attacks lasted about 10 seconds and were extremely distressing..." [58]

"sensation of quivering in the right side of the face, spreading to the right arm, index finger, and thumb...last for a few seconds...highly unpleasant" [58]

"warning sensation of 'dullness,' quickly followed by diplopia, difficulty pronouncing words...stiffness and unsteadiness of legs" [63]

"Lose color in one eye" [34]

"sensation of 'heaviness' and 'stiffness' right leg and arm. Almost simultaneously she experienced double vision, ataxia and dysarthria...a few moments later she felt a sensation of heat in the left forearm" [56]

Other types of transient neurological events are as noted in Table 21.3, which is by no means exhaustive. What characterize these events are their brevity, repetition, and stereotypy. Table 21.3 lists some descriptions of episodes from the neurological literature which emphasize the variation of symptomatology across individuals.

One study [55] looked at MRI in 2 patients with unilateral painful tonic limb spasms. They found focal lesions in the cerebral peduncle and upper pons in these cases.

Spissu et al. reviewed 5 cases of tonic spasms and found lesions in the posterior limb of the internal capsule in 4 and of the cerebral peduncle in 2 [62].

Treatment of tonic spasms and other transient neurological events has been described in either case studies or case series. Anecdotally, many patients do not require treatment once symptoms are explained, but for others, particularly when events are uncomfortable or affect function, intervention may be necessary. Twomey et al. described using carbamazepine with "good response" in 5 of 7 treated patients among a series of 14 patients with paroxysmal symptoms [64]. Osterman described multiple patients treated with carbamazepine with reduction or cessation of episodes [56]. In Matthews's case series of 28 episodes of paroxysmal symptoms, 12 stopped spontaneously, phenobarbital or phenytoin "appeared to arrest the paroxysms" in 6, and carbamazepine was used "effectively" in 6. In 4 patients there was no response to these medicines [58]. Sakurai et al. described treating patients with "positive MS symptoms" with orally administered mexiletine with reduction of episodes [65]. Symptoms which patients described included paroxysmal Lhermitte's sign, paroxysmal pain or itching. Solaro et al. in 1998 described an open label trial of gabapentin in doses ranging from 600 to 1200 mg/day in 21 patients with a variety of paroxysmal events [66]. Eighteen experienced resolution or amelioration of their symptoms during this uncontrolled trial. Restivo et al. in 2003 described the use of botulinum toxin for painful tonic spasms in 5 patients not obtaining relief from a variety of anticonvulsant medicines and reduced pain scores at 30 day follow-up after botulinum injection [67]. Importantly, these syndromes are often confused with spasticity and treated with baclofen and other antispasticity medications, typically without beneficial response.

Treating tonic spasms and other transient neurological events in MS patients can be the most rewarding of therapeutic exercises. The patient often presents having up to hundreds of episodes per day, have defied diagnosis and treatment by others, and are cured within hours of starting an antiepileptic medication. Initial treatment has traditionally involved carbamazepine or phenytoin, although new antiepileptic therapies may be similarly effective. Serum drug levels are rarely needed, as dosing is guided by treatment response and side effects.

REFERENCES

1. Kelley BJ, Rodriguez M. Seizures in patients with multiple sclerosis. *CNS Drugs.* 2009;23:805–815.

2. Koch M, Uyttenboogaart M, Polman S, De Keyser J. Seizures in multiple sclerosis. *Epilepsia.* 2008;49:948–953.

3. Catenoix H, Marignier R, Ritleng C, et al. Multiple sclerosis and epileptic seizures. *Mult Scler.* 2011;17(1):96–102.

4. Newman P, Saunders M. A unique case of musicogenic epilepsy. *Arch Neurol.* 1980;37(4):244–245.

5. Spatt J, Goldenberg G, Mamoli B. Simple dysphasic seizures as the sole manifestation of relapse in multiple sclerosis. *Epilepsia.* 1994;35(6):1342–1345.

6. Hess DC, Sethi KD. Epilepsia partialis continua in multiple sclerosis. *Int J Neurosci.* 1990;50(1–2):109–111.

7. Martinez-Juarez IE, Lopez-Meza E, Gonzalez-Arragon MD, et al. Epilepsy and multiple sclerosis: Increased risk among progressive forms. *Epilepsy Res.* 2009;84:250–253.

8. Spatt J, Chaix R, Mamoli B. Epileptic and non-epileptic seizures in multiple sclerosis. *J Neurol.* 2001;248(1):2–9.

9. Kinnunen E, Wilkström J. Prevalence and prognosis of epilepsy in patients with multiple sclerosis. *Epilepsia.* 1986;27:729–733.

10. Nyquist PA, Cascino GD, Rodriguez M. Seizures in patients with multiple sclerosis seen at Mayo Clinic, Rochester, Minn, 1990–1998. *Mayo Clin Proc.* 2001;76:983–986.

11. Truyen L, Barkhof F, Frequin ST, et al. Magnetic resonance imaging of epilepsy in multiple sclerosis: A case control study. *Mult Scler.* 1996;1:213–217.

12. Calabrese M, De Stefano N, Atzori M, et al. Extensive cortical inflammation is associated with epilepsy in multiple sclerosis. *J Neurol.* 2008;255:581–586.

13. Geurts JJ, Bo L, Pouwels PJ, et al. Cortical lesions in multiple sclerosis: Combined postmortem MR imaging and histopathology. *Am J Neuroradiol.* 2005;26:572–577.

14. Ciccarelli O, Chen JT. MS cortical lesions on double inversion recovery: Few but true. *Neurology.* 2012;78:296–297.

15. Luchinetti CF, Bogdan FG, Popescu MD, et al. Inflammatory cortical demyelination in early multiple sclerosis. *N Engl J Med.* 2011;365:2188–2197.

16. Peterson JW, Bo L, Mork S, et al. Transected neurites, apoptotic neurons, and reduced inflammation in cortical multiple sclerosis lesions. *Ann Neurol.* 2001;50:389–400.

17. Schuele SU, Kellinghaus C, Shook SJ, et al. Incidence of seizures in patients with multiple sclerosis treated with intrathecal baclofen. *Neurology.* 2005;64:1086–1087.

18. Goodman AD, Brown TR, Edwards KR, et al. A phase 3 trial of extended release oral dalfampridine in multiple sclerosis. *Ann Neurol.* 2010;68:494–502.

19. Koch MW, Polman SK, Uyttenboogaart M, De Keyser J. Treatment of seizures in multiple sclerosis. *Cochrane Database Syst Rev.* 2009 Jul 8;(3):CD007150.

20. Waxman SG. Axonal conduction and injury in multiple sclerosis: The role of sodium channels. *Nat Rev Neurosci.* 2006;7:932–941.

21. Dan P. The role of ion channels in neurodegeneration. *Modulator.* 2008;22:14–17.

22. Solaro C, Brichetto G, Battaglia MA, et al. Antiepileptic medications in multiple sclerosis: Adverse effects in a three-year follow-up study. *Neurol Sci.* 2005;25:307–310.

23. Sotgiu S, Murrighile MR, Constantin G. Treatment of refractory epilepsy with natalizumab in a patient with multiple sclerosis. Case report. *BMC Neurol.* 2010;10:84.

24. Krupp LB, Alvarez LA, LaRocca NG, Scheinberg LC. Fatigue in MS. *Arch Neurol.* 1988;11:78–83.

25. Clark CM, Fleming JA, Li D, et al. Sleep disturbance, depression and lesion site in patients with multiple sclerosis. *Arch Neurol.* 1992;49:641–643.

26. Tachibana N, Howard RS, Hirsch NP, et al. Sleep problems in multiple sclerosis. *Eur Neurol.* 1994;34:320–323.

27. Ferini-Strambi L, Filippi M, Martinelli V, et al. Nocturnal sleep study in multiple sclerosis: Correlations with clinical and brain magnetic resonance imaging findings. *J Neurol Sci.* 1994;125:194–197.

28. Stanton BR, Barnes F, Silber E. Sleep and fatigue in multiple sclerosis. *Mult Scler.* 2006;12:481–486.

29. Veauthier C, Radbruch H, Gaede G, et al. Fatigue in multiple sclerosis is closely related to sleep disorders: A polysomnographic cross-sectional study. *Mult Scler.* 2011;17(5):613–622.

30. Attarian HP, Brown KM, Duntley SP, et al. The relationship of sleep disturbances and fatigue in multiple sclerosis. *Arch Neurol.* 2004;61:525–528.

31. Barner AM, Johnson KL, Amtmann D, Kraft GH. Prevalence of sleep problems in individuals with multiple sclerosis. *Mult Scler.* 2008;14:1127–1130.

32. Kaminska M, Kimoff RJ, Benedetti A, et al. Obstructive sleep apnea is associated with fatigue in multiple sclerosis. *Mult Scler.* 2012;18(8):1159–1169.

33. Fleming WE, Pollak CP. Sleep disorders in multiple sclerosis. *Semin Neurol.* 2005;25:64–68.

34. Rae-Grant AD, Eckert NJ, Bartz S, et al. Sensory symptoms of multiple sclerosis: A hidden reservoir of morbidity. *Mult Scler.* 1999;5:179–183.

35. Amarenco G, Kerdraon J, Denys P. Bladder and sphincter disorders in multiple sclerosis: Clinical, urodynamic and neurophysiological study of 225 cases (in French). *Rev Neurol (Paris).* 1995;151:722–730.

36. Onen SH, Alloui A, Gross A, et al. The effects of total sleep deprivation, selective sleep interruption and sleep recovery on pain tolerance thresholds in health subjects. *J Sleep Res.* 2001;10:35–42.

37. Dauvilliers Y, Montplaisir J, Molinari N. Age at onset of narcolepsy in two large populations of patients in France and Quebec. *Neurology.* 2001;57(11):2029–2033.

38. Berg O, Hanley J. Narcolepsy in two cases of multiple sclerosis. *Acta Neurol Scand.* 1963;39(3):252–257.

39. Ekbom K. Familial multiple sclerosis with narcolepsy. *Arch Neurol.* 1966;15(4):337–344.

40. Schrader H, Gotlibsen OB, Skomedal GN. Multiple sclerosis and narcolepsy/cataplexy in a monozygotic twin. *Neurology.* 1980;30:105–108.

41. Younger DS, Pedley TA, Thorpy MJ. Multiple sclerosis and narcolepsy: Possible similar genetic susceptibility. *Neurology.* 1991;41:447–448.

42. Kanbayashi T, Shimohata T, Nakashima I, et al. Symptomatic narcolepsy in patients with neuromyelitis optica and multiple sclerosis. *Arch Neurol.* 2009;66(12):1563–1566.

43. Testa S, Oppotuno A, Gallo P, Tavolato B. A case of multiple sclerosis with an onset mimicking the Klein-Levin syndrome. *Ital J Neurol Sci.* 1987;8:151–155.

44. Plazzi G, Montagna P. Remitting REM sleep behavior disorder as the initial sign of multiple sclerosis. *Sleep Med.* 2002;3(5):437–439.

45. Tippmann-Peikert M, Boeve BF, Keegan BM. REM sleep behavior disorder initiated by acute brainstem multiple sclerosis. *Neurology.* 2006;66:1277–1279.

46. Gomez-Choco MJ, Iranzo A, Blanco Y, et al. Prevalence of restless legs syndrome and REM sleep behavior disorder in multiple sclerosis. *Mult Scler.* 2007;13:805–808.

47. Auer RN, Rowlands CG, Perry SF, et al. Multiple sclerosis with medullary plaques and fatal sleep apnea (Ondine's curse). *Clin Neuropathol.* 1996;15:101–105.

48. Baker M, Bostock H. Ectopic activity in demyelinated spinal root axons of the rat. *J Physiol.* 1992;451:539–552.

49. Smith KJ, McDonald WI. The pathophysiology of multiple sclerosis? The mechanisms underlying the production of symptoms and the natural history of the disease. *Phil Trans R Soc Lond B.* 1999;354:1649–1673.

50. Felts PA, Kapoor R, Smith KJ. A mechanism for ectopic firing in central demyelinated axons. *Brain.* 1995;118:1225–1231.

51. Davis FA, Becker FO, Michael JA, Sorensen E. Effect of intravenous sodium bicarbonate, disodiumedetate and hyperventilation on visual and oculomotor signs in multiple sclerosis. *J Neurol Neurosurg Psychiatry.* 1970;33:723–732.

52. Burke D. Microneurography, impulse conduction, and paresthesias. *Muscle Nerve.* 1993;16:1025–1032.

53. Burchiel KJ. Abnormal impulse generation in focally demyelinated trigeminal roots. *J Neurosurg.* 1980;53:674–688.

54. Raminsky M. Hyperexcitability of pathologically myelinated axons and positive symptoms in multiple sclerosis. In: Waxman SG, Ritchie JM, eds. *Demyelinating Diseases: Basic and Clinical Electrophysiology.* New York: Raven Press; 289–297.

55. Rose MR, Ball JA, Thompson PD. Magnetic resonance imaging in tonic spasms of multiple sclerosis. *J Neurol.* 1993;241:115–117.

56. Osterman PO, Westerberg C-E. Paroxysmal attacks in multiple sclerosis. *Brain.* 1975;98:189–202.

57. Andermann F, Cosgrove JBR, Lloyd-Smith D, et al. Paroxysmal dysarthria and ataxia in multiple sclerosis. *Neurology.* 1959;9:211–215.

58. Mathews WB. Paroxysmal symptoms in multiple sclerosis. *J Neurol Neurosurg Psychiatry.* 1975;38:617–623.

59. Roos RA, Wintzen AR, Vielvoye G, Polder TW. Paroxysmal kinesigenic choreoathetosis as a presenting symptom of multiple sclerosis. *J Neurol Neurosurg Psychiatry.* 1991;54:657–658.

60. Postert T, McMonagle U, Buttner T, et al. Paroxysmal convergence spasm in multiple sclerosis. *Acta Neurol Scand.* 1996;94:35–37.

61. Matthews WB. Tonic seizures in disseminated sclerosis. *Brain.* 1958;81:193–201.

62. Spissu A, Cannas A, Ferrigno P, et al. Anatomic correlates of painful tonic spasms in multiple sclerosis. *Mov Disord.* 1999;14:331–335.

63. Espir MLE, Watkins SM, Smith HV. Paroxysmal dysarthria and other transient neurological disturbances in disseminated sclerosis. *J Neurol Neurosurg Psychiatry.* 1966;29:323–330.

64. Twomey JA, Espir MLE. Paroxysmal symptoms as the first manifestations of multiple sclerosis. *J Neurol Neurosurg Psychiatry.* 1980;43:296–304.

65. Sakurai M, Kanazawa I. Positive symptoms in multiple sclerosis: Their treatment with sodium channel blockers, lidocaine, and mexiletine. *J Neurol Sci.* 1999;162:162–168.

66. Solaro C, Lunardi GL, Capello E, et al. An open-label trial of gabapentin treatment of paroxysmal symptoms in multiple sclerosis patients. *Neurology.* 1998;51:609–611.

67. Restivo DA, Tinazzi M, Patti F, et al. Botulinum toxin treatment of painful tonic spasms in multiple sclerosis. *Neurology.* 2003;61:719–720.

22

Eye Symptoms, Signs, and Therapy in Multiple Sclerosis

COLLIN McCLELLAND
STEVEN GALETTA

KEY POINTS FOR CLINICIANS

- Demyelinating optic neuritis (DON) is a hallmark manifestation of multiple sclerosis (MS) and is marked by acute or subacute onset of vision loss, eye pain, and a relative afferent pupillary defect (RAPD) in unilateral cases.

- Intravenous steroids do not alter the long-term visual outcome of isolated DON but expedite visual recovery and show a protective effect against MS development for 2 years.

- Neuromyelitis optica (NMO)-associated optic neuritis may present similar to DON. Providers should maintain a low threshold for serum NMO antibody testing in cases of DON as NMO requires a different long-term treatment.

- Maculopathies, including fingolimod-associated macular edema, often have subtle fundus findings and can mimic DON. Unlike DON, they characteristically lack pain and often do not demonstrate an RAPD.

- Demyelination rarely causes isolated ocular motor (cranial nerve [CN] III, IV, and VI) palsies. Alternative etiologies should always be carefully evaluated.

Multiple sclerosis (MS) frequently affects both the afferent visual system and the efferent ocular motor system. An estimated 27% to 37% of MS patients develop demyelinating optic neuritis (DON) during their disease course, while 40% to 76% suffer from abnormalities of ocular movement. A basic understanding of neuroophthalmology is important for all providers who manage MS patients.

The neuroophthalmic sequelae of MS include highly characteristic features such as DON and internuclear ophthalmoplegia (INO), as well as other manifestations such as nystagmus, cranial nerve palsies, uveitis, and saccadic abnormalities. Vision loss may also arise from treatment complications including fingolimod-associated macular edema (ME), corticosteroid-induced central serous chorioretinopathy (CSR),

and natalizumab-associated progressive multifocal leukoencephalopathy (PML). This chapter reviews high-yield clinical knowledge pertinent to the diagnosis and management of MS-associated visual impairment.

EVALUATION: AFFERENT PATHOLOGY

A hallmark feature of MS, DON occurs in about one-third of MS patients and is the presenting feature in about 15% to 20%. While the term *optic neuritis* is often used as a synonym for demyelinating optic neuritis associated with MS, the term *optic neuritis* also refers to optic nerve inflammation that complicates other inflammatory and infectious conditions. Referring to MS-associated optic neuritis as idiopathic DON lessens the ambiguity.

The optic neuritis treatment trial (ONTT) defined the presenting characteristics [1], optimal treatment [2], visual prognosis [3], and long-term risk of MS in patients with DON [4]. MS and DON share similar patient demographics; DON is common in young patients (mean age = 31.8), whites (85%), and females (F:M = 3:1) [1]. The diagnosis of DON remains clinical and is characterized by vision loss over hours to days, eye pain, and the presence of a relative afferent pupillary defect (RAPD) in unilateral cases. Visual impairment can affect central vision, peripheral vision, and color vision; a thorough exam for suspected DON should assess all these aspects of visual function. In most clinical settings, visual acuity is tested on a high-contrast distance Snellen acuity chart or a near card using the patient's optimal refractive correction for the distance tested. Presenting visual acuity in DON ranges from normal to no light perception, with severe vision loss occurring in a minority of patients (Table 22.1) [1].

> DON is characterized by acute vision loss, eye pain, and a relative afferent pupillary defect (in unilateral cases).

Dyschromatopsia, or abnormal color perception, occurs in most DON cases (88% to 94%) and can be tested easily in clinic using pseudoisochromatic color plates or

TABLE 22.1
Presenting Features of Vision Loss in DON [1]

VISION	PERCENTAGE (%)
VA: 20/20 or greater	10.5
VA: 20/25 to 20/40	24.8
VA: 20/50 to 20/190	28.8
VA: 20/200 to 20/800	20.3
VA: Finger counting or lesser	15.6
Dyschromatopsia (color plate testing)	88.2
VF: Diffuse depression	44.8
VF: Altitudinal defect	28.8
VF: 3 quadrant defect	14.0
VF: 1 quadrant defect	11.8
VF: Cecocentral scotoma	8.7
VF: Hemianopic defect	8.3
VF: Peripheral rim defect	7.0
VF: Arcuate scotoma	7.4
VF: Central scotoma	7.0
VF: Enlarged blind spot	2.6
VF: Nasal step defect	1.3
VF: Other focal defects	3.0

VA, visual acuity; VF, visual fields.

subjective red desaturation testing using a red bottle top [1]. Visual field loss occurs universally in DON. While confrontational testing techniques are helpful for large visual field defects, more subtle defects require formal visual field testing. Automated static threshold perimetry (eg, Humphrey visual field testing) was used in the ONTT, which found that the most common pattern (45%) was diffuse depression [1]. Patterns of focal visual field loss varied widely (Table 22.1). Unfortunately, the presenting features of vision loss in DON are nonspecific and occur in many other optic neuropathies and retinopathies. Diagnosis, therefore, often relies on more distinguishing features such as eye pain, fundus appearance, and the presence of visual recovery.

Eye pain is described in about 92% of DON cases and is typically worse with eye movement [1]. The pain may precede or follow vision loss and usually subsides in 3 to 5 days. DON without eye pain is atypical and raises concern for alternative diagnoses (Table 22.2). Almost all DON cases will exhibit an RAPD on the swinging flashlight test (Video 22.1; to view the video, please visit http://www.demosmedpub. com/video/?vid=597). The absence of an RAPD raises concern (Table 22.2) for bilateral DON, retinopathy-mimicking DON, or prior insult to the contralateral optic nerve. About two-thirds of DON cases have normal-appearing optic nerves, while the other one-third typically show only mild optic disc edema [1]. Peripapillary hemorrhages and retinal exudates associated with severe disc edema occur in about 5% of cases and suggest "atypical optic neuritis" related to infectious or nondemyelinating inflammatory disorders (Table 22.2). While laboratory tests for DON mimics are rarely helpful in classic presentations of DON, the presence of peripapillary hemorrhages, retinal exudates, or severe disc edema should prompt a targeted evaluation. Optic disc edema accompanied by macular exudates forming a sunburst-like pattern surrounding the fovea (Figure 22.1) is highly suggestive of neuroretinitis, a diagnosis not associated with MS. While most cases of neuroretinitis are idiopathic, specific etiologies (Table 22.2) should be considered and tested for depending on clinical context.

> Most cases of DON (two-thirds) have normal-appearing optic nerves. The other one-third usually shows mild disc edema.

While neuro-imaging is not usually necessary to diagnose DON, MRI of the brain is indicated to assess for characteristic white matter lesions in patients without known MS (see the section on management). In cases when DON is difficult to distinguish clinically from nonarteritic anterior ischemic optic neuropathy (NAION), dedicated orbital MRI sequences may be beneficial [5]. DON demonstrates optic nerve enhancement in nearly all cases (greater than 90%) while it is rarely seen in NAION (about 7%) [5]. In cases with acute painful vision loss, RAPD, and orbital signs (eg, proptosis, conjunctival injection/chemosis, or restricted motility), MRI of the orbits may be helpful to rule out orbital pseudotumor, or idiopathic orbital inflammatory syndrome. Usually

TABLE 22.2
Clues to Alternative Diagnoses in Presumed DON

ATYPICAL FEATURE	ALTERNATIVE DIAGNOSES TO CONSIDER
Severe disc swelling (including peripapillary hemorrhages or exudates)	"Atypical optic neuritis": Autoimmune-associated (Lupus, Sjogren's, sarcoid, inflammatory bowel disease), infectious (syphilis, HIV, Lyme, tuberculosis), papilledema, hypertensive retinopathy, anterior ischemic optic neuropathy (nonarteritic and giant cell arteritis)
Macular star of exudates	Neuroretinitis (cat scratch disease, Lyme, syphilis, toxoplasmosis, sarcoid, tuberculosis, numerous viral etiologies)
Lack of expected visual recovery	Neuromyelitis optica-associated optic neuritis, compressive lesions (malignancy or aneurysm), sarcoidosis, ischemic optic neuropathy, maculopathies (CSR, ME, choroidal neovascular membrane, retinal vascular occlusion, etc.), nutritional/toxic (B_{12} deficiency, vitamin A deficiency, folate deficiency, cigarette smoking), metabolic (Leber hereditary optic neuropathy)
Severe photophobia	Nondemyelinating optic neuritis associated with uveitis: Sarcoid-, syphilis-, Lyme disease-, Behcet-, tuberculosis-, and inflammatory bowel disease-associated optic neuritis
Optic nerve sheath enhancement on MRI	"Optic perineuritis": Orbital pseudotumor, sarcoid, inflammatory bowel disease, Lyme disease, Syphilis, Wegener's disease, and optic nerve sheath meningioma
Lack of pain	Ischemic optic neuropathy, neuromyelitis optica-associated optic neuritis, Leber hereditary optic neuropathy, numerous maculopathies (CSR, ME, choroidal neovascular membrane, retinal vascular occlusion, etc.). Consider retrochiasmatic visual loss
Lack of a relative afferent pupillary defect	Numerous maculopathies (CSR, ME, choroidal neovascular membrane, retinal vascular occlusion, etc.), bilateral optic neuropathy (including bilateral DON), media opacities (eg, posterior subcapsular cataract, corneal pathology, vitreous hemorrhage, etc.)
Metamorphopsia	Numerous maculopathies (CSR, ME, choroidal neovascular membrane, retinal vascular occlusion, etc.)

CSR, central serous chorioretinopathy; DON, demyelinating optic neuritis; ME, macular edema.

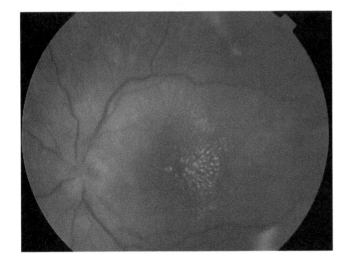

FIGURE 22.1
Color fundus photograph of the left eye demonstrating characteristic features of neuroretinitis in a patient with cat scratch fever. There is moderate to severe optic nerve swelling with macular exudates forming a "star" pattern. The patient with typical papillitis may have a similar disc appearance, without the retinal exudates.

idiopathic and considered within the spectrum of orbital pseudotumor, optic perineuritis is primarily a radiographic diagnosis characterized by peripheral enhancement of the optic nerve [6]. Peripheral vision loss tends to predominate in optic perineuritis, although central acuity can be affected and mimic DON. Distinction from DON is important because optic perineuritis is exquisitely sensitive to steroids (intravenous or oral) and is not associated with MS.

Some maculopathies may mimic DON. Fingolimod (Gilenya) has been shown to cause ME in 0.5% to 0.6% of patients [7]. ME is associated with painless central vision loss in one or both eyes, typically with normal pupillary function (no RAPD). The result of a breakdown of the blood retinal barrier, ME frequently occurs in association with diabetes, uveitis, and retinal vein occlusions. The fundus findings of ME are often subtle, and diagnosis relies heavily on ocular coherence tomography (OCT) (Figure 22.2) and fluorescein angiography (FA). The greatest risk for ME occurs in the first 3 to 4 months of fingolimod treatment. Patients should receive a baseline pretreatment ophthalmic exam followed by a repeat exam 3 to 4 months after starting fingolimod [7]. Patients with risk factors for ME (such as diabetes and uveitis) may require closer follow-up.

> Fingolimod-associated macular edema usually causes painless central vision loss and occurs in the first 4 months of treatment.

CSR is a maculopathy marked by painless detachment of the neurosensory retina [8]. CSR causes subacute

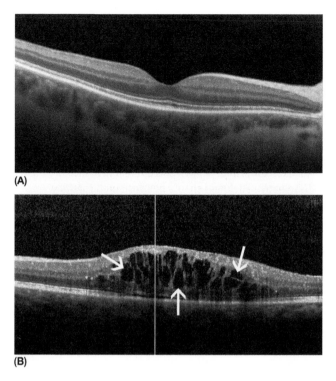

(A)

(B)

FIGURE 22.2
Spectral domain ocular coherence tomography (SD-OCT) slice demonstrating normal macular contour with the foveal pit located centrally (A). SD-OCT slice showing cyst-like spaces of fluid within the retina (arrows) characteristic of ME, which can be associated with fingolimod (Gilenya) therapy (B).

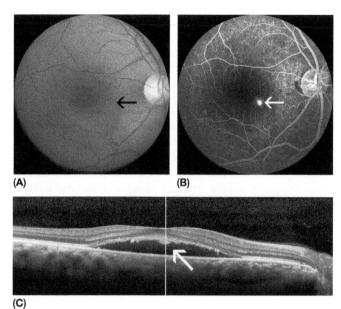

(A)   **(B)**

(C)

FIGURE 22.3
Color fundus photograph of the right eye showing subtle findings of a neurosensory retinal detachment including a hyperpigmented macular patch (arrow) that would be slightly elevated on stereoscopic view (A). Arteriovenous phase FA image showing a hyperfluorescent "dot" inferonasal to the fovea (arrow). The complete FA sequence (not shown) reveals an "expansile dot" pattern of leakage diagnostic of CSR (B). SD-OCT slice demonstrating macular subretinal fluid (arrow) consistent with serous retinal detachment due to CSR (C).

onset of central vision loss that may mimic DON. CSR is important to MS providers because it can be triggered by glucocorticoid administration and, unlike DON, will worsen with prolonged steroid therapy [9]. Patients are classically middle aged (mean = 41 years), predominantly male (M:F = 6:1), and exhibit type A personalities [8]. Exam findings are often subtle (Figure 22.3A) and include mild elevation of the detached macula, an absence of the normal foveal light reflex, and abnormal macular coloration. Diagnosis is facilitated by FA (Figure 22.3B) and OCT (Figure 22.3C).

Both CSR- and fingolimod-associated ME are maculopathies most easily distinguished from unilateral DON by the lack of pain and absence of an RAPD. Metamorphopsia, or the wavy distortion of straight lines, is a specific symptom of maculopathies not usually described in optic neuropathies.

> Maculopathies, unlike DON, are usually painless and may lack an RAPD. OCT and FA often aid in the diagnosis of maculopathies.

EVALUATION: EFFERENT PATHOLOGY

The symptoms of MS-related eye movement abnormalities include visual fatigue, blurred vision, diplopia (double

vision), and oscillopsia (subjective movement of visual targets). In most cases, these abnormalities reflect demyelinating lesions of the brain stem and cerebellum. The motility disturbance INO is highly characteristic of MS and indicates disruption of interneurons traveling through the medial longitudinal fasciculus (MLF) from the abducens nucleus in the pons to the contralateral medial rectus oculomotor subnucleus in the midbrain. INO is detectable clinically in up to 34% of patients with MS [10]. Findings of INO include ipsilateral impairment of adduction often combined with a compensatory jerk nystagmus of the contralateral eye in abduction (Video 22.2; to view the video, please visit http://www.demosmedpub.com/video/?vid=596). Subtle cases of INO may be symptomatic yet easily missed on exam, demonstrating only a delay in adducting saccades in the eye ipsilateral to the MLF lesion. Patients with MS who complain of transient double vision or blurring upon quick lateral gaze may harbor a subtle INO. Asking patients to repeatedly alternate fixation from a target in far left gaze to a target in far right gaze helps to expose the slow adducting saccades of INO.

> Patients with transient double vision or blurring upon quick lateral gaze may have a subtle INO.

In most cases of INO, the eyes are horizontally aligned in primary gaze. Not unusual in MS, bilateral INO may lead to a large exotropia in primary gaze called "wall-eyed" bilateral INO (WEBINO). Another INO variant seen in MS, the "one-and-a-half syndrome," essentially combines an INO from an MLF lesion with a conjugate horizontal gaze palsy from a lesion of the paramedian pontine reticular formation (PPRF) and/or the abducens nucleus. Patients with "one-and-a-half syndrome" have markedly abnormal horizontal eye movements with only intact abduction in the eye contralateral to the pontine lesion. MS patients with INO commonly suffer from concomitant skew deviation causing vertical or diagonal binocular diplopia in primary gaze [11]. Skew deviation results from disruption of vestibular input to the vertical ocular motor nuclei traveling in the MLF. Skew deviation may be either comitant (ocular deviation is the same in all positions of gaze) or incomitant (ocular deviation is different in various positions of gaze).

MS accounts for about 34% of INO cases and is the second most common cause after ischemia. INO due to stroke is more commonly unilateral and is less apt to recover compared to demyelinating INO which recovers completely in about 60% of cases [12]. Proton density imaging (PDI) MRI sequences may be more sensitive than either T2-weighted or fluid-attenuated inversion recovery (FLAIR) sequences for detecting MLF lesions [13].

Nystagmus, or abnormal rhythmic eye movements, occurs in about 30% of MS patients. The underlying pathophysiology is complex but can be simplified to the failure of one or more gaze-stabilizing systems including visual fixation, vestibular function, and gaze-holding mechanisms [14]. Visual fixation provides afferent input to the brain, allowing ocular stabilization. Many forms of nystagmus are exacerbated when fixation is disrupted by visual impairment. Pendular nystagmus, characterized by a back-and-forth slow phase of equal velocity in the absence of a fast corrective phase, can occur in MS and may be dissociated with more prominent nystagmus in the eye with worse acuity. Pendular nystagmus can occur in association with lesions throughout the brain stem or cerebellum affecting neural integrator feedback, although pontine lesions are the most commonly implicated on MRI [15].

Gaze-holding in eccentric gaze relies on normal function of the horizontal gaze and vertical gaze neural integrators. These complex networks in the brain stem and cerebellum permit ocular stability in eccentric gaze despite orbital viscoelastic forces pulling the eyes back toward primary position. Impairment of the neural integrator network causes gaze-evoked nystagmus in up to 26% of MS patients [16]. Gaze-evoked nystagmus is characterized by a jerk nystagmus that beats in the direction of attempted eccentric gaze. Fortunately, this nystagmus does not typically manifest in primary gaze, so it is less debilitating than pendular nystagmus.

Isolated ocular motor cranial nerve palsies occur infrequently in MS patients. Demyelination of either the nuclei or fascicles of CN III, IV, and VI can present with binocular diplopia. MS patients with a new onset isolated CN III, IV, or VI palsy should be considered for other etiologies including compressive lesions, diabetes, hypertension, stroke, and infection. This is particularly true in patients with isolated CN III palsy, which may be a harbinger of impending rupture of a posterior communicating artery aneurysm. Only about 1% of CN III palsies are attributable to MS [17]. Demyelinating CN IV palsies occur even less frequently comprising an estimated 0.06% of all CN IV palsies [18]. MS-associated CN VI palsy is more common than CN III or CN IV palsy and responsible for about 7% of all CN VI palsies [19]; the estimated rate is higher (24%) when considering younger patients (aged 15 to 50) without trauma [20].

> Isolated CN III and IV nerve palsies are rare in MS. Alternative etiologies should be considered carefully before attributing these deficits to MS.

Saccadic dysmetria, a common finding in MS and associated with cerebellar dysfunction, occurs when the eyes undershoot (hypometria) or overshoot (hypermetria) the target of fixation and can result in subjective complaints of difficulty focusing or tracking. Testing for saccades can be performed by asking the patient to alternate fixation repeatedly from a target in left gaze to a target in right gaze; dysmetria is evident when small corrective saccades are necessary to fixate the target after it was missed on initial attempts. Within the cerebellum, the dorsal vermis and caudal fastigial oculomotor region play important roles in making saccades accurate. Other saccadic abnormalities, such as delay and intrusions, also occur in MS patients.

MANAGEMENT: AFFERENT DEMYELINATION

Most cases of DON recover well without treatment. Intravenous (IV) methylprednisolone 250 mg 4 times daily followed by oral prednisone 1 mg/kg a day for 11 days has been shown to expedite visual recovery in DON. In practice, most clinicians use a dose of 1,000 mg a day for 3 days followed by the oral prednisone taper. There is no evidence, however, that corticosteroids change long-term visual outcomes [2]. In most cases, visual improvement in DON begins after 2 to 3 weeks and maximal recovery usually occurs within months. Ten years following DON, the majority of patients have excellent vision with 74% retaining 20/20 vision and 90% retaining 20/40 or even better vision [3]. Failure to abide by this timeline for progression and recovery should raise suspicion for alternative diagnoses including neuromyelitis optica (NMO). NMO presents with unilateral optic neuritis in up to 63% of cases and is often indistinguishable from MS-associated DON [21]. A common theme differentiating NMO and MS relapses, NMO-associated optic neuritis tends to be more severe at onset and less apt to recover compared to MS-associated DON [22]. Only about 43% of NMO-associated optic neuritis cases experience complete recovery. The combination of limited recovery and high recurrence rate leads to a dismal visual prognosis. About 60% to 70% of patients with NMO have severe unilateral vision loss (less than 20/200) in 7 to 11 years [21,23]. A recent study found that about 32% of apparent DON cases with severe vision loss (less than 20/200) at presentation were NMO antibody positive [24]. Treatment for NMO frequently requires immunosuppressive therapy and preliminary evidence suggests that interferon beta may exacerbate NMO, making early distinction important [22]. For these reasons, NMO testing should be considered in all apparent idiopathic DON cases, especially cases with bilateral, recurrent, or severe presentation and in cases with poor visual recovery.

> Serum NMO antibody testing should be considered in all idiopathic DON cases.

While vision usually recovers well, many patients with prior DON complain of persistent "faded" vision. Common permanent findings of prior DON include optic atrophy, OCT nerve fiber layer thinning, diminished contrast sensitivity, visual field defects, color vision deficits, and prolonged latency on visual evoked potential (VEP) testing. In both active and recovered DON, patients may complain of temporary visual blurring related to body temperature elevation. Coined "Uhthoff's phenomenon," visual loss occurs owing to heat-related slowing of impulse conduction in ganglion cell axons. Upon normalization of body temperature, the vision recovers within minutes to hours. Despite patient fears, Uhthoff's phenomenon will not precipitate recurrent DON nor result in additional optic nerve damage.

> Temporary vision loss related to elevated body temperature is called Uhthoff's phenomenon and is a nonspecific feature of DON.

In addition to expediting recovery, the ONTT suggested that sequential IV and oral steroid treatment for acute DON is protective against the development of MS for 2 years (7.5% of treated patients versus 16.7% of untreated controls developed MS) [25]. Accordingly, either IV steroids or observation may be considered in low-risk patients with acute DON and a normal brain MRI depending on the severity of vision loss and the patient's functional needs. In DON patients with characteristic white matter changes of MS on MRI, however, IV steroids should be administered for the potential protective effect. While controversial, oral steroids are avoided by most clinicians for the first episode of DON after the ONTT found that they incur a higher risk of optic neuritis recurrence than no treatment at the 5 year mark [26].

The risk for MS development in patients with isolated DON can be predicted by the presence of characteristic white matter changes on MRI (see Chapter 8). According to the ONTT, the long-term risk of MS in DON patients with a normal brain MRI is 25% while the risk is 72% with an abnormal MRI [4]. While other risk factors for MS development after clinically isolated syndrome have been identified, MRI remains the most utilized predictor (see Chapters 8 and 9). Early recognition of high-risk patients is important considering the proven safety and efficacy of platform MS

medications in preventing the development of MS (see Chapter 11). Patients with DON and characteristic white matter changes should be considered for preventive MS therapy.

While most patients with DON recover well, relapses and incomplete recovery can lead to debilitating, permanent vision loss. Management in these cases focuses on symptom relief and maximizing residual visual function. Low vision specialists assist patients with moderate to severe vision loss and often substantially improve quality of life by offering individualized guidance on vision-enhancing tools such as hand-held magnifiers, telescopes, and glare-reducing glasses.

MANAGEMENT: EFFERENT DEMYELINATION

Acute onset diplopia or nystagmus is debilitating and warrants corticosteroid therapy similar to other MS relapses (see Chapters 11 and 12). The management of permanent efferent sequelae is challenging and symptom dependent.

Medical treatment for nystagmus remains suboptimal. Nevertheless, some patients will enjoy dampening of nystagmus and visual improvement with medication. While numerous medications have been reported to help MS-associated pendular nystagmus, controlled trials suggest that gabapentin and memantine are the most promising [14]. Gabapentin is also reported to be effective in many other nystagmus forms. Other nystagmus forms seen occasionally in MS have been shown to benefit from the following treatments: baclofen for acquired periodic alternating nystagmus; 3,4-diaminopyridine or 4-aminopyridine for downbeat nystagmus; and clonazepam for seesaw nystagmus [14]. Prisms can dampen nystagmus that improves with convergence, although this feature is more typical of infantile nystagmus rather than MS-related nystagmus. While eye muscle surgery has an important role in patients with infantile nystagmus, there is little evidence to support its use in acquired MS-related nystagmus. In the future, an experimental electrooptical device using image stabilization optics to neutralize oscillopsia in pendular nystagmus may become widely available [27].

> Gabapentin and memantine are first-line medications for the treatment of MS-associated pendular nystagmus.

Chronic diplopia is a debilitating MS manifestation. Single binocular vision in primary-gaze and down-gaze is most important for daily function and is the goal of both prism therapy and strabismus surgery. Occasionally, the motility disturbance is complex and patching one eye is the only reasonable solution.

Prisms bend light entering the eye to varying amounts, creating single vision for patients with small angle strabismus. For incomitant strabismus, where the ocular misalignment varies depending on gaze direction, prisms help to create a window of single vision (typically in primary gaze) but may not correct diplopia in all directions. Temporary "stick on" prisms are inexpensive, lightweight, and easy to apply. Owing to mild visual blurring, however, they are poorly tolerated as a long-term solution. Prisms may also be "ground in" to glasses, providing excellent visual clarity, but are considerably more expensive than temporary prisms. Increased visual distortion and weight inherent with higher power prism glasses (more than 10 to 15 prism diopters of total prismatic correction) limit patient satisfaction.

For patients who have chronic large ocular deviations and are dissatisfied with prisms, strabismus surgery may be considered to improve both appearance and binocular function. Similar to prism therapy, strabismus surgery may only achieve a window of single binocular vision in a particular gaze (usually primary gaze). In practice, strabismus surgery is rarely performed in MS patients because of the risk of subsequent events that may produce diplopia again.

SPECIAL CONSIDERATIONS

Retrochiasmatic Demyelination

Demyelination less commonly affects the retrochiasmal visual pathways and is typically asymptomatic. Rarely large plaques can cause visual field defects. As opposed to DON, retrochiasmatic lesions will present with painless homonymous visual field defects (in both eyes), normal visual acuity, and often occur concomitantly with other neurological deficits. Similar to other MS relapses, recovery of visual field loss is expected. Because visually symptomatic retrochiasmal disease is rare, other MS mimics should be considered including neurosarcoidosis, Lyme disease, syphilis, malignant glioma, and PML. A brain infection attributed to the John Cunningham (JC) virus and occurring mostly in the immunocompromised, PML frequently involves the retrogeniculate visual pathway. Homonymous hemianopia was the presenting feature in 35% to 45% of PML cases before the HIV epidemic and decreased to an estimated 17% since [28,29]. PML is associated with natalizumab use with an approximate incidence of 2 in 1,000. The risk of PML in this population increases with the number of natalizumab infusions, previous immunosuppressive medications, and the presence of serum JC virus antibodies (see Chapter 11). While natalizumab-associated PML most commonly presents with cognitive, motor, and language deficits, 1 study showed that visual impairment and hemianopia were presenting features in 8 of 28 (29%) and 5 of 28 (18%), respectively [30]. Given these trends, new onset homonymous field defects in MS patients on recent or active natalizumab therapy should raise immediate concerns for PML.

New onset homonymous field defects in MS patients on natalizumab is highly suspicious for PML.

TABLE 22.3
Referral Guidelines for Vision Problems in MS*

COMPLAINT OR FINDING	APPROPRIATE SPECIALIST	EXPECTED INTERVENTION
Monocular diplopia	General ophthalmologist	Evaluation and treatment for dry eye, cataract, uncorrected astigmatism, and epiretinal membrane
Acute binocular diplopia (if diagnosis unclear)	Neuroophthalmologist	Diagnosis and treatment is case specific
Chronic binocular diplopia with ocular misalignment	Pediatric ophthalmologist or neuroophthalmologist	Alignment measurements for possible prism therapy or rarely strabismus surgery
Acute eye pain, redness, photophobia, and/or new floaters	General ophthalmologist or retinal specialist	Evaluation and treatment for uveitis, posterior vitreous detachment, or retinal detachment
Atypical fundus findings in presumed DON (eg, severe disc edema or macular pathology)	Neuroophthalmologist, general ophthalmologist, or retinal specialist	Careful dilated examination evaluating for intraocular causes of vision loss including maculopathies
Absence of a relative afferent pupillary defect in presumed DON	Neuroophthalmologist, general ophthalmologist, or retinal specialist	Careful dilated examination evaluating for intraocular causes of vision loss including maculopathies
Metamorphopsia	Neuroophthalmologist, general ophthalmologist, or retinal specialist	Careful dilated examination evaluating for intraocular causes of vision loss including maculopathies
Failure of visual recovery in presumed DON (if diagnosis unclear)	Neuroophthalmologist	Evaluation for DON mimics
Any patient with moderate or severe permanent vision loss limiting activities	Low vision specialist	Low vision refraction and patient-tailored education on low-vision aides
Mild insidious blurred vision that improves with pinhole	Optometrist or general ophthalmologist	Refraction and glasses prescription

*These are guidelines. Specialists may vary considerably in scope of practice.

Uveitis in MS

Intraocular inflammation, or uveitis, occurs 10 times more commonly in MS patients than in the general population. There is an estimated incidence of 1% to 2% in the MS population [31,32]. Uveitis may precede or follow the diagnosis of MS. While MS-associated uveitis may affect any segment of the eye, idiopathic intermediate uveitis, or pars planitis, is the most characteristic form [33]. Up to 15% of pars planitis cases are associated with MS, and the 2 share an associated human leukocyte antigen (HLA) type (HLA-DR15). Most MS-associated pars planitis is bilateral and occurs in young (aged 20 to 50) white females. Symptoms of uveitis, in general, include photophobia, eye pain, blurred vision, and conjunctival injection, or redness. Pars planitis, in contrast, tends to present with a slow, painless increase in floaters and blurred vision. Complications of pars planitis include retinal neovascularization, cystoid ME, epiretinal membrane, cataracts, and retinal detachment. Topical, local, and oral steroids are the mainstay of therapy and allow most patients to retain good vision.

> Photophobia, new floaters, and eye irritation are characteristic symptoms of uveitis.

KEY POINTS FOR PATIENTS AND FAMILIES

- Eye symptoms in MS include loss of vision in 1 eye (optic neuritis), double vision, a rare red eye due to inflammation of the eye (uveitis), and other visual symptoms.

- Optic neuritis is often treated by a course of high-dose steroids. While this does not affect the long-term outcome, it does speed recovery of visual function.

- Double vision and nystagmus (eye "jumpiness") usually resolves over time but when chronic, it may improve by placing prisms in the glasses or with certain medications.

- Careful ophthalmological screening and follow-up is important for patients using fingolimod (Gilenya) for MS to avoid possible visual changes due to a condition known as macular edema.

REFERENCES

1. The clinical profile of optic neuritis. Experience of the Optic Neuritis Treatment Trial. Optic Neuritis Study Group. *Arch Ophthalmol.* 1991;109(12):1673–1678.

2. Beck RW, Cleary PA. Optic neuritis treatment trial. One-year follow-up results. *Arch Ophthalmol.* 1993;111(6):773–775.

3. Beck RW, Trobe JD, Moke PS, et al. High- and low-risk profiles for the development of multiple sclerosis within 10 years after optic neuritis: Experience of the optic neuritis treatment trial. *Arch Ophthalmol.* 2003;121(7):944–949.

4. Optic Neuritis Study Group. Multiple sclerosis risk after optic neuritis: Final optic neuritis treatment trial follow-up. *Arch Neurol.* 2008;65(6):727–732.

5. Rizzo JF 3rd, Andreoli CM, Rabinov JD. Use of magnetic resonance imaging to differentiate optic neuritis and nonarteritic anterior ischemic optic neuropathy. *Ophthalmology.* 2002;109(9):1679–1684.

6. Purvin V, Kawasaki A, Jacobson DM. Optic perineuritis: Clinical and radiographic features. *Arch Ophthalmol.* 2001;119(9):1299–1306.

7. Jain N, Bhatti MT. Fingolimod-associated macular edema: Incidence, detection, and management. *Neurology.* 2012;78(9):672–680.

8. Ross A, Ross AH, Mohamed Q. Review and update of central serous chorioretinopathy. *Curr Opin Ophthalmol.* 2011;22(3):166–173.

9. Bouzas EA, Karadimas P, Pournaras CJ. Central serous chorioretinopathy and glucocorticoids. *Surv Ophthalmol.* 2002;47(5):431–448.

10. Muri RM, Meienberg O. The clinical spectrum of internuclear ophthalmoplegia in multiple sclerosis. *Arch Neurol.* 1985;42(9):851–855.

11. Liu GT, Volpe NJ, Galetta S. *Neuro-ophthalmology: Diagnosis and Management*, 2nd ed. Philadelphia: Elsevier; 2010: xiv, 706.

12. Keane JR. Internuclear ophthalmoplegia: Unusual causes in 114 of 410 patients. *Arch Neurol.* 2005;62(5):714–717.

13. Frohman EM, Frohman TC, O'Suilleabhain P, et al. Quantitative oculographic characterisation of internuclear ophthalmoparesis in multiple sclerosis: The versional dysconjugacy index Z score. *J Neurol Neurosurg Psychiatry.* 2002;73(1):51–55.

14. Thurtell MJ, Leigh RJ. Therapy for nystagmus. *J Neuroophthalmol.* 2010;30(4):361–371.

15. Lopez LI, Bronstein AM, Gresty MA, et al. Clinical and MRI correlates in 27 patients with acquired pendular nystagmus. *Brain.* 1996;119(Pt 2):465–472.

16. Serra A, Derwenskus J, Downey DL, Leigh RJ. Role of eye movement examination and subjective visual vertical in clinical evaluation of multiple sclerosis. *J Neurol.* 2003;250(5):569–575.

17. Keane JR. Third nerve palsy: Analysis of 1400 personally-examined inpatients. *Can J Neurol Sci.* 2010;37(5):662–670.

18. Thomke F, Lensch E, Ringel K, Hopf HC. Isolated cranial nerve palsies in multiple sclerosis. *J Neurol Neurosurg Psychiatry.* 1997;63(5):682–685.

19. Patel SV, Mutyala S, Leske DA, et al. Incidence, associations, and evaluation of sixth nerve palsy using a population-based method. *Ophthalmology.* 2004;111(2):369–375.

20. Peters GB 3rd, Bakri SJ, Krohel GB. Cause and prognosis of nontraumatic sixth nerve palsies in young adults. *Ophthalmology.* 2002;109(10):1925–1928.

21. Merle H, Olindo S, Bonnan M, et al. Natural history of the visual impairment of relapsing neuromyelitis optica. *Ophthalmology.* 2007;114(4):810–815.

22. Morrow MJ, Wingerchuk D. Neuromyelitis optica. *J Neuroophthalmol.* 2012;32(2):154–166.

23. Wingerchuk DM, Hogancamp WF, O'Brien PC, Weinshenker BG. The clinical course of neuromyelitis optica (Devic's syndrome). *Neurology.* 1999;53(5):1107–1114.

24. Lai C, Tian G, Takahashi T, et al. Neuromyelitis optica antibodies in patients with severe optic neuritis in China. *J Neuroophthalmol.* 2011;31(1):16–19.

25. Beck RW, Cleary PA, Trobe JD, et al. The effect of corticosteroids for acute optic neuritis on the subsequent development of multiple sclerosis. The Optic Neuritis Study Group. *N Engl J Med.* 1993;329(24):1764–1769.

26. The 5-year risk of MS after optic neuritis. Experience of the optic neuritis treatment trial. Optic Neuritis Study Group. *Neurology.* 1997;49(5):1404–1413.

27. Smith RM, Oommen BS, Stahl JS. Application of adaptive filters to visual testing and treatment in acquired pendular nystagmus. *J Rehabil Res Dev.* 2004;41(3A):313–324.

28. Brooks BR, Walker DL. Progressive multifocal leukoencephalopathy. *Neurol Clin.* 1984;2(2):299–313.

29. Berger JR, Pall L, Lanska D, Whiteman M. Progressive multifocal leukoencephalopathy in patients with HIV infection. *J Neurovirol.* 1998;4(1):59–68.

30. Clifford DB, De Luca A, Simpson DM, et al. Natalizumab-associated progressive multifocal leukoencephalopathy in patients with multiple sclerosis: Lessons from 28 cases. *Lancet Neurol.* 2010;9(4):438–446.

31. Chen L, Gordon LK. Ocular manifestations of multiple sclerosis. *Curr Opin Ophthalmol.* 2005;16(5):315–320.

32. Edwards LJ, Constantinescu CS. A prospective study of conditions associated with multiple sclerosis in a cohort of 658 consecutive outpatients attending a multiple sclerosis clinic. *Mult Scler.* 2004;10(5):575–581.

33. Zein G, Berta A, Foster CS. Multiple sclerosis-associated uveitis. *Ocul Immunol Inflamm.* 2004;12(2):137–142.

23

Bulbar and Pseudobulbar Dysfunction in Multiple Sclerosis

DEVON S. CONWAY

KEY POINTS FOR CLINICIANS

- Corticobulbar and pseudobulbar pathology can be seen in multiple sclerosis (MS) and often go unrecognized.

- Neurogenic dysphagia can put patients at risk for aspiration pneumonia or other life-threatening complications.

- Noninvasive techniques are available for dysphagia management, but physicians may also want to consider surgical myotomy of the cricopharyngeal muscle, or chemical myotomy with botulinum toxin.

- Selective serotonin reuptake inhibitors, amitriptyline, and levodopa have all shown promise in treating pseudobulbar affect (PBA) in MS patients, but the data is limited.

- Dextromorphan/Quinidine was shown to be an effective treatment for PBA in MS in a large, randomized, placebo-controlled trial.

The corticobulbar tracts originate in the motor cortex and innervate the motor nuclei of cranial nerves V, VII, IX, X, XI, and XII. Corticobulbar dysfunction can occur in a variety of neurological conditions, including amyotrophic lateral sclerosis, stroke, and multiple sclerosis (MS). Common symptoms of corticobulbar dysfunction in neurological disease are listed in Table 23.1.

Pseudobulbar affect (PBA) refers to pathological displays of emotion and can affect the MS patient. Other names commonly used to refer to PBA include pathological laughter and crying, emotional lability, and emotional incontinence. Although the exact anatomic etiology of PBA is unknown, a recent MRI study found patients with PBA were more likely to have lesions affecting the brain stem, bilateral medial inferior frontal regions, and the bilateral inferior parietal regions [1]. It is thought that such lesions may result in impaired inhibition of emotional display, thereby resulting in the characteristic features of PBA.

Corticobulbar and pseudobulbar dysfunction often go unrecognized in MS patients. It is important to remain mindful of these complications, as there are a number of possible interventions that may improve quality of life.

DYSPHAGIA

Swallowing is a complex motor task that involves moving food from the oral cavity to the stomach while simultaneously providing airway protection from aspiration. It is typically described as comprising 4 phases based on the location of the bolus: oral preparatory, oral, pharyngeal, and esophageal. Neurogenic dysphagia can occur in MS

TABLE 23.1
Corticobulbar Symptoms in Neurological Disease

- Dysphagia
- Dysarthria
- Laryngospasm
- Weakness of the facial muscles and tongue

and can result in a number of complicating factors such as weight loss and decreased quality of life. Of special concern in MS patients with dysphagia is the risk of aspiration pneumonia. In 1 study, 62% of patients dying from a known complication of MS died from pneumonia [2].

> Neurogenic dysphagia can cause life-threatening complications.

A number of brain structures are involved in the process of chewing and swallowing. These include the sensorimotor and premotor cortex, which project through the corticobulbar tracts to the nuclei of the trigeminal, facial, glossopharyngeal, vagal, and hypoglossal cranial nerves [3]. The nucleus tractus solitarius and the nucleus ambiguus are the most important portions of the brain stem in the facilitation of normal swallowing. Proper swallowing depends on the interaction of sensory and motor functions as well as the interaction of voluntary and involuntary aspects of the process [4].

A number of groups have attempted to quantify the prevalence of dysphagia in MS patients. An early study of 525 patients (Expanded Disability Status Scale [EDSS] scores from 0 to 9.5) found that 43% had neurogenic dysphagia [5]. A later study of 143 MS patients by Calcagno et al. found dysphagia in 49 of them (34.3%) [6]. Interestingly, severe brain stem involvement from MS was associated with increased risk of dysphagia (OR = 3.24, CI = 1.44–7.31). Also, those with an EDSS score above 6.5 had increased risk of dysphagia compared to less affected patients (OR = 2.99, CI = 1.36–6.59). In the 46 patients with mild or moderate dysphagia, compensatory strategies such as postural changes and modifying the volume quantity and the speed of food presentation were sufficient to avoid aspiration.

> Brain stem involvement and greater disability levels are associated with dysphagia.

Thomas and Wiles surveyed 79 MS patients admitted to the hospital (24 at the diagnostic admission and 55 with established disease) [7]. A standardized water swallowing test was administered and 43% of the MS patients were found to have abnormal swallowing. This constituted 29% of the newly diagnosed patients and 49% of those with

established MS. While certain survey questions strongly predicted the presence of dysphagia (eg, "episodes of coughing after eating or drinking" or "food going down the wrong way"), there were a number of false negative responses as well, suggesting that some patients might be unaware of their swallowing dysfunction.

A more recent study enrolled 308 consecutive patients with relapsing-remitting (RR), secondary progressive (SP), and primary progressive (PP) MS [8]. Participants were only considered dysphagic if they had permanent dysphagia, meaning dysphagia outside of an acute relapse. Permanent dysphagia was detected in 73 (24%) patients. Again, patients with greater disability were more likely to have dysphagia. It was present in 35.4% of those with an EDSS of 8.0 and 95% of those with an EDSS of 9.0. However, permanent dysphagia was observed in patients with an EDSS as low as 2.0.

> Dysphagia prevalence in MS has been estimated between 24% and 43%.

Poorjavad et al. attempted to determine the prevalence of different types of swallowing disorders in MS patients [9]. Participants were screened with the Northwestern Dysphagia Patient Check Sheet, which can be used to differentiate between pharyngeal or oral stage disorders and can detect aspiration and pharyngeal delay [10]. In their cohort of 101 consecutive MS patients, 32 (31.7%) were found to have dysphagia. Pharyngeal stage disorders were found in 28.7% of the cohort, aspiration in 6.9%, oral stage disorders in 5%, and pharyngeal delay in 1%. Dysphagia was significantly more prevalent in patients with a longer disease duration, more cerebellar dysfunction, and in those with higher EDSS scores.

Potential interventions for patients with dysphagia are summarized in Table 23.2. A number of noninvasive techniques are available that may be of use in MS patients with dysphagia. For instance, repetitive exercises that focus on important aspects of swallowing such as mastication, cheek tonization, and movements of the tongue and larynx may be helpful with regard to restitution of the swallowing function [11]. Postural changes and swallowing techniques are also available that facilitate swallowing and protection of the airway. For instance, holding the breath

TABLE 23.2
Management Options for Dysphagia in MS

- Repetitive exercises focusing on important aspects of swallowing
- Postural changes
- Swallowing techniques that facilitate airway protection
- Diet modification
- Cricopharyngeal muscle myotomy
- Chemical myotomy of the cricopharyngeal muscle with botulinum toxin

while swallowing and exhaling strongly immediately afterward helps to close the vocal cords and prevent aspiration. Finally, modification of the diet may also be useful. For instance, soft textured foods can be used in patients with difficulty in the oral preparation phase of swallowing. Also, use of cooled drinks or thickened liquids may be helpful in those who have choking with thin liquids [11].

> Speech therapists can teach noninvasive techniques that may improve neurogenic dysphagia.

More invasive options are also available. As indicated, the most prevalent cause of dysphagia in MS patients is incomplete relaxation or defective opening of the upper esophageal sphincter. This can lead to hypopharyngeal retention of the food bolus, putting the patient at risk for aspiration [4]. Myotomy of the cricopharyngeal muscle of the upper esophageal sphincter has been described as an effective method of management in patients with neurogenic dysphagia from causes other than MS [12].

A less invasive approach to upper esophageal sphincter dysfunction is chemical myotomy of the cricopharyngeal muscle with botulinum toxin (BTX). One study identified 25 MS patients with dysphagia [13]. Video fluoroscopy was performed and demonstrated that 14 of them had signs of upper esophageal sphincter hyperactivity, such as reduced pharyngeal clearance and incomplete cricopharyngeal opening. Following BTX injection, patients were reassessed using video fluoroscopy and other tools. Dysphagia completely resolved in 10 of the patients and significantly improved in the remaining 4. Injections were repeated every 3 to 4 months with sustained benefit. Work has also been done suggesting that EMG can predict which patients with neurogenic dysphagia are most likely to respond to cricopharyngeal muscle BTX injections [4].

DYSARTHRIA

Dysarthria is dysfunction in the initiation, control, or coordination of speech. Its prevalence in MS has not been well studied. Shibasaki et al. characterized the initial neurological symptoms of 204 British and 60 Japanese patients with probable MS at the time of presentation [14]. In this series, 3% of the patients presented with a speech disturbance.

A later study was conducted with 77 MS patients including a mix of PPMS, SPMS, and RRMS [15]. EDSS scores varied between 1.0 and 9.0. Participants underwent the clinical dysarthria test procedure, which assesses respiration, phonation, oral motor performance, articulation, prosody, and intelligibility [16]. The study found that no patients had profound dysarthria, 8% had moderate to severe dysarthria, 37% had mild or moderate dysarthria, and 55% had none or minimal speech deviation. After correcting for dropouts, the true prevalence of dysarthria in MS patients was estimated to be 51%.

Unfortunately, there is scarce evidence about the value of interventions for dysarthria in MS. However, as with other neurological diseases that can cause dysarthria, expert opinion favors early speech and language therapy [17].

> Dysarthria may have a prevalence as high as 51% in MS.

Patients with MS are also at risk for developing paroxysmal dysarthria [18]. Paroxysmal dysarthria typically lasts for a few seconds, and can occur frequently throughout the day. It is often accompanied by episodic ataxia, in which case it is referred to as paroxysmal dysarthria and ataxia (PDA). Most case reports of these conditions have described a midbrain lesion, which is the presumed etiology [18,19].

Paroxysmal events in MS are poorly understood but are thought to be secondary to ephaptic spread affecting the damaged neurons. Given this, membrane stabilizers such as carbamazepine have been used to treat PDA. One case series of 3 patients with paroxysmal dysarthria or PDA showed resolution of attacks after administration of carbamazepine 200 to 400 mg daily [18]. Another case series with 2 patients found a similar benefit for carbamazepine [19]. However, in both case series, the resolution occurred on the order of weeks to months and may simply reflect repair of the causative lesion.

> MS patients may develop paroxysmal dysarthria and ataxia, which may respond to carbamazepine or lamotrigine.

Finally, a similar case of a 36-year-old woman with a 14 year history of MS has been reported [20]. The patient developed paroxysmal dysarthria that became more frequent despite treatment with methylprednisolone. After treatment with carbamazepine 600 mg per day for 10 days led to no improvement, the patient was converted to lamotrigine 100 mg per day. Lamotrigine led to substantial reduction in her paroxysmal events and nearly complete resolution in 2 weeks.

PSEUDOBULBAR AFFECT

PBA is characterized by involuntary and inappropriate outbursts of emotional expression that do not properly align with the patient's emotional state. It is observed in a number of neurological conditions including stroke, amyotrophic lateral sclerosis (ALS), traumatic brain injury, and MS [21]. The pathophysiology of PBA is incompletely understood. According to 1 prominent theory, dysfunction in a corticopontinecerebellar circuit is the cause of PBA symptoms [22]. Via this circuit, emotional expression is controlled by the cerebellum, which appropriately modulates the level of emotional response according to the situation. Disruption of the corticopontinecerebellar connections lowers the threshold for emotional response, and can predispose the individual to inappropriate outbursts [23].

Few studies have investigated the prevalence of PBA in MS. Further, comparison between studies can be confounded by inconsistent definitions of what constitutes PBA. The most commonly cited investigation enrolled 152 consecutive outpatients that were screened by 2 neurologists for the presence of pathological laughter and crying (PLC) [24]. To receive this diagnosis, patients had to display a sudden loss of emotional control on multiple occasions in response to nonspecific stimuli and without a matching mood state. Fifteen of the subjects had PLC, a point prevalence of 9.9%. The patients with PLC were more likely to be in the progressive phase of MS and to have more physical disability (mean EDSS 6.0 vs. 4.7, $P = .03$). Also, patients with PLC were not more likely than controls to have a premorbid or a family history of mental illness.

> PBA is believed to have a prevalence of about 10% in MS patients.

A number of treatments have been proposed for PBA in patients with neurological disease, including selective serotonin reuptake inhibitors (SSRIs). One case series followed 10 patients: 4 with ALS, 4 with MS, and 2 with stroke [25]. All included patients had more than 30 affective outbursts daily prior to study entry. The patients were treated with 100 mg of the SSRI fluvoxamine daily. Within 2 to 6 days, all patients' affective outbursts had decreased to 5 or less per day.

Levodopa has also been considered for the treatment of PLC in neurological disease. One study enrolled 25 patients with pathological crying, pathological laughing, or both [26]. The cause was cerebrovascular disease in 23 patients and brain trauma in the remaining 2. In 10 of the 25 patients treated with levodopa, there was complete resolution of PLC. All but 4 of the remaining patients had a partial response to the levodopa.

Finally, amitriptyline has been compared to placebo in a double-blind crossover trial. Seventeen MS patients with PLC were enrolled but only 12 completed the study [27]. Patients were randomly assigned to receive 30 days of placebo or amitriptyline at a goal dose of 75 mg. This was followed by a 1 week washout period and then 30 days of the alternative option. A spouse or close family member kept a daily count of the number of episodes of inappropriate emotional outbursts. In 8 patients the number of episodes of pathological laughter or crying was reduced to 0 while on active treatment, while 4 patients had more episodes on drug than off.

> Case series have shown efficacy of SSRIs, levodopa, and amitriptyline in treating MS-associated PBA.

While these and similar studies provide promising preliminary results for the treatment of PBA/PLC in neurological disease, they suffer from a number of methodological problems. Most studies have had a limited sample size that includes patients with neurological diseases other than MS. Also, for the most part, the studies were not randomized placebo-controlled trials and instead involved a pre–post analysis. Hence, the results may not be specific to MS and the studies are prone to bias.

The largest randomized controlled trial of a PBA treatment in an exclusively MS population involved dextromethorphan/quinidine (DMQ) [28]. A prior study of DMQ showed it to be effective in a combined sample of 326 MS and ALS patients [21]. Dextromethorphan is a sigma-1 receptor agonist as well as a noncompetitive antagonist of the N-methyl-D-aspartate receptor [28]. Through its activity, glutamate influence is attenuated. Dextromethorphan is rapidly metabolized to dextrorphan by cytochrome P450 2D6. Quinidine is a cytochrome P450 2D6 inhibitor, and is included to allow for steady concentrations of dextromethorphan.

The inclusion criteria included a diagnosis of MS and a clinical diagnosis of PBA. Participants were also required to have a score of 13 or more on the Center for Neurologic Study—Lability Scale (CNS-LS). This scale provides a score for PBA ranging from 7 to 35 and has been validated in MS [29].

A total of 150 participants were enrolled and were randomized 1:1 to either dextromethorphan/quinidine or placebo. The primary efficacy variable was mean reduction in the CNS-LS score, which was assessed 4 times between 15 and 85 days from treatment initiation. The mean reduction was 7.7 points for the active treatment group and 3.3 points for the placebo group ($P < .0001$). Secondary outcomes included quality of life, quality of relationships, and pain intensity, all assessed using visual analog scales. There was significant benefit in all 3 of these outcomes for the active treatment group versus placebo.

> Dextromethorphan/quinidine was shown to be an effective treatment for PBA in MS in a large, randomized, placebo-controlled trial.

A summary of treatment options for PBA in MS is provided in Table 23.3, along with the level of evidence supporting each medication.

TABLE 23.3
Treatment Options and Evidence Level for PBA in MS

MEDICATION	GOAL DOSE	EVIDENCE LEVEL
Fluvoxamine	100 mg daily	Level 3
Levodopa	0.6 to 1.5 grams daily	Level 3
Amitriptyline	75 mg daily	Level 3
Dextromethorphan/ Quinidine	30 mg/30 mg twice daily*	Level 1

*The commercially available formulation, Nuedexta, contains dextromethorphan 20 mg and quinidine 10 mg and is dosed twice daily.

PATIENT CASE

A 24-year-old woman with no significant medical history comes to the clinic complaining of 1 week of transient episodes of slurred speech. She has never had a neurological episode previously.

Question: What evaluation is needed?

Answer: The case is concerning for transient ischemic attack. An MRI/MRA of the brain would be recommended both to rule out stroke and evaluate for any flow limiting stenoses. Given the patient's age, the MRI would also be helpful in evaluating for demyelinating disease and it would be reasonable to administer gadolinium.

Question: The MRI is negative for stroke and the MRA is normal. However, the MRI does show a mild to moderate lesion burden of ovoid periventricular lesions and juxtacortical lesions. There is an enhancing midbrain lesion near the right red nucleus. What should the next step be?

Answer: The patient appears to have MS and is likely experiencing paroxysmal dysarthria as a result of her midbrain lesion. Given the active enhancement, a course of IV methylprednisolone, 1,000 mg daily for 3 to 5 days followed by a prednisone taper would be reasonable.

Question: After treatment with corticosteroids, the patient continues to experience paroxysmal dysarthria. What management options are available?

Answer: Treatment with carbamazepine or lamotrigine may help to resolve the episodes.

REFERENCES

1. Ghaffar O, Chamelian L, Feinstein A. Neuroanatomy of pseudobulbar affect: A quantitative MRI study in multiple sclerosis. *J Neurol.* 2008;255(3):406–412.

2. Sadovnick AD, Eisen K, Ebers GC, Paty DW. Cause of death in patients attending multiple sclerosis clinics. *Neurology.* 1991;41(8):1193–1196.

3. Tassorelli C, Bergamaschi R, Buscone S, et al. Dysphagia in multiple sclerosis: From pathogenesis to diagnosis. *Neurol Sci.* 2008;29(Suppl 4):S360–S363.

4. Alfonsi E, Merlo IM, Ponzio M, et al. An electrophysiological approach to the diagnosis of neurogenic dysphagia: Implications for botulinum toxin treatment. *J Neurol Neurosurg Psychiatry.* 2010;81(1):54–60.

5. Abraham S, Scheinberg LC, Smith CR, LaRocca NG. Neurologic impairment and disability status in outpatients with multiple sclerosis reporting dysphagia symptomatology. *J Neuro Rehab.* 1997;11:7–13.

6. Calcagno P, Ruoppolo G, Grasso MG, et al. Dysphagia in multiple sclerosis—prevalence and prognostic factors. *Acta Neurol Scand.* 2002;105(1):40–43.

7. Thomas FJ, Wiles CM. Dysphagia and nutritional status in multiple sclerosis. *J Neurol.* 1999;246(8):677–682.

8. De Pauw A, Dejaeger E, D'Hooghe B, Carton H. Dysphagia in multiple sclerosis. *Clin Neurol Neurosurg.* 2002;104(4):345–351.

9. Poorjavad M, Derakhshandeh F, Etemadifar M, et al. Oropharyngeal dysphagia in multiple sclerosis. *Mult Scler.* 2010;16(3):362–365.

10. Logemann JA, Veis S, Colangelo L. A screening procedure for oropharyngeal dysphagia. *Dysphagia.* 1999;14(1):44–51.

11. Prosiegel M, Schelling A, Wagner-Sonntag E. Dysphagia and multiple sclerosis. *Int MS J.* 2004;11(1):22–31.

12. Duranceau A. Cricopharyngeal myotomy in the management of neurogenic and muscular dysphagia. *Neuromuscul Disord.* 1997;7(Suppl 1):S85–S89.

13. Restivo DA, Marchese-Ragona R, Patti F, et al. Botulinum toxin improves dysphagia associated with multiple sclerosis. *Eur J Neurol.* 2010;18(3):486–490.

14. Shibasaki H, McDonald WI, Kuroiwa Y. Racial modification of clinical picture of multiple sclerosis: Comparison between British and Japanese patients. *J Neurol Sci.* 1981;49(2):253–271.

15. Hartelius L, Runmarker B, Andersen O. Prevalence and characteristics of dysarthria in a multiple-sclerosis incidence cohort: Relation to neurological data. *Folia Phoniatr Logop.* 2000;52(4):160–177.

16. Hartelius L, Svensson P. *Dysarthria Test.* Stockholm: Psykologiforlaget; 1990.

17. Langhorne P, Bernhardt J, Kwakkel G. Stroke rehabilitation. *Lancet.* 2011;377(9778):1693–1702.

18. Blanco Y, Compta Y, Graus F, Saiz A. Midbrain lesions and paroxysmal dysarthria in multiple sclerosis. *Mult Scler.* 2008;14(5):694–697.

19. Li Y, Zeng C, Luo T. Paroxysmal dysarthria and ataxia in multiple sclerosis and corresponding magnetic resonance imaging findings. *J Neurol.* 2010;258(2):273–276.

20. Valentino P, Nistico R, Pirritano D, et al. Lamotrigine therapy for paroxysmal dysarthria caused by multiple sclerosis: A case report. *J Neurol.* 2011;258(7):1349–1350.

21. Pioro EP, Brooks BR, Cummings J, et al. Dextromethorphan plus ultra low-dose quinidine reduces pseudobulbar affect. *Ann Neurol.* 2010;68(5):693–702.

22. Parvizi J, Coburn KL, Shillcutt SD, et al. Neuroanatomy of pathological laughing and crying: A report of the American Neuropsychiatric Association Committee on Research. *J Neuropsychiatry Clin Neurosci.* 2009;21(1):75–87.

23. Miller A, Pratt H, Schiffer RB. Pseudobulbar affect: The spectrum of clinical presentations, etiologies and treatments. *Expert Rev Neurother.* 2011;11(7):1077–1088.

24. Feinstein A, Feinstein K, Gray T, O'Connor P. Prevalence and neurobehavioral correlates of pathological laughing and crying in multiple sclerosis. *Arch Neurol.* 1997;54(9):1116–1121.

25. Iannaccone S, Ferini-Strambi L. Pharmacologic treatment of emotional lability. *Clin Neuropharmacol.* 1996;19(6):532–535.

26. Udaka F, Yamao S, Nagata H, et al. Pathologic laughing and crying treated with levodopa. *Arch Neurol.* 1984;41(10):1095–1096.

27. Schiffer RB, Herndon RM, Rudick RA. Treatment of pathologic laughing and weeping with amitriptyline. *N Engl J Med.* 1985;312(23):1480–1482.

28. Panitch HS, Thisted RA, Smith RA, et al. Randomized, controlled trial of dextromethorphan/quinidine for pseudobulbar affect in multiple sclerosis. *Ann Neurol.* 2006;59(5):780–787.

29. Smith RA, Berg JE, Pope LE, et al. Validation of the CNS emotional lability scale for pseudobulbar affect (pathological laughing and crying) in multiple sclerosis patients. *Mult Scler.* 2004;10(6):679–685.

24

Pain Management in Multiple Sclerosis

JOHN F. FOLEY
KARA MENNING
CORTNEE ROMAN

KEY POINTS FOR THE CLINICIAN

- Pain is a common symptom in multiple sclerosis (MS).

- Pain may occur with primary demyelination as well as indirect musculoskeletal compromise.

- Acute MS relapses may produce pain (eg, optic neuritis, dysesthesia, or Lhermitte's sign).

- Central neuropathic pain (CNP) occurs in up to 28% of MS patients, and most commonly involves the lower extremities.

- CNP is often associated with spinal cord plaque and is most often amenable to treatment similar to that used to treat peripheral neuropathic pain.

- Trigeminal neuralgia is related to demyelination in the trigeminal nerve root entry zone, and is amenable to medical and surgical interventions.

PREVALENCE AND IMPACT OF PAIN IN MULTIPLE SCLEROSIS

Once thought to be an uncommon symptom in multiple sclerosis (MS), we now know that pain is frequently reported by patients living with this disease. Pain may occur as a result of an acute relapse, or on a chronic daily basis as a result of long-standing neurological insult. It may represent the central presenting symptom of MS, or it may develop much later in the disease course. The estimated prevalence of pain in MS patients reported in the literature is as high as 86% [1–3]. It has been reported that almost one-half of MS patients report chronic pain, with some studies showing that its occurrence increases with age and disease duration [4]. One study found pain to be present twice as often in women with relapsing-remitting MS (RRMS) compared to healthy women, with pain intensity over 7 days twice as high [5]. In a large multicenter cross-sectional Italian study, the authors interviewed 1,672 patients and found that pain was present in 43% of them, categorized as follows: back pain 16%, dysesthetic pain 18%, painful spasm 11%, trigeminal neuralgia (TN) 2%, visceral pain 3%, Lhermitte's sign 9% [3]. This is reflected in clinical practice, as well, with many office visits centering on evaluating and treating a patient's pain.

There is no doubt that pain adversely affects quality of life. For many MS patients, pain is often widespread, chronic, severe, and frequently interferes with sleep, occupational performance, and recreation [1,4]. There also appears to be a connection between higher pain levels and worsened fatigue and depression [5]. Pain also creates an economic burden resulting from direct medical expenses and productivity loss. One year's financial expenditure for patients with neuropathic pain is up to 3 times higher than those without pain, with far more frequent office visits per year [6].

MECHANISMS OF PAIN IN MS AND CLINICAL PRESENTATIONS

Multiple potential pain generators exist with MS. Pain can occur as a primary result of demyelination along the neuraxis, and is often mediated by dorsal root neurons radiating via the spinothalamic tract to the thalamus. Projections from the thalamus include the medial system with radiations to the locus coeruleus, periaquaductal gray matter, thalamic nuclei, insula, secondary somatosensory cortex hippocampus, amygdala, and hypothalamus [7]. This system processes the emotional and cognitive aspects of pain. The lateral system processes the sensory discriminative elements of the signal and flows through the lateral thalamus, somatosensory cortex, parietal operculum, and insula [7].

Abnormal amplification of normal axon nociception responders can produce pain. MS plaque may interrupt descending inhibitory pain fibers [8]. The immune process may also directly produce a central pain response [9,10]. Generation of pain produced by activation of non pain sensory receptors is called *allodynia*. Exaggeration of painful stimuli is known as *hyperalgesia*. This central sensitization phenomenon is poorly understood. Secondary pain syndromes can be related to asymmetric load carrying or hypertonicity-producing musculoskeletal or nociception pain with activation of peripheral pain receptors. Headache seems to also occur with increased frequency in MS. Recognition of pain type by the clinician is important for appropriate intervention, keeping in mind that different pain types often coexist in the same patient. Specific pain syndromes are listed in Table 24.1.

TABLE 24.1
Pain Syndromes Associated With Multiple Sclerosis

PAIN SYNDROME	CHARACTERISTICS
Central neuropathic pain	Associated with relapse
Dysesthetic extremity pain	Generally chronic
Trigeminal/Glossopharyngeal/ Occipital neuralgia	Generally paroxysmal
Lhermitte's phenomenon	Paroxysmal
Pseudoradicular pain	Chronic or paroxysmal
Musculoskeletal	Chronic
Visceral pain	Chronic or paroxysmal
Headache	Chronic or paroxysmal
Optic neuritis pain*	Associated with relapse
Painful tonic spasm*	Generally paroxysmal

*Discussed in other chapters.

ASSESSMENT OF PAIN IN MS

The management of MS-related pain can be a challenge, and often requires patient-specific tailoring, trial and error, and frequent reassessment. When assessing pain severity in patients, quantification is helpful, even if the responses obtained are ultimately subjective. A number of pain scales exist to help with the quantification of a patient's pain perception and consequences of pain, such as the pain Visual Analogue Scale (VAS), the Brief Pain Inventory, the McGill Pain Assessment Questionnaire [11], the Medical Outcomes 36-Item Short-Form Health Survey (SF-36), and the Hospital Anxiety and Depression Scale (HADS) [12]. The Pain Effects Scale (PES) is a 6-item self-report questionnaire that can be completed by the patient within a few minutes (see Figure 24.1). Patients with upper extremity or visual impairments can have the PES administered as an interview. This scale provides insight into the way pain interferes with mood, mobility, sleep, activities of daily living, and quality of life and can be readministered over time [13].

CENTRAL NEUROPATHIC PAIN

The prevalence of central neuropathic pain (CNP) in the MS population may be as high as 28% [14]. In a study of 429 patients, CNP localized to the lower extremities in 87%, the upper extremities in 31%, with at least some bilateral involvement in 76%, occurring daily in 88%, but rarely (2%) was paroxysmal [14]. Dysesthesias are described as a constant, burning discomfort which can be symmetric or asymmetric, usually affecting the lower limbs, and can also present as increased sensitivity to touch. Paresthesias are most often described as a "pins and needles" sensation, but can also present as aching, throbbing, stabbing, shooting, tightness, or numbness [12,15]. Dysesthesias and paresthesias are most commonly felt in the limbs, but may also occur elsewhere.

CNP management requires frequent assessments, managing expectations, and finding a regimen that is effective without causing too many treatment-related debilitating side effects. Nonpharmacological interventions may also be beneficial. Physical therapy, regular exercise, relaxation, stretching, massage therapy, hypnotherapy, and psychological intervention should be introduced where felt appropriate. Two reviews of neuropathic pain comprehensively evaluate the evidence-based data available [11,16]. Class 1 clinical trials for pharmacological intervention on CNP in MS do not exist. Most therapeutic agents utilized for treatment of CNP have been coopted from the peripheral pain trials, or from studies in other central nervous system conditions. Dysesthesias and paresthesias can usually be treated with antiepileptics or tricyclic antidepressants. Sometimes, combinations of medications with different mechanisms of action are needed to adequately control pain symptoms without causing side effects such as sedation [11]. Figure 24. 2 describes the treatment algorithm utilized by our clinic.

INSTRUCTIONS

Individuals with MS can sometimes experience unpleasant sensory symptoms as a result of their MS (eg, pain, tingling, burning). The next set of questions covers pain and other unpleasant sensations, and how they affect you. Please circle the one number (0, 1, 2, ...) that best indicates the extent to which your sensory symptoms (including pain) interfered with that aspect of your life during the past 4 weeks. If you need help in marking your responses, tell the interviewer the number of the best response (or what to fill in). Please answer every question. If you are not sure which answer to select, please choose the one answer that comes closest to describing you. The interviewer can explain any words or phrases that you do not understand.

During the past 4 weeks,
how much did these symptoms
interfere with your...

		Not at all	A little	Moderately	Quite a bit	To an extreme degree
1.	mood	1	2	3	4	5
2.	ability to walk or move around	1	2	3	4	5
3.	sleep	1	2	3	4	5
4.	normal work (both outside your home and at home)	1	2	3	4	5
5.	recreational activities	1	2	3	4	5
6.	enjoyment of life	1	2	3	4	5

FIGURE 24.1
MOS pain effects scale (PES).

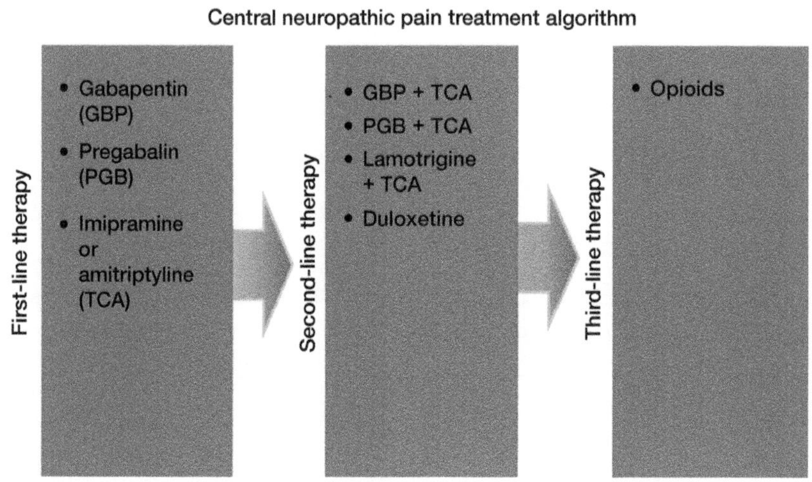

Central neuropathic pain treatment algorithm

First-line therapy
• Gabapentin (GBP)
• Pregabalin (PGB)
• Imipramine or amitriptyline (TCA)

Second-line therapy
• GBP + TCA
• PGB + TCA
• Lamotrigine + TCA
• Duloxetine

Third-line therapy
• Opioids

FIGURE 24.2
Algorithm for the pharmacological management of CNP in MS.

TRIGEMINAL NEURALGIA

Trigeminal neuralgia (TN) occurs more frequently (typically 2% to 4 %) [3,17] and more often is bilateral (up to 18%) [18] in the MS population. TN may be the presenting symptom at the time of MS diagnosis. Lesions in the region of the trigeminal nerve root entry zone (REZ), and possibly the nerve nucleus itself, are felt to be causal to the condition, and vascular compression may further complicate the pathophysiology. Lesions in the REZ may also remain asymptomatic or produce only dysesthesia or hyperalgesia without classic TN [19]. Clinical symptoms

Trigeminal neuralgia treatment algorithm

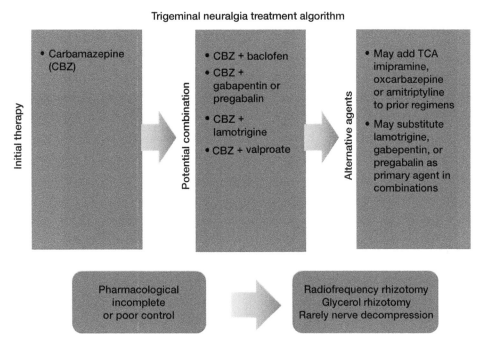

FIGURE 24.3
Algorithm for the management of TN in MS.

of TN may include hyperesthesia or hyperalgesia of one or several facial nerve segments. The pain occurs unilaterally along the path of the trigeminal nerve (V1–V3 distribution), and is described as lancinating, burning, shock-like, stabbing, or electrical pain. It is often precipitated by an external stimulus such as a puff of air to the face, chewing, drinking, shaving, brushing one's teeth, or touching the affected side. The pain is typically extremely short in duration, although lower level dysesthesia may persist in the same distribution as the more severe shock-like sensations. TN is one of the most severe pain syndromes of MS.

The mainstay of pharmacological treatment remains carbamazepine. TN pain is often completely controlled at moderate to high doses. If partial control is achieved, the addition of baclofen, imipramine, or valproate to the regimen is sometimes useful. Alternative therapies may include oxcarbamazepine, phenytonin, or benzodiazepines. In patients refractory to pharmacological therapy, the options of radiofrequency or glycerol rhizotomy can sometimes provide lasting relief [19]. In very unusual cases, nerve decompression may also be of benefit (see Figure 24.3).

LHERMITTE'S SIGN

Jean Lhermitte presented the review paper on this phenomenon to the Neurological Society of Paris entitled *Pain of an Electric Character Discharge Following Head Flexion in Multiple Sclerosis* [20]. Lhermitte's sign is described as a brief, electric, shock-like sensation extending down the spine, sometimes into the lower extremities, typically triggered by forward flexion of the head. The sensation is often described as shock-like or electrical with brief duration. It is a common complaint in the MS population, occurring with a frequency of 9% to 41% [3,21,22]. It is generally felt to be related to a lesion of the ascending spinothalamic tract at the cervical level, with MRI showing a cervical spinal cord plaque in more than 95% of patients [22]. An increase in pressure on the dorsal columns with neck flexion is postulated to produce a transient conduction block, resulting in the dysesthetic sensation radiating down the spine. Therapy involves treatment of the primary MS cervical plaque with steroids if the plaque is acute or subacute, and treatment of the disease with immunomodulators. Symptomatic therapy is generally of limited utility.

PSEUDORADICULAR PAIN

A diagnosis of pseudoradiculopathy related to MS is a diagnosis of exclusion. Careful radiographic evaluation of the spine to rule out root compression is essential. The clinical syndrome in presentation is very similar to that of acute disc herniation. It occurs most typically in lumbar root transition zones, but has been noted in both cervical and thoracic regions [23]. It may occur as the first manifestation of MS or years after the diagnosis. It may be constant or paroxysmal, and may be associated with trauma. Intravenous methylprednisolone may help ameliorate symptoms in acute or subacute presentations. CNP modulators are sometimes of assistance in more chronic presentations.

HEADACHE

Headache appears to occur more commonly in the MS population, with the studies done to date recently summarized by O'Conner [6]. Rolak and Brown [24] found that 52% of MS patients reported headache, with 31% classified as muscle contraction headache and 21% as migraine. Generally, headaches did not correlate with MS relapse. Headache can rarely occur as the presenting symptom in MS. MS-related headache is treated in the same fashion as idiopathic headache and is not further addressed in this chapter.

MUSCULOSKELETAL PAIN

Musculoskeletal pain can present as lower back, joint, or neck pain and is most often a secondary manifestation of the disease process, exacerbated by poor posture and body mechanics. If a patient has weakness of one limb, pain can be caused by inadequate attempts to stabilize the trunk with the opposite leg or either the knee or hip joint [11]. Wheelchair-bound patients may present with chronic neck or back pain due to immobilization, spasticity, osteoporosis, or malposition. Increased biomechanical stress as well as a shifting of weight to accommodate a weak limb can cause sore muscles, joint pain, neuralgic pain such as occipital neuralgia, or radiculopathy. Orthopedic conditions such as osteoarthritis and osteoporosis, to which MS can indirectly contribute, should be ruled out and managed adequately. Spasticity is another problem frequently seen in this patient population and is addressed in another chapter.

In general, musculoskeletal pain is first treated with physical therapy [11] including exercise routines that contain frequent stretching and strengthening activities. Consultation with a physical therapist who is familiar with MS is generally immensely helpful in assessing each patient's needs. Use of durable medical equipment such as limb braces, canes, walkers, and electrical stimulation devices may improve energy conservation and reduce strain. Pharmacological treatment of musculoskeletal pain usually consists of nonsteroidal anti-inflammatory drugs (NSAIDS). Antidepressants and opioids have some support from randomized controlled trials but their long-term efficacy is not widely agreed upon [3]. Local infiltrations of steroids and analgesics can be helpful. Orthopedic surgery can be performed if needed (eg, for severe osteoarthritis), but indications and goals should be carefully assessed, ideally by concertation between the orthopedic

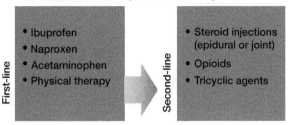

FIGURE 24.4
Algorithm for the management of musculoskeletal pain in MS.

surgeon, rehabilitation professionals, and the neurological team (see Figure 24.4).

VISCERAL PAIN

Visceral pain is an infrequent manifestation of MS, occurring in up to 2% of the population, and generally described as aching, bloating, or cramping generally related to constipation [17]. This is a diagnosis of exclusion, and standard medical evaluation of the abdomen should be completed prior to settling on this diagnosis. Standard anticonstipation regimens will sometimes improve this problem (see Chapter 25).

IATROGENIC PAIN

Treatment-related pain is common. Interferon-related pain may include myalgias, headache, and/or spasticity. By increasing hydration, administering anti-inflammatory medications pre and postinjection, some discomfort may be minimized or even avoided. Subcutaneous injections can cause site pain, including swelling, tenderness, and bruising. Medications used for symptom management can be contributing factors to secondary pain, mainly headache and gastrointestinal pain, and may require medication adjustment or additional intervention.

SUMMARY

Pain is a pervasive symptom in MS and often is a major issue compromising quality of life. It is often undertreated and can present in many different fashions. It often is amplified in the setting of comorbid psychiatric disease, frequently seen with MS, and may occur at any stage in the disease. Adequate management requires precise characterization of the pain, realistic goal setting, periodic assessments, and a standardized treatment approach that optimizes pain control and minimizes polypharmacy.

PATIENT CASE

A 44-year-old white female presented with a history of MS since 2003. At that time, she developed a sensation of spiders crawling on her feet and scalp, followed shortly thereafter by severe left-sided facial pain. The pain in the lower extremities evolved to a sensation of "stabbing and burning." The facial pain was described as "knife-like," very brief in duration, recurring multiple times. She had previously been treated with gabapentin, which had produced excessive fatigue. She was started on carbamazepine which proved partially effective. Dose escalation failed to control the problem. Baclofen and valproate were tried with little efficacy. She was started on oxycarbamazepine 300 mg 3 times daily with generally fair control. In 2010, she had a relapse of trigeminal pain requiring intravenous (IV) hydromorphone in the emergency room, then oxycodone. She received 3 days of IV methylprednisolone with good improvement. CNP in the lower extremities persisted but was attenuated with lamotrigine. In 2008, she experienced significant worsening in her left facial pain and underwent glycerol neurolysis. This resulted in pain freedom until 2010 when she noted electrical jolting pain into the left maxilla. Light touch to the face could bring on the pain. A repeat glycerol neurolysis was undertaken with excellent pain amelioration. She is currently stable with both her lower extremity pain and trigeminal neuralgia.

REFERENCES

1. Hirsch AT, Turner AP, Ehde DM, Haselkorn JK. Prevalence and impact of pain in multiple sclerosis: Physical and psychologic contributors. *Arch Phys Med Rehabil.* 2009;90(4):646–651.

2. Piwko C, Desjardins OB, Bereza BG, et al. Pain due to multiple sclerosis: Analysis of prevalence and economic burden in Canada. *Pain Res Manage.* 2007;12(4):259–265.

3. Solaro, C, Brichetto G, Amato MP, et al. The prevalence of pain in multiple sclerosis. *Neurology.* 2004;63:919–921.

4. Stenager E, Knudsen L, Jensen K. Acute and chronic pain syndromes in multiple sclerosis. *Acta Neurol Scand.* 1991;84(3):197–200.

5. Newland PK, Naismith RT, Ullione M. The impact of pain and other symptoms on quality of life in women with relapsing remitting multiple sclerosis. *J Neurosci Nurs.* 2009;41(6):322–328.

6. O'Conner AB. Neuropathic pain: Quality of life impact, cost and cost effectiveness of therapy. *Pharmacoeconomics.* 2009;27(2):95–112.

7. Scherder E, Wolters E, Polman C, et al. Pain in Parkinson's disease and multiple sclerosis; its relation to the medial and lateral pain systems. *Neurosci Biobehav Rev.* 2005;29(7):1047–1056.

8. White SR, Vyas D, Bieger D, Samathanam G. Monoamine-containing fiver plexus in spinal cord of guinea pigs during paralysis, recovery and relapse stages of chronic relapsing experimental allergic encephalomyelitis. *J Neuroimmunol.* 1989;22(3):211–221.

9. Zhang JH, Huang YG, The immune system: A new look at pain. *Chin Med J.* 2006;119:930–938.

10. Wieseler F, Maier SF, Watkins LR. Central proinflammatory cytokines and pain enhancement. *Neurosignals.* 2005;14(4):166–174.

11. Pollmann W, Fenneberg W. Current management of pain associated with multiple sclerosis. *CNS Drugs.* 2008;22(4):291–324.

12. Kenner M, Menon U, Elliot DG. Multiple sclerosis as a painful disease. *Int Rev Neurobiol.* 2007;79:303–321.

13. Ritvo P, Fischer J, Miller D, et al. MSQLI: Multiple Sclerosis Quality of Life Inventory: A Users Manual. 1997. Retrieved from www.nationalmssociety.org/for-professionals/researchers/clinical-study-measures/pes/index.aspx

14. Osterberg A, Boivie J, Thuomas KA. Central pain in multiple sclerosis-prevalence and clinical characterisitics. *Euro J Pain.* 2005;9(5):531–542.

15. Pain in MS. (June, 2008). Retrieved June 2012, from www.msif.org/en/about_ms/ms_by_topic/pain/index.html

16. Dworkin RH, O'Conner AB, Backonja M, et al. Pharmacologic management of neuropathic pain: Evidence-based recommendations. *Pain.* 2007;132:237–251.

17. Moulin D. Pain in central and peripheral demyelinating disorders: Multiple sclerosis and Guillain-Barre syndrome. *Neuropathic Pain Syndromes.* 1998 November;16(4):889–893.

18. Zorro O, Lobato-Polo J, Kano H, et al. Gamma knife radiosurgery for multiple sclerosis-related trigeminal neuralgia. *Neurology.* 2009 Oct 6;73(14):1149–1154.

19. Hooge JP, Redekop WK. Trigeminal neuralgia in multiple sclerosis. *Neurology.* 1995 July; 45(7):1294–1296.

20. Lhermitte, J, et al. Les douleurs à type de décharge électrique à la flexion céphalique dans la sclérose en plaques. *Rev Neurol (Paris).* 1924;2:36–52.

21. Kanchandani R, Howe JG. Lhermitte's sign in multiple sclerosis: A clinical survey and review of the literature. *J Neurol Neurosurg Psychiatry.* 1982;45:308–312.

22. Al-Araji A, Oger J. Reappraisal of Lhermitte's sign in multiple sclerosis. *Mult Scler.* 2005;11:398–402.

23. Ramirez-Lassepas M, Tulloch JW, Quinones MR, Snyder BD. Acute radicular pain as a presenting symptom in multiple sclerosis. *Arch Neurol.* 1992;49(3):255–258.

24. Rolak L, Brown S. Headaches in multiple sclerosis: A clinical study and review of the literature. *J Neurol.* 1990;237:300–302.

25

Bladder and Bowel Dysfunction in Multiple Sclerosis

BOGDAN ORASANU
SANGEETA T. MAHAJAN

KEY POINTS FOR CLINICIANS

- Bladder symptoms are very common among multiple sclerosis (MS) patients (reported by 80% of patients at the time of diagnosis and up to 96% by 10 years after diagnosis).

- The first line of treatment for urinary incontinence symptoms in MS is behavioral modification, once infection and urinary retention have been ruled out. However, many patients will require pharmacotherapy.

- Intra-detrusor botulinum toxin A injections have greatly improved the management of overactive bladder symptoms in patients with neurogenic bladder who failed anticholinergic medication, and have recently obtained FDA approval for this indication.

- Up to 25% of patients with MS will experience urinary retention and require urinary catheterization of some form for voiding during the course of their disease. In general, a postvoid residual more than 150 mL is considered abnormal.

- Detrusor areflexia or impaired contractility with detrusor sphincter dyssynergia are the most common reasons for urinary retention in patients with MS. Medications are generally not helpful for these conditions.

- Bowel complaints are also common among MS patients, with 53% to 41% reporting chronic constipation and 29% to 51% fecal incontinence. Many patients may vary between the 2 extremes at times or may report mixed symptoms.

- Medications should be carefully screened as potential causes of bowel complaints.

- Constipation can often be treated with fluid intake and dietary modifications, aggressive fiber supplementation, a regular time of evacuation, and over-the-counter medications.

- Fecal incontinence may be treated with dietary changes, over-the-counter medications to slow bowel motility, and physical therapy to improve patient mobility.

Multiple sclerosis (MS) is well known to have significant detrimental effects on bowel and bladder function. Urinary symptoms remain one of the most frequent complaints among men and women with MS, and are reported by 80% of patients at the time of MS diagnosis, and up to 96% 10 years after diagnosis [1]. Bowel complaints are common, with constipation occurring in 53% to 54% of MS patients and fecal incontinence in 29% to 51% [2]. Owing to the sensitive nature of these topics, many patients and their caregivers often avoid discussing bowel and bladder symptoms, letting the patients and their family cope with these disabling problems as "par for the course" with little to no intervention.

Attention to the care of bowel and bladder issues is an important component of the care of all MS patients.

Often, starting the conversation may be the hardest part of caring for these complaints. In general, bowel and bladder symptoms can be treated with behavioral changes and medications, while surgery is rarely utilized.

BLADDER DYSFUNCTION IN MS

Pathophysiology and Symptoms

Bladder function is significantly affected by abnormalities in neurological function. In normal micturition, mechanoreceptors in the bladder wall are stimulated by stretch as the bladder fills (Figure 25.1). With increasing bladder filling

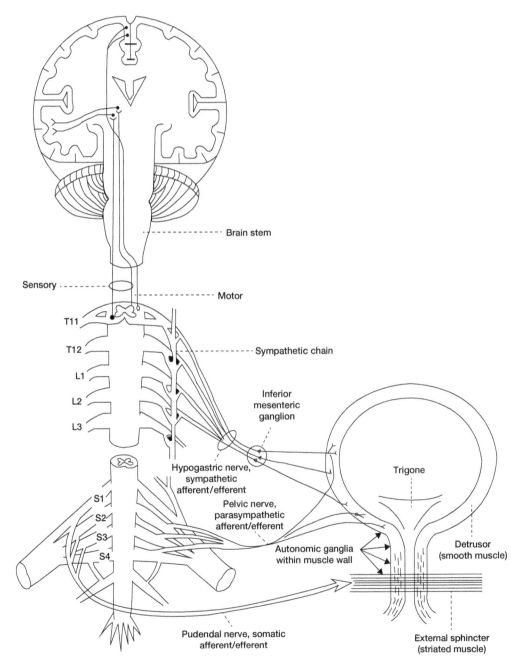

FIGURE 25.1
Diagram of the neuroanatomy of normal bladder function. *From [4].*

volume, pressure in the bladder remains low via accommodation. Information regarding bladder filling is relayed to the brain via the posterior and lateral white matter of the spinal cord, terminating in the pontine micturition center (PMC) [3,4]. As bladder filling continues, increased afferent neuron firing occurs, eventually resulting in the PMC triggering 1 of 2 responses: storage or voiding. With storage, the PMC then triggers further relaxation and storage of the bladder via activation of beta-receptors in the bladder and alpha-stretch receptors in the urethra, thereby relaxing the bladder and closing the urethra, via sympathetic control through the pudendal nerve [4]. Once the bladder reaches significant capacity, the PMC then triggers detrusor contraction and urethral relaxation, resulting in relaxation of the bladder outlet through the hypogastric nerve, via the parasympathetic nervous system, thereby resulting in urine flowing out of the bladder and urethra as the act of coordinated voiding [5].

Among the general U.S. population, 1 in 3 women suffer from some form of urinary incontinence [6]. Rates of bladder dysfunction are much higher among MS patients with most patients developing urinary symptoms during their disease course. Symptoms of bladder dysfunction tend to occur more frequently with increasing disease duration, generally starting 6 to 8 years after symptom onset, but they may be present earlier [7,8]. Up to 14% of patients will report acute urinary complaints as their initial symptom of MS [9].

Bladder complaints may range from urinary retention to urinary incontinence (Table 25.1). Overactive bladder (OAB) is a syndrome characterized by the presence of any 1 of 4 symptoms (urgency, urge incontinence, frequency, nocturia), and is the primary cause of urinary incontinence in MS patients [10]. Dysfunctional voiding and/or urinary retention may result from bladder outlet obstruction (ie, detrusor-sphincter dyssynergia [DSD]), detrusor hypoactivity, or detrusor acontractility. In general, a postvoid residual of more than 150 mL is considered abnormal. Mixed symptoms are common, with up to 70% of respondents reporting both urinary incontinence and retention symptoms in 1 recent study. In another series, symptomatic voiding dysfunction was present in 97% of patients, urgency and frequency in 32%, incontinence in 49%, and urinary hesitancy and retention in 19% [11].

Marrie et al. surveyed over 16,000 participants in the North American Research Committee on Multiple Sclerosis (NARCOMS) database and found that 80% of their respondents had complaints of bowel or bladder symptoms, often moderate to severe in nature, and 50% or more reported at least mild disability resulting from these symptoms [12]. A follow-up study by Mahajan et al. demonstrated at least 1 moderate to severe urinary symptom of OAB in 65% of respondents and significant correlations between increased prevalence of urinary symptoms and longer disease duration, increased physical disability, and reduced quality of life [13].

Evaluation and Clinical Findings

Bladder and bowel function are integrally related to the patient's mental, cognitive, and functional status. The evaluation of patients with MS and urinary symptoms should commence with a detailed physical examination. Many of the causes of pelvic floor complaints are modifiable and should be assessed carefully [14] (Table 25.2).

Functional status plays an important role, not only as a cause of incontinence when mobility is limited, but also for its impact on treatment decisions. For example, significant hand ataxia would interfere with self-catheterizing and would call for an alternative approach. Common treatable causes of urinary incontinence should be screened for and can be remembered using the DIAPPERS acronym (Table 25.3). Special attention should be paid to screening for infection, hematuria, and urinary retention. All patients

TABLE 25.1
Possible Bladder Symptoms Experienced by Patients With MS

SYMPTOMS	DEFINITION
Urgency	The sudden strong desire to urinate that cannot be deferred
Frequency	A complaint by the patient that he or she voids too often
Urge incontinence	Involuntary urine leakage accompanied by an urgent desire to urinate
Nocturia	The complaint of needing to wake up 1 or more times a night to urinate
Urinary retention	A painful or nonpainful bladder, that remains palpable or percussable after the patient has passed urine; may be associated with incontinence; generally a postvoid residual volume of more than 150 mL
Hesitancy	Difficulty initiating a urine stream resulting in the delay in onset of voiding
Straining	Requiring additional muscular effort to initiate, maintain, or accelerate the urine stream

TABLE 25.2
Important Factors to Assess at the Time of Patient Interview Regarding Bladder Complaints [14]

- Mental status/cognitive function
- Functional status (activities of daily living, walking, transfer ability)
- Diet
- Fluid intake habits
- Incontinence
- Recurrent urinary tract infections
- Postvoid residual
- Urinary frequency and urgency symptoms
- Medications (type and timing)
- Concurrent medical problems

TABLE 25.3
DIAPPERS: Potentially Treatable/Reversible Causes of Incontinence [14]

Delirium: May be related to infection of metabolic disorder

Infection: Screen for infection with clean catch or straight-catheterized specimen, checking urinalysis and culture and sensitivity when indicated. Gross hematuria or persistent microhematuria (2 samples with more than 3 to 5 RBCs per high power field) should be referred to urology for evaluation

Atrophic vaginitis: Modifies vaginal pH and increases susceptibility to UTI; should be treated with transvaginal estrogen supplementation

Pharmaceuticals: Drugs that may cause urinary complaints including: (a) retention: alpha-agonists, opioids, anticholinergics; (b) incontinence: alpha blockers; muscle relaxants; (c) urgency and frequency: diuretics, alcohol

Psychological: Assess for depression or cognitive impairment

Excess excretion: Causes of fluid accumulation in the body, including: peripheral edema, congestive heart failure, vascular disease, excessive oral fluid intake, diuretic usage

Restricted mobility: Difficulty ambulating to commode, problems with transfer, lack of assistance, distance to bathroom facilities, etc.

Stool impaction: Refer to gastroenterology if dietary modification and common oral fiber and laxatives are not sufficient

RBCs, red blood cells; UTI, urinary tract infection.

with urinary complaints should have postvoid residual volume measurement and urinalysis testing, with a urine culture when indicated. A postvoid residual volume below 150 mL is considered normal.

A simple bladder diary, often for 24 hours or up to 3 days (including day and night), can be very helpful, not only in characterizing symptoms, but also in identifying potential areas for intervention. A basic bladder diary consists of simply keeping a record of times and volumes of daily fluid intake, voided urine, and any leakage episodes, to allow a provider to understand patients' habits and symptoms (Figure 25.2).

A variety of screening questionnaires are available to assess urinary and pelvic floor complaints, including the Medical, Epidemiological, and Social aspects of Aging (MESA) questionnaire, Urogenital Distress Inventory (UDI-6), and Pelvic Floor Impact Questionnaire (PFIQ) [15,16]. Currently, no MS-specific questionnaire exists to assess urinary symptoms in detail.

Urodynamic testing may be recommended for patients with an unclear urological diagnosis and commonly involves filling the bladder while observing for changes in bladder, abdominal, and urethral pressures. During testing, changes in pressures with bladder filling, the presence or absence of urine leakage with or without provocation, and bladder function during voiding are observed. Special attention should be made to determine if patient-reported symptoms correlate with urodynamic diagnoses to enable a treatment plan (Table 25.4).

Treatment

Significant advances have been made in increasing awareness of pelvic floor dysfunction among patients and care providers. However, these benefits do not always extend to patients with neurogenic bladder dysfunction, especially patients with MS. On review of the evaluation and treatment history of patients participating in the NARCOMS data base, Mahajan et al. demonstrated that only 43% of participants with moderate to severe bladder symptoms had ever been evaluated by urology, and only 51% had received any anticholinergic medications for these symptoms. Among those who had been treated, older medications with significant side effects were commonly used and not consistent with the newer less problematic options offered to the general population [13].

The first-line of treatment for urinary incontinence symptoms in MS is behavioral modification, once infection and urinary retention have been ruled out. Our unit has a series of simple patient information sheets that we routinely distribute to patients outlining these treatments (Table 25.5). Most patients with non-neurogenic dysfunction will generally experience a 50% improvement in their urinary complaints with these simple lifestyle changes. Although they are also beneficial in patients with neurogenic dysfunction, the majority of patients will note less significant symptom improvement, and will likely need to go on to pharmacotherapy.

Pharmacotherapy is commonly utilized as a second-line therapy for neurogenic patients. A variety of medications are currently available in oral and topical forms, although the use of all of these medicines is limited by the potential side effects of constipation, dry mouth, and sometimes mental status changes (Table 25.6). Patients with urinary retention may find some improvement with alpha-blocking agents, but their use is limited by dizziness, drowsiness, hypotension, and even syncope, all requiring bedtime dosing. For all medications, patients should be started on the lowest possible dose and titrated based on tolerability and efficacy.

For patients with OAB symptoms refractory to multiple medications and behavioral changes, urodynamic testing can be very useful. Many patients will exhibit detrusor overactivity on urodynamic testing, qualifying them for more potent and invasive therapies, including: (a) intra-detrusor botulinum toxin injections; (b) sacral neuro-modulation; (c) percutaneous nerve stimulation (PNS); (d) chronic catheterization or urinary diversion. Intra-detrusor botulinum toxin A injections have excellent efficacy in both neurogenic and idiopathic OAB patients. Botulinum toxin A

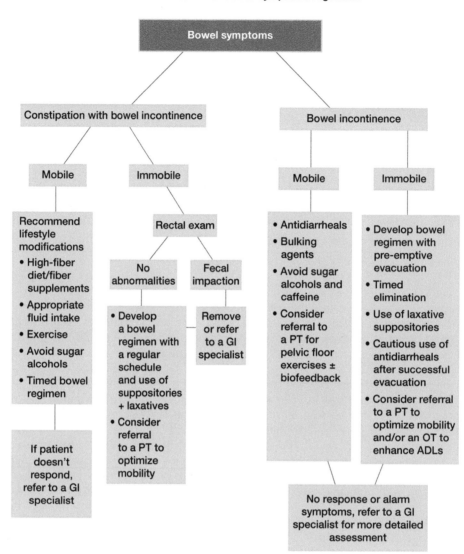

FIGURE 25.2

Treatment algorithm for patients with MS and bowel symptoms. ADLs, activities of daily living; GI, gastrointestinal; OT, occupational therapy; PT, physical therapy.

TABLE 25.4

Common Findings on Urodynamic Testing and Associated Symptoms [4,10]

URODYNAMIC FINDING	DEFINITION	ASSOCIATED SYMPTOMS
Detrusor overactivity without obstruction	Involuntary detrusor contractions during bladder filling with or without leakage	Urgency, frequency, urge incontinence, and nocturia
Detrusor sphincter dyssynergia	Detrusor contraction concurrent with an involuntary contraction of the urethral or periurethral striated muscle (may block urine outflow)	Urinary hesitancy, straining, or obstruction
Detrusor overactivity with outlet obstruction	Detrusor overactivity plus detrusor sphincter dyssynergia (defined above). May occasionally obstruct urine flow altogether	Urinary urgency with hesitancy, straining, or obstruction
Detrusor overactivity with impaired contractility	Detrusor overactivity with reduced strength and/or duration of bladder contraction, resulting in prolonged bladder emptying and/or inability to completely empty in a timely fashion	Slow bladder emptying and/or urinary retention
Detrusor areflexia	Inability of the bladder to contract with routine filling at normal physiological volumes to elicit bladder emptying	Urinary retention

TABLE 25.5
Behavioral Modifications for Urinary Symptoms in MS

Fluid titration	Patients are instructed to moderate drinking habits, focusing on no more than 4 to 6 ounces of fluid per hour
Reduce bladder irritant intake	Includes: Alcohol, caffeine, citrus juices, artificial sweeteners
Cut off oral fluids 2 to 3 hours before bedtime	Minimize the need for night time voiding and potential nocturia
Change medication timing	Do not take diuretics in evening; move bedtime medications 2 to 3 hours earlier
Scheduled voiding	Voiding by the clock to prevent bladder overfilling and potential incontinence episodes
Bladder retraining	Teaching patients who void too frequently methods to control urinary urge and extend time between voids
Kegel exercises	Teaching patients to improve voluntary control of pelvic floor muscles to control urinary urge and incontinence

TABLE 25.6
Medications for the Treatment of Bladder Dysfunction

GENERIC NAME	BRAND NAME	ROUTE	DOSE	FREQUENCY
Anticholinergic medications for the treatment of overactive bladder symptoms				
Fesoterodine	Toviaz	Oral	4 or 8 mg	Daily
Oxybutynin	Ditropan	Oral	5, 10, 15 mg	Up to 3 times a day
	Dirtropan XL	Oral	5, 10, 15 mg	Daily
	Oxytrol Patch	Topical	3.9 mg/day	One patch twice weekly
	Gelnique	Topical	10%	Daily
Solifenacin	Sanctura	Oral	20 mg	Twice a day
	Sanctura XR	Oral	60 mg	Daily
Darifenacin	Enablex	Oral	7.5, 15 mg	Daily
Tolterodine	Detrol	Oral	2, 4 mg	Twice a day
	Detrol LA	Oral	2, 4 mg	Daily
Alpha-adrenergic blockers for the treatment of impaired bladder emptying				
Tamsulosin	Flomax	Oral	0.4 mg	At bedtime
Alfuzosin	Uroxatral	Oral	10 mg	At bedtime
Doxazosin	Cardura	Oral	1, 2, 4, 8 mg	At bedtime
	Cardura XL	Oral	4, 8 mg	At bedtime
Silodosin	Rapaflo	Oral	4, 8 mg	At bedtime
Terazosin	Hytrin	Oral	1, 2, 5, 10 mg	At bedtime

is currently available in the United States as onabotulinum toxin A (Botox), abobotulinum toxin A (Dysport), or incobotulinum toxin A (Xeomin), and acts by blocking acetylcholine release at the neuromuscular junction, thereby causing a reversible, temporary, flaccid paralysis of the treated muscle, resulting in diminished detrusor contraction and associated urge sensation. Onabotulinum toxin A was recently approved by the FDA for the treatment of neurogenic detrusor overactivity, thereby greatly improving insurance coverage [17–19]. Whereas Xeomin was less studied, both Botox and Dysport have shown excellent efficacy for the treatment of neurogenic OAB, with 58% to 100% of treated patients reporting complete continence after treatment [20,21]. The effects of intra-detrusor injections last

6 to 12 months on average [22]. Owing to a risk of temporary urinary retention (which varied widely between 0% and 30%, depending on the study [23]), patients need to be willing and able to catheterize after the injections, if they are not already performing intermittent catheterization. Other potential but rare side effects include generalized weakness, dysphagia, diplopia, and blurred vision. However, to date there have been no reports of respiratory paralysis after lower urinary tract injection of botulinum toxin [23].

Sacral neuromodulation (Interstim) is another option for patients with refractory OAB symptoms. The metal parts of the device preclude the ability to undergo MRI studies, limiting its use in MS patients. However, in some patients, Interstim may be a useful alternative, with 50% of patients reporting significant symptomatic improvement, and another 25% moderate improvement after implantation [24]. Interstim is FDA-approved for the treatment of refractory OAB symptoms, and most recently has demonstrated utility for the treatment of fecal incontinence.

PNS uses intermittent stimulation of the tibial nerve at the ankle with no permanent lead or pulse generator implanted, and is provided in the outpatient clinic setting. A large randomized, double-blinded, sham-controlled study, showed marked improvement in bladder symptoms in patients receiving PNS therapy (54.5% PNS patients vs. 20.9% sham). Adverse events associated with PNS are mild, transient, and relatively uncommon (1%–2%), including bruising or bleeding at the needle site, tingling, and mild pain [25].

Up to 25% of patients with MS will experience urinary retention and require urinary catheterization or some form for voiding during the course of their disease [26]. Detrusor areflexia or impaired contractility and DSD are the most common reasons for urinary retention in patients with MS. Medications are generally not helpful for this condition. Intermittent catheterization tends to be the preferred method of bladder emptying in both men and women (Mahajan, unpublished). Long-term use of indwelling catheters can be complicated by chronic infection, catheter-bypassing incontinence (leakage around the catheter due to detrusor overactivity), and necrosis of the bladder neck with potential fistula formation. Antibiotic prophylaxis may be considered in patients using catheterization and developing recurrent infections. Suprapubic catheters may also be useful as a minimally invasive option. Bladder augmentation and urinary diversion with or without catheterizable stomas remain treatments of last resort and should be performed only after less invasive therapies have failed. Urethral sphincterotomy may be helpful in patients with DSD, but can be complicated by significant stress urinary incontinence afterward, and is generally avoided.

BOWEL DYSFUNCTION IN MS

Bowel symptoms are thought to occur in more than 50% of patients with MS. Both constipation and fecal incontinence are common, with constipation being, by far, more prevalent. Based on the Rome Criteria, constipation is defined as any 2 of the following criteria: (a) less than 3 bowel movements per week; (b) hard stool more than 25% of the time; (c) a feeling of incomplete bowel emptying more than 25% of the time; (d) excessive straining with bowel movements more than 25% of the time; and (e) the need to manually disimpact or manipulate stool to help evacuation [14]. A recent survey from the NARCOMS Patient Registry found significant rates of bowel symptoms in 502 participants, with 39% reporting constipation, 11% fecal incontinence, and 36% mixed constipation and incontinence [27]. Bowel complaints significantly impact quality of life and can lead to serious social impairment, in some cases more than other impairments from MS [28]. The impact of symptoms often depends on the patient's level of activity, with more active patients desiring more complete fecal continence.

The etiology of bowel dysfunction in MS is multifactorial. Bowel complaints may precede the onset of MS by many years or be unrelated to MS, therefore a temporal relationship should be established [28]. Sacral spinal cord lesions may affect neurological control of intestines and sphincter function, thereby slowing gastric emptying, increasing colonic transit time, and causing paradoxical puborectalis muscle contraction, potentially exacerbating constipation. Weakened abdominal muscles (creating more difficulty in "bearing down" during defecation), decreased activity, or constipating medications used to treat other MS symptoms, may also worsen constipation [14,29]. In contrast, laxatives used to treat constipation, impaired function of the external anal sphincter (inadequate voluntary contractions of the anal sphincter), and increased thresholds of conscious rectal sensation (making the patient unaware of rectal feeling) may result in fecal incontinence [14,29].

Evaluation and Clinical Findings

The assessment of bowel symptoms may be performed during an office visit or by asking patients to complete validated questionnaires at home or in the waiting area. However, periodic assessments are absolutely necessary to determine treatment efficacy and detect changes in the patient's disease status that could aggravate bowel symptoms. Suggested general questions useful to ask during a patient evaluation, and additional questions triggered by specific responses, are presented in Table 25.7. Also, during the interview, mental, cognitive, and functional status (mobility, spasticity, hand coordination, sexual activity) should be carefully assessed [14].

The Bowel Function Questionnaire for Persons with MS (BFQ-MS) is a self-administered questionnaire consisting of 15 items pertaining to constipation, 13 items pertaining to fecal incontinence, and 20 items pertaining to both constipation and fecal incontinence. It is useful to differentiate symptoms and treatments between the 3 types of bowel dysfunction [30]. Several other validated patient-administered questionnaires are available, including the Quality of Life Scoring Tool Relating to Bowel Management (QOL-BM), the Constipation Symptom Assessment Instrument (PAC-SYM), and the Brief Fecal Incontinence questionnaire [30].

Secondary causes of bowel dysfunction must be excluded prior to treatment. Patients should be asked about prior history of bowel inflammatory diseases (eg, Crohn's disease or ulcerative colitis) and, if suspected, should be further investigated. Prior surgical procedures (especially rectal, anal, or perineal surgeries) or difficult deliveries with large perineal lacerations (in women) must be carefully investigated as they could manifest with similar bowel dysfunctions. Many patients with MS have associated medical comorbidities and are taking numerous drugs. Therefore, current medications should be reviewed carefully to identify those with constipating or diarrheal side effects (Table 25.8).

A focused physical examination should be performed in conjunction with the interview questions, including

TABLE 25.7
Screening Questions for Bowel Symptoms in Patients With MS

How are your bowel movements?

How many times do you move your bowels during a typical week?

What is the consistency of your bowel movements?

    If constipated: do you strain to pass stool?

                  do you have the sensation of incomplete emptying of the bowels?

Did you notice any changes in your bowel habits?

    If yes: what changes and for how long?

            what have you done to control the symptoms (behavioral changes, medications, etc.)?

Did you experience pain or discomfort when passing stool?

Did you have bowel accidents?

    If yes: did you leak stool or flatus?

            how much does it bother you?

            do you need to wear protective garments?

            are there any warning signs prior to an accident (urgency)?

            did you do anything to make the problem better?

What does your diet consist of? (ask especially about fluid and fiber intake)

TABLE 25.8
Medications That Can Precipitate or Exacerbate Bowel Dysfunction

Medications promoting constipation	Anticholinergics (fesoterodine, darifenacin, oxybutynin, solifenacin, tolterodine, trospium chloride) Antihypertensives (calcium channel blockers and central alpha agonists) Analgesics/narcotics (including nonsteroidal anti-inflammatory drugs, morphine, codeine) Antidepressants (selective serotonin reuptake inhibitors) Antipsychotics (chlorpromazine, clozapine, risperidone, olanzapine) Antihistamines (diphenhydramine, doxylamine, promethazine) Tricyclic antidepressants (amitriptyline, nortriptyline, imipramine, desipramine) Sedatives/tranquilizers (barbiturates, benzodiazepines, zolpidem) Antacids (aluminum and calcium compounds) Diuretics (triamterene, indapamide, hydrochlorothiazide) Iron supplements
Medications with diarrheal side effects	Antihypertensives (enalapril, metoprolol) Antiarrhythmics (quinidine) Antibiotics (penicillins, cephalosporins, carbapenems, antituberculosis agents, macrolides, sulfonamides, tetracyclines, quinolones) Antineoplastics (5-fluorouracil, capecitabine, irinotecan) Protease inhibitors (saquinavir, ritonavir, indinavir) Some diuretics (furosemide, indapamide, bumetanide) Antacids (magnesium hydroxide) Laxatives (bisacodyl, senna, lactulose, docusate, methylcellulose)

abdominal, pelvic, and rectal examinations. The clinician should look for masses and/or tenderness, pelvic organ prolapse, hemorrhoids, anal fissures, and anal sphincter tone. A rectal digital examination is necessary to assess the resting anal tone and external sphincter pressures, and to collect a stool sample for occult blood testing. Bloodwork should include blood glucose, electrolytes, calcium, and if necessary, thyroid function tests [30].

Treatment of Constipation

The Consortium of MS Centers (CMSC) Consensus Panel on Elimination Disorders recommended dividing patients with MS-related bowel dysfunction into 2 groups, constipation with incontinence and incontinence only, and further dividing by mobility status (mobile and immobile). The CMSC then formulated treatment algorithms for each

TABLE 25.9
Medications to Relieve Constipation

Bulk-forming	Methylcellulose (Citrucel)
	Psyllium hydrophilic mucilloid (Metamucil)
	Polycarbophil (FiberCon)
	Guar gum (Benefiber)
	Malt soup extract (Maltsupex)
Stool softeners	Docusate (Colace, Surfak, Correctol, Dok)
Stimulant laxatives	Senna (Senokot, Ex-Lax, Senexon, Senna-Gen)
	Bisacodyl (Bisac-Evac, Biscolax, Dulcolax, Dacodyl, Fleet Bisacodyl Enema/Suppository)
	Cascara sagrada
	Castor oil
Osmotic laxatives	Lactulose (Constulose, Enulose, Generlac, Kristalose)
	Sorbitol
	Polyethylene glycol solution (Miralax)
	Glycerin suppository
Combination of stimulant laxative and stool softener	Senna concentrate and docusate (Peri-Colace, Dok Plus, Senokot-S)
Saline laxatives	Magnesium hydroxide (Phillips Milk of Magnesia, Fleet Pedia-Lax)
	Magnesium citrate (Citroma)
	Magnesium sulfate
Lubricant laxatives	Mineral oil (Fleet, Kondremul)

group (Figure 25.2) [14]. A minimum trial period of at least 4 weeks is recommended with each treatment regimen prior to determining efficacy. Also, in patients with associated bladder complaints, bladder symptoms should be addressed prior to bowel complaints [31].

Lifestyle modification is the first line of treatment for patients with MS and constipation. A high fiber diet (25 g/day for females and 38 g/day for males according to the Institute of Medicine) is recommended to increase stool volume, and to make stools softer and easier to eliminate [14]. Good sources of fiber include fruits and vegetables; grains, cereal, and pasta; legumes, nuts, and seeds. Patients should be instructed to avoid consuming constipating and gas-producing aliments such as sugar alcohols/substitutes (lactitol, maltitol, sorbitol, and xylitol), caffeine, and alcohol.

Bulk-forming laxatives could also be used in addition to a high fiber diet. Each dose of a bulk-forming laxative should be taken with at least 8 ounces of fluid for full benefit and the total fluid intake should be increased to 2000 mL clear liquids per day [31]. Many other over-the-counter constipation-relieving products are commercially available and could be successfully used with minimal side effects (Table 25.9). However, the CMSC Consensus Panel recommends using gentler laxatives such as stool softeners, saline laxatives, or osmotic laxatives, and avoiding, or at least using with caution, harsher products such as stimulant laxatives [14].

Digital rectal stimulation and abdominal massages can also be effective ways of stimulating bowel function and can be performed by the patient or caregiver. During a rectal stimulation, a gloved and lubricated finger is inserted into the rectum and slowly rotated in a circular

motion, being careful not to traumatize the rectal mucosa. It is thought to stimulate the rectal stool evacuation by activating the anorectal colonic reflexes [32]. Similarly, researchers showed a significant improvement of constipation after 4 weeks of daily abdominal massages in patients with MS [33].

Although there is no agreement regarding the beneficial effects of exercise on constipation, it is thought to promote peristalsis, increase the transit time, and decrease water absorption, and therefore help prevent the occurrence of a hard, dry, and painful stool [32]. The CMSC Consensus Panel recommends walking for 10 to 30 minutes a day, or even more intense aerobic activity (like swimming, dancing, running) if patient mobility allows [14]. For some patients, a physical therapy (PT) consult may be necessary to improve mobility.

All patients with MS and bowel symptoms should be instructed to eat regular meals and plan to try having a bowel movement 20 to 30 minutes after a warm meal, when the gastrocolic reflex produces an urge to defecate. The patients should be able to sit in an upright position for at least 15 to 30 minutes on a commode or toilet with their feet on the floor or a stool, and to lean forward to increase the abdominal pressure and facilitate defecation [14,30].

In patients with limited mobility and more advanced disease, an initial rectal examination is recommended to screen for fecal impaction. If no abnormalities are detected, the patients should be treated as previously described and considered for a referral to PT to improve their mobility. If fecal impaction is noted during the rectal examination, the impacted stool should be manually removed by a health care provider with specialized training.

If the patient does not respond or symptoms worsen after the treatment, or when a defecatory disorder is suspected, the patient should be referred to a gastroenterologist for further management. Anorectalmanometry, the balloon expulsion test, defecography, and colonic transit studies, are the most common objective tests for bowel dysfunction [30].

Treatment of Fecal Incontinence

In mobile patients with fecal incontinence, dietary irritants (such as sugar substitutes, alcohol, and caffeine) should be eliminated and muscle relaxant medications (baclofen, tizanidine) should be avoided or, if they are necessary, their dose adjusted [31]. If diarrhea is present, fecal impaction must be excluded and antidiarrheal medications can be prescribed. Treatment with loperamide (Imodium, Kaopectate II, NeoDiaral, Diaraid), up to 4 to 5 tablets daily, or codeine phosphate, is very effective in patients with mild to moderate symptoms, slowing down bowel motility and preventing stool leakage episodes [28].

Anticholinergic drugs taken for overactive bladder may also be an effective treatment for fecal incontinence due to bowel hyperactivity. By increasing stool mass and promoting fecal consistency, bulking agents are often efficient in decreasing diarrhea and improving the incontinence. PT with biofeedback may increase the strength of pelvic floor muscles and rectal sensory perception. Anal plugs can be used as a last resort in patients with refractory fecal incontinence, and consists of disposable cone-shaped, compressed foam devices with a removal cord on one side. Once introduced into the anus they expand to their maximum size, closing off the anus [32,34]. If these therapeutic measures fail, or the patient has concerning symptoms (acute onset of symptoms, diarrhea with dehydration, weight loss, or rectal bleeding), a gastroenterology consult should be obtained.

In patients with impaired mobility, a toileting regimen with daily time for defecation should be emphasized. Referral to physical and occupational therapy to help improve mobility should be considered. Incontinence pads are used by approximately one-third of MS patients with fecal incontinence. They are particularly useful if the quantity of lost stool is small, but need to be changed frequently to prevent skin irritation that can result in incontinence dermatitis and/or pressure ulcers [30]. Recent data suggests that sacral neuromodulation might be effective in neurological patients with refractory severe fecal incontinence.

CONCLUSION

Bladder and bowel symptoms greatly impact the quality of life of persons with MS, yet they too often go unrecognized or untreated. Screening for these symptoms is relatively simple and can be facilitated by a variety of questionnaires and simple physical exam. Bowel and bladder complaints can be significantly improved with simple behavioral changes and common over-the-counter or prescription medications. In more complex cases, specialty consultation and paraclinical testing help guide the use of more advanced treatment options.

REFERENCES

1. Foster H. Bladder symptoms and multiple sclerosis. *MS Quaterly Report.* 2002;21(Spring).

2. Crayton H, Heyman R, Rossman H. A multimodal approach to managing the symptoms of multiple sclerosis. *Neurology.* 2004;63(Suppl 5):S12–S18.

3. Andrews K, Husmann D. Bladder dysfunction and management in multiple sclerosis. *Mayo Clin Proc.* 1997;72:1176–1183.

4. Fernández O. Mechanisms and current treatments of urogenital multiple sclerosis. *J Neurol.* 2002;249:1–8.

5. Blaivas J, Holland NJ, Giesser B, et al. Multiple sclerosis bladder: Studies and care. *Ann NY Acad Sci.* 1984;436:328–346.

6. Burgio K, Matthews K, Engel B. Prevalence, incidence, and correlates of urinary incontinence in healthy middle aged women. *J Urol.* 1991;146:1255–1259.

7. Betts C, D'Mellow M, Fowler C. Urinary symptoms and neurologic features of bladder dysfunction in multiple sclerosis. *J Neurol Neurosurg Psychiatry.* 1993;56:245–250.

8. deSeze M, Ruffion A, Denys P, et al. The neurogenic bladder in multiple sclerosis: Review of the literature and proposal of management guidelines. *Mult Scler.* 2007;13:915–928.

9. Phadke J. Clinical aspects of multiple sclerosis in North-East Scotland with particular reference to course and prognosis. *Brain.* 1990;113:1597–1628.

10. Abrams P, Cardozo L, Fall M, et al. The standardisation of terminology of lower urinary tract dysfunction: Report from the standardisation sub-committee of the international continence society. *Neurourol Urodyn.* 2002;21:167–178.

11. Goldstein I, Siroky MB, Sax DS, Krane RJ. Neurologic abnormalities in multiple sclerosis. *J Urol.* 1982;128:541–545.

12. Marrie R, Cutter G, Tyry T, et al. Disparities in the management of multiple sclerosis-related bladder symptoms. *Neurology.* 2007;68:1971–1978.

13. Mahajan S, Patel P, Marrie R. The undertreatment of overactive bladder symptoms in women with multiple sclerosis: An ancillary analysis of the NARCOMS Patient Registry. *J Urol.* 2010;183:1432–1437.

14. Namey M, Halper J. Elimination dysfunction in multiple sclerosis: Proceedings of a consensus conference held October 28–29, 2011 in Short Hills, New Jersey. *Int J MS Care.* 2011;14(Suppl 1):1–26.

15. Uebersax J, Wyman JF, Shumaker SA, et al. Short forms to assess life quality and symptom distress for urinary incontinence in women: The incontinence impact questionnaire and the urogenital distress inventory. *Neurourol Urodyn.* 1995;14:131–139.

16. Barber M, Kuchibhatla MN, Pieper CF, Bump RC. Psychometric evaluation of 2 comprehensive condition-specific quality of life instruments for women with pelvic floor disorders. *Am J Obstet Gynecol.* 2001;185(6):1388–1395.

17. Schurch B, Stöhrer M, Kramer G, et al. Botulinum-A toxin for treating detrusor hyperreflexia in spinal cord injured patients: A new alternative to anticholinergic drugs? Preliminary results. *J Urol.* 2000;164:692–697.

18. Karsenty G, Denys P, Amarenco G, et al., Botulinum toxin-A (BTA) in the treatment of neurogenic detrusor overactivity incontinence (NDOI)—A prospective randomized study to compare 30 vs. 10 injection sites, in 35th Annual Meeting of the International Continence Society. Montreal; 2005.

19. Brubaker L, Richter HE, Visco A, et al. Refractory idiopathic urge urinary incontinence and botulinum A injection. *J Urol.* 2008;180:217–222.

20. Ghalayini I, Al-Ghazo M, Elnasser Z. Is the efficacy of repeated intradetrusorbotulinum neurotoxin type A (Dysport) injections dose dependent? Clinical and urodynamic results after four injections in patients with drug-resistant neurogenic detrusor overactivity. *Int Urol Nephrol.* 2009;41:805–813.

21. Giannantoni A, Conte A, Proietti S, et al. Botulinum toxin type A in patients with Parkinson's disease and refractory overactive bladder. *J Urol.* 2011;186:960–964.

22. Kuo H. Will suburothelial injection of small dose of botulinum A toxin have similar therapeutic effects and less adverse events for refractory detrusor overactivity? *Urology.* 2006;68(5): 993–998.

23. Smaldone MC, Ristau BT, Leng WW. Botulinum toxin therapy for neurogenic detrusor overactivity. *Urol Clin North Am.* 2010;37(4):567–580.

24. Bosch J. Electrical neuromodulatory therapy in female voiding dysfunction. *BJU Int.* 2006;98(Suppl 1):43–48.

25. Staskin DR, Peters KM, Macdiarmid S, et al. Percutaneous tibial nerve stimulation: A clinically and cost effective addition to the overactive bladder algorithm of care. *Curr Urol Rep.* 2012;13(5):327–334.

26. James R, Mahajan S. The prevalence of urinary catheterization among men and women with MS. (In Press).

27. Gulick E. Comparison of prevalance, related medical history, symptoms, and interventions regarding bowel dysfunction in persons with multiple sclerosis. *J Neurosci Nurs.* 2010;42: E12–E23.

28. Wiesel P, Norton C, Glickman S, Kamm MA. Pathophysiology and management of bowel dysfunction in multiple sclerosis. *Eur J Gastroenterol Hepatol.* 2001;13(4):441–448.

29. Awad R. Neurogenic bowel dysfunction in patients with spinal cord injury, myelomeningocele, multiple sclerosis and Parkinson's disease. *World J Gastroenterol.* 2011;17(46):5035–5048.

30. Gulick E, Namey M. Bowel dysfunction in persons with multiple sclerosis. In: Catto-Smith A, ed. *Constipation – Causes, Diagnosis and Treatment.* InTech; 2012.

31. Holland N, Kennedy P. Bowel management in multiple sclerosis. Clinical Bulletin: Information for Health Professionals; 2012.

32. Paris G, Gourcerol G, Leroi A. Management of neurogenic bowel dysfunction. *Eur J Phys Rehabil Med.* 2011;47(4):661–676.

33. McClurg D, Hagen S, Lowe-Strong A. Abdominal massage for the alleviation of constipation symptoms in people with multiple sclerosis: A randomized controlled feasibility study. *Mult Scler.* 2011;17(2):223–233.

34. Bywater A, While A. Management of bowel dysfunction in people with multiple sclerosis. *Br J Comm Nurs.* 2006;11(8):333–334.

26

Sexual Dysfunction and Other Autonomic Disorders in Multiple Sclerosis

ELIZABETH CRABTREE-HARTMAN

KEY POINTS FOR CLINICIANS

- Sexual dysfunction (SD) is common in both male and female patients with multiple sclerosis (MS), and SD occurs early in a substantial proportion of patients.

- Decreased libido is the most commonly reported SD among male and female MS patients.

- Primary SD refers to challenges that are a direct consequence of neurological dysfunction due to MS. Secondary SD refers to symptoms due to MS that in turn negatively affect one's sexual response. Tertiary SD refers to disability-related psychological, social, and cultural influences upon sexual functioning.

- MS patients with SD show greater pontine pathology on MRI.

- Data regarding sildenafil for erectile dysfunction in male MS patients are conflicting.

- Treatment of SD should employ a biopsychosocial construct. Likely, the neurologist will recruit input from other professionals.

- MS can cause cardiovascular abnormalities. This should be kept in mind when prescribing and managing disease-modifying therapies such as mitoxantrone or fingolimod.

The most common clinical manifestations of multiple sclerosis (MS) include visual, motor, sensory, and cognitive impairments. However, impact upon the autonomic nervous system is not uncommon, and can affect the urogenital tract, the gastrointestinal tract, and the cardiovascular system. Fatigue is also considered an autonomic feature of MS by some. While a comprehensive review is not possible in this setting, this chapter focuses on the diagnosis and management of sexual dysfunction (SD) and cardiovascular changes in MS.

SEXUAL DYSFUNCTION

Prevalence and Clinical Presentations

MS typically affects sexually active adults. SD is rare as a presenting feature in MS (5.6%) but commonly transpires during the course of the disease. SD is a common symptom for both sexes with prevalence rates varying from 40% to 80% in women and from 50% to 90% in men [1,2]. Prevalence appears to depend on the type of disease course, again with some variability. Estimates range from 68% to 77% of patients with relapsing-remitting MS (RRMS), 78% of patients with secondary progressive MS (SPMS), and 23% to 100% of patients with primary progressive MS (PPMS) reporting at least 1 form of SD [3,4]. While some evidence suggests a correlation with disease duration and increased age [2], substantial support exists for early onset of SD, and over 50% of women report SD 2 to 5 years after diagnosis [5]. Most data indicate a higher rate of SD among patients with MS compared to other chronic diseases and to healthy age-matched controls [6]. Furthermore, men report SD more than women in most cohorts [6,7], but not all data sets have demonstrated a significant difference between sexes [1]. While considerable overlap occurs in symptoms between MS patients and non-MS patients, and between male and female MS patients, distinct challenges are also appreciated (Table 26.1).

> MS patients have a higher rate of sexual dysfunction when compared to the general population and to other chronic diseases.

> Men report sexual dysfunction more than women in most cohorts.

SD in MS is sometimes regarded as primary, secondary, or tertiary. Primary SD refers to challenges that are a direct consequence of neurological dysfunction due to MS. Secondary SD refers to MS symptoms that in turn negatively affect the sexual response. Tertiary SD refers to disability-related psychological, social, and cultural influences on sexual functioning (Table 26.2).

Typically, the most common report among women with MS is decreased libido, reported by 60% to 80% [1,3]. Other common concerns include decreased vaginal lubrication, changes in vaginal sensation, difficulty reaching orgasm, and anorgasmia. Diminished sensation in erogenous zones may be a concern specific to the MS population (Table 26.1). Interestingly, the presence of decreased libido, decreased vaginal lubrication, and difficulty with reaching orgasm may not be different from age-matched patients with other chronic diseases [6]. This likely infers a causality that is multifactorial, rather than solely implicating the underlying pathophysiology of MS.

The most commonly reported concerns related to SD among men are decreased libido, impotence, incomplete erections, erectile dysfunction, and ejaculatory dysfunction. All of these symptoms are more common in patients with MS compared to healthy controls and age-matched patients with other chronic disease [6].

As noted, decreased libido is the most commonly reported symptom of SD by both men and women with MS. Libido, or sexual interest or drive, can be affected by a number of spheres outside of biology (Table 26.3). Libido can be affected by: partner availability, personal

> Many MS symptoms can negatively impact sexual relationships.

TABLE 26.1
SD in MS

	VERSUS THE	
GENERAL POPULATION	FEMALE MS PATIENTS	MALE MS PATIENTS
• Higher rate SD • Less masturbation • Diminished sensation	• Decreased libido • Less activity • Decreased sensation • Decreased lubrication • Delayed orgasm or anorgasmia	• Decreased libido • Erectile dysfunction • Ejaculatory dysfunction

TABLE 26.2
Primary, Secondary, and Tertiary SD

PRIMARY	SECONDARY	TERTIARY
Altered genital sensation	Fatigue	Altered self-image
Decreased libido	Muscle weakness	Low self-esteem
Problems with arousal and orgasm	Spasticity	Depression
Decreased vaginal lubrication	Impaired mobility	Anger
Erectile dysfunction	Tremor	Fear of rejection
	Incoordination	Feeling less attractive
	Sphincteric dysfunction	Guilt
	Cognitive problems	Shift in gender roles

TABLE 26.3

Factors Affecting Libido

- Partner availability
- Personal well-being/depression
- Socioeconomic circumstances
- Performance anxiety
- Medications

TABLE 26.4

MS Symptoms That May Negatively Affect Sexual Relationships

Fatigue
Depression
Spasticity
Motor weakness
Muscle spasms
Loss of sensation/dysesthesia
Pain
Anxiety regarding urinary/fecal incontinence
Side effects from medications

well-being/depression, socioeconomic circumstances, performance anxiety, and medications. Thus, MS may affect libido biologically, but it should also be noted that MS can negatively impact each of the domains listed.

In addition, many aspects of MS can negatively affect sexual relationships (Table 26.4). For both sexes, progressive symptoms rather than a relapsing-remitting course, disability measured by the Expanded Disability Status Scale, depression, anxiety, and fatigue correlate with more pronounced SD as measured by the Szaz Sexual Functioning Scale [1]. In this study, only men demonstrated a correlation between the Szaz Sexual Functioning Scale and employment status, as well as age. Women had a distinct correlate with cognitive impairment. Clinically, SD in patients with MS strongly correlates with bladder dysfunction [2,3]. Evidence is less robust for a correlation with pyramidal involvement [8] or with cerebellar dysfunction [9,10].

> Sexual dysfunction in patients with MS strongly correlates with bladder dysfunction.

MRI correlates for SD have been based on small numbers but interestingly show convergent evidence for pontine pathology as represented by atrophy measures and T1 lesion volume. In both studies, T2 lesion volume was not different between MS patients with SD and those without SD [11,12].

Several studies have demonstrated that patients with MS have a lower level of quality of life than healthy controls. Analysis of the impact of SD in patients with

MS on quality of life measures has been performed by 3 groups. These studies have differed in the patient populations studied in terms of geography, numbers, and disease duration. Nonetheless, all have disclosed a negative impact of SD in MS on multiple quality of life measures [1,5].

Treatment

A handful of queries have assessed pharmacological intervention for SD, specifically for male and female patients with MS. Evidence for the efficacy of sildenafil for the treatment of female SD in MS has thus far been negative [13] and data regarding sildenafil for erectile dysfunction in male MS patients are conflicting. An earlier trial studying 217 men (105 treatment, 113 placebo) disclosed 89% of patients reporting improved erections compared to 24% in the placebo group [14]. More recently, 33% of patients with MS receiving sildenafil and 18% receiving placebo reported improved erections, but this did not reach statistical significance [15]. Good data regarding pharmacological treatment of SD in MS are sadly thin. Therefore, formal recommendations regarding pharmacological address of SD specifically in the MS population are lacking. Furthermore, most cohorts have been largely heterosexual, and sexual function in gay, bisexual, transsexual, and transgender patients with MS has not undergone meaningful systematic study.

> Evidence regarding the efficacy of sildenafil for SD in women with MS has been negative so far.

Sexual function is a complex product of biological, psychological, societal, and interpersonal factors, and MS can negatively affect each of these arenas. Also, changes caused by perimenopause, menopause, and andropause will transpire for many patients with MS and can alter sexual function. Therefore, SD in the patient with MS likely represents a multifactorial process. As with non-MS patients, SD may be most appropriately approached with a biopsychosocial construct that addresses the interdependent aspects of sexuality.

Patients with SD may benefit from individual or couple counseling. Most neurologists and neurorehabilitation physicians have not had formal training in counseling and treatment of sexuality issues. However, the role of the caring physician in the management of SD in patients with MS is multifaceted (Table 26.5). A challenging but essential

> Although most neurologists do not have formal training in sexual dysfunction and the issues surrounding it, the neurologist plays an essential role in managing SD in MS patients.

TABLE 26.5
The Role of the Physician in Managing SD in MS Patients

Open the dialog regarding SD
Maximize disease-modifying therapy
Identify and address contributing MS symptoms (bladder,
 fatigue)
Streamline/minimize medication with untoward side effects on
 sexual function
Appropriate referral (urologist, gynecologist, couples counseling)

component is opening a dialog with patients regarding SD. Thereafter, the physician must identify areas of concern regarding sexual function, maximize address of disease activity and of contributing symptoms, streamline medications with an untoward impact on sexual function, and refer to appropriate consultation (urology, gynecology, counseling/psychology).

CARDIOVASCULAR CHANGES

Orthostatic hypotension may be present in up to 25% of patients, but is rarely a presenting feature in MS [16]. Management approaches specifically for MS have not been studied. Generic interventions such as adequate fluid intake and a diet with sufficient sodium may be of benefit.

> Specific management strategies for cardiovascular changes occurring with MS have not been studied.

Decreased heart rate variability and decreased blood pressure response to tilt table testing are common features of autonomic dysfunction in MS patients. The dysregulation correlates with MS lesion load in the brain stem as well as in the cerebral hemispheres, and is thought to manifest through brain stem reflex pathways. Baroreflex dysfunction in MS patients has been shown to be mediated through the cardiovagal limb of the baroreflex as well as sympathetic tone on blood vessels [17].

In a small study of 9 patients, POTS (postural orthostatic tachycardia syndrome) in MS patients most commonly was associated with symptoms of fatigue and dizziness. Therapeutic intervention included nonpharmacological interventions, such as increased dietary salt and fluid intake, aerobic exercise, and resistance training to improve lower extremity strength. Medications used included fludrocortisones, midodrine, pyrodostigmine, selective serotonin reuptake inhibitors, and modafinil. Two-thirds of patients experienced improvement in symptoms after therapeutic intervention in this small series [18].

Disease-modifying therapies such as mitoxantrone and fingolimod can affect cardiac function. Cardiovascular abnormalities may preclude the use of these agents or should warrant close monitoring of cardiac function during treatment.

Edema, limb discoloration, and acrocyanosis frequently accompany weakness, particularly in the lower extremities. Nonpharmacological address includes elevation of the affected limb(s), compression stockings, and regular exercise/movement of the affected limbs. Doppler studies may be indicated to rule out peripheral vascular insufficiency. Cilostazol, a platelet inhibitor, has been noted as a potential treatment, but has not been studied in MS [19].

Autonomic Dysreflexia

Autonomic dysreflexia is excessive sympathetic output that can occur in patients who have experienced myelitis at or above the sixth thoracic neurological level. An afferent stimulus, most commonly from the lower urinary tract, triggers a peripheral sympathetic response which results in vasoconstriction and hypertension. Normally, descending inhibitory signals would counteract the rise in blood pressure, but these are disrupted at the level of injury. Treatment of autonomic dysreflexia in other settings, such as traumatic spinal cord injury, includes the use of alpha adrenergic blockers. Therapeutics specific to MS patients have not been studied [20].

Sudomotor Changes

Sudomotor changes in MS include subclinical changes in sweating responses, as well as static changes in the limbs. Qualitative and quantitative data regarding sweating is convergent, and discloses decreased sweating responses in MS patients compared to healthy controls [21].

CONCLUSION

Autonomic dysfunction is not uncommon in MS, but often relies upon the physician to initiate a dialog regarding certain symptoms. Symptoms are often interdependent in MS, and this applies to autonomic features as well. Responsible symptom management must always begin with careful history taking, evaluation for contributing etiologies outside of MS, including medications, and strategizing to use pharmacological and nonpharmacological interventions that are individually tailored to each patient.

PATIENT CASE

A 42-year-old male patient with RRMS presents to clinic reporting erectile dysfunction. He is taking glatiramer acetate and has been without clinical relapse for over 1 year. On physical exam, he displays mild weakness in a pyramidal distribution in his legs accompanied by increased tone, hyperreflexia, and bilateral Babinski sign. Since his last visit, there have been subtle interval clinical changes (decreased strength and increased 25 foot walk time). How should his management be approached?

In general, new or escalating symptoms in an MS patient generate a differential of new MS activity, pseudoexacerbation, or pathology other than MS. This patient's exam suggests spinal cord involvement with recent worsening. His management should include a screen for typical triggers such as urinary tract infection (UTI), thyroid dysfunction, and a liver panel if on polypharmacy. If labs are negative, MR imaging can be considered and would include the brain and spinal cord. Disease-modifying therapy should be maximized and may be guided by test results. A testosterone level can also be sent. If found to be low, replacement should be guided by a urologist. Testosterone replacement can benefit erectile dysfunction and may have a positive effect upon MS. It should be noted that there is in vitro data suggesting a deleterious effect of testosterone upon induced excitotoxicity in oligodendrocytes, and testosterone replacement should be approached with caution. Small studies have shown that male patients with MS and erectile dysfunction can benefit from pharmacological address with sildenafil.

KEY POINTS FOR PATIENTS

- SD affects many men and women with MS.

- The most common symptom of SD in men and women with MS is decreased libido (sexual drive). Other problems include decreased sensation and lubrication in women, and erectile dysfunction in men.

- Many MS symptoms can interfere with sexual relationships, as well as other factors such as depression and side effects from medications.

- In addition to treating contributing symptoms, the management of SD often involves counseling.

- Medications used to treat erectile dysfunction have been used in men with MS with variable results.

- The effects of MS on blood circulation are not well understood. For example, swelling and discoloration of the skin can occur along with muscle weakness, particularly in the legs and feet.

REFERENCES

1. Tepavcevic DK, Kostic J, Basuroski ID, et al. The impact of sexual dysfunction on the quality of life measured by MSQoL-54 in patients with multiple sclerosis. *Mult Scler.* 2008;14(8):1131–1136.

2. Zivadinov R, Zorzon M, Bosco A, et al. Sexual dysfunction in multiple sclerosis, II: Correlation analysis. *Mult Scler.* 1999;5(6):428–431.

3. Demirikiran M, Sarica Y, Uguz S, et al. Multiple sclerosis patients with and without sexual dysfunction: Are there any differences? *Mult Scler.* 2006;12(2):209–214.

4. Zorzon M, Zivadinov R, Monti Bragadin L, et al. Sexual dysfunction in multiple sclerosis: A 2-year follow-up study. *J Neurol Sci.* 2001;187(1–2):1–5.

5. Nortvedt MW, Riise T, Frugard J, et al. Prevalence of bladder, bowel and sexual problems among multiple sclerosis patients two to five years after diagnosis. *Mult Scler.* 2007;13(1):106–112.

6. Zorzon M, Zivadinov R, Bosco A, et al. Sexual dysfunction in multiple sclerosis: A case-control study, I: Frequency and comparison of groups. *Mult Scler.* 1999;5(6):418–427.

7. Stenager E, Stenager EN, Jensen K. Sexual function in multiple sclerosis: A 5-year follow-up study. *Ital J Neurol Sci.* 1996;17(1):67–69.

8. Barak Y, Achiron A, Elizur A, et al. Sexual dysfunction in relapsing-remitting multiple sclerosis: Magnetic resonance imaging, clinical, and psychological correlates. *J Psychiatry Neurosci.* 1996;21(4):255–258.

9. Hulter BM, Lundberg PO. Sexual function in women with advanced multiple sclerosis. *J Neurol Neurosurg Psychiatry.* 1995;59(1):83–86.

10. Gruenwald I, Vardi Y, Gartman I, et al. Sexual dysfunction in females with multiple sclerosis: Quantitative sensory testing. *Mult Scler.* 2007;13(1):95–105.

11. Zivadinov R, Zorzon M, Locatelli L, et al. Sexual dysfunction in multiple sclerosis: A MRI, neurophysiological and urodynamic study. *J Neurol Sci.* 2003;210(1–2):73–76.

12. Zorzon M, Zivadinov R, Locatelli L, et al. Correlation of sexual dysfunction and brain magnetic resonance imaging in multiple sclerosis. *Mult Scler.* 2003;9(1):108–110.

13. Dasgupta R, Wiseman OJ, Kanabar G, et al. Efficacy of sildenafil in the treatment of female sexual dysfunction due to multiple sclerosis. *J Urol.* 2004;171(3):1189–1193.

14. Fowler CJ, Miller JR, Sharief MK, et al. A double blind, randomized study of sildenafil citrate for erectile dysfunction in men with multiple sclerosis. *J Neurol Neurosurg Psychiatry.* 2005;76(5):700–705.

15. Safarinejad MR. Evaluation of the safety and efficacy of sildenafil citrate for erectile dysfunction in men with multiple sclerosis: A double-blind, placebo controlled, randomized study. *J Urol.* 2009;181(1):252–258.

16. Merlelbach S, Dilmann U, Kolmel C, et al. Cardiovascular autonomic dysregulation and fatigue in multiple sclerosis. *Mult Scler.* 2001;7(5):327–334.

17. Sanya EO, Tutaj M, Brown CM, et al. Abnormal heart rate and blood pressure responses to baroreflex stimulation in multiple sclerosis patients. *Clin Auton Res.* 2005;15:213–218.

18. Kanjwal K, Karabin B, Kanjwal Y, Grubb B. Autonomic dysfunction presenting as postural orthostatic syndrome in patients with multiple sclerosis. *Int J Med Sci.* 2010;7(2):62–67.

19. Frohman TC, Castro W, Shah A, et al. Symptomatic therapy in MS. *Ther Adv Neurol Disord.* 2011;4(2):83–98.

20. Haensch C, Jorg J. Autonomic dysfunction in MS. *J Neurol.* 2006;253(Suppl 1):1/3–1/9.

21. Saari A, Tolonen U, Paakko E, et al. Sweating impairment in patients with multiple sclerosis. *Acta Neurol Scand.* 2009;120:358–363.

27

Spasticity Management in Multiple Sclerosis

FRANCOIS BETHOUX
MARY ALISSA WILLIS

KEY POINTS FOR CLINICIANS

- Spasticity, a component of the upper motor neuron syndrome, is a movement disorder characterized by a velocity-dependent increase in resistance to passive muscle stretch.

- Multiple sclerosis (MS) frequently causes spasticity, but the impact of spasticity in terms of discomfort and loss of function can be difficult to assess owing to other impairments (eg, paresis, neuropathic pain, ataxia).

- Spasticity can help maintain function by compensating for loss of motor control (eg, lower extremity extensor hypertonia and spasms facilitate standing).

- Spasticity treatment planning involves taking into account patient symptoms (eg, muscle stiffness/tightness, muscle spasms) and examination findings (eg, resistance to passive movement, range of motion limitations, observed spasms and clonus), and defining realistic goals.

- Muscle stretching and rehabilitation (physical/occupational therapy) must be considered when treating spasticity, alone or in combination with other treatments.

Spasticity is a movement disorder characterized by a velocity-dependent increase in resistance to passive muscle stretching related to increased tonic and phasic stretch reflexes [1]. The presumed pathophysiological mechanism is a lack of descending inhibitory control on spinal cord neurons due to central nervous system (CNS) damage. Spasticity is a component of the upper motor neuron syndrome, which also includes weakness, loss of selective voluntary motor control, loss of dexterity, muscle spasms, synkinesis, and hyperreflexia.

The prevalence of spasticity in multiple sclerosis (MS) is high, with objective signs of spasticity noted in close to 60% of patients [2]. Symptoms of spasticity were reported by 84% of responders in a survey from the North American Research Committee on MS (NARCOMS), with 34% of responders rating the symptoms as moderate, severe, or total [3].

EVALUATING SPASTICITY

Symptoms reported by the patient or a caregiver are essential in screening for spasticity (see Table 27.1). Beyond the basic symptoms, information should be sought about how spasticity impacts the patient's (and caregivers') activities and quality of life, asking for precise examples. For instance, painful spasms at night may disrupt sleep and cause increased fatigue the next day; stiffness in the hip adductors may interfere with hygiene and with the ability to perform intermittent catheterization; stiffness in the arms may interfere with the ability to get dressed, either independently or with the help of a caregiver. However, the description of symptoms can be misleading. For example, a patient may report that a limb is "stiff" because of difficulty voluntarily moving the affected limb, which is actually related to weakness without increase in tone. Paresthesias and neuropathic pain can be associated with a sensation of spasms, without involuntary muscle contraction on examination. Pain in MS is often multifactorial (neuropathic pain, musculoskeletal from abnormal posture and movement, pain from spasticity). A detailed interview, and the response to empirical symptomatic therapies, can help determine if the pain is likely to be primarily related to spasticity.

Examination is key in confirming the presence of spasticity, assessing its severity, and identifying other pertinent neurological impairments (see Table 27.2). Dynamic phenomena ("spastic catch," abnormal movement patterns, spasms, clonus) are related to hyperexcitable reflexes, while static phenomena (decreased range of motion, fixed deformity) are related to changes in the rheological properties of musculoskeletal structures. In some patients, hypertonia is minimal at rest and becomes severe and bothersome with voluntary movement; therefore, spasticity should be assessed at rest (sitting or lying down) and with activity. Spasticity must be distinguished from other causes of abnormal muscle tone, particularly dystonia and extrapyramidal hypertonia (both more rarely encountered in MS). A complete neurological examination is warranted, as other impairments are likely to contribute to the patient's functional limitations.

> Although screening for spasticity relies on patient-reported symptoms, the diagnosis must be confirmed by physical examination.

Spasticity is most often evaluated by recording the signs and symptoms listed during a standard neurological examination. More standardized, quantitative clinician- or patient-reported measures are available to enhance outcome assessment (see Table 27.2). The Ashworth Scale, in its standard or modified versions, is widely used despite known limitations [4,5]. Proper training is required to ensure inter and intrarelater reliability. Other measures of impairment and activity are important to consider, depending on the treatment goals (eg, range of motion, muscle strength, pain, walking performance tests, upper extremity function tests, generic quality of life measures).

MANAGEMENT OF SPASTICTY

While spasticity management does not alter MS disease activity, the use of disease therapies and treatment of spasticity-related symptoms are complementary in the overall management of patients with MS. The goals of spasticity management include:

- providing relief of symptoms;
- improving posture;
- improving function and/or ease of care (sometimes called "passive function");
- preventing long-term complications (eg, fixed contractures, decubiti).

Realistic goals should be discussed with patients and care providers early on.

A summary of treatment modalities is provided in Table 27.3. Muscle stretching must be a part of the treatment plan (except in rare cases where it is contraindicated). Although the rationale for the use of rehabilitation in the

TABLE 27.1
Symptoms and Signs Commonly Associated With Spasticity and the Upper Motor Neuron Syndrome

Symptoms

Muscle stiffness or tightness
Difficulty performing voluntary movement
Clonus (sometimes described by patients as "shaking" or "tremor")
Muscle spasms
Pain (associated with spasms, stiffness, or passive movement)
Limb deformity
Difficulty attaining or maintaining adequate trunk and limb posture
Reported by caregivers: difficulty moving the limbs passively, difficult performing hygiene and care

Clinical Findings

Velocity-dependent resistance to passive mobilization
"Clasp-knife" phenomenon (initial resistance to passive movement followed by sudden relaxation as the
    muscle continues to be stretched)
Abnormal limb or trunk posture, musculoskeletal deformity
Decreased passive range of motion
Hyperreflexia with or without clonus
Spastic cocontraction of agonist and antagonist muscles
Synergistic movement patterns
Flexor or extensor muscle spasms
Weakness
Loss of dexterity

TABLE 27.2
Outcome Measures for Spasticity Management

NAME	PURPOSE	MEASUREMENT SCALE AND COMMENTS
Clinical Measures		
Ashworth Scale (and modified versions)	To assess spasticity via resistance to passive movement	Applied to individual muscle groups; from 0 = no resistance to 4 = limb rigid in flexion or extension for each muscle or muscle group tested
Tardieu Scale	To assess spasticity via resistance to passive movement at 3 different speeds	R1: angle to first point of resistance during a fast stretch R2: angle to maximum range of motion during slow passive movement within physiological limits R2–R1 defines "dynamic tone"
Resistance to passive movement (REPAS) Scale	To assess spasticity via resistance to passive movement	Same rating scale as the Ashworth Scale, but examination and rating instructions are more standardized Predefined list of 26 passive movements to be tested Total score from 0 to 104
Patient Self-Report Measures		
Spasm Frequency Scale (SFS)	To assess spasticity via spasm frequency	Ordinal scale from 0 = no spasm to 4 = more than 10 spontaneous spasms per hour
Spasticity Numeric Rating Scale (NRS)	To assess the overall severity of spasticity	Ordinal scale from 0 = no spasticity, to 10 = worst possible spasticity
MS Spasticity Scale-88 (MSSS-88)	To assess the impact of spasticity (how much patients are bothered by consequences of spasticity)	For each of 88 items, from 1 = not at all bothered, to 4 = extremely bothered Total score from 88 to 352

management of spasticity is mostly empirical, skilled rehabilitation strategies should be considered, particularly when improvement of active function is sought. Management frequently involves a combination of complementary modalities to achieve the desired outcome. The Multiple Sclerosis Council for Clinical Practice Guidelines published evidence-based recommendations for the management of spasticity in MS and proposed a decision algorithm [6].

> Stretching should be taught to all patients with spasticity or their caregivers, and should be performed daily.

Oral antispasticity agents (Table 27.4) are widely used, although clinical trial evidence to support the efficacy of these medications in MS is limited [7]. Some of these symptomatic medications are used off label. The Multiple Sclerosis Council guidelines recommend baclofen and tizanidine as effective, first-line medications for spasticity. Monotherapy, in conjunction with stretching, is often at least partially effective for mild to moderate spasticity, although side effects can be a limiting factor, even with low doses. Dose escalation and combination of medications for severe spasticity are often limited by worsening sedation, increased weakness, or cognitive symptoms. Other considerations in choosing pharmacotherapy include cost, medication interactions, comorbidities, and the patient's ability to follow instructions and to follow-up with the care provider. Antispasticity medications are usually started at a low dose and gradually titrated to limit side effects. Some of these medications should not be abruptly discontinued

(eg, baclofen). Table 27.4 summarizes the dosing and considerations for the most commonly used medications. It should be kept in mind that some other medications commonly used in MS can cause worsening of spasticity (eg, interferon beta, selective serotonin re-uptake inhibitors [SSRIs]). Many other symptomatic medications may cause sedation or weakness (eg, amitriptyline, anticholinergics for bladder management).

> When prescribing oral medications for spasticity, slow dose titration is recommended to minimize side effects.

Local treatments such as injection of anesthetic agents, chemical neurolysis, or botulinum toxin (BT) may facilitate stretching, improve comfort, and improve function by relaxing specific muscles or muscle groups. Owing to their transient effects, local anesthetics (lidocaine, etidocaine, bupivacaine) are sometimes used to evaluate the potential benefit of longer lasting procedures such as chemical neurolysis (eg, phenol blocks) or chemodenervation (eg, BT injections). Chemical neurolysis produces a much longer lasting (up to 36 months) nerve block by damaging nerve structures. Potential side effects include chronic dysesthesias.

Three formulations of BT-A (abobotulinum toxin A, onabotulinum toxin A, incobotulinum toxin A) and 1 formulation of BT-B (rimabotulinum toxin B) are available in the United States. Intramuscular BT injections are widely used to treat spasticity, despite the fact that only onabotulinum toxin A has obtained FDA approval on a limited number of upper extremity muscles (therefore, BT injections in the lower

TABLE 27.3
Summary of Treatment Modalities for Spasticity

TREATMENT	INDICATIONS	POTENTIAL ADVERSE EFFECTS/COMMENTS
Rehabilitation/exercise (eg, stretching, serial casting, splinting, orthotics, electrical stimulation, functional training)	Can be used across the spectrum of spasticity severity Should be considered in combination with all other treatment modalities	Tolerance to exercise and rehabilitation can be limited in MS
Oral medications (eg, baclofen, tizanidine, dantrolene sodium, benzodiazepines)	Can be used across the spectrum of spasticity severity Starting at a low dose and titrating slowly is advised Medications can be combined, with close attention to cumulative side effects	Side effects include sedation, weakness, cognitive slowing, and liver toxicity for some medications
Local treatments (phenol/alcohol injections, BT injections)	To treat focal spasticity, or to address a focal problem related to diffuse spasticity Duration of effect: up to 36 months with phenol, usually 3 months with BT	Phenol/alcohol injections: local side effects (pain, chronic dysesthesia) BT injections: local side effects (pain, weakness, atrophy); systemic side effects (nausea, fatigue, respiratory infections, dysphagia, development of neutralizing antibodies, rare severe generalized side effects)
Neuromodulation (intrathecal baclofen therapy)	To treat severe diffuse spasticity refractory to oral medications and stretching A screening test should be performed to help with decision making and to refine expectation	Complications from surgery and anesthesia, wound dehiscence, pseudomeningocele, infection around the device, catheter malfunction, pump malfunction, baclofen withdrawal or overdose
Orthopedic surgery (tendon release, tendon transfer, osteotomy)	To address contractures and deformities resulting from spasticity These procedures are rarely used in MS	Complications include delayed healing and infection. A period of immobilization is usually required It is important to optimize spasticity control before performing orthopedic surgery
Neurosurgery (neurotomy, selective dorsal rhizotomy)	To decrease spasticity by decreasing nerve input These procedures are rarely used in MS	Sensory loss, paresthesias, weakness

TABLE 27.4
Oral Antispasticity Agents

MEDICATION	DOSE	ADVERSE EFFECTS	COMMENTS
Baclofen	Start: 5 to 10 mg/day Max: 80 mg/day in 3 to 4 divided doses per FDA recommendation, higher doses are used in practice as tolerated	Sedation, increased fatigue, confusion, dizziness, muscle weakness	Withdrawal: muscle stiffness, paresthesias, hallucinations, confusion, fever, seizures Overdose: hypotonia, respiratory depression, hypotension, coma Reduce dose in patients with impaired renal function
Tizanidine	Start: 2 to 4 mg/day Max: 36 mg/day in 3 to 4 divided doses	Sedation, dry mouth, dizziness, hypotension, elevated liver enzymes, hallucinations, muscle weakness	May potentiate effects of antihypertensive agents Reduce dose when given with fluoroquinolones (ie, ciprofloxacin)
Benzodiazepines	Diazepam: Start: 2 mg qhs Max: 30 mg/day in 3 to 4 divided doses Clonazepam: Start: 0.5 mg qhs Max: 2 mg/day	CNS depression, muscle weakness	Withdrawal: anxiety, tremor, agitation, insomnia, seizures Overdose: respiratory depression, coma Often prescribed to relieve nocturnal spasms Frequently used to treat baclofen withdrawal
Gabapentin	Start: 100 to 300 mg/day Max: 3600 mg/day in 3 to 4 divided doses	Nystagmus, diplopia, somnolence, ataxia, dizziness, peripheral edema, depression, and suicidal ideation	Secondary antispasticity agent Most useful in patients with paresthesias or neuropathic pain in addition to spasticity Reduce dose in patients with impaired renal function
Dantrolene sodium	Start: 25 mg/day Max: 400 mg/day in 4 divided doses	Sedation, GI symptoms, muscle weakness, hepatotoxicity	Potential for severe liver toxicity and the risk of weakness limit clinical use Fatal hepatitis in 0.3%. Follow liver function periodically Use lowest effective dose
Levetiracetam	Start: 250 mg/day Max: 3000 mg/day. Usually given twice daily	Sedation, confusion, nausea, depression, and suicidal ideation	Secondary antispasticity agent Was found to be effective on phasic signs of spasticity (spasms) but not on tonic signs of spasticity (resistance to passive movement) in a retrospective chart review of 12 MS patients Reduce dose in patients with impaired renal function
Clonidine	Start: 0.1 mg/day Max: 0.2 mg twice daily Transdermal patch is available	Bradycardia, hypotension, drowsiness, dry mouth, constipation, dizziness, pedal edema, depression	Secondary antispasticity agent Use with caution in patients with dysautonomia Avoid abrupt cessation because of possible rebound autonomic symptoms
Cyproheptadine	Start: 4 mg/day Max: 24 mg/day in 3 divided doses	Sedation, dry mouth, dizziness, weight gain	Cyproheptadine is used to alleviate the symptoms of baclofen withdrawal Reduce dose in patients with renal impairment

221

extremities are off label). The Therapeutics and Technology Assessment Subcommittee of the American Academy of Neurology concluded that BT is effective on upper and lower limb spasticity in reducing muscle tone and improving passive function (level A recommendation), and probably effective in improving active function (level B recommendation) in adults [8]. BT is injected into a spastic muscle, preferably with electromyography (EMG) or electrical stimulation guidance (more rarely with ultrasound guidance), even though there is no published evidence showing that guidance leads to improved outcomes [8]. There are few publications reporting on the efficacy and tolerability of BT therapy in MS, but data from other patient populations is consistent with clinical experience with MS patients. The therapeutic effect typically appears after 24 to 72 hours, peaks at 2 to 4 weeks, and usually lasts 10 weeks or more. Injections are typically repeated at 12 weeks. More frequent injections and use of high doses have been linked to the development of anti-BT antibodies with loss of clinical efficacy. It is estimated that BT diffuses approximately 30 mm around the injection site. Systemic side effects are uncommon, usually non-life threatening (eg, nausea, fatigue, dysphagia), and reversible, although severe complications (including generalized weakness, diplopia, severe dysphagia, urinary incontinence, respiratory compromise, in some cases leading to death) from spread of toxin effect have been reported. In addition, in recent trials of onabotulinum toxin A for upper extremity spasticity in the United States, more frequent respiratory infections were reported with active treatment compared to placebo.

> Intramuscular injections of BT can help with focal spasticity, or when focal areas are targeted (eg, difficulty opening the hand due to finger flexor spasticity, foot drop, hip adductor spasticity).

Intrathecal baclofen (ITB) is approved by the FDA for the treatment of severe spasticity of spinal or cerebral origin refractory to oral antispasticity medications or when such medications are not tolerated. Administration of ITB reduces the incidence of CNS sedation compared to oral baclofen by allowing effective cerebrospinal fluid (CSF) concentrations to be achieved with much smaller doses of baclofen. The medication is delivered directly into the intrathecal space via a programmable infusion system consisting of a battery-powered pump implanted subcutaneously in the lower abdominal wall and an intraspinal catheter (tip at the lower thoracic level usually) tunneled subcutaneously to the pump. The total daily dose and rate of administration of baclofen can be adjusted noninvasively via an external programming device. The benefits of ITB therapy in MS were reported in several publications [9–11]. Potential complications were also well documented, and include complications from surgery, wound dehiscence, pseudomeningocele and CSF leak, infection, system malfunction, and baclofen withdrawal and overdose. In order to optimize outcomes, best practices should be followed [12]. A bolus test injection (usually 25 to 100 mcg of ITB), should be performed in all patients (continuous infusion trials via an externalized intraspinal catheter are less commonly performed). It is critical that the patient and

proxies understand their role in communicating with health care providers, the importance of routine follow-up visits for refills, the symptoms and signs of baclofen withdrawal and overdose, and instructions for emergency situations.

> Intrathecal baclofen therapy is approved for severe spasticity refractory to first-line spasticity treatments. Thorough patient evaluation and education is warranted to optimize outcomes.

OTHER CONSIDERATIONS

Spasticity increases with stress and noxious stimuli (eg, pain, decubiti, urinary tract infection, and even ingrown toenail), and usually exhibits spontaneous fluctuations (typically increasing at night). Variations in ambient and core body temperature have been anecdotally reported to affect spasticity. For example, colder temperatures are often associated with increased spasticity.

It is important to remember that spasticity can also have beneficial consequences. For example, a patient may use extensor tone to stand and perform pivot transfers, which would otherwise be compromised by severe paraparesis. It is also believed that spasticity may decrease the risk of deep venous thrombosis and pressure ulcers by maintaining muscle tone in paralyzed muscles.

> The role of spasticity in compensating for weakness must be taken into account when planning spasticity management.

CONCLUSION

Spasticity is a common cause of discomfort and functional limitation in patients with multiple sclerosis. Successful spasticity management requires thorough assessments, a realistic treatment plan, and often multidisciplinary care. Key considerations before designing a spasticity management plan include:

- severity of resistance to passive movement;
- severity of spasms and clonus;
- pain with passive or active movement, or with spasms;
- dynamic versus resting spasticity;
- other neurological impairments (particularly weakness) that can impact function;
- degree of reliance on spasticity to perform critical functions (eg, transfers);
- complications related to spasticity (eg, contractures, maceration, skin breakdown);
- other factors contributing to spasticity (eg, recurrent urinary tract infections);
- patient's human and physical environment;
- patient/caregiver goals.

PATIENT CASE 1

Ms. D, a 31-year-old right-handed mother of 3 young children, presents with left spastic hemiparesis in the context of relapsing-remitting MS. She walks with no assistive device. Her main complaint is muscle spasms in the left toes, which are painful, and interfere with her ability to walk (she needs to stop and stretch her toes when the spasms occur). She also reports muscle stiffness in the left leg, and to a lesser degree in the left arm. On examination, there is left-sided weakness, mild in the left upper extremity (muscle testing 4 to 5/5), moderate in the left lower extremity (muscle testing 3 to 4/5). There is mild resistance to passive movement in the left upper and lower extremities, with the exception of the left ankle plantarflexors, where resistance to passive movement is severe (3/4 on the Modified Ashworth Scale [5]) with decreased range of motion in the left ankle/foot. Gait is hemiparetic with decreased left foot clearance due to foot drop and decreased active hip and knee flexion. Constant flexion of the toes upon standing and walking quickly becomes painful and forces the patient to rest. She walks 25 feet in 12 seconds.

Question: Does the patient need an intervention on her spasticity, and if so, what could be the main goals?

Answer: Based on the patient's complaints and examination findings, it appears that spasticity management could be beneficial, with the following broad goals: to reduce discomfort and pain associated with muscle spasms in the toes, and to facilitate walking. These goals should be discussed with the patient, along with the fact that weakness also contributes to the gait disturbance.

Question: Which first-line interventions can be offered?

Answer: The patient needs to start on a stretching regimen to improve or preserve range of motion in the left upper and lower extremities. She may benefit from wearing a left ankle-foot orthosis (AFO), and needs strengthening and gait training. To implement these interventions, a referral to physical therapy should be considered. It is also reasonable to discuss a symptomatic medication for spasticity (such as baclofen or tizanidine), starting with a low dose and with slow titration, as sedation and increased weakness could interfere with daytime activities.

Question: The patient attends several physical therapy sessions. She now stretches several times per day and exercises on a regular basis. She was unable to tolerate a left AFO owing to her toe spasms. She started on baclofen, but could not increase the dose beyond 10 mg twice daily because of sedation. At that dose, her stiffness and spasms were not controlled so she discontinued the medication. Neurological examination is stable. The patient is frustrated because the spasms and pain in her toes prevent her from walking long distances and interfere with her ability to take care of her children. The physical therapist states that the patient is not able to fully perform the exercises because of her spasticity. Can other treatment options be offered?

Answer: Because the main problems related to spasticity are focal in the distal left lower extremity, it is reasonable to consider BT therapy (off-label use). Physical therapy should be continued after BT injections to allow further gait training.

Question: BT injections are administered in the left gastrocnemius, tibialis posterior, and toe flexor muscles. Toe spasms and pain "improved 85%" for 6 weeks, then gradually returned. She has been able to wear a left AFO, and does not catch her left foot as much. On examination, strength is stable; resistance to passive movement is improved in the ankle plantarflexors (from 3/4 to 2/4 on the Modified Ashworth Scale). Gait is improved with better left foot clearance. She walks 25 feet in 10 seconds (20% improvement). What is the next step?

Answer: The response from the first injection session is encouraging, but the duration of effect was relatively short, and there was only partial relief of toe spasms and pain. We recommend repeat BT injections with a higher dose, to continue with stretching and exercise, and to continue wearing the AFO. At this point, it is important to continue spasticity management, in the context of a chronic disease with high risk of worsening of disability over time.

PATIENT CASE 2

Ms. H. is a 37-year-old woman with primary progressive MS. She was diagnosed with MS when leg stiffness and weakness failed to improve after cervical decompression and fusion. After a period of physical exertion, she develops low back pain, increased stiffness in the legs and spasms in the left leg. Her left knee is "locked up in a bent position." Examination shows spastic paraparesis, worse in the left leg than the right. Stiffness and spasms persist despite treatment with oral baclofen and tizanidine.

Question: Ms. H. describes symptoms of spasticity that limit function and produce significant discomfort despite maximally tolerated doses of two oral antispasticity agents. What modalities could be added to help reduce pain and possibly improve function?

Answer: She should start a stretching regimen to preserve and improve range of motion. A referral for physical therapy evaluation would also be appropriate. Injection of BT in the left hamstrings (off label) may reduce spasms and when combined with physical therapy, improve the passive and active extension of the left knee.

Question: BT injections administered in the left hamstrings reduced pain by 50% and facilitated extension of the left knee. One month later, however, she develops severe extensor spasms in both legs, and her left knee is "locked up in an extended position." She complains of pain when she moves her legs, rated 8/10. On examination, there is severe resistance to passive movement in the legs, rated 3/4 on the Modified Ashworth Scale. Muscle testing is difficult to perform, but shows moderate diffuse weakness most severe at the hip flexors (3/5) and the tibialis anterior (3/5). She performs the timed 25 foot walk (T25FW) in 42 seconds using a rollator. She continues physical therapy and oral antispasticity agents. What other options should be considered?

Answer: Ms. H. now has severe diffuse spasticity with worsening pain and marginal ambulation. The examination does not reveal any obvious targets for local injections. Discussion of ITB therapy is appropriate.

Question: A test injection of ITB 50 mcg is performed. The following pre- and postinjection measures are reported. Is the patient a good candidate for ITB therapy?

	PREINJECTION		POSTINJECTION	
Pain	8/10		2/10	
T25FW	42 s		25.6 s	
Manual Muscle Testing*				
Hip flexors	4	2	3	2
Knee flexors	3	1	4	2
Knee extensors	3	3	3	4
Dorsiflexors	4	2	4	2
Spasticity (Modified Ashworth Scale)**				
Hip adductors	3	3	2	2
Knee flexors	3	3	1	3
Knee extensors	3	3	1	1
Plantarflexors	3	3	2	3

*Range 0 to 5, with higher scores indicating better strength.
**Range 0 to 4, with higher scores indicating more severe spasticity.

Answer: She chose to proceed with ITB pump surgery after the successful test injection. Following surgery, she experienced marked relief of spasticity, and after intensive rehabilitation her gait pattern improved. One year after pump placement, she reports that comfort and walking are significantly improved. She still has difficulty abducting the legs and discomfort on the inside of the thighs. Examination reveals mild to moderate spasticity in the legs with the exception of a Modified Ashworth Scale score of 3 in the hip adductors on both sides. She walks 25 feet in 17.6 seconds using a rollator and a left AFO. Her gait has a scissoring appearance.

Question: This patient has overall good results with ITB therapy, physical therapy, and orthotics. Is there a role for other modalities in fine-tuning her spasticity management?

Answer: The dose of ITB was increased to address the residual spasticity in the hip adductors, but this caused increased leg weakness and difficulty walking, so was returned to the previous dose. BT injections were performed in the hip adductors bilaterally, which helped decrease pain, improve range of motion, and improve gait pattern. She continues to stretch and swim daily.

KEY POINTS FOR PATIENTS AND FAMILIES

- Many people with MS have spasticity, a type of muscle tightness that affects the control of movement.

- Other symptoms associated with spasticity include muscle spasms and a repetitive involuntary "shaking" called clonus which often happens in the ankle.

- Spasticity does not equal weakness, though these often come together.

- Spasticity may cause discomfort and difficulty with usual activities.

- Treatment for spasticity begins with physical measures such as stretching and physical therapy.

- Certain medicines may reduce spasticity, although side effects may limit the ability to increase the dose.

- Botulinum toxin A is an injection treatment which is FDA-approved for the treatment of spasticity in the upper extremity (arm and hand), although it is also used off label in the lower extremity.

- Implanting a programmable pump under the skin to deliver baclofen in the spinal fluid may be useful for hard-to-treat severe spasticity.

REFERENCES

1. Lance J. Symposium synopsis. In: Feldman RG, Young RR, Koella WP, eds. *Spasticity: Disordered Motor Control.* Chicago: Year Book Medical Publishers; 1980:485–494.

2. Matthews B. Symptoms and signs of multiple sclerosis. In: Compston A, Ebers G, Lassmann H, et al. eds. *Mc Alpine's Multiple Sclerosis.* London: Churchill Livingstone; 1998.

3. Rizzo M, Hadjimichael O, Preiningerova J, Vollmer T. Prevalence and treatment of spasticity reported by multiple sclerosis patients. *Mult Scler.* 2004;10:589–595.

4. Ashworth B. Preliminary trial of carisoprodol in multiple sclerosis. *Practitioner.* 1964;192:540–542.

5. Bohannon R, Smith M. Inter-rater reliability of a modified Ashworth scale of muscle spasticity. *Phys Ther.* 1987;67:206–207.

6. Multiple Sclerosis Council for Clinical Practice Guidelines. Spasticity management in multiple sclerosis. Consortium of Multiple Sclerosis Centers; 2003.

7. Shakespeare D, Young C, Boggild M. Anti-spasticity agents for multiple sclerosis. *Cochrane Database Syst Rev.* 2009;4.

8. Simpson DM, Gracies JM, Graham HK, et al. Assessment: Botulinum neurotoxin for the treatment of spasticity (an evidence-based review): Report of the Therapeutics and Technology Assessment Subcommittee of the American Academy of Neurology. *Neurology.* 2008;70:1691–1698.

9. Stempien L, Tsai T. Intrathecal baclofen pump use for spasticity. *Am J Phys Med Rehab.* 2000;79:536–541.

10. Azouvi P, Mane M, Thiebaut J, et al. Intrathecal baclofen administration for control of severe spinal spasticity: Functional improvement and long-term follow-up. *Arch Phys Med Rehab.* 1996;77:35–39.

11. Zahavi A, Geertzen JHB, Middel B, et al. Long term effect (more than five years) of intrathecal baclofen on impairment, disability, and quality of life in patients with severe spasticity of spinal origin. *J Neurol Neurosurg Psychiatry.* 2004;75:1553–1557.

12. Ridley B, Korth Rawlins P. Intrathecal baclofen therapy: Ten steps towards best practice. *J Neurosci Nursing.* 2006;38:72–82.

28

Multiple Sclerosis and Ambulation

FRANCOIS BETHOUX
KEITH McKEE

KEY POINTS FOR CLINICIANS

- Ambulation limitations are a frequent consequence of MS, affecting up to 75% of persons with MS over the course of the disease.

- Gait abnormalities may occur early in the disease, even before a gait disturbance can be identified on examination.

- Ambulation limitations have a profound impact on an individual's ability to function and quality of life.

- Ambulation is affected by multiple neurological impairments and comorbidities, sometimes making it difficult to identify targets for intervention.

- A variety of tools are available to assess ambulation in patients with MS. Timed tests such as the timed 25 foot walk are useful in a clinical setting.

- There is a growing body of evidence showing the effects of rehabilitation/exercise, medications, and assistive devices on walking performance.

MULTIPLE SCLEROSIS AND AMBULATION

Health care providers involved in the care of patients with multiple sclerosis (MS) are well aware that MS frequently affects ambulation. Indeed, the tests and scales most commonly used to monitor the disease course involve some aspect of walking, including walking speed in the timed 25 foot walk (T25FW), walking distance and use of an assistive device in the Expanded Disability Status Scale (EDSS). Walking limitations are one of the most visible consequences of the disease. Only recently have more detailed data on the prevalence and impact of walking limitations in MS become available. An estimated 75% of persons with MS (PwMS) experience a limitation of their ability to walk or of their mobility over the course of the disease [1,2]. In

a recent survey among over 1,000 PwMS, 41% reported having difficulty walking [3].

Several publications underscore the importance of walking limitations, and their profound impact on the lives of PwMS. Lower limb function was ranked first among 12 bodily functions within a population of 162 PwMS, whether the duration of their disease was under 5 years or over 15 years [4]. Abnormal gait parameters are correlated with patient-reported ability to perform activities of daily living [5]. Walking limitations have been linked to unemployment [6]. However, in the large survey mentioned above, 39% of PwMS stated that they rarely or never discussed this problem with their physician, suggesting that walking limitations are not always addressed in the health care setting [3].

What Causes Ambulation Limitations in MS?

There are multiple causes to walking limitations in MS. The primary etiology is the damage caused to the central nervous system (CNS) by the disease process. Among neurological impairments, abnormal motor control (paresis, spasticity, ataxia) in the lower extremities is the most obvious offender. Indeed, studies have reported a correlation between gait limitations and muscle weakness [7] or spasticity [8]. Often, other impairments contribute to the problem, such as loss of sensation in the lower extremities, motor and sensory loss in the upper extremities (impacts gait pattern and interferes with the ability to use assistive devices), visual disturbance, and cognitive impairment.

The impact of cognitive impairment is demonstrated through the common deterioration in walking performance while performing a cognitive task, more so than in healthy controls [9]. Dual-tasking also leads to deterioration of spatiotemporal parameters of gait [10], even at the early stage of the disease [11]. These observations suggest that MS patients with gait disturbance need to consciously "focus on their legs" to preserve their ability to walk and to avoid falling.

> Cognitive impairment and comorbidities should be assessed when managing ambulation limitations.

The relationship between walking performance and fatigue is more complex. Even though some studies report a correlation between self-reported fatigue and altered gait parameters [12], other studies failed to demonstrate a significant change in walking performance on timed tests over the course of the day, despite a worsening in self-reported fatigue [13]. This observation may indicate that motor fatigue is not always correlated with the subjective sensation of fatigue.

> The sensation of fatigue does not always correlate with changes in walking performance.

The role of comorbidities in walking limitations should not be overlooked. As they age, patients with MS may develop the same musculoskeletal disorders as the general population (osteoarthritis, back pain, osteoporosis). Moreover, MS can indirectly increase the risk of musculoskeletal comorbidities. For example, an abnormal gait pattern may cause early osteoarthritis of the lower extremities and low back pain because of abnormal body mechanics, and osteoporosis may develop as a consequence of decreased mobility. Addressing these problems may result in significant improvement of walking performance, even if neurological impairments remain unchanged. Conversely, addressing abnormal gait patterns early is important in limiting the risk of musculoskeletal complications.

Other comorbidities may also have an impact. Marrie et al. analyzed data on 8,983 individuals with MS in the North American Research Committee on Multiple Sclerosis Registry and found that the presence of cardiovascular comorbidities increased the risk of ambulatory disability [14]. Even depression, a frequent comorbidity in MS, may impact ambulation by decreasing a patient's motivation to walk and to exercise.

Walking and Falls

The issue of imbalance and falls cannot be overlooked in a discussion about walking and MS. The incidence of falls is high in MS. Cattaneo et al. reported that 54% of individuals in a convenience sample of 50 MS patients had experienced a fall in the past year, and 32% of those had fallen 2 or more times [15]. Other studies reported comparable numbers [16]. Many risk factors for falling have been identified, including a higher level of disability, impaired mobility, imbalance, cognitive impairment, bladder dysfunction, and fear of falling [17]. The use of an assistive device is associated with an increased risk of falling [15], but this is seen as an indication that a higher level of disability is a risk factor for falling, rather than a direct adverse effect of assistive devices. The main concern related to falls is the occurrence of injuries, particularly fractures [18,19], which are more frequent in patients with a higher level of disability, but may also occur early in the disease course [20]. Since decreased mobility is also associated with an increased risk of osteoporosis, it is essential to perform bone density testing and initiate interventions to reduce fall risk in patients who report falls or are at high risk of falling.

> Patients with MS and ambulation limitations should be asked systematically about falls.

ASSESSING AMBULATION

In order to address walking limitations, it is helpful for health care professionals to identify the problem and assess its severity. A variety of measures are available, although only some have been fully validated in MS (Table 28.1) [21].

Simple questions such as "How is your walking?" are a great way to start the conversation, but are usually not enough to determine the extent of the problem and develop a treatment plan. Specific information should be sought about the amount of walking actually performed (eg, "Do you walk every day?"; "Do you walk outside your home?"; "How far can you walk without stopping?"), including the use of assistive devices or other support, and safety indicators ("Do you ever fall?"; "When was the last time you fell?"; "Did you sustain any injuries from falling?"). Validated questionnaires, such as the MS Walking Scale-12 (MSWS-12) are now available to gather patient feedback

TABLE 28.1
Assessment Tools for Ambulation in MS

ASSESSMENT TOOL	PURPOSE	DESCRIPTION
Interview	Screen for ambulation limitations and obtain pertinent history	Presence and severity of limitations Pertinent neurological symptoms and comorbidities Safety issues (falls) Interventions tried in the past and results
Physical examination	Assess impairments and observe gait	Neurological impairments (eg, weakness, spasticity, sensory loss, ataxia, visual loss, cognitive impairment) Other contributing impairments (eg, musculoskeletal problems) Describe gait pattern (includes effort needed to walk, need for assistive device, safety issues)
Walking performance tests	Quantify walking performance via direct observation	Timed tests on short distance (eg, T25FW, 10 meter walk, timed up and go) Timed tests on long distance (eg, 2 minute walk, 6 minute walk) Tests of walking distance (eg, walking distance from EDSS) Six Spot Step Test (walking as quickly as possible along a rectangular field while kicking 5 cylinder blocks out of their marked circles)
Rating scales of walking	Rate walking performance via direct observation	Ambulation Index (combination of need for assistive device and time to walk 25 feet) Dynamic Gait Index (rates the degree of impairment on various maneuvers that involve walking and balance) Rivermead Visual Gait Assessment (quantification of gait disturbance rates deviations from normal postures and movements while walking)
Self-report questionnaires	Assess the patient's perception of walking limitations	MSWS-12 (assesses how MS affected various aspects of walking in the past 2 weeks) Patient-Determined Disease Steps (assesses the level of walking limitations) Rivermead Mobility Index (assesses various aspects of mobility, including walking)
Instrumented measurement of walking in daily life	Quantify walking in daily life via a device worn by the patient	Pedometry Accelerometry Global positioning system (GPS)
Quantitative gait analysis	Quantify various components of gait	Spatiotemporal parameters of gait Kinetics of gait Kinematics of gait Energy expenditure

EDSS, Expanded Disability Status Scale; MSWS-12, MS Walking Scale-12; T25FW, timed 25 foot walk.

about walking performance in daily activities in a standardized manner [22]. These questionnaires can be filled in by the patient before an office visit; the responses to each item facilitate the interview, and the total score can be monitored over time. Since health care providers rarely observe patients walking in their own home environment, self-report measures are a useful complement to clinical tests performed in the office.

> Validated questionnaires such as the MSWS-12 provide information that can guide the assessment of ambulation limitations.

Clinical examination allows the characterization of a gait abnormality and provides information on the underlying impairments: neurological impairments such as paresis,

spasticity, cerebellar ataxia, sensory loss, and other contributing impairments such as osteoarthrosis of lower extremity joints or other musculoskeletal problems. Gaining an understanding of the causal factors is essential in designing an appropriate treatment plan.

Walking tests performed in the clinic or gait laboratory allow the provider to gather quantitative information about walking performance and gait disturbance. Among timed walking tests, the T25FW [23], a test of maximum (but safe) walking speed on a short distance, is the most frequently used in clinical and research settings. The T25FW is both easy to administer and validated, and a 20% change in performance is thought to be clinically significant [24].

> The T25FW and the 6 minute walk are the most commonly used tests of walking performance in MS.

TABLE 28.2
Common Gait Abnormalities in MS

- Decreased walking speed
- Decreased (in some cases increased) cadence
- Decreased step and stride length
- Increased step width
- Increased double support time
- Decreased swing phase
- Increased step variability

The 6 minute walk (6MW) [25] is considered a measure of endurance, but is not as often administered, mostly because of feasibility issues (administration time, need for a long hallway, and in some patients need for recovery time). In addition to providing a number that can be monitored over time, these tests give an opportunity for the clinician to observe the patient's gait pattern.

Ambulation rating scales are generally used in a rehabilitation setting and allow the provider to attribute scores to observed gait deviations, including the use of assistive devices. The Dynamic Gait Index assesses performance on 8 walking tasks designed to challenge the patient's balance (eg, walking with horizontal or vertical head movements), and is correlated with reported falls [26].

Quantification of gait disturbance via gait analysis is traditionally performed in research settings and in some clinical centers, as a full gait analysis system is costly, requires a large space and specialized staff to run the tests and to interpret the data, and testing is time consuming. Less cumbersome, more affordable, and more user-friendly systems allow the measurement of spatiotemporal parameters of gait in the clinic [27]. Abnormalities of gait pattern in MS have been described in several publications (Table 28.2) and can be detected early in the disease, before a gait disturbance is noted on examination [28]. The energetic cost of walking (measured with the rate of oxygen consumption) is increased in patients with MS compared to healthy controls.

More recently, pedometers, accelerometers, and less frequently GPS systems, have been used in research studies to measure walking and activity in the patient's own environment. While these devices may provide a more accurate picture of ambulation in daily activities, the clinical significance and psychometric properties (validity, reliability, sensitivity to change) of the results, usually expressed in step counts or activity counts, have not been fully determined. Published data to date suggest that step counts and activity counts are reduced in those with MS compared to healthy subjects, and that the reduction is greater when the level of walking disability is greater, as it would be expected [29].

IMPROVING AMBULATION

There is a growing body of evidence supporting the use of various interventions to improve ambulation in MS (Table 28.3).

Rehabilitation and Exercise

Rehabilitation and exercise should be considered as first-line interventions when trying to improve ambulation, and carried out concomitantly with other interventions. Routine exercise is encouraged in MS, alone or in a group, at home or in a gym, on a regular basis. Exercise was shown to have a beneficial effect on aerobic capacity, walking speed, walking endurance, and functional performance in MS [30,31], in addition to improving fatigue, mood, and health-related quality of life [32]. Many MS patients have difficulty initiating an exercise routine on their own, therefore a referral to a physical therapist (preferably with experience in MS) to develop an individualized home exercise program is often helpful. Gait rehabilitation is a more thorough and intense training performed by a physical therapist and usually includes stretching and range of motion exercises, strengthening exercises, and task-specific training (eg, gait and balance training, training to climb stairs, etc.). In addition, physical therapists help determine the need for assistive devices and orthoses, and train patients to use them properly and safely. Body weight supported treadmill training (BWSTT) was shown to be effective at improving walking performance in MS [33] and can be performed with the help of 1 or 2 physical therapists to move the legs or with the assistance of a robotic device. However, this training may not be more effective than traditional gait training [34].

> Rehabilitation and exercise are the first line of treatment for ambulation limitations in MS.

Assistive Devices and Orthoses

Assistive devices include canes, crutches, and walkers, all of which are routinely recommended when MS compromises gait efficiency and/or gait safety. These devices are meant to improve the efficiency of gait, to decrease the musculoskeletal stress due to gait deviations, and to decrease the risk of falling. Despite extensive empirical experience, there is very little published evidence on the efficacy of these assistive devices. Although these devices are prescribed by a physician, it is strongly recommended to involve a physical therapist for evaluation and training, as mentioned earlier. Ankle foot orthoses (AFOs) are commonly used to correct foot drop, but their effect on gait may be limited and needs to be better studied [35]. Heavier orthoses such as knee ankle foot orthoses (KAFO) can be helpful in controlling hyperextension of the knee, but are often too heavy for routine use.

> Assistive devices should be considered to improve the efficiency and safety of walking, and to preserve mobility in nonambulatory patients.

TABLE 28.3
Interventions to Improve Ambulation

TYPE OF INTERVENTION	DESCRIPTION	COMMENTS
Exercise	Stretching (with assistance if needed) Aerobic exercise Resistance training Aquatic exercise Walking exercise (with appropriate assistive devices and orthoses for safety)	Exercise program often needs to be initiated under the guidance of a physical therapist. Exercise regimen needs to be adjusted as the patient's functional capacity changes. Involving family members or care partners, or involvement in group exercise sessions, may improve adherence as well as safety and quality of exercise. Improvement of walking performance was demonstrated after exercise programs.
Rehabilitation	Stretching performed by physical therapist Exercise supervised by physical therapist Traditional gait and balance training Training to the use of assistive devices and orthoses Periodic re-evaluation is needed Training to home exercise program Technology-assisted gait training BWSTT FES-assisted BWSTT or cycling Robotic-assisted BWSTT	A referral to neurologic physical therapy should be systematically considered when ambulation is impaired. Physical therapy can and should be used in combination with other interventions to optimize outcomes. Published evidence showing the efficacy of rehabilitation interventions on walking is limited. Improvement of walking performance was demonstrated with traditional gait training. Robot-assisted BWSTT may not be superior to traditional gait training, based on 1 publication. Periodic re-evaluation is needed.
Assistive devices and orthoses	Unilateral support: Cane, crutch, walking stick Bilateral support: Bilateral canes or crutches Walker: standard, 2-wheel, 4-wheel (with hand brakes, basket, and seat) Foot FlexR, Foot Up, Dictus Band AFO Plastic, solid or articulated ankle Usually custom-molded as opposed to off-the-shelf Carbon fiber KAFO KO HFAD FES devices for foot drop	There is limited evidence showing the efficacy of assistive devices and orthoses in MS. An uncontrolled pilot study of the HFAD showed significant improvement of walking performance and leg strength at 8 and 12 weeks.

Medications	DMTs (to help prevent worsening of walking limitations due to disease activity)
	Dalfampridine (approved to improve walking in patients with MS, based on improvement of walking speed in phase 3 clinical trials)
	Symptomatic medications:
	  For spasticity (see Chapter 27)
	  For pain (see Chapter 24)
	  For other symptoms as indicated
	Treatments for comorbidities (eg, cardiovascular, respiratory, musculoskeletal)
		Slowing of disability progression was demonstrated with some DMTs.
		
		The efficacy of dalfampridine was established using the T25FW with a responder analysis, and more recently with the 6-MW test.
		The effects of symptomatic medications and treatments for comorbidities on ambulation in MS are rarely assessed.

Surgical treatments	Orthopedic surgery
	  For musculoskeletal injuries related to falls
	  For contractures and limb deformity (eg, tendon release, osteotomy) related to spasticity
	  For severe osteoarthritis or other musculoskeletal comorbidity
	Neurosurgical interventions for spasticity
	  ITB therapy
	  Selective dorsal rhizotomy
	  Tibial nerve neurotomy
		Decision making is often difficult, because of a lack of evidence to guide decision making, and because of uncertainty regarding the functional results of surgical interventions.
		
		ITB therapy is approved for the treatment of severe spasticity refractory to oral medication in a variety of conditions including MS. Published data suggest that ambulation can be preserved in carefully selected ambulatory MS patients treated with ITB.

6-MW, 6 minute walk; AFO, ankle foot orthosis; BWSTT, body weight supported treadmill training; DMT, disease-modifying therapy; FES, functional electrical stimulation; HFAD, hip flexion assist device; ITB, intrathecal baclofen; KAFO, knee ankle foot orthosis; KO, knee orthosis; T25FW, timed 25 foot walk.

Recently, "active" devices promoting active movement (instead of immobilizing a limb segment) have become available. For example, functional electrical stimulation (FES) devices using peroneal nerve stimulation can trigger active dorsiflexion to correct foot drop during specific portions of the gait cycle. These FES devices consist of a cuff worn on the proximal lower leg containing the electrodes, and a mechanism (heel switch or tilt sensor) to trigger the stimulation at the appropriate time in the gait cycle (ie, from the time the foot is lifted off the floor to the time it makes contact with the floor again). Although FES devices for foot drop have received extensive publicity, published evidence in MS is scarce and sometimes contradictory [36,37]. Also, the hip flexion assist device (HFAD), which consists of 2 elastic bands attached proximally to a waist belt and distally to the shoe, significantly improved walking performance in a pilot study on 21 MS patients [38].

In patients who walk only in their home ("household ambulators"), and in those who lose the ability to ambulate altogether, mobility can be preserved by using a wheelchair. Power mobility devices (ie, power wheelchairs and scooters) are considered when upper extremity function is impaired. It is essential to customize these devices to the abilities and needs of the patient, and to their environment. For example, custom seating may be needed in patients with poor trunk control, and the size of the wheelchair should be compatible with the space available within the home. This requires a thorough evaluation by qualified rehabilitation professionals.

Medications

Dalfampridine (also called fampridine in other parts of the world), an extended-release formulation of 4-aminopyridine, was approved in the United States and other countries as a symptomatic medication to improve walking in patients with MS, based on improved walking speed (on T25FW testing) in 2 phase 3 placebo-controlled clinical trials [39,40]. Dalfampridine is prescribed at the dose of 10 mg twice daily (12 hours apart). Higher doses showed no added efficacy, but caused an increased frequency of serious adverse events (particularly seizures) in a phase 2 dose-ranging study. The risk of seizures is a significant concern, and patients should be educated to take the medication as prescribed, to not cut or crush the tablets, and to not try to "catch up" if they think they have missed a dose. Common side effects include urinary tract infections, insomnia, dizziness, headache, nausea, and paresthesias. Anaphylactic reactions temporally related to dalfampridine dosing have been reported in the post-marketing experience. Since this medication is excreted predominantly in the urine, estimated creatinine clearance should be known before initiating treatment and monitored at least annually, and it should be used with caution in individuals over age 50 years owing to more common occurrence of mild renal impairment in this subgroup of patients. Dalfampridine is contraindicated in patients

> Dalfampridine is approved by the FDA to improve walking in patients with MS, based on an improvement in walking speed in clinical trials.

with a history of seizure or with moderate or severe renal impairment (creatinine clearance of 50 mL/min or less).

Other medications can contribute directly or indirectly to improve or preserve walking. Medications targeting symptoms that interfere with walking, such as spasticity (see Chapter 27) and pain, may enhance walking performance, although the functional effects of these drugs are rarely tested, or the functional tests used are not consistent [41].

It is worth noting that some medications may cause worsening of gait disturbance and imbalance because of side effects such as somnolence, dizziness, or weakness. Therefore, in the presence of an abrupt deterioration of walking performance, it is important to review a current medication list, along with other potential factors such as MS exacerbation or progression, infection, or other acute illness.

Surgical Treatments

Two types of surgical treatment can be contemplated to improve ambulation in MS: neurosurgical interventions to control spasticity, and orthopedic surgery.

Among neurosurgical interventions for spasticity, intrathecal baclofen (ITB) therapy is the most common. Two case series in MS patients showed that ambulation is usually preserved after the implantation of a baclofen pump [42,43], but improvement of gait pattern has not been demonstrated. Although selective dorsal rhizotomy or tibial nerve neurotomy are sometimes used in MS on the basis of their effects on gait in patients with cerebral palsy and stroke, there is no published evidence in MS to our knowledge.

Musculoskeletal comorbidity has been shown to impact the level of disability in MS (see Chapter 33). Conversely, gait deviations from neurological impairments cause stress on the musculoskeletal system, severe spasticity can cause contractures and limb deformity, and falls can cause fractures, sprains, and other musculoskeletal injuries. It is therefore important to recognize and treat musculoskeletal problems in the presence of MS. Unfortunately, there is little evidence to guide clinical decision making, especially when surgery is considered. Even if MS does not contraindicate surgery, the functional results are less

> Although surgery is not contraindicated in MS, the use of surgical treatments to improve ambulation requires careful patient selection and intensive rehabilitation.

predictable than in the general population, and prolonged rehabilitation is often needed. Disease management and spasticity control should be optimized before elective musculoskeletal surgery. One publication recommended the use of prophylactic corticosteroids at the time of surgery [44], but this remains controversial owing to a possible negative effect of corticosteroids on healing and infectious risk and the lack of evidence that surgery or anesthesia increases the risk of MS exacerbation [45].

CONCLUSION

Preserving the ability to ambulate can be an uphill battle in MS, involving patients, family, personal care providers, and health care providers. Considering the physical, psychological, and socioeconomic consequences of loss of mobility, it is essential to identify, understand, and address walking limitations as early as possible, often starting with simple and safe interventions such as exercise, physical therapy, symptomatic medications, and the use of assistive devices. Ambulation should be monitored periodically in the comprehensive management of MS, using validated tools such as the T25FW, 6-MW, and MS Walking Scale-12. Further research is needed to better understand the pathophysiology of gait impairments, to validate outcome measures for mobility, and to further test the efficacy and safety of various interventions (and combination of interventions) in subgroups of patients.

REFERENCES

1. Swingler RJ, Compston DA. The morbidity of multiple sclerosis. *Q J Med.* 1992;83:325–337.

2. Hobart JC, Lamping DL, Fitzpatrick R, et al. The Multiple Sclerosis Impact Scale (MSIS-29): A new patient-based outcome measure. *Brain.* 2001;124:962–973.

3. La Rocca N. Impact of walking impairment in multiple sclerosis: Perspectives of patients and care partners. *Patient.* 2011;4:189–201.

4. Heesen C, Böhm J, Reich C, et al. Patient perception of bodily functions in multiple sclerosis: Gait and visual function are the most valuable. *Mult Scler.* 2008;14:988–991.

5. Paltamaa J, Sarasoja T, Leskinen E, et al. Measures of physical functioning predict self-reported performance in self-care, mobility, and domestic life in ambulatory persons with multiple sclerosis. *Arch Phys Med Rehabil.* 2007;88:1649–1657.

6. Edgley K, Sullivan MJ, Dehoux E. A survey of multiple sclerosis: II. Determinants of employment status. *Can J Rehabil.* 1991;4:127–132.

7. Thoumie P, Lamotte D, Cantalloube S, et al. Motor determinants of gait in 100 ambulatory patients with multiple Sclerosis. *Mult Scler.* 2005;11:485–491.

8. Sosnoff JJ, Gappmaier E, Frame A, Motl RW. Influence of spasticity on mobility and balance in persons with multiple sclerosis. *JNPT.* 2011;35:129–132.

9. Yogev-Seligmann G, Hausdorff JM, Giladi N. The role of executive function and attention in gait. *Mov Disord.* 2007;23: 329–342.

10. Hamilton F, Rochester L, Paul L, et al. Walking and talking: An investigation of cognitive-motor dual tasking in multiple sclerosis. *Mult Scler.* 2009;15:1215–1227.

11. Kalron A, Dvir Z, Achiron A. Walking while talking: Difficulties incurred during the initial stages of multiple sclerosis disease process. *Gait Posture.* 2010;32:332–335.

12. Huisinga JM, Filipi ML, Schmid KK, Stergiou N. Is there a relationship between fatigue questionnaires and gait mechanisms in persons with multiple sclerosis? *Arch Phys Med Rehabil.* 2011;92:1594–1601.

13. Feys P, Gijbels D, Romberg A, et al. Effect of time of day on walking capacity and self-reported fatigue in persons with MS: A multi-center trial. *Mult Scler.* 2012;18(3):351–357.

14. Marrie RA, Rudick R, Horwitz R, et al. Vascular comorbidity is associated with more rapid disability progression in multiple sclerosis. *Neurology.* 2010;74:1041–1047.

15. Cattaneo D, De Nuzzo C, Fascia T, et al. Risks of falls in subjects with multiple sclerosis. *Arch Phys Med Rehabil.* 2002;83:864–867.

16. Kasser SL, Jacobs JV, Foley JT, et al. A prospective evaluation of balance, gait, and strength to predict falling in women with multiple sclerosis. *Arch Phys Med Rehabil.* 2011;92:1840–1846.

17. Finlayson ML, Peterson EW, Cho CC. Risk factors for falling among people aged 45 to 90 years with multiple sclerosis. *Arch Phys Med Rehabil.* 2006;87:1274–1279.

18. Cameron MH, Poel AJ, Haselkorn JK, et al. Falls requiring medical attention among veterans with multiple sclerosis: A cohort study. *J Rehabil Res Dev.* 2011;48:13–20.

19. Peterson EW, Cho CC, von Koch L, Finlayson ML. Injurious falls among middle aged and older adults with multiple sclerosis. *Arch Phys Med Rehabil.* 2008;89:1031–1037.

20. Moen SM, Celius EG, Nordsletten L, Holmoy T. Fractures and falls in patients with newly diagnosed clinically isolated syndrome and multiple sclerosis. *Acta Neurol Scand Suppl.* 2011;(191):79–82.

21. Bethoux F, Bennett S. Evaluating walking in patients with multiple sclerosis: Which assessment tools are useful in clinical practice? *Int J MS Care.* 2011;13(1):4–14.

22. Hobart JC, Riazi A, Lamping DL, et al. Measuring the impact of MS on walking ability: The 12-item MS Walking Scale (MSWS-12). *Neurology.* 2003;60:31–36.

23. Rudick RA, Cutter G, Reingold S. The multiple sclerosis functional composite; a new clinical outcome measure for multiple sclerosis trials. *Mult Scler.* 2002;8:359–365.

24. Kragt JJ, van der Linden FA, Nielsen JM, et al. Clinical impact of 20% worsening on Timed 25-foot Walk and 9-hole Peg Test in multiple sclerosis. *Mult Scler.* 2006;12:594–598.

25. Goldman M, Marrie RA, Cohen JA. Evaluation of the six-minute walk in multiple sclerosis subjects and healthy controls. *Mult Scler.* 2007;14:383–390.

26. Cattaneo D, Regola A, Meotti M. Validity of six balance disorders scales in persons with multiple sclerosis. *Disabil Rehabil.* 2006;28:789–795.

27. Givon U, Zeilig G, Achiron A. Gait analysis in multiple sclerosis: Characterization of temporal-spatial parameters using GAITRite functional ambulation system. *Gait Posture.* 2009;29:138–142.

28. Martin CL, Phillips BA, Kilpatrick TJ, et al. Gait and balance impairment in early multiple sclerosis in the absence of clinical disability. *Mult Scler.* 2006;12:620–628.

29. Gijbels D, Alders G, Van Hoof E, et al. Predicting habitual walking performance in multiple sclerosis: Relevance of capacity and self-report measures. *Mult Scler.* 2010;16:618–626.

30. Rampello A, Franceschini M, Piepoli M, et al. Effect of aerobic training on walking capacity and maximal exercise tolerance in patients with multiple sclerosis: A randomized crossover controlled study. *Phys Ther.* 2007;87(5):545–559.

31. Dalgas U, Stenager E, Jakobsen J, et al. Resistance training improves muscle strength and functional capacity in multiple sclerosis. *Neurology.* 2009;73(18):1478–1484.

32. Dalgas U, Stenager E, Jakobsen J, et al. Fatigue, mood and quality of life improve in MS patients after progressive resistance training. *Mult Scler.* 2010;16:480–490.

33. Pilutti LA, Lelli DA, Paulseth JE, et al. Effects of 12 weeks of supported treadmill training on functional ability and quality of life in progressive multiple sclerosis: A pilot study. *Arch Phys Med Rehabil.* 2011;92:31–36.

34. Vaney C, Gattlen B, Lugon-Moulin V, et al. Robotic-assisted step training (lokomat) not superior to equal intensity of over-ground rehabilitation in patients with multiple sclerosis. *Neurorehabil Neural Repair.* 2012;26(3):212–221.

35. Sheffler LR, Hennessey MT, Knutson JS, et al. Functional effect of an ankle foot orthosis on gait in multiple sclerosis: A pilot study. *Am J Phys Med Rehabil.* 2008;87(1):26–32.

36. Barrett CL, Mann GE, Taylor PN, Strike P. A randomized trial to investigate the effects of functional electrical stimulation and therapeutic exercise on walking performance for people with multiple sclerosis. *Mult Scler.* 2009;15(4):493–504.

37. Paul L, Rafferty D, Young S, et al. The effect of functional electrical stimulation on the physiological cost of gait in people with multiple sclerosis. *Mult Scler.* 2008;14(7):954–961.

38. Sutliff M, Naft J, Stough D, et al. Efficacy and safety of a hip flexion assist orthosis in ambulatory multiple sclerosis patients. *Arch Phys Med Rehabil.* 2008;89(8):1611–1617.

39. Goodman AD, Brown TR, Krupp LB, et al. Sustained-release oral fampridine in multiple sclerosis: A randomised, double-blind, controlled trial. *Lancet.* 2009;373:732–738.

40. Goodman AD, Brown TR, Edwards KR, et al. A phase 3 trial of extended release oral dalfampridine in multiple sclerosis. *Ann Neurol.* 2010;68:494–502.

41. Shakespeare D, Young C, Boggild M. Anti-spasticity agents for multiple sclerosis. *Cochrane Database of Syst Rev.* 2003;(4):CD001332.

42. Sadiq SA, Wang GC. Long-term intrathecal baclofen therapy in ambulatory patients with spasticity. *J Neurol.* 2006;253: 563–569.

43. Bethoux F, Stough D, Sutliff M. Treatment of severe spasticity with intrathecal baclofen therapy in ambulatory multiple sclerosis patients: 6-month follow-up. *Arch Phys Med Rehab.* 2004;84:A10.

44. Dickerman RD, Schneider SJ, Stevens QE, et al. Prophylaxis to avert exacerbation/relapse of multiple sclerosis in affected patients undergoing surgery. *J Neurosurg Sci.* 2004;48:135–137.

45. D'hooghe MB, Nagels G, Bissay V, De Keyser J. Modifiable factors influencing relapses and disability in multiple sclerosis. *Mult Scler.* 2010;16(7):773–785.

29

General Health and Wellness in Multiple Sclerosis

MARY R. RENSEL

KEY POINTS FOR CLINICIANS

- Multiple sclerosis (MS) patients need to have a primary care provider.
- Treat vitamin D deficiency.
- Encourage regular exercise, smoking cessation, and good nutrition for health promotion and to lessen comorbidities.
- Consider mind-body therapies such as meditation and yoga to help MS symptoms.
- It is crucial that our MS patients also have a primary care physician (PCP).
- Preventive medicine is important in all stages of MS to lessen the risk of comorbidities.
- Comorbidities increase the risk of physical disability in MS.
- MS patients may have various barriers to primary care providers.

COMORBIDITIES IN MULTIPLE SCLEROSIS

Multiple sclerosis (MS) patients need monitoring and treatment by a neurologist with experience in MS. In addition to this, we now know that age-appropriate health screens, vascular risk management, immunizations, and management of other health conditions are equally important, but are not routinely addressed by neurologists. There is increasing evidence that other medical conditions such as hypertension and hypercholesterolemia may influence the level of disability from MS. Therefore, another health provider is needed. These services can be provided by a primary care physician (PCP).

There are various special barriers to primary care faced by people with MS. First, it may be difficult for MS patients to go to certain types of facilities because of physical limitations. Second, some MS patients require

frequent visits to deal with MS-related problems, so additional health care visits for preventive services may seem burdensome for practical and financial reasons. Third, many PCPs defer to the neurologist to manage medical problems and are less proactive or aggressive in dealing with general health issues, simply because the person has MS.

Despite these potential barriers, wellness and preventive medical care are extremely important for people with MS, and strong efforts should be made to ensure they are provided for.

COMMON PRIMARY CARE ISSUES IN MS PATIENTS

There are primary care issues that are common in MS patients, such as osteoporosis, vitamin D deficiency, depression, fatigue, and sleep disorders. Osteoporosis in MS patients may be related to the use of steroids, due to limited ambulation [1], or perhaps related to the MS disease itself. Vitamin D deficiency is common in MS patients and common in the higher latitudes of the globe. There is some evidence that vitamin D deficiency may play a role in triggering MS, or even in disease activity once a person has been diagnosed with MS [2]. This is not certain at present, but is another important reason to maintain recommended vitamin D levels (see section on vitamin D for more information). Managing vascular risk factors or comorbidities: hypertension, cholesterol, obesity, diabetes, and smoking are not only important for cardiovascular health, but recent data show that risk factor modification may be important in limiting MS disease severity including physical disability [3,4]. Depression, fatigue, and sleep disorders are very common in MS patients and are addressed separately in this text.

Factors that have been shown to be possible predictors of physical disability in MS include social support, emotional health, health behaviors, smoking, obesity, and vascular comorbidities [5–7]. Comorbidities and adverse lifestyle factors (smoking) affect the following factors in various ways: the clinical phenotype of the disease, delay in diagnosis, worsen disability progression, and negatively affecting health-related quality of life. MS patients will need a cane earlier if they have a single physical comorbidity and even earlier with multiple comorbidities. The prevalence of smoking in MS patients is similar to the general population. Smokers have an increased risk of autoimmune conditions and developing MS as well as having higher levels of disability [8]. MS patients should quit smoking for health promotion. MS patients should be referred to a smoking cessation program in their community.

The level of alcoholism in MS patients is similar to the general population. Patients should discuss their alcohol intake in detail with their care team. Excess alcohol should be avoided, and if there is alcohol dependency or abuse, it should be aggressively addressed. Alcohol intake should be limited with various medications including interferons, antiepileptic medications, and benzodiazepines.

Owing to the many general health issues with relevance to MS, it is imperative that MS patients have primary care doctors to perform preventive care as well as to treat known conditions. It is also our role to encourage regular visits with a PCP, smoking cessation, healthy eating, and adequate physical activity to help promote general wellness and lessen the risk of comorbidities.

Health Promotion

Health promotion includes setting goals and establishing health-enhancing behaviors, such as regular exercise, good nutrition, and stress management. Health promotion has been shown to improve employment,

physical conditioning and strength, quality of life, and even lessen the severity of MS [9–11]. There is good evidence that regular exercise is important in MS, so we encourage specific planning for exercise programming in the MS population. MS patients can benefit from having access to physical therapy (PT) and occupational therapy (OT) to help map out a home exercise plan, improve strength, balance, and enrich activities of daily living. MS patients should also have access to mental health professionals as part of their care team to help with stress management, emotional health, goal setting, and coexisting psychiatric disorders.

As health practitioners, we want to give our patients all the opportunities to enhance their general wellness and give them tools to cope with MS. At this time there are many avenues for a patient to tap into to improve their overall health. Health promoting tools include the plethora of technical resources; for example, applications (apps) for smart phones and online information on the Internet. Smart phone apps can help the patient obtain health information, improve exercise, gain access to information on health and nutrition and modifying lifestyle behaviors, such as smoking cessation. The Internet is another vast source of information and guidance for coping with the illness for MS patients. The Internet has served as a source of advice on health care information and has enhanced the opportunities for patients to be more engaged and active in coping with their disease. While the Internet can be useful to attain information, one must be reminded that the Internet is not a neutral technology, it is highly commercialized [12]. Eighty percent of patients looking for information online will find what they are looking for and the common users of the Internet are patients with long-standing illnesses. It is our role to point the patients to web sites and apps with accurate information.

Pearls

Encourage MS patients to set goals and promote healthy behaviors:

1. Follow a healthy diet
2. Perform regular exercise
3. Regular visits with their PCPs to prevent and manage comorbidities
4. Smoking cessation
5. Moderation of alcohol intake
6. Manage stress
7. Correct vitamin D deficiency

GENERAL HEALTH AND WELLNESS IN MS

Wellness is the quality or state of being in good health especially as an actively sought goal [13]. People with

MS, like everyone else, should seek optimal health and wellness. The pursuit of wellness is a continuous process throughout life. MS presents special challenges to this, however, and the means to achieve this goal will differ for each MS patient.

Exercise in MS

Exercise can be helpful and safe for an MS patient. MS patients, with most level of abilities, can work with PT and OT to help improve physical functioning and to maintain a home exercise program for conditioning. Exercise can improve the MS patient's quality of life, including improvement of both physical and emotional health [14]. MS patients typically report a sedentary lifestyle; this is not always related to the level of disability but is related to the severity of MS symptoms reported. Fatigue, mood, and quality of life have been shown to be positively affected by exercise [15]. Yoga and aerobic exercise have been shown to improve fatigue in MS [16]. Therefore, regular aerobic activity should be encouraged to help MS fatigue. There have been studies showing an increase in brain-derived neurotrophic factors (BDNF) and insulin-like growth factor (IGF) with aerobic activity suggesting the potential enhancement for neuronal repair and brain plasticity due to exercise [17]. Studies have shown that a higher level of cardiopulmonary fitness was associated with faster physical performance and greater brain activation on defined tasks, providing evidence that exercise may help cognition [18]. A safe, regular exercise program should be encouraged in MS patients to improve cardiopulmonary fitness, fatigue, and emotional health. Many patients find that a combination of aerobic activity and stretching helps manage MS symptoms and improve stamina. PT and OT can help in establishing a home exercise program.

Pearls

The effects of exercise in MS patients include:

1. Lessening MS symptoms such as fatigue
2. Decreasing risk of vascular comorbidities
3. Increasing conditioning and strength
4. Improving quality of life—both physical and emotional
5. Possibly promoting nerve repair (theoretical)

Vitamin D and MS

An increasing number of studies support a positive role for vitamin D in MS. Low sunlight and UV radiation exposure, as well as low vitamin D levels and intake, are inversely correlated with the risk of developing MS [2]. Lower vitamin D levels have been associated with an increase in MRI activity [19] and an increase in risk of relapse [20].

These studies may explain the findings that MS relapses are typically in the fall and spring when vitamin D levels fall. Calcium and vitamin D pretreatment resulted in the inability to induce experimental allergic encephalomyelitis (EAE), an animal model of MS. There have been pediatric MS studies showing that low vitamin D levels increased the risk of relapses in a clinically isolated syndrome (CIS) [21]. Vitamin D appears to play a role in the risk of acquiring and the severity of MS. The majority of MS patients are deficient in vitamin D. The recommended dose of calcium and vitamin D for the adult population is 1,200 mg a day of calcium and at least 600 mg a day of vitamin D. Additional doses of vitamin D_3 in the 2 to 4,000 IU per day ranges, or higher, may be needed depending on the level of vitamin D; target is near 50. One should also encourage regular exposure to the sun, 10 minutes daily or 30 minutes a few times a week, and then use sunscreen for extended periods in the sun. There are ongoing studies to determine the most efficacious level of vitamin D and if vitamin D is a potential treatment and prevention for MS.

Pearls

1. MS patients should be on at least 2000 IU vitamin D_3 daily.
2. Maintain vitamin D_{25} OH levels near 50.
3. MS patients should take calcium with the vitamin D at doses as recommended by their PCP.

Osteoporosis and MS

Patients with MS have multiple risk factors for osteoporosis: impaired gait, sedentary lifestyle, and the use of steroids [1]. Daily long-term steroid use has been associated with an increased risk of osteoporosis; yet, pulse steroids given every few months has not been associated with bone degradation. In general, we avoid daily oral steroids in the treatment of MS. It has been shown that MS patients have a high risk of osteoporosis even with a normal gait. Bone loss can be prevented by proper nutrition, weight bearing exercise as able, and calcium and vitamin D supplementation. MS patients should be on calcium and vitamin D supplementation if they have had a fracture, gait impairment, low vitamin D levels, and or frequent steroids usage. Patients can be referred to their PCP for management of bone health as there are multiple prescription medications and various approaches available to promote bone health.

Pearls

1. To maintain healthy bones, follow healthy nutrition, stop smoking, moderate alcohol intake, and perform regular exercise with weight bearing.

2. If there have been fractures, frequent steroid usage or limited mobility patients should be on calcium and vitamin D orally.
3. Healthy vitamin D levels need to be maintained.

MS and Fatigue

Fatigue is a common symptom of MS. Patient should be educated to the importance of sleep hygiene, regular exercise, healthy nutrition, and limiting caffeine intake. There are medications for fatigue in MS but generally working on the factors listed above help sleep efficacy and can remarkably help the patient's energy levels. A good sleep history should be taken to assure there is no consequent sleep disorders. Sleep disorders in MS are be discussed in Chapter 21.

INTEGRATIVE MEDICINE AND MS

Integrative Medicine (IM) combines treatments from conventional medicine and complementary medicine for which there is some high quality evidence of safety and effectiveness [22].

MS Patients and IM

Nearly 60% of MS patients have tried IM; the rate has increased over the past decade [23]. The types of IM that have been reported to be used by MS patients include reflexology, massage therapy, yoga, meditation, diet, omega-3 fatty acid supplements, acupuncture, Reiki, tai chi, and vitamins and supplements [24]. The reasons that MS patients use IM include dissatisfaction with conventional medicine, having more control over their disease management, improved sense of well-being, and to help their MS symptoms. MS patients with a longer course of MS, higher educational levels, female sex, and high level of fatigue tend to use IM more than others [25].

Nutritional Issues in Relation to MS

At this time, there is no direct evidence of a nutritional etiology related to the development of MS. Nonetheless, there are studies linking high intake of saturated fats, high calorie and animal product intake with an increased risk of MS [26]. Conversely, high fish intake and lowered saturated fat diets have been associated with lessening the risk of MS [27]. Polyunsaturated fatty acids are thought to encourage a healthy immune system. Linolenic acid was tested in the 1960s as a possible treatment for MS, and the results were mixed [28]. We recommend a diet high in omega-3 fatty acids greater

than omega-6 fatty acids. Omega-3 fatty acids are found in various sources: flaxseed, soy, soybean oil, canola oil, walnuts, fish, and fish oils. There are some findings that suggest that fish oils are well tolerated with the disease-modifying medications of MS although they did not consistently act to influence the relapse rate of MS [29]. We can educate the patient in ways to reduce the intake of saturated fats and optimize the diet such as by limiting meats, eating fish a few times a week, and increasing whole grains, fruits, and vegetables. Dietary modifications can also help with various MS symptoms, such as constipation and fatigue. A healthy diet with fewer sugars and processed foods may increase the energy of the MS patient. MS patients have high rates of constipation, so patients should be educated on the need to eat 3 regular meals, eat high fiber meals, have adequate water intake, and eat fruits and vegetables regularly.

General dietary recommendations include: Each day eat at least 5 servings of fresh or cooked vegetables and fruits and at least 2 servings of whole grain products. The recommended goal for daily fiber intake is 25 to 35 g. The recommended daily fluid intake is 8, 8 oz glasses of water or noncarbonated noncaffeinated fluids a day. The daily fluid intake recommendations may need to be adjusted according to the daily caffeine intake, medical conditions, and activity level. Nutritional therapy consultation can help to educate the patient on a healthy diet. There have been multiple studies looking at isolated nutritional supplement to help the MS patient, and to date no particular consistent positive findings occurred when patients added an isolated supplement of vitamin E, vitamin C, fish oils, evening primrose oil, or vitamin A (Table 29.1).

MS patients are obese more frequently than the general population. The Department of Veterans Affairs series showed that veterans with MS are more likely to be obese than non-MS patients [30]. Higher body mass

TABLE 29.1
Outcomes of Studies of IM in MS patients

POSITIVE FINDINGS	NEGATIVE FINDINGS
Fish Oil	Antioxidant vitamins
St John's Wort	Ginkgo
Omega-3 fatty acids	Vitamin C
Coenzyme Q10	Vitamin E
Cannabis	Vitamin B_{12}
Low dose naltrexone	Ginseng
Meditation	Vitamin A
Therapeutic touch	Prolonged fasting
Aerobic exercise	Inosine
Reflexology	Bee venom
Music therapy	
Yoga	

index (BMI) was found in patients who were married, male, employed, and had diabetes or arthritis. One study found that 60% of MS patients were overweight and this was associated with an increase in the amount of physical disability; even a mild level of disability had a higher risk of being overweight [31]. Importantly, obesity is associated with hypertension, hypercholesterolemia, and type 2 diabetes, and these conditions are associated with increased risk of physical disability from MS. Obesity has been found commonly in the pediatric population [32]. It is the role of the MS care provider to encourage a PCP, as part of their health care team, to insure preventive medicine is practiced, including nutritional education.

To promote wellness, we have recommended the following suggestions for our MS patients:

1. Follow a low-fat diet while avoiding high intake of saturated fats.
2. Eat vegetables for at least 2 meals per day, 5 to 7 servings a day. Serving size varies, low starch vegetables serving size is ½ cup cooked or 1 cup raw vegetables as a serving. It is important to eat a variety of colorful vegetables.
3. Eat 3 to 5 servings daily of a colorful variety of fruits.
4. Eat proteins daily. Proteins include meat, poultry, fish, eggs, beans, and nuts.
5. Increase intake of whole grains in your cereals, breads, and pastas.
6. Eliminate simple carbohydrates such as white flour and white sugar.
7. At this time there is no known necessity to avoid gluten to help treat MS.
8. Fish may be helpful for the immune system, tuna or salmon have high levels of omega-3 oils.
9. Follow the ChooseMyPlate.gov recommendations on the balance of food products and portion sizes on your plate. Choose more vegetables and proteins than grains or fruit on your plate.
10. Maintain a healthy weight.

Supplements and MS

There is no known combination of supplements that helps to treat MS. That being said, there are multiple trials of over-the-counter products to help MS symptoms or disease management. The goal of supplementation is to promote a healthy immune system. MS patients may want to avoid immune system stimulating supplements such as Echinacea, oral garlic tabs, zinc, Astralagus, Cat's claw, maitake mushroom, mistletoe, and stinging nettle. There is a theoretical risk of stimulating the immune system in an MS patient thereby worsening the disease. Fish oils studies have had a mixed result as a therapy for MS. Evening primrose or flaxseed oil will increase the daily intake of omega-3 which may help the immune system

although at this time there is no conclusive evidence to this effect. There are clinical trials from years ago showing that Linoleic acid can help relapses and possibly disability progression in 2 of 3 clinical trials [28]. Vitamin B complex and Coenzyme Q10 tablets may help improve fatigue in MS. Urinary tract infections (UTI) are common in MS patients and can lead to worsening of MS symptoms. Vitamin C and cranberry tablets may help protect against UTIs. (See above section in relation to the vitamin D and bone health literature).

Recommended supplements to consider:

1. Multivitamin daily
2. Vitamin D
3. Calcium supplement to help bone health
4. B Complex for fatigue
5. Coenzyme Q10 for fatigue
6. Vitamin C to prevent UTIs
7. Cranberry capsules to prevent UTIs
8. Avoid "immune boosters"

Mind-Body Therapies and Healing Touch in MS

There are various mind-body therapies available to our patients; yet there have been few controlled trials that demonstrate their efficacy in MS. Mind-body therapies include meditation, yoga, biofeedback, and Acupuncture. There is level 3 evidence that MS patients can benefit from mind-body therapies including meditation [33]. Meditation, including Qigong, tai chi, and walking meditation were shown to help MS patients with quality of life, depression, pain, and fatigue [34–36]. Yoga can be helpful for MS patients with various levels of isability and it may help with fatigue [16]. Music therapy has been shown to help with depression and gait disorder. Acupuncture is a component of traditional Chinese medicine. Although up to 20% of MS patients have tried acupuncture [45], clinical trials with acupuncture are too limited to provide definitive information regarding MS symptoms. There are studies of acupuncture helping spinal cord injury pain [37]. There are reports of mind-body therapies helping particular symptoms of MS. One such study is with biofeedback improving refractory bowel symptoms [39]. Self hypnosis was compared to progressive muscle relaxation for MS pain; it showed self hypnosis helped pain intensity and interference [40].

There is another practice called *Healing Touch* that is a hands-mediated therapy where a practitioner lays hands near or on the body to direct healing energy. Healing Touch has potential clinical effectiveness in improving health-related quality of life in chronic disease management. Healing Touch is generally safe, with no serious adverse effects having been reported [40]. There are various types of Healing Touch, and some have been studied in clinical trials in MS patients. Reflexology is an alternative medicine technique involving activating pressure points with the hands on various parts of the body. There is a study showing reflexology helping MS symptoms: motor, sensory, and bladder symptoms [41]. There are other studies showing that sham massage and Reflexology both help MS symptoms equally; therefore, this is another practice that needs further research in MS [42]. Reiki is an ancient Japanese healing method that involves "laying on the hands." It has been reported to help stress, depression, and pain in various other medical conditions

[38]. There are multiple systematic reviews of controlled trials of Reiki and this was not found to be effective in various outcomes including pain and anxiety in various settings including diabetic peripheral neuropathy (PN) and fibromyalgia pain [44]. There is inconclusive evidence of Reiki's effectiveness in MS [43].

Healing Touch practices can be a potential source of help for our patients with little potential of side effects or harm. There are generally many community-based options for learning these techniques that are readily accessible with low cost to the patient.

KEY POINTS FOR PATIENTS AND FAMILIES

- See a primary care provider regularly to prevent and or treat other conditions that can affect the level of physical disability of MS.

- Exercise regularly, see a PT and OT to help with MS symptoms and to set up and maintain a home exercise program.

- Healthy nutrition is important, see a nutritionist if you need help starting or modifying your food plan.

- Take supplementary vitamin D and calcium; keep vitamin D level at 50 ng/mL or higher.

- Maintain a healthy weight

- Stop smoking

- Moderate alcohol intake

- Consider mind-body therapies like meditation to help with feeling better.

- Manage stress

KEY WEBSITES FOR PATIENTS WITH MS

National MS Society: www.NMSS.org
Mellen Center: my.clevelandclinic.org/multiple_sclerosis_center/default.aspx
FDA: www.fda.gov
NIH: information on current and past clinical trials in MS: nih.gov
NCCAM The National Center for Complementary and Alternative Medicine: nccam.nih
.gov/health/decisions/practitioner.htm

REFERENCES

1. Hearn AP, Silber E. Osteoporosis in multiple sclerosis. *Mult Scler.* 2010;16:1031–1043.

2. Wingerchuk D. Supplementing our understanding of vitamin D and multiple sclerosis. *Neurology.* 2010;74:1846–1847.

3. Marrie RA, Horwitz R, Cutter G, et al. Comorbidity delays diagnosis and increases disability at diagnosis in MS. *Neurology.* 2009;72:117–124.

4. Sundstrom P, Nystrom L. Smoking worsens the prognosis in multiple sclerosis. *Mult Scler.* 2008;14:1031–1035.

5. Marrie RA, Rudick R, Horwitz R, et al. Vascular comorbidity is associated with more rapid disability progression in multiple sclerosis. *Neurology.* 2010 Mar 3;74:1041–1047.

6. Marrie RA, Horwitz RI, Cutter G, et al. Association between co morbidity and clinical characteristics of MS. *Acta Neurol Scand.* 2011;124(2):135–141.

7. Mohr DC. Psychological stress and the subsequent appearance of new brain MRI lesions in MS. *Neurology.* 2000;55:55–61.

8. Healy BC, Ali EN, Guttmann CR, et al. Smoking and disease progression in multiple sclerosis. *Arch Neurol.* 2009 Jul;66(7):858–864.

9. Watt D, Verma S, Flynn L. Wellness programs: A review of the evidence. *Can Med Assoc J.* 1998;158:224–230.

10. Ennis M, Thain J, Boggild M, et al. A randomized controlled trial of a health promotion education program for people with multiple sclerosis. *Clin Rehab.* 2006;20:783–792.

11. Stuifbergen AK, Becker H, Blosis S. A randomized clinical trial of wellness intervention for women with multiple sclerosis. *Arch Phys Med Rehab.* 2003;84:467–476.

12. Korp P. Health on the Internet: Implications for health promotion. *Health Educ Res.* 2006 Feb;21(1):78–86.

13. http://dictionary.reference.com/browse/webster

14. Petajan JH, Gappmaier E, White AT, et al. Impact of aerobic training on fitness and quality of life in MS. *Ann Neurol.* 1996;39(4):432–441.

15. Stenager E, Jakobsen J, Petersen T, et al. Fatigue, mood and quality of life improve in MS patients after progressive resistance training. *Mult Scler.* 2010 Apr;16(4):480–490.

16. Oken BS, Kishiyama S, Zajdel D, et al. Randomized controlled trial of yoga and exercise in multiple sclerosis. *Neurology.* 2004 Jun 8;62(11):2058–2064.

17. Gold S, Schulz K, Hartmann S, et al. Basal serum levels and reactivity of nerve growth factor and brain-derived neurotrophicfactor to standardized acute exercise in multiple sclerosis and controls. *J Neuroimmunol.* 2003 May;138(1-2):99–105.

18. Prakash R, Snook E, Erickson, K, et al. Cardiorespiratory fitness: A predictor of cortical plasticity in multiple sclerosis. *Neuroimage.* 2007 Feb 1;34(3):1238–1244.

19. Løken-Amsrud KI, Holmøy T, Bakke SJ, et al. Vitamin D and disease activity in multiple sclerosis before and during interferon-β treatment. *Neurology.* 2012 Jul 17;79(3):267–273.

20. Runia TF, Hop WC, de Rijke YB, et al. Lower serum vitamin D levels are associated with a higher relapse risk in multiple sclerosis. *Neurology.* 2012 Jul 17;79(3):261–266.

21. Mowry EM, Krupp LB, Milazzo M, et al. Vitamin D status is associated with relapse rate in pediatric-onset multiple sclerosis. *Ann Neurol.* 2010;67:618–624.

22. http://nccam.nih.gov/health/whatiscam

23. Berkman C, Pignotti M, Cavallo P, Holland N. Use of alternative treatments by people with multiple sclerosis. *Neurorehabil Neural Repair.* 1999;13:243–254.

24. Bowling A. Complementary and alternative medicine in MS. *Continuum Lifelong Learning Neurol.* 2010;16(5):78–89.

25. Marrie RA, Hadjimichael O, Vollmer T. Predictors of alternative medicine use by MS patients. *Mult Scler.* 2003;9(5):461–466.

26. Ghadirian P, Jain M, Ducic S, et al. Nutritional factors in the aetiology of multiple sclerosis. *Int J Epidemiol.* 1998;27:845–852.

27. Alter M, Yamoor M, Harshe M. Multiple sclerosis and nutrition. *Arch Neurol.* 1974;31:267–272.

28. Dworkin RH, Bates D, Millar JH, Paty DW. Linoleic acid and multiple sclerosis: A reanalysis of three double-blind trials. *Neurology.* 1984 Nov;34(11):1441–1445.

29. Bates D, Cartlidge NE, French JM, et al. A double-blind controlled trial of long chain n-3 polyunsaturated fatty acids in the treat.ment of multiple sclerosis. *J Neurol Neurosurg Psychiatry.* 1989;52:18–22.

30. Marrie RA, Horwitz RI. Emerging effects of comorbidities on multiple sclerosis. *Lancet Neurol.* 2010;9:820–828.

31. Khurana SR, Bamer AM, Turner AP, et al. The prevalence of overweight and obesity in veterans with multiple sclerosis. *Am J Phys Med Rehabil.* 2009 Feb;88(2):83–91.

32. Yeh A. Obesity as a risk factor in pediatric demyelinating disorders. *Neurology.* 2011:76(Suppl 4):A131.

33. Tavee J, Stone L. Healing the mind: Meditation and multiple sclerosis. *Neurology.* 2010 Sep 28;75(13):1130–1131.

34. Grossman P, Kappos L, Gensicke H, et al. MS quality of life, depression, and fatigue improve after mindfulness training: A randomized trial. *Neurology.* 2010;75:1141–1149.

35. Tavee J, Rensel M, Planchard S, Stone L. Effects of meditation on pain and quality of life in multiple sclerosis and peripheral neuropathy: A controlled study. *Neurology.* 2010 Mar 2;74(Suppl 2).

36. Wahbeh H, Elsas S-M, Oken BS. Mind–body interventions: Applications in neurology. *Neurology.* 2008 Jun 10;70:2321–2328.

37. Nayak S, Shiflett S, Schoenberger N, et al. Is acupuncture effective in treating chronic pain after spinal cord injury? *Arch Phys Med Rehabil.* 2001 Nov;82(11):1578–1586.

38. Lee MS, Pittler, MH, Ernest E. Effects of Reiki in clinical practice: A systematic review of randomised clinical trials. *Int J Clin Prac.* 2008 Jun;62(6):947–954.

39. Giuseppe P, Raptis D, Storrie S, et al. Bowel biofeedback treatment in patients with multiple sclerosis and bowel symptoms. *Dis Col Rectum.* 2011 Sep;54(9):1114–1121.

40. Jensen MP, Barber J, Romano JM, et al. A comparison of self hypnosis versus progressive muscle relaxation in patients with multiple sclerosis and chron pain. *Int J Clin Exp Hypn.* 2009 Apr;57(2):198–221.

41. Anderson J, Taylor AG. Effects of healing touch in clinical practice. *J Holist Nurs.* 2011 Sep;29(3):221–228.

42. Siev-Ner I, Gamus D, Lerner-Geva L, Achiron A. Reflexology treatment relieves symptoms of multiple sclerosis: A randomized controlled study. *Mult Scler.* 2003 Aug;9(4):356–361.

43. Hughes CM, Smyth S, Lowe-Strong AS. Reflexology for the treatment of pain in people with multiple sclerosis: A double-blind randomised sham-controlled clinical trial. *Mult Scler.* 2009 Nov;15:1329–1338.

44. Wang MY, Tsai PS, Lee PH, et al. The efficacy of reflexology: Systematic review. *J Adv Nurs.* 2008 Jun;62(5):512–520.

45. Schwartz CE, Laitin E, Brotman S, LaRocca N. Utilization of unconventional treatments by persons with MS: Is it alternative or complementary? *Neurology.* 1999;52(3):626–629.

ADDITIONAL READING

Bowling AC, Stewart TM. *Dietary Supplements and Multiple Sclerosis: A Health Professional's Guide.* Demos Medical Publishing; 2004.

Bourdette D, Shinto L, Yadav V. CAM for the treatment of MS. *Exp Rev Clin Immunol.* 2010 May;6(3):381.

Tremlett HL, Wiles CM, Luscombe DK. Nonprescription medicine use in a multiple sclerosis clinic population. *Brit J Clin Pharm.* 2000;50:55–60.

30

Complementary and Alternative Medicine: Practical Considerations

ALLEN C. BOWLING

KEY POINTS FOR CLINICIANS

- Conventional health care providers may not discuss complementary and alternative medicine (CAM) therapies with their patients even though the majority of MS patients use some form of CAM and these CAM therapies exhibit a wide range of risk–benefit profiles.

- CAM therapies that are low risk and possibly therapeutic and thus might be worth consideration by some MS patients include acupuncture, cooling, cranberry, ginkgo biloba, mindfulness, low dose naltrexone, tai chi, vitamin B_{12}, vitamin D, and yoga.

- CAM therapies that are less worthy of consideration because they are low risk but have unknown efficacy in MS include fish oil, the Swank diet, and gluten-restricted diets.

- CAM therapies that should be approached with caution or avoided owing to lack of efficacy, uncertain efficacy, or potential risks include antioxidants, bee venom therapy, Chinese herbal medicine, echinacea (and other "immune-stimulating" supplements), and marijuana.

- Clinicians who provide objective information about CAM therapies to their patients may provide a valuable role in informed decision making about CAM and may thereby facilitate the appropriate use of CAM. Likewise, clinicians who do not discuss CAM issues may silently endorse CAM and indirectly perpetuate the misuse of CAM in patients who are under their care.

The use of unconventional medicine, also known as complementary and alternative medicine (CAM), is popular among multiple sclerosis (MS) patients yet may not be openly discussed at clinic visits. In the general population, CAM is used by 30% to 50%, while among those with MS it is used by 50% to 75% [1–3]. Conventional health care providers may not address CAM with their MS patients for a variety of reasons, including limited time and limited CAM knowledge or experience. The remarkable advances in disease-modifying therapies over the past several years have greatly improved treatment options, but the increased complexity of decision making and monitoring associated with some of these therapies may make it even more challenging for clinicians to interact with MS patients about CAM issues. This chapter is aimed at providing busy clinicians with an easy-to-use, concise guide to CAM therapies they are likely to encounter in practice. There are several key points that provide context for the wide range of CAM therapies. Specific CAM therapies that are discussed in this chapter are shown in Table 30.1. More detailed, comprehensive, and critical reviews of MS-relevant CAM therapies may be found elsewhere [1,2].

TABLE 30.1
MS-Relevant CAM Therapies

Acupuncture, Chinese herbal medicine, and traditional Chinese medicine	"Gluten sensitivity"
Antioxidants	Low dose naltrexone
Bee venom therapy	Marijuana
Cooling therapy	Mindfulness
Cranberry	Tai chi
Echinacea and other "immune-stimulating" supplements	Vitamin B$_{12}$
Fish oil and the Swank diet	Vitamin D
Ginkgo biloba	Yoga

TABLE 30.2
National Institutes of Health (NIH) Classification of CAM

Natural Products
Vitamin and mineral supplements, herbs

Manipulative and Body-Based Practices
Chiropractic manipulation, massage

Mind and Body Medicine
Meditation, yoga, guided imagery

Movement Therapies
Feldenkrais, pilates

Traditional Healing
Native American medicine

Energy Medicine
Healing touch, Reiki, magnet therapy

Whole Medical Systems
Naturopathy, traditional Chinese medicine, Ayurveda

DEFINITIONS AND CLASSIFICATION SCHEMES

In the CAM field, there are a variety of terms. The broadest term, *unconventional medicine*, is often defined as therapies that are not typically taught in medical schools or generally available in hospitals. The way in which these unconventional therapies are used is the basis for *complementary and alternative medicine (CAM)*: *complementary* indicates that the unconventional therapies are used in conjunction with conventional medicine, while *alternative* indicates that they are used instead of conventional medicine. The National Institutes of Health (NIH) has developed a classification scheme that divides CAM therapies into 7 different categories (Table 30.2) [1,2].

CAM Therapies

Acupuncture, Chinese Herbal Medicine, and Traditional Chinese Medicine

Acupuncture is the most widely known and, among MS patients, perhaps most widely practiced component of the ancient, multimodal healing method known as traditional Chinese medicine (TCM). Other components of TCM include herbs, nutrition, tai chi, exercise, stress reduction, and massage [1,2]. Studies of MS and acupuncture are extremely limited [4]. Studies in other conditions indicate that acupuncture is effective for pain, nausea, and vomiting [1,2]. There are no well-conducted studies of Chinese herbal medicine in MS. In terms of safety, acupuncture is generally well tolerated. In contrast, Chinese herbal medicine, which is often provided in conjunction with acupuncture, poses theoretical risks. Many of the commonly used herbs (including Asian ginseng, astragalus, and maitake and reishi mushrooms) may activate immune cells and could thereby worsen MS or antagonize the effects of MS disease-modifying medications [1,2].

If patients are using acupuncture, be sure to directly ask whether they are receiving Chinese herbal medicine along with acupuncture.

Acupuncture is generally safe and may alleviate pain. In contrast, for disease-modifying effects or symptomatic relief in MS, Chinese herbal medicine is of unknown efficacy and carries theoretical risks.

Antioxidants

Various antioxidant supplements are touted for MS. There is theoretical evidence that by inhibiting free radical-induced damage antioxidants could decrease myelin and axonal injury. In addition, studies in the animal model of MS indicate that antioxidants are therapeutic. However, several antioxidants "activate" immune cells and thus could worsen MS or antagonize the effects of disease-modifying medications. Clinical trials of antioxidants in MS are limited and inconclusive. Some of these trials have not been powered adequately. MS trials with 1 antioxidant, inosine, have shown mixed results [5,6].

Common antioxidants include coenzyme Q10, selenium, and vitamins A, C, and E.

There is a theoretical basis and animal model evidence to suggest that antioxidants could be therapeutic in MS, but antioxidants also carry theoretical risks in MS and there are not any MS clinical trials that provide definitive evidence of safety and efficacy.

Bee Venom Therapy

Bee venom therapy (BVT) involves the use of bee stings for possible medical benefits. There is a long history of BVT use in MS [2]. However, studies of BVT in MS are limited. In the most rigorous clinical trial to date, BVT in 26 patients with relapsing-remitting and secondary-progressive MS did not produce therapeutic effects on multiple outcome measures, including relapse rate, disability, MRI activity, quality of life, and fatigue [7]. Another study of 9 progressive MS patients did not find any therapeutic effects—4 of the 9 patients were withdrawn due to neurological worsening during the study [8]. BVT is generally safe, but anaphylactic reactions occur rarely. Also, periorbital bee stings, which are sometimes claimed to treat optic neuritis, may actually cause optic neuritis and should be avoided [1,2].

In MS, BVT has not been shown to produce any clear therapeutic effects and it may rarely cause serious side effects.

Cooling Therapy

The aim of cooling therapy is to make therapeutic use of the long-recognized temperature sensitivity that occurs in MS. It is known that MS symptoms frequently worsen with body warming and may improve with cooling. Various cooling strategies have been developed [2]. Simple methods include drinking cold beverages, avoiding exposure to warm environments, and staying in air-conditioned areas. More sophisticated approaches utilize specially designed cooling garments. MS clinical trials of variable quality have reported improvement in multiple symptoms with cooling [2,9,10]. The most rigorous study, which was randomized, blinded, and controlled, found objective improvement in walking and visual function and subjective improvement in cognition, strength, and fatigue [10]. Cooling is generally safe. The garments may be awkward to use. Cooling may provoke neurological worsening in the small fraction of MS patients who, paradoxically, are cold-sensitive [2].

> Cooling is a simple strategy that may be underutilized in the MS community.

Cooling is a simple, inexpensive approach that has little risk and multiple potential symptomatic benefits.

Cranberry

Cranberry is relevant to MS because MS-induced urinary retention increases the risk of urinary tract infections (UTIs) and the fruit of the cranberry plant may prevent UTIs. Some, but not all, clinical trials of cranberry indicate that it may prevent UTIs [2,11,12]. The UTI prevention effect may actually be less in those with underlying neurological conditions [12]. Importantly, cranberry is not effective for treating UTIs. Although cranberry is generally well tolerated, chronic use may increase the risk of kidney stones and cranberry use has rarely been associated with bleeding and

> Cranberry's likely mechanism of action—inhibition of bacterial adhesion to uroepithelium—is different from the mechanism of action of any conventional UTI medication.

prolongation of the international normalized ratio (INR) in those on warfarin [12]. Cranberry may be taken in the form of tablets, capsules, or juice.

Cranberry is usually well tolerated and may prevent UTIs. It should not be used to treat UTIs.

Echinacea and Other "Immune-Stimulating" Supplements

It is claimed erroneously in some lay publications that as MS is an immune condition, MS patients should take "immune-stimulating" supplements such as echinacea. Lists of various supplements that are known to activate T cells and macrophages are then provided and recommended for MS patients. This information is incorrect, and the recommendations are potentially dangerous. These supplements could actually worsen MS or antagonize the effects of disease-modifying medications. Based on animal models or in vitro studies, multiple herbs, vitamins, and minerals are associated with T cell or macrophage activation (Table 30.3) [1,2,11].

There is no evidence that "immune-stimulating" supplements provide any therapeutic effects in MS. In fact, owing to theoretical risks, these supplements should actually be avoided or used with caution.

Fish Oil and the Swank Diet

For decades, it has been hypothesized that polyunsaturated fatty acids (PUFAs), such as fish oil, may have disease-modifying effects in MS. Fatty acids exist in saturated and polyunsaturated forms. PUFAs include omega-3 and omega-6 fatty acids. Fish oil contains omega-3 fatty acids [2,13,14].

In the 1940s, a dietary approach known as the "Swank diet" was developed. This diet was low in saturated fat and high in PUFAs. It was claimed to have disease-modifying effects in MS, but the studies of this diet are inconclusive because they were not randomized, controlled, or blinded [13,14].

There have been several clinical trials of omega-3 fatty acid supplementation in MS. These studies have been inconclusive [13,14]. One large, controlled, randomized, double-blind trial of fish oil supplements did not report statistically significant effects, but there was a trend that favored the treatment group ($P < .07$) [15]. A recent rigorous, MRI-based study of fish oil as monotherapy or as combination therapy with interferon beta-1a did not

TABLE 30.3

Herbs, Vitamins, and Minerals With Possible "Immune-Stimulating" Effects

Alfalfa	Melatonin
Antioxidants	Maitake mushroom
Ashwagandha (*Withania somnifera*)	Mistletoe
Asian ginseng	Shiitake mushroom
Astragalus	Siberian ginseng
Cat's claw	Stinging nettle
Echinacea	Zinc
Garlic	

find an effect of fish oil on its primary outcome measure of MRI activity or on multiple secondary outcome measures, including relapse rate, disability progression, fatigue, and quality of life [16]. Since this trial was relatively small ($n = 92$) and of short–moderate duration (6 months for monotherapy, 18 months for combination therapy), it may not have been long enough and may have lacked statistical power to be absolutely definitive. However, there were no clear "trends" that favored fish oil for the multiple outcome measures. Fish oil is usually well tolerated. The clinical trials of fish oil in MS have not indicated any significant safety issues or antagonism of interferon effects. The FDA classifies fish oil as "generally regarded as safe" ("GRAS"). Fish oil may have mild anticoagulant effects. Also, PUFAs, especially in high doses, may produce vitamin E deficiency and thus supplementation with modest doses of vitamin E (100 international units [IU] daily) may be reasonable [2,12,16].

> Fish oil (and other dietary approaches) should not be used instead of conventional disease-modifying medications.

Fish oil is generally well tolerated. However, clinical trials of fish oil in MS have been inconclusive. Similarly, the clinical trial of the Swank diet has significant flaws and is inconclusive.

Ginkgo biloba

Ginkgo biloba has been used for centuries as an herbal therapy. It contains chemical constituents with a wide range of potential pharmacological activities, including anti-inflammatory and antioxidant effects. Through these actions, ginkgo could, in theory, exert symptom-relieving and disease-modifying actions in MS. One large study of ginkgo found that it was *not* effective for treating MS attacks. Limited MS clinical trials for possible symptomatic effects found improvement in fatigue and cognitive dysfunction [17,18]. Ginkgo is usually well tolerated, but there are some potential drug interactions and side effects. It may rarely cause seizures and produce anticoagulant effects. Mild side effects include headaches, rashes, dizziness, nausea, vomiting, and diarrhea [1,11].

> Ginkgo should probably be avoided in those with seizures and those who are undergoing surgery, have coagulopathies, or take antiplatelet or anticoagulant medications.

Limited clinical trials suggest that ginkgo improves fatigue and cognitive dysfunction but is ineffective for MS attacks. Ginkgo has limited side effects.

"Gluten Sensitivity"

Over the past several years, there has been a dramatic increase in interest in "gluten sensitivity" which has been paralleled by an increase in the availability of gluten-free foods. "Celiac disease," also known as "celiac sprue" and "gluten-sensitive enteropathy," is a well characterized form of gluten sensitivity that affects about 1% of the general population. This condition may cause significant malabsorption and is diagnosed on the basis of symptoms, antibody testing, and small-bowel biopsy. It is treated with a gluten-free diet [19,20].

It has been proposed that there is a milder and much more common variant of celiac disease that is known by several terms, including "gluten sensitivity," "non-celiac gluten sensitivity," and "celiac lite." With this condition, it is claimed that gluten may cause intestinal symptoms (diarrhea, abdominal pain, bloating) as well as extraintestinal symptoms (headache, lethargy, ataxia). It is also claimed that chronic neurological symptoms may be provoked in MS patients who have "gluten sensitivity." At this time, "gluten sensitivity" is difficult to diagnose or study as there are not any established diagnostic criteria. This condition has not been studied specifically in the MS population. It is a fairly benign experiment to limit or eliminate gluten from the diet of MS patients who believe they may have this condition, but this may be laborious and expensive. Also, this "casual," self-treatment approach may delay diagnosis and lead to inappropriate or inadequate management and treatment in those who actually have celiac disease [19–22].

"Gluten sensitivity" is a poorly defined condition that has not been fully characterized in MS or in the general population. Diagnostic testing for celiac disease should be considered in those who have significant gastrointestinal symptoms that are provoked by gluten.

Low Dose Naltrexone

Treatment with low doses of oral naltrexone, an opiate antagonist used for opiate and alcohol addiction, has been claimed to be therapeutic for many medical conditions, including MS. It is claimed that in MS, low dose naltrexone (LDN) relieves symptoms and also modifies the disease course by decreasing the attack rate and slowing disability progression. Much of the lay writing about LDN is based on anecdotal reports. Three clinical trials of LDN in MS have produced mixed results. One study in primary progressive MS reported improved spasticity, worsened pain, and no effect on other outcome measures, including fatigue, depression, and quality of life [23]. Two other studies used similar clinical trial designs to evaluate LDN in relapsing and progressive forms of MS. One of these studies found improvement in pain and mental health [24], while the other did not report any therapeutic effects [25]. Based on available evidence, LDN appears to be generally well tolerated. In one of the clinical trials, 1 patient with progressive MS experienced neurological worsening. In patients who are treated with opiates, LDN could provoke withdrawal.

> LDN should probably be avoided in patients who are treated with opiates.

LDN appears to be generally well tolerated. Therapeutic effects have been inconsistent in the studies of LDN in MS.

Marijuana

Marijuana contains tetrahydrocannabinol (THC) and other compounds known as cannabinoids (CBs). CBs have a wide range of biochemical effects that could, in theory, exert symptomatic and disease-modifying effects in MS. However, clinical trials of CBs in MS have produced variable results. Some, but not all, studies have shown improvement in spasticity [1,2,26–28]. In the largest and most rigorous study in MS, CBs produced subjective, but not objective, evidence for relief of pain and spasticity [27]. A 12 month extension of this study found that THC produced a small improvement in spasticity and a possible effect on disability [28]. A cannabinoid oromucosal spray (Sativex) is licensed for use outside the United States. Sativex has produced variable results in clinical trials evaluating multiple MS symptoms, including pain, spasticity, bladder dysfunction, and sleeping difficulties [29,30]. Marijuana may cause multiple adverse effects, including sedation, nausea, vomiting, impaired driving, seizures, incoordination, and poor pregnancy outcomes. Smoked marijuana may impair pulmonary function and increase the risk of cancer of the lung as well as the head and neck. In the United States, marijuana use is illegal at the federal level, but some states have legalized "medical marijuana" for those with MS and multiple other conditions [1,2,11].

States in which "medical marijuana" is legal for use in MS, patients may mistakenly assume that as it is legal, marijuana has been proven to be safe and effective in MS.

Clinical trials of marijuana use in MS have produced variable results for symptomatic and disease-modifying effects. Marijuana may produce significant side effects, and its use is illegal in many states and countries.

Mindfulness

Mindfulness refers to the psychological quality of bringing one's complete attention to the present moment in a nonjudgmental way. Training people to use this approach has been studied especially for the relief of stress and anxiety in an approach known as "Mindfulness Based Stress Reduction." Mindfulness approaches have also been studied in many other medical and psychological conditions. In MS, mindfulness was studied in an 8 week, randomized trial of 150 patients who received either mindfulness training or usual care [31]. Health-related quality of life improved immediately after the intervention and also at 6 months follow-up. Subgroup analysis also indicated improvement in fatigue, depression, and anxiety. Mindfulness is

Although mindfulness has undergone extensive clinical study over the past 30 years, it may be unfamiliar to many conventional health providers.

usually well tolerated. This approach should be taught by those who are able to recognize serious psychological or psychiatric issues for which mindfulness is not appropriate. In some cases, meditation and other relaxation methods may cause spasms and produce anxiety ("relaxation-induced anxiety"), fear of losing control, and disturbing thoughts [2].

Mindfulness is a low-risk approach that may relieve anxiety and other symptoms in MS.

Tai Chi

Tai chi is an ancient healing approach. Like acupuncture, tai chi is a component of the multimodal healing method of traditional Chinese medicine. Two small clinical trials of tai chi in MS reported improvement in walking, spasticity, and social and emotional functioning [32,33]. Tai chi is generally well tolerated. It may cause strained muscles and joints. Modified forms of tai chi are available for those with disabilities [2].

Tai chi is a generally safe therapy that has been reported as a low-risk therapy that has produced improvement in multiple MS symptoms in limited clinical trial testing.

Vitamin B_{12}

Lay publications sometimes claim that vitamin B_{12} supplements produce therapeutic effects in MS. There is no strong clinical evidence to support such an approach. Several studies indicate that there is a small fraction of MS patients who have vitamin B_{12} deficiency. MS patients who are vitamin B_{12}-deficient should be supplemented. Vitamin B_{12} supplements are generally well tolerated. Rarely, these supplements may cause rashes, diarrhea, and itching [1,2,11].

Since vitamin B_{12} deficiency may mimic MS and a subgroup of MS patients are vitamin B_{12}-deficient, MS patients should have a vitamin B_{12} level determined at least once.

Vitamin B_{12} supplements are generally safe. Supplementation with vitamin B_{12} is only indicated in those with vitamin B_{12} deficiency.

Vitamin D

Vitamin D has many potential effects on MS. It has been known for years that MS patients are at risk for developing osteopenia and osteoporosis, and vitamin D is important for maintaining bone density. In addition to these effects on bones, studies over the past decade have raised the possibility that, through immune-regulating effects, vitamin D might have disease-modifying (and preventive) actions in MS, and, possibly by improving leg function and gait stability, vitamin D could improve neurological function in MS [1,34].

Observational studies have shown that low blood levels and low intake of vitamin D are associated with a higher risk for developing MS. Low blood levels are also associated with a higher risk of converting from clinically isolated syndrome (CIS) to MS and with a higher risk for attacks, MRI activity, and disability progression in those with MS. Interventional studies of vitamin D in MS have been published but these are of variable quality and have reported mixed results to date. High quality intervention studies are needed [34–36].

Vitamin D is usually well tolerated. The recommended daily amount (RDA) is 600 to 800 IU. The daily tolerable upper intake level (UL) is 4,000 IU daily. High doses may cause nausea, vomiting, fatigue, hypertension, and renal damage. Emerging evidence indicates that high doses (greater than 4,000 IU daily) or high blood levels (greater than 55 ng/mL) of vitamin D could *increase* the risk of fractures, falls, cardiovascular disease, all-cause mortality, and some cancers, including pancreatic [1,2,11,37].

In reasonable doses, vitamin D is generally safe. Limited studies indicate that vitamin D could have preventive, disease-modifying, and symptomatic effects in MS. Further studies are needed in this area. Vitamin D supplementation should be considered in MS patients with low vitamin D levels.

Yoga

Yoga is a component of Ayurveda, an ancient healing approach developed in India. Although yoga is widely used in some MS communities, it has undergone limited investigation in MS. There is 1 rigorous clinical trial of yoga in MS [38]. This study examined 2 different interventions, yoga and conventional exercise, and found that, relative to a control group, fatigue was lower with either yoga or conventional exercise. Smaller and less rigorous clinical trials of yoga and MS have reported improvement in fatigue, balance, walking endurance, spasticity, and cognitive function [39,40]. Yoga is generally well tolerated and may be modified for those with disabilities [2].

Yoga is a generally well-tolerated approach that may improve fatigue and multiple other symptoms in MS.

CONCLUSION

CAM use is common among MS patients, yet CAM may not be discussed with MS patients in some health care settings. Conventional health care providers may provide a valuable role in the care and education of their MS patients by providing guidance about CAM use. It may be especially helpful to provide general information about CAM and also specific, MS-relevant information about the risks and benefits of CAM therapies.

KEY POINTS FOR PATIENTS AND FAMILIES

- When trying to decide about using some form of CAM, discuss this with a health care provider. The risks and benefits of the CAM therapy should be obtained and reviewed before making a decision.

- If no objective information is available about a CAM therapy, it should be approached with caution.

- Vitamins, minerals, and herbs should be used with caution as they, like drugs, have the potential to worsen medical conditions or interact with other medications. There is limited information about the safety and effectiveness of dietary supplements in MS and when used in combination with MS medications.

- There are *no* CAM approaches that have been proven to be disease modifying and there are *many* conventional medications that have been proven to have this effect. CAM approaches should be used in conjunction with disease-modifying therapy rather than as an alternative.

- Information about CAM and MS is ever-changing. As a result, it is important to have ongoing discussions with a health care provider about CAM therapies that are being used or are being considered.

REFERENCES

1. Bowling AC. Complementary and alternative medicine and multiple sclerosis. *Neurol Clin.* 2011;29:465–480.

2. Bowling AC. *Complementary and Alternative Medicine and Multiple Sclerosis.* New York: Demos Medical Publishing; 2007.

3. O'Connor K, Weinstock-Gutmann B, Carl E, et al. Patterns of dietary and herbal supplement use by multiple sclerosis patients. *J Neurol.* 2012;259:637–644.

4. Donnelan CP, Shanley J. Comparison of the effect of two types of acupuncture on quality of life in secondary progressive multiple sclerosis: A preliminary single-blind randomized controlled trial. *Clin Rehabil.* 2008;22:195–205.

5. Markowitz CE, Spitsin S, Zimmerman V, et al. The treatment of multiple sclerosis with inosine. *J Altern Compl Med.* 2009;15:619–625.

6. Gonsette RE, Sindic C, D'hooge MB, et al. Boosting endogenous neuroprotection in multiple sclerosis: The association of inosine and interferon-beta in relapsing-remitting multiple sclerosis (ASIIMS) trial. *Mult Scler.* 2010;16:455–462.

7. Wesselius T, Heersema DJ, Mostert JP, et al. A randomized crossover study of bee sting therapy for multiple sclerosis. *Neurology.* 2005;65:1764–1768.

8. Castro HJ, Mendez-Inocencio JI, Omidvar B, et al. A phase I study of the safety of honeybee venom extract as a possible treatment for patients with progressive forms of multiple sclerosis. *Allergy Asthma Proc.* 2005;26:470–476.

9. Meyer-Heim A, Rothmaier M, Weder M, et al. Advanced lightweight cooling-garment technology: Functional improvements in thermosensitive patients with multiple sclerosis. *Mult Scler.* 2007;13:232–237.

10. NASA/MS Cooling Study Group. A randomized controlled study of the acute and chronic effects of cooling therapy for MS. *Neurology.* 2003;60:1955–1960.

11. Jellin JM, Gregory PJ, Batz F, et al. *Pharmacist's Letter/Prescriber's Letter Natural Medicines Comprehensive Database,* 8th ed. Stockton, CA: Therapeutic Research Faculty; 2010.

12. Guay DRP. Cranberry and urinary tract infections. *Drugs.* 2009;69:775–807.

13. Stewart TM, Bowling AC. Polyunsaturated fatty acid supplementation in MS. *Int MS J.* 2005;12:88–93.

14. Mehta LR, Dworkin RH, Schwid SR. Polyunsaturated fatty acids and their potential therapeutic role in multiple sclerosis. *Nature Clin Pract Neurol.* 2009;5:82–92.

15. Bates D, Cartlidge N, French J, et al. A double-blind controlled trial of long chain n-3 polyunsaturated fatty acids in the treatment of multiple sclerosis. *J Neurol Neurosurg Psychiatry.* 1989;52:18–22.

16. Torkildsen O, Wergelend S, Bakke S, et al. Omega-3 fatty acid treatment in multiple sclerosis (OFAMS study). *Arch Neurol.* 2012;69(8):1044–1051. doi:10.101/archneurol.2012.283.

17. Lovera J, Bagert B, Smoot K, et al. Ginkgo biloba for the improvement of cognitive performance in multiple sclerosis: A randomized, placebo-controlled trial. *Mult Scler.* 2007;13:376–385.

18. Johnson SK, Diamond BJ, Rausch S, et al. The effect of Ginkgo biloba on functional measure in multiple sclerosis: A pilot randomized controlled trial. *Explore (NY).* 2006;2:19–24.

19. Troncone R, Jabri B. Coeliac disease and gluten sensitivity. *J Intern Med.* 2011;269:582–590.

20. Sapone A, Bai JC, Ciacci C, et al. Spectrum of gluten-related disorders: Consensus on new nomenclature and classification. *BMC Medicine.* 2012;10:13.

21. DiSabatino A, Corazza GR. Nonceliac gluten sensitivity: Sense or sensibility? *Ann Intern Med.* 2012;156:309–311.

22. Hadjivassiliou M, Sanders DS, Grünewald RA, et al. Gluten sensitivity: From gut to brain. *Lancet Neurol.* 2010;9:318–330.

23. Gironi M, Martinelli-Boneschi F, Sacerdote P, et al. A pilot trial of low-dose naltrexone in primary progressive multiple sclerosis. *Mult Scler.* 2008;14:1076–1083.

24. Cree BA, Kornyeyeva E, Goodin DS. Pilot trial of low-dose naltrexone and quality of life in multiple sclerosis. *Ann Neurol.* 2010;68:145–150.

25. Sharafaddinzadeh N, Moghtaderi A, Kashipazha D, et al. The effect of low-dose naltrexone on quality of life of patients with multiple sclerosis: A randomized placebo-controlled trial. *Mult Scler.* 2010;16:964–969.

26. Corey-Bloom J, Wolfson T, Gamst A, et al. Smoked cannabis for spasticity in multiple sclerosis: A randomized, placebo-controlled trial. *Can Med Assoc J.* 2012;184(10):1143–1150. doi:10.1503/cmaj.110837.

27. Zajicek J, Fox P, Sanders H, et al. Cannabinoids for treatment of spasticity and other symptoms related to multiple sclerosis (CAMS study): Multicentre randomised placebo-controlled trial. *Lancet.* 2003;362:1517–1526.

28. Zajicek J, Sanders HP, Wright DE, et al. Cannabinoids in multiple sclerosis (CAMS) study: Safety and efficacy data for 12 months follow-up. *J Neurol Neurosurg Psychiatry.* 2005;76:1664–1669.

29. Barnes MP. Sativex: Clinical efficacy and tolerability in the treatment of symptoms of multiple sclerosis and neuropathic pain. *Exp Opin Pharmacother.* 2006;7:607–615.

30. Centonze D, Mori F, Koch G, et al. Lack of effect of cannabis-based treatment on clinical and laboratory measures in multiple sclerosis. *Neurol Sci.* 2009;30:531–534.

31. Grossman P, Kappos L, Gensicke H, et al. MS quality of life, depression, and fatigue improve after mindfulness training. *Neurology.* 2010;75:1141–1149.

32. Husted C, Pham L, Hekking A. Improving quality of life for people with chronic conditions: The example of t'ai chi and multiple sclerosis. *Altern Ther Health Med.* 1999;5:70–74.

33. Mills M, Allen J. Mindfulness of movement as a coping strategy in multiple sclerosis. A pilot study. *Gen Hosp Psychiatry.* 2000;22:425–431.

34. Simon KC, Munger KL, Ascherio A. Vitamin D and multiple sclerosis: Epidemiology, immunology, and genetics. *Curr Opin Neurol.* 2012;25:246–251.

35. Kampman MT, Steffensen LH, Mellgren SI, Jørgensen L. Effect of vitamin D3 supplementation on relapses, disease progression, and measures of function in persons with multiple sclerosis: Exploratory outcomes from a double-blind randomised controlled trial. *Mult Scler.* 2012;18(8):1144–1151. doi:10.1177/1352458511434607.

36. Soilu-Hanninen M, Aivo J, Lindstrom BM, et al. A randomised, double-blind, placebo controlled trial with vitamin D3 as an add on treatment to interferon beta-1b in patients with multiple sclerosis. *J Neurol Neurosurg Psychiatry.* 2012;83:565–571.

37. Ross AC, Taylor CL, Yaktine AL, et al., eds. *Dietary Reference Intakes for Calcium and Vitamin D.* Washington DC: The National Academies Press; 2010.

38. Oken BS, Kishiyama S, Zajdel D, et al. Randomized controlled trial of yoga and exercise in multiple sclerosis. *Neurology.* 2004;62:2058–2064.

39. Velikonja O, Curic K, Ozura A, et al. Influence of sports climbing and yoga on spasticity, cognitive function, mood and fatigue in patients with multiple sclerosis. *Clin Neurol Neurosurg.* 2010;112:597–601.

40. Ahmadi A, Nikbakh M, Arastoo AA, et al. The effects of a yoga intervention on balance, speed and endurance of walking, fatigue, and quality of life in people with multiple sclerosis. *J Hum Kinetics.* 2010;23:71–78.

Part V. Special Issues

31

Pediatric Multiple Sclerosis

LINDSEY STULL
AMY T. WALDMAN

KEY POINTS FOR CLINICIANS

- Pediatric and adult multiple sclerosis (MS) have similar clinical symptoms.

- The presence of encephalopathy and a polysymptomatic presentation or diffuse central nervous system (CNS) involvement are required for a diagnosis of acute disseminated encephalomyelitis (ADEM). A history of infection or vaccination is not required for ADEM.

- For children presenting with transient neurological symptoms such as paresthesias, the diagnosis of MS may not be recognized by a pediatrician or other health care professional, especially if the symptoms self-resolve, the neurological examination is normal, or limited imaging is performed. Therefore, a high index of suspicion for pediatric MS is required.

- In children meeting the clinical criteria for a clinically isolated syndrome, the MRI criteria for dissemination in space and dissemination in time proposed by the 2010 revisions to the McDonald Criteria are applicable to children, especially those greater than 11 years of age.

- Children with MS have more frequent relapses early in the disease course and a greater T2 lesion volume at disease onset than adults; however, they generally have a slower progression to disability.

- Primary progressive MS is exceedingly rare in children and should prompt consideration of alternative diagnoses such as metabolic, mitochondrial, or neurodegenerative disorders (including leukodystrophies).

- In pediatric MS, relapse management is similar to adult MS, typically beginning with high-dose corticosteroids, 20 to 30 mg/kg per day (maximum of 1,000 mg) for 3 to 5 days, followed by an oral prednisone taper.

- Adult dosing of disease-modifying therapy (interferon beta and glatiramer acetate) is generally prescribed, although interferons should be titrated up to the full dose to minimize potential side effects.

- While disability can be minimal in pediatric MS, cognitive evaluation is a key aspect of care.

Pediatric multiple sclerosis (MS) was first described in 1922. Thirty-six years later, one of the first retrospective studies on pediatric MS, which enrolled 40 children with MS between 1920 and 1952, concluded that children and adults with MS have similar clinical profiles including symptoms and physical and laboratory (cerebral spinal fluid [CSF]) findings. Shortly thereafter, pediatric MS was recognized by the first expert panel organized to establish a definition of clinically definite MS. In 1961, Dr. George Schumacher and colleagues permitted the inclusion of children (greater than 10 years of age) in their clinical description of the disease [1].

Although pediatric MS has been recognized for almost a century, dedicated pediatric MS centers, facilitated by national collaborative programs, have been established mostly over the past decade. Pediatric MS research has also grown substantially. Although many similarities exist between pediatric- and adult-onset MS, the differences between the groups are of considerable interest to investigators. Such differences, which have raised questions about the impact of age, genetic susceptibility, and environmental exposures on the developing immune system, will hopefully lead to a greater understanding of the pathophysiology of the disease. This chapter highlights these unique issues relevant to the diagnosis and prognosis for MS in our youngest patients.

DEFINITIONS OF ACQUIRED DEMYELINATING SYNDROMES IN CHILDREN

Perhaps the greatest challenge in diagnosing MS in children is the overlap between acute disseminated encephalomyelitis (ADEM) and pediatric MS. More common in children than adults, ADEM is an inflammatory demyelinating disease of the brain and spinal cord. ADEM is typically a monophasic illness; however, relapses of ADEM have occurred in children who do not meet the criteria for MS. In 2007, the International Pediatric MS Study Group proposed working definitions to allow for greater consistency in the diagnosis of ADEM, pediatric MS, and other acquired demyelinating syndromes in childhood (see Table 31.1) [2]. By creating a uniform language, the group hoped for more accurate diagnostic and prognostic data from future research.

According to the International Pediatric MS Study Group definitions, a first demyelinating event in childhood meets the criteria for ADEM if encephalopathy is present and the child has a multifocal/polysymptomatic presentation. In the absence of one or both of these criteria, the child has a clinically isolated syndrome (CIS), which can be monofocal or multifocal based on the clinical symptoms. For example, optic neuritis with asymptomatic brain lesions at the time of the initial presentation is considered a monofocal CIS.

As in adults, pediatric MS is a chronic disease defined by neurological events separated in time and space affecting any age (including those under 10 years). The consensus definitions, published in 2007, allow for the diagnosis of MS

using MRI scans and spinal fluid to confirm dissemination in time and space. The definitions of the latter were based on the 2005 McDonald Criteria. The 2010 McDonald Criteria are applicable to children (see Diagnosis and MRI section in this chapter). Ninety-five percent of children have relapsing-remitting MS [3]; secondary progression rarely occurs during childhood or adolescence. Primary progressive MS is exceedingly rare in children; therefore, a progressive clinical course in a child should prompt consideration of genetic, metabolic, mitochondrial, neoplastic, and other disorders.

Neuromyelitis optica (NMO) is diagnosed in children who have optic neuritis and myelitis and the presence of either a longitudinally extensive lesion (measuring 3 vertebral segments or more) on an MRI of the spinal cord or NMO-IgG antibody positivity [2]. An MRI of the brain may also reveal lesions, especially in the deep gray matter or brain stem. Large, diffuse subcortical white matter lesions can also occur.

INCIDENCE OF PEDIATRIC MS

Approximately 3% to 5% of adults with MS experience their first attack prior to 18 years of age [4]. The incidence of pediatric MS in the United States is 0.5 per 100,000 children, or 379 new cases each year according to a recent study performed using a large health maintenance organization database in southern California [5]. The same study estimated the incidence of all demyelinating diseases (including ADEM, optic neuritis, and transverse myelitis) to be 1.6 per 100,000 or 1,246 new cases per year [5]. In comparison, a prospective national Canadian study reported an incidence of an initial demyelinating syndrome of 0.9 per 100,000 children [6]. Another prospective national study determined the incidence of pediatric MS (less than 16 years) in Germany to be 0.3 per 100,000 children [7]. The variation between studies may reflect different methodologies or may be due to different environmental and genetic factors. For example, age, race, ethnicity, and residence may alter susceptibility for pediatric MS.

> 3% of MS patients experience their first symptom in childhood.

DEMOGRAPHICS

The risk of pediatric MS increases with age. Multiple studies have shown an increased risk in pediatric MS after 10 to 11 years of age [7–9] (see section on Risk of MS after a first demyelinating event) whereas ADEM commonly occurs between 3 and 8 years of age [10–12]. While younger

> The risk of pediatric MS increases after 11 years of age.

TABLE 31.1
Definitions

ACQUIRED DEMYELINATING SYNDROMES	PROPOSED CONSENSUS DEFINITIONS	COMMENTS
ADEM (monophasic)	• A first clinical event with a presumed inflammatory or demyelinating cause, with acute or subacute onset that affects multifocal areas of the CNS • The clinical presentation must be polysymptomatic and must include encephalopathy, which is defined as 1 or more of the following: • Behavioral change, eg, confusion, excessive irritability • Alteration in consciousness, eg, lethargy, coma • Event should be followed by improvement, either clinically, on MRI, or both, but there may be residual deficits • New or fluctuating symptoms, signs, or MRI findings occurring within 3 months of the inciting ADEM event are considered part of the acute event • Neuroimaging shows focal or multifocal lesion(s), predominantly involving white matter, without radiological evidence of previous destructive white matter changes • Brain MRI, with FLAIR or T2-weighted images, reveals large (1 to 2 cm in size) lesions that are multifocal, hyperintense, and located in the supratentorial or infratentorial white matter regions; gray matter, especially basal ganglia and thalamus, is frequently involved • In rare cases, brain MR images show a large single lesion (1 to 2 cm), predominantly affecting white matter • Spinal cord MRI may show confluent intramedullary lesion(s) with variable enhancement, in addition to abnormal brain MRI findings	• A single clinical event of ADEM can evolve over a period of 3 months, with fluctuations in clinical symptoms and severity • MRI findings alone are insufficient for the diagnosis of ADEM • Documentation of a prior infection and isolation of an infectious agent are not required for diagnosis
Recurrent ADEM	• New event of ADEM with a recurrence of the initial symptoms and signs, 3 or more months after the first ADEM event, without involvement of new clinical areas by history, examination, or neuroimaging • Event does not occur while on steroids, and occurs at least 1 month after completing therapy • Lesions seen on the original MRI may have enlarged; however, no new areas of the CNS are affected on MRI.	
Multiphasic ADEM	• ADEM followed by a new clinical event also meeting criteria for ADEM, but involving new anatomic areas of the CNS as confirmed by history, neurological examination, and neuroimaging • The subsequent event must occur (a) at least 3 months after the onset of the initial ADEM event and (b) at least 1 month after completing steroid therapy • The subsequent event must include a polysymptomatic presentation including encephalopathy, with neurological symptoms or signs that differ from the initial event (mental status changes may not differ from the initial event) • The brain MRI must show new areas of involvement but also demonstrate complete or partial resolution of those lesions associated with the first ADEM event	• The new event must meet the clinical criteria for ADEM, including the presence of encephalopathy. Serial MRIs of patients with multiphasic ADEM, obtained following resolution of the second demyelinating event, should ultimately show a complete or partial resolution in the MRI lesions, in contrast to serial MRI findings in patients with MS that typically demonstrate ongoing accrual of asymptomatic lesions
Neuromyelitis Optica (modified criteria from 2005)	• Must have optic neuritis and acute myelitis as major criteria • Must have either a spinal MRI lesion extending over 3 or more segments or be NMO-positive on antibody testing	• Brain lesions, located in the hypothalamus, brain stem, or diffuse cerebral white matter, have been described in children who have typical features of NMO

CIS	• A CIS is a first acute clinical episode of CNS symptoms with a presumed inflammatory demyelinating cause for which there is no prior history of a demyelinating event. This clinical event may either be monofocal or multifocal, but usually does not include encephalopathy (except in cases of brain stem syndromes) • Examples include optic neuritis (unilateral or bilateral), transverse myelitis (typically partial), and brain stem, cerebellar, and/or hemispheric dysfunction	• The term CIS is applied to the first clinical demyelinating event (ie, isolated in time). In contrast to ADEM, there is no encephalopathy or fever • The Study Group elected to define CIS as multifocal if the clinical features could be attributed to more than one CNS site and monofocal if the clinical symptoms could be attributed to a single CNS lesion. These distinctions are based solely on clinical findings. The term multifocal cannot be applied to a clinically monofocal presentation in which the MRI shows multiple asymptomatic lesions
Pediatric MS	• Pediatric MS requires multiple episodes of CNS demyelination separated in time and space as specified for adults, however, eliminating any lower age limit (eg, includes those under age 10) • The MRI can be used to meet the dissemination in space criterion • The combination of an abnormal CSF and 2 lesions on the MRI, of which 1 must be in the brain, can also meet dissemination in space criterion; the CSF must show either oligoclonal bands or an elevated IgG index • MRI can be used to satisfy the criterion for dissemination in time following the initial clinical event, even in the absence of a new clinical demyelinating event; new T2 or gadolinium-enhancing lesions must develop 3 months following the initial clinical event • An episode consistent with the clinical features of ADEM cannot be considered as the first event of MS	• The dissemination in space criterion can be satisfied in the neurological evaluation if the history and findings are consistent with multifocal disease. Failure to meet MRI criterion of dissemination in space does not preclude the subsequent diagnosis of MS • In the special circumstance of a child whose initial clinical demyelinating event was diagnosed as ADEM, a second non-ADEM demyelinating event alone is not sufficient for the diagnosis of MS

ADEM, acute disseminated encephalomyelitis; CIS, clinically isolated syndrome; CNS, central nervous system; CSF, cerebrospinal fluid; FLAIR, fluid attenuated inversion recovery; NMO, neuromyelitis optica. *Source:* [2].

children are more likely to present with ADEM and older children have monofocal or multifocal CISs, there are exceptions, and the proposed International Pediatric MS Study Group criteria, not age, should be used to diagnose acquired demyelinating syndromes in children.

Overall, the proportion of males and females presenting with all demyelinating diseases is approximately equal; however, the female:male ratio is approximately 2:1 in pediatric MS whereas there is perhaps a male predominance in ADEM [10,11].

Many pediatric studies have demonstrated a lower proportion of white/Caucasian race among pediatric-onset MS compared to adult-onset disease [4,13–15]. While referral bias may influence the proportion of minorities at some centers, there is growing evidence to suggest that the risk of MS is increased in African American and Asian children as well as those with a Hispanic background. The influence of race and ethnicity on disease severity is addressed later in the chapter (see section on Relapses).

The difference in demographics between children and adults with MS may be due to differences in susceptibility among different races and ethnicities in children or may reflect more diverse populations living in areas of higher MS risk. In fact, a Canadian study demonstrated a higher proportion of patients with Caribbean, Asian, or Middle Eastern ancestry than the adult MS population from the same area, suggesting that risk of MS is determined in part by disease risk in the place of residence during childhood regardless of ancestry [15].

OTHER RISK FACTORS

Environmental risk factors for MS have been the subject of much research. As noted earlier, the place of residence during childhood influences the risk of MS. The prevalence of MS increases proportionate to distance from the equator, perhaps owing to decreased sun exposure. Lower serum levels of vitamin D increase the risk of pediatric and adult MS [8,16] and have been linked to an increased relapse rate in pediatric MS (see subsequent section on Relapses) [17]. Large-scale retrospective analyses have also shown an increased risk for MS in children of mothers with lower levels of exposure to UV radiation in the first trimester of pregnancy [18].

Other factors contributing to adult MS have also been investigated in children. The *HLA-DRB1*1501/1503* allele linked to increased susceptibility in adult MS has been shown to confer similarly increased risk upon pediatric patients of European ancestry presenting with acquired demyelinating syndromes [19]. A remote Epstein–Barr virus (EBV) infection is also associated with an increased risk of MS. The presence of antibodies against EBV nuclear antigen along with the presence of the *HLA-DRB1*1501* allele markedly increases MS risk in adults [20]. However, a genetic–environmental interaction has not been shown in children. Rather, the *HLA-DRB1*15* genotype, remote EBV infection, and vitamin D insufficiency (defined as less than 75 nmoL/L which corresponds to 30 ng/mL), are

independent risk factors for pediatric MS [8]. Absence of these 3 risk factors is associated with a low risk of MS (5%) [8]. In a national prospective study, approximately 57% of the children with all 3 factors have been diagnosed with MS [8]. Additional national collaborative studies to further investigate potential interactions are currently underway.

While the *HLA-DRB1* allele and Epstein–Barr nuclear antigen-1 seropositivity are independent risk factors, the *HLA-DRB1* allele may be implicated in the role of herpes simplex virus (HSV) in MS. One study showed that HSV played a protective role against MS in children with the *HLA-DRB1* allele, and that the risk of MS was increased in those with HSV that did not have the allele [21]. The same study demonstrated a decreased risk of MS in children previously exposed to cytomegalovirus (CMV) [21].

A French study linked parental smoking at home to increased risk (adjusted RR = 2.12) of pediatric-onset MS as compared to controls. The investigators also found that the risk was higher still (RR = 2.49) with longer duration of exposure in children over the age of 10 [22]. Though several studies pointed to a possible relationship between Hepatitis B vaccination and subsequent development of pediatric MS, more stringent analyses have found the vaccination to have no effect on risk [23].

> The presence of the *HLA-DRB1* allele, remote EBV infection, vitamin D deficiency, and parental smoking increase the risk of pediatric MS.

CLINICAL FEATURES

Signs and Symptoms

The clinical symptoms in pediatric MS are very similar to adult-onset disease. CNS demyelination may result in visual disturbances, sensory manifestations, weakness or spasticity, balance difficulties, gait abnormalities, or bowel and bladder dysfunction localizing to the brain or spinal cord. Lhermitte's sign and Uhthoff's phenomenon also occur in children.

One of the most common presenting symptoms of MS in both children and adults is optic neuritis, characterized by decreased visual acuity, red color desaturation, and visual field deficits. Compared to adults, children are more likely to have bilateral involvement, especially children under 10 years of age. Children often present with significant vision loss (visual acuities of 20/200 or worse); however, the visual recovery is favorable as most achieve a visual acuity of 20/40 or better [24,25]—many of the children in these studies received intravenous corticosteroids (see section on Relapses). Children with bilateral optic

> Bilateral optic neuritis is more common in children under 10 years of age.

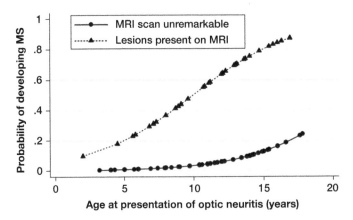

FIGURE 31.1
Probability of developing MS versus age at presentation of optic neuritis in children. The probability of developing pediatric MS, adjusted for the presence (defined as 1 or more T2-weighted and FLAIR signal abnormalities outside the visual system) or absence of MRI lesions, is presented. *Source: [9].*

neuritis are not at higher risk for MS compared to those presenting with unilateral optic neuritis. Rather, risk of MS after optic neuritis increases with age at presentation, regardless of whether the child has unilateral or bilateral disease. The presence of asymptomatic MRI lesions outside the visual system markedly increases the risk of MS [9] (see Figure 31.1 and section on Risk of MS after a first demyelinating event).

Laboratory Studies

Cerebrospinal Fluid
A lumbar puncture is routinely recommended for nearly all children presenting with demyelinating disease, although some physicians are less inclined to order a spinal tap for isolated optic neuritis [26]. Approximately 70% of physicians routinely obtain CSF studies in isolated optic neuritis [26].

> Oligoclonal bands are present in about 60% of children with MS and are more common in children over 11 years of age.

The presence of oligoclonal bands (OCB) in the CSF is not as high in children with MS as suggested in adult studies: approximately 60% of children with MS have OCB [8] compared to 85% of adults with MS [27] (see Chapter 9). Once again, age is a key factor as age influences the CSF profile, with younger children (under 11 years of age) more likely to have a greater CSF white blood cell (WBC) count with a higher number of polynuclear cells (neutrophils), although a lymphocytic predominance is present in all ages [28]. In the same study, OCBs were present in 63% of older children (11 years

of age or older) but only 43% of younger children with MS. Similarly, an elevated IgG index was seen in 68% of older children versus 35% of younger children. In adults, the presence of OCB during a first demyelinating event increases the risk of having a second clinical attack within a year [29,30]. While children with a positive IgG profile and the absence of neutrophils in the CSF independently had shorter times to their second attack in 1 study, further data is needed to determine whether the CSF profile influences the risk and timing of attacks [28].

Other Laboratory Investigations
The evaluation of a child with any demyelinating disease should include a complete blood count, erythrocyte sedimentation rate, and antinuclear antibody [31]. In addition, a basic metabolic panel, angiotensin-converting enzyme, C-reactive protein, thyroid stimulating hormone, B_{12} level, and folate are typically ordered by a majority of physicians to exclude mimics of CNS demyelination [26]. A serum vitamin D_{25} (OH) level is commonly obtained as vitamin D deficiency may increase susceptibility to MS and influence relapse rate. Further laboratory studies are often selected on the basis of the clinical phenotype, such as NMO IgG in a patient presenting with optic nerve and spinal cord symptoms or a metabolic work-up or lysosomal enzymes in a child with a history of developmental regression.

MRI

MRI of the brain and/or spinal cord is the standard of investigation for children with suspected demyelinating disease. As in adults, T2/fluid attenuated inversion recovery (FLAIR) hyperintensities are found in children with MS throughout the supra- and infratentorial brain and spinal cord. In order of decreasing frequency, brain lesions can be found in the deep white matter, juxtacortical white matter, periventricular white matter, corpus callosum, internal capsule, cortical gray matter, deep gray nuclei, brain stem, and cerebellum [32]. Most lesions in children measure less than 1 cm axially (and 1.5 cm longitudinally). However, larger lesions are also common in pediatric MS, as 65% of a pediatric MS cohort had at least one lesion measuring more than 2 cm [32].

Brain lesion volumes were compared between children with CISs and adults with MS. At the time of a first demyelinating event, children have similar supratentorial lesion volumes but increased infratentorial lesion volumes compared to adults with established MS [33]. Comparing the first MRI scan of the brain between children and adults, another study also demonstrated an increased number of T2 lesions (more than 3 mm²), large T2 lesions (more than 1 cm), posterior fossa lesions, and gadolinium-enhancing lesions in children compared to adults [34]. With follow-up imaging, the same study also showed that children had more new T2 hyperintensities and more gadolinium-enhancing lesions compared to adults [34].

The MRI scan in prepubertal children (under 11 years of age) presents additional challenges. While the number of T2 lesions on the initial MRI scan is similar between children under 11 years and 11 years or older, younger children have fewer discrete ovoid lesions and more large lesions (larger than 1 cm) [35]. Additional trends in the younger group included fewer enhancing lesions and more deep gray matter involvement. On follow-up imaging, a reduction in the number of T2 hyperintensities was observed in the prepubertal group with MS. ADEM is often diagnosed in these patients because of their age and MRI appearance (see the section on Differential Diagnosis).

Diagnosis

As in adults, pediatric MS is diagnosed after 2 events, separated in time and space. The 2010 revisions to the McDonald criteria (discussed in Chapter 7) specifically addressed the application of these criteria to the pediatric population. The McDonald Criteria were designed and validated in adults presenting with a CIS. The McDonald MRI Criteria for dissemination in time and space are appropriate for children with CISs, especially those over the age of 11 years.

> The 2010 McDonald Criteria can be used to demonstrate dissemination in time and space, especially in children over 11 years of age.

The original McDonald Criteria for dissemination in space (3 of the following 4: (a) 1 gadolinium-enhancing lesion or 9 or more T2 hyperintense lesions in the absence of a gadolinium-enhancing lesion, (b) 1 or more infratentorial lesion(s), (c) 1 or more juxtacortical lesion(s), (d) 3 or more periventricular lesions) were not sensitive for children with clinically definite MS [36]. To date, the most sensitive MRI criteria for a diagnosis of pediatric MS are the Callen MS criteria. The criteria include at least 2 of the following 3: (a) 5 or more T2 lesions in the brain, (b) 2 or more periventricular lesions, and (c) 1 or more brain stem lesion(s). These criteria, established in a cohort of children with clinically definite MS compared to healthy controls and children with other neurological diseases (migraine, CNS Lupus), have a sensitivity of 85% and a specificity of 98%.

> The Callen MS criteria include the presence of at least 2 of the following: (a) 5 or more T2 lesions, (b) 2 or more periventricular lesions, and (c) 1 or more brain stem lesion(s). These criteria have a sensitivity of 85% and a specificity of 98% for a diagnosis of pediatric MS.

Differential Diagnosis

Clinicians must take care to exclude a number of other conditions that may present with CNS involvement, including other acquired demyelinating disorders (NMO, transverse myelitis, fulminant demyelinating diseases) as well as metabolic, infectious, vascular, genetic, neoplastic, mitochondrial, and systemic inflammatory disorders.

One of the biggest diagnostic challenges is differentiating between ADEM and a first attack of MS. ADEM is clinically distinguished if encephalopathy and multifocal deficits are present (see Table 31.1); however, exceptions occur. Some neurologists have questioned the inclusion of encephalopathy for a diagnosis of ADEM. As stated by the International Pediatric MS Study Group, the inclusion of encephalopathy improves specificity for ADEM.

> ADEM is characterized by encephalopathy and multifocal deficits.

MRI has also been used to differentiate ADEM from MS. ADEM is typically associated with multiple large asymmetric lesions in the white matter and deep gray nuclei; the brain stem, cerebellum, and spinal cord may also be affected. The following criteria can be used with a sensitivity of 81% and specificity of 95% to distinguish a first attack of MS from ADEM. At the time of an initial demyelinating event, the diagnosis of MS is likely if 2 of the following are present: (a) 2 or more periventricular lesions, (b) the presence of black holes (enhancing or nonenhancing), or (c) the absence of a diffuse bilateral lesion pattern

> Using MRI to differentiate between ADEM and MS, the presence of 2 of the following favors a diagnosis of MS: (a) 2 or more periventricular lesions, (b) the presence of 1 or more T1 hypointensities, or (c) the absence of a diffuse bilateral lesion pattern.

Traditionally, ADEM is considered a monophasic illness; however, relapses do occur. A relapse within 3 months of the initial event or one that occurs within 1 month of the withdrawal of steroids is not considered a new attack but rather part of the original event. However, relapses occurring more than 3 months after the initial event and more than 1 month after steroids may be diagnosed as relapsing ADEM, or multiphasic ADEM, depending whether the same CNS site or new CNS sites are affected (see Table 31.1). Encephalopathy must also be present for these diagnoses.

The International Pediatric MS Study Group proposed that a relapse without encephalopathy after a first attack meeting the criteria for ADEM should not be considered as MS. Rather, after a first event consistent with ADEM, 2 additional attacks (not meeting the ADEM criteria) are used for a clinical diagnosis of MS. However, some have questioned whether a single relapse without encephalopathy after a first attack meeting the criteria for ADEM should be diagnosed as MS [26]. Similar to improving the specificity by including encephalopathy in the criteria for an ADEM diagnosis, this restricted definition was proposed to decrease the number of false positive diagnoses of MS in children with transient demyelinating diseases. However, it is possible to be diagnosed with MS after ADEM. In a national prospective Canadian study, 5% of children meeting criteria for ADEM developed MS using the International Pediatric MS Study Group definitions (2 non-ADEM attacks after an initial event consistent with ADEM) [8]. There are a number of children, especially prepubertal, who may not neatly fit these definitions, and it is the Study Group's expectations that these definitions will be further validated or updated by collaborative prospective studies.

Aside from demyelinating diseases, there are a number of other disorders that mimic CNS demyelination. The differential diagnosis is similar to adults (as discussed in Chapter 10). Especially relevant to the pediatric population, metabolic diseases or leukodystrophies should be considered in some children. Children with these diseases often have a progressive decline without clear relapses. Such a clinical presentation is unlikely to be primary progressive MS, which is extremely rare in children. Other organ involvement (eye, skin, liver, heart, etc.) should prompt consideration for such diagnoses. Also, bilateral deep gray matter involvement is common in ADEM or even NMO but can also be present in other conditions, such as metabolic disorders, toxic encephalopathies, or hypoxic-ischemic injury.

Risk of MS After a First Demyelinating Event

MRI is a useful tool in predicting the risk of MS after a CIS. In children with a normal MRI of the brain at the time of their initial event, the risk of developing MS is approximately 2% (Figure 31.2) [8]. Accordingly, while a normal brain MRI is prognostically favorable, it does not exclude the possibility of a relapse (recurrent optic neuritis without brain lesions or recurrent transverse myelitis) [8]. For those children with T2/FLAIR hyperintensities in the brain at the time of their first attack, the risk of MS is increased if nonenhancing T1 hypointense lesions and/or 1 or more periventricular lesion(s) are present. This risk is further increased with persistent T1 lesions on serial images [37].

> At the time of a first demyelinating event, the presence of 1 or more T1 hypointense lesion(s) and/or 1 or more periventricular lesion(s) is associated with an increased risk of MS.

As noted previously, the risk of MS increases with age. In children (under 18 years of age) with optic neuritis, the risk of MS increases by 32% for every 1 year increase in age over 2 years, after adjusting for the presence or absence of asymptomatic brain lesions on MRI (see Figure 31.1) [9]. Another study also examined the relation between age and MRI lesions and their influence on MS risk after a first demyelinating event (including ADEM, transverse myelitis, etc.). After stratifying by the presence of T2 lesions on MRI, the risk is further defined by the age, which doubles in children over 11.85 years [8] (see Figure 31.2).

Relapses

Similar to adults, a relapse is typically defined by the presence of symptoms localizing to the CNS that are present

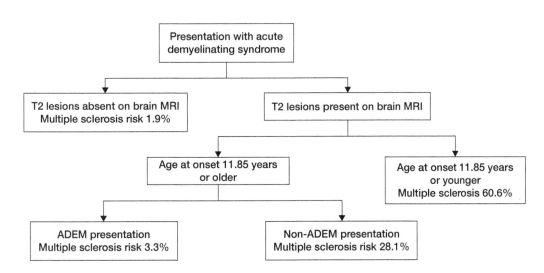

FIGURE 31.2
MS risk stratification algorithm for children presenting with an acute demyelinating syndrome. This classification scheme predicts the diagnosis in children presenting with an acute demyelinating syndrome with 83.7% accuracy. *Source: [8].*

for at least 24 hours and not related to a fever or illness [38]. The onset of symptoms should be separated from the onset of a previous attack by at least 30 days. The clinical presentation of MS attacks in children resembles that seen in adults, though attacks are often more severe. Investigators at 1 center categorized roughly one-half of pediatric attacks as severe, with only 10% to 17% of adult exacerbations filling the same criteria. They also found more pediatric attacks involving the brain stem/cerebellum and cerebral hemispheres [38].

> A higher relapse rate is seen in children compared to adults. Low serum 25OH vitamin D levels and non-white race are also associated with a higher relapse rate.

Three specific factors have been associated with a greater relapse rate: younger age at onset, lower serum vitamin D levels, and non-white race. Compared to adults, children have a significantly higher annualized relapse rate, which was demonstrated repeatedly with multiple statistical models and methodologies (such as including and excluding a first attack and comparing the annualized relapse rate both pre- and post-disease-modifying therapy [DMT]) [39]. A retrospective study observed a correlation between serum 25-hydroxyvitamin D3 level, adjusted for time of year, and relapse rate [17]. The same study also demonstrated an increased relapse rate in Hispanic children [17], a finding that concurs with another study's conclusion that Hispanic children are more likely to experience breakthrough disease with first-line DMT [13]. African American patients also had more relapses than white patients in a Detroit cohort [14]. Pediatric patients do seem to recover more completely from exacerbations—1 study found that 66% of children with severe initial demyelinating events recovered fully, as opposed to 46% of adults from the same center. Incomplete recovery from one event predicted the same in later relapses [38]. Moreover, the rate of disability progression in children increases with each relapse in the first 2 years [40].

> Pediatric MS attacks are generally treated with intravenous methylprednisolone at 20 to 30 mg/kg a day for 3 to 5 days, and 50% of physicians prescribe an oral prednisone taper.

Pediatric MS attacks are managed similar to adults. Intravenous corticosteroids are used as a first-line therapy, although an expert panel agreed that not every flare requires treatment [26]. Rather, the clinical presentation with respect to the severity of the attack influences the decision to treat. While adults are often treated with 1 g/day of intravenous methylprednisolone, children generally receive 20 to 30 mg per kilogram of body weight per day (maximum of 1 g per day) for 3 to 5 days, with 50% of the panel routinely using a subsequent oral steroid taper [26]. For patients who do not improve with methylprednisolone, intravenous immunoglobulin and plasmapheresis have also been used to treat acute attacks in children; however, the expert panel did not reach a consensus with respect to the definition of treatment failure or protocol for initiation of a second-line acute relapse treatment.

MANAGEMENT

The management of pediatric MS is a complex undertaking driven by the child's clinical course and often requiring the participation of a multidisciplinary team including, but not limited to, neurologists, neuro-ophthalmologists, neuropsychologists, urologists, physiatrists, physical and occupational therapists, school nurses, and teachers. Education of patient, family (both parents and siblings), caregivers, and school as to the nature of the disease and its management should be thorough and ongoing to ensure that each child receives the best care possible. Frequent evaluations, such as clinical examinations every 3 months, and regular MRI scans (every 3 to 6 months) for the first year may be necessary to assess for disease progression, assess for medication compliance/adherence and side effects, and counsel the family.

Generally, treatment of pediatric MS closely resembles that of adult MS—clinicians commonly recommend long-term use of DMT and management of more severe attacks with corticosteroids (see earlier section on Relapses). While they are not FDA-approved for children under 18 years of age, interferon beta-1a and beta-1b and glatiramer acetate have similar safety and efficacy as in adults and should be initiated in children with established MS and those identified as high risk (ie, CIS with asymptomatic brain lesions). Interferons should be initiated at lower doses and titrated up to adult dosing to decrease side effects (such as flu-like symptoms) [41]. Otherwise, the dosing is not weight-based or reduced owing to age alone. Neutralizing antibodies to interferons are infrequently seen in children [42].

> Although they are not FDA-approved for children, interferon beta and glatiramer acetate should be initiated in children with MS and CIS (at high risk for MS).

There are no guidelines to determine treatment failure, with most clinicians using their global clinical impression to decide when to change or escalate therapy [26]. Multiple treatments have been proposed, such as switching DMT or adding corticosteroids, intravenous immunoglobulin, or plasma exchange at regular intervals [26]. Natalizumab has been used in selected children with MS who have failed first-line therapy [43–45].

Immunosuppressive agents, such as cyclophosphamide, azathioprine, mycophenolate, and mitoxantrone, have also been used in children failing first-line therapy.

As in adult MS, other therapies may be required for disabling symptoms. Physical, occupational, and speech therapy may be offered as needed. Spasticity may require baclofen or dantrolene. Benzodiazepines and botulinum toxin may also be used but do not have FDA indications for spasticity in children. The commonly used medications for fatigue in adults (amantadine and modafinil) do not have indications for MS fatigue in children but have been used. Oxybutynin and hyoscyamine have pediatric indications for neurogenic bladder; hyoscyamine can also be used for neurogenic bowel. Tolterodine does not have FDA-recommended pediatric dosing. Gabapentin and pregabalin have been tried for neuropathic pain (although they are also off-label for pediatrics). Antidepressants may be required for some children; however, given the FDA boxed-warnings on the use of antidepressants in children, these medications are often best initiated and titrated by a psychiatrist. While many of the symptomatic medications are not specifically approved by the FDA for MS-related symptoms, they have been studied in children with other etiologies (such as cerebral palsy, traumatic brain injury, etc.), and dosing is often extrapolated from such studies or adult data.

PROGNOSIS

A major goal of MS therapy is to slow the progression of physical and cognitive disability. Generally, pediatric-onset MS patients maintain lower Expanded Disability Status Scale (EDSS) scores for a longer period of time after disease onset as compared to adult-onset patients. In a longitudinal study, the interval between onset and conversion to secondary progressive MS and irreversible disability was about 10 years longer in pediatric-onset patients. However, conversion occurred when childhood-onset patients were approximately 10 years younger than their adult counterparts [40].

Cognitive decline may occur both more frequently and at an accelerated rate in pediatric patients, perhaps owing to the effects of demyelination on brains that have not yet reached the final stages of maturation. In a group of 63 Italian children, a neuropsychological test battery

> MS is more slowly progressive in children; however, children reach irreversible disability at younger ages compared to adults.

classified 31% as cognitively impaired, with 15 found to have an IQ score of under 90; follow-up 2 years later placed 70% of the same cohort in the cognitive impairment group [46,47]. Pediatric MS patients scored lowest on tests at both sessions involving verbal comprehension, complex attention, and memory. The authors found that a younger age at onset correlated with cognitive impairment at the first assessment, while older age and higher educational level at the time of testing correlated with cognitive impairment at the time of follow-up. Other studies with smaller cohorts have similarly found cognitive impairment in approximately one-third of children with MS. Commonly affected functions include attention and processing speed as well as verbal abilities. Younger age of onset and/or longer disease length predicted impairment in several independent studies [48,49], indicating perhaps a need for close surveillance and/or early interventions in these cases.

CONCLUSION

In general, pediatric and adult MS share similar clinical symptoms, CSF profiles, and lesion characteristics on MRI scans. The mechanisms influencing the age of onset are poorly understood. Genetic and environmental risk factors are currently being studied in both groups, and exposure to viruses in the pediatric years may influence the biological onset of disease. While similarities exist between pediatric- and adult-onset MS, there are a number of interesting differences between the groups. Children have higher relapse rates and greater T2 lesion volumes yet slower progression of disability. Hypotheses for this paradox have included greater edema with less myelin damage or better remyelination and repair [34,38]. Perhaps MS in children is associated with primary inflammation and less axonal destruction. The unique characteristics that may influence the disease progression in children are the subject of considerable pediatric MS research. Moreover, pediatric clinical trials of DMTs are on the immediate horizon and will hopefully elucidate the optimal MS therapy for our youngest patients.

ACKNOWLEDGMENT

The authors would like to thank Dr. Brenda Banwell for her review of the chapter and thoughtful suggestions.

Ms. Stull is supported by the Swaiman Medical Scholarship Program from the Child Neurology Foundation (USA).

Dr. Waldman is supported by K23NS069806-01A1 from the National Institutes of Health (USA).

PATIENT CASE 1

A 5-year-old presents to the emergency department with a 2 week history of intermittent headaches and hypersomnolence. There was no recent fever, illness, or vaccination. After school, she would often fall asleep, which was unlike her. On the day of admission, the child awoke with left-sided weakness. She had difficulty hopping on the left side and had some balance issues. There was also an episode of incontinence. She was brought to the emergency department where the above symptoms were confirmed on neurological examination. In addition, she aroused with stimulation but would quickly fall back to sleep when not continually stimulated. She was also noted to have bidirectional nystagmus, an ataxic gait, and extensor plantar responses.

Question: What evaluation is needed?

Answer: The clinical picture of encephalopathy (manifesting as hypersomnolence and difficulty maintaining wakefulness) and multifocal neurological signs and symptoms is consistent with ADEM. Laboratory studies should include a complete blood count, basic metabolic panel, erythrocyte sedimentation rate, antinuclear antibody, angiotensin-converting enzyme, C-reactive protein, thyroid stimulating hormone, B_{12} level, folate, and vitamin D 25(OH). A lumbar puncture should be performed and assessed for white and red blood cell counts, protein, glucose, culture, CSF immunoglobulin index and synthesis rate, and OCBs. An MRI of the brain, C-, and T-spine, without and with gadolinium, should be obtained.

The spinal tap revealed 57 white blood cells and 8 red blood cells with a differential of 21% neutrophils, 15% monocytes, and 64% lymphocytes. The CSF glucose was 62 with a protein of 32. OCBs were absent. The CSF immunoglobin G index and synthesis rate were normal. The remainder of the laboratory tests was unremarkable. An MRI of the brain revealed multiple large, asymmetric T2/FLAIR hyperintense signal abnormalities within the supratentorial white matter, deep gray matter, and brain stem. The post contrast images demonstrated no abnormal enhancement. There were no areas of restricted diffusion. She also had an MRI of the cervical and thoracic spine which revealed 3 extensive areas of increased T2 signals in the spinal cord. The most prominent was seen from C4 to C7 where the cord was widened at this level. A second area was present from C2 to C3 through the mid C5 vertebral body, as well as an increased area in the distal spinal cord and conus.

Question: What do you do now?

Answer: It is reasonable to treat her at this point with a course of high-dose corticosteroids (ie, 20 to 30 mg/kg per day of intravenous methylprednisolone for 3 to 5 days). Some physicians will follow intravenous methylprednisolone by a prednisone taper, typically lasting 2 to 4 weeks. Information about the side effects of corticosteroids and expectation of treatment response should be reviewed with her.

She steadily improves with the administration of steroids. Approximately 9 days after the prednisone was stopped, she had an episode in which she "looked off" and was tired after dinner. She then "looked like she was drunk" while she was walking. The next morning she fell a few times and had emesis as well as pain in her head and legs.

Question: What do you do now?

Answer: As in adults presenting with a relapse, it is important to exclude infection, and the child had considerable spinal cord involvement, so a urinalysis would be appropriate, even without urinary symptoms. If symptoms are mild, further treatment may not be necessary. For moderate to severe symptoms, a repeat course of high-dose corticosteroids may be indicated (ie, 3 to 5 days of 20 to 30 mg/kg per day intravenous methylprednisolone, which may be followed by a longer taper, perhaps 4 to 6 weeks or longer depending on her initial response).

Urinalysis was normal and no infectious etiology was found on routine examination. She improved with 3 days of intravenous methylprednisolone and was discharged on a longer steroid taper.

Question: What is the diagnosis?

Answer: The diagnosis remains ADEM. Her symptoms recurred within 4 weeks of steroid withdrawal; therefore, this is not considered a new attack or relapse (as in recurrent ADEM or multiphasic ADEM).

Question: What is her long-term risk of MS?

Answer: The risk of MS is approximately 5%.

After a diagnosis of ADEM, 2 additional relapses (not meeting criteria for ADEM) are required for a diagnosis of pediatric MS.

PATIENT CASE 2

A 14-year-old female presents to the emergency department after waking up this morning with blurry vision in the left eye. She complained of pain behind her left eye. Her examination was notable for a left relative afferent pupillary defect, visual acuity of 20/200 OS, blurred disc margin in the left eye, and decreased color vision on the left using Ishihara color plates.

Question: What evaluation is needed?

Answer: The child should be assessed by a neurologist and neuro-ophthalmologist to determine the extent of the CNS involvement. An MRI of the brain without and with gadolinium is the standard of care to evaluate for asymptomatic lesions outside the visual system. As noted in the previous case, laboratory studies and a lumbar puncture may be obtained. An MRI of the C- and T-spine may be necessary, especially if the neurological examination is abnormal.

Formal neuro-ophthalmological examination confirmed the above findings. No clinical abnormalities were appreciated in the right eye. The remainder of the neurological examination was normal. MRI of the brain revealed a T2/FLAIR hyperintensity in the left optic nerve. Three additional T2/FLAIR hyperintensities were seen in the periventricular region, and 1 discrete lesion was present in the juxtacortical white matter. None of the lesions enhanced after the administration of gadolinium.

Question: What is the diagnosis?

Answer: The diagnosis is unilateral optic neuritis, or, in this case, a monofocal CIS. While the presence of lesions in the periventricular and juxtacortical white matter does meet McDonald Criteria for dissemination in space, she has not demonstrated dissemination in time (which requires the presence of enhancing and nonenhancing lesions simultaneously to diagnosis dissemination in time on a single MRI scan).

Question: What do you do now?

Answer: It is reasonable to treat her at this point with a course of high-dose corticosteroids (ie, 3 days of 20 to 30 mg/kg per day, maximum 1 g per day, intravenous methylprednisolone, followed by a prednisone taper). Information about the side effects of corticosteroids and expected treatment response should be addressed. She will also require regular neurological examinations and repeat MRI scans to assess for disease progression.

Question: What is her risk for MS?

Answer: She is considered at high-risk for MS given her age and the presence of asymptomatic T2/FLAIR hyperintensities in the brain. She should be offered DMT (interferon beta or glatiramer acetate) even though she does not meet diagnostic criteria for MS.

Question: How should DMT be initiated?

Answer: The physician should present the family with all of the current first-line therapies (interferon beta-1a and 1b and glatiramer acetate) with a review of the differences in route, frequency, and side effects for each medication. In general, the dosing is similar for children and adults, although the interferons should all be titrated upward to decrease side effects. Not all children and families accept initiation of DMT at the first attack and the advantages and disadvantages should be thoroughly reviewed.

Question: What is the long-term prognosis for pediatric MS?

Answer: While many children have more frequent relapses early in the disease course, children have slower disease progression. Children should be encouraged to fully participate in their usual activities. Frequent neurological examinations and serial imaging are important to monitor disease progression.

KEY POINTS FOR PATIENTS AND FAMILIES

- MS affects children as well as adults; however, the course of the illness and symptoms are different in each person, regardless of age.

- Children with MS should see a neurologist regularly and repeat MRI scans even when they feel well.

- Goals of treatment include controlling acute inflammation, reducing the frequency of relapses and accrual of new MRI lesions, slowing physical and cognitive decline, and maximizing quality of life for the affected child.

- Children should be encouraged to participate in activities they enjoy, and regular exercise is encouraged.

- Children may require an individualized education plan through their school if they have difficulties with coursework or miss school because of medical appointments or hospitalizations.

REFERENCES

1. Poser CM, Brinar VV. Diagnostic criteria for multiple sclerosis: An historical review. *Clin Neurol Neurosurg.* 2004;106:147–158.

2. Krupp LB, Banwell B, Tenembaum S. Consensus definitions proposed for pediatric multiple sclerosis and related disorders. *Neurology.* 2007;68:S7–S12.

3. Polman CH, Reingold SC, Banwell B, et al. Diagnostic criteria for multiple sclerosis: 2010 revisions to the McDonald criteria. *Ann Neurol.* 2011;69:292–302.

4. Chitnis T, Glanz B, Jaffin S, Healy B. Demographics of pediatric-onset multiple sclerosis in an MS center population from the Northeastern United States. *Mult Scler.* 2009;15:627–631.

5. Langer-Gould A, Zhang JL, Chung J, et al. Incidence of acquired CNS demyelinating syndromes in a multiethnic cohort of children. *Neurology.* 2011;77:1143–1148.

6. Banwell B, Kennedy J, Sadovnick D, et al. Incidence of acquired demyelination of the CNS in Canadian children. *Neurology.* 2009;72:232–239.

7. Pohl D, Hennemuth I, von Kries R, Hanefeld F. Paediatric multiple sclerosis and acute disseminated encephalomyelitis in Germany: Results of a nationwide survey. *Eur J Pediatr.* 2007;166:405–412.

8. Banwell B, Bar-Or A, Arnold DL, et al. Clinical, environmental, and genetic determinants of multiple sclerosis in children with acute demyelination: A prospective national cohort study. *Lancet Neurol.* 2011;10:436–445.

9. Waldman AT, Stull LB, Galetta SL, et al. Pediatric optic neuritis and risk of multiple sclerosis: Meta-analysis of observational studies. *J AAPOS.* 2011;15:441–446.

10. Tenembaum S, Chamoles N, Fejerman N. Acute disseminated encephalomyelitis: A long-term follow-up study of 84 pediatric patients. *Neurology.* 2002;59:1224–1231.

11. Tenembaum S, Chitnis T, Ness J, Hahn JS. Acute disseminated encephalomyelitis. *Neurology.* 2007;68:S23–S36.

12. Dale RC, de Sousa C, Chong WK, et al. Acute disseminated encephalomyelitis, multiphasic disseminated encephalomyelitis and multiple sclerosis in children. *Brain.* 2000;123(Pt 12): 2407–2422.

13. Yeh EA, Waubant E, Krupp LB, et al. Multiple sclerosis therapies in pediatric patients with refractory multiple sclerosis. *Arch Neurol.* 2011;68:437–444.

14. Boster AL, Endress CF, Hreha SA, et al. Pediatric-onset multiple sclerosis in African-American black and European-origin white patients. *Pediatr Neurol.* 2009;40:31–33.

15. Kennedy J, O'Connor P, Sadovnick AD, et al. Age at onset of multiple sclerosis may be influenced by place of residence during childhood rather than ancestry. *Neuroepidemiology.* 2006;26:162–167.

16. Munger KL, Levin LI, Hollis BW, et al. Serum 25-hydroxy-vitamin D levels and risk of multiple sclerosis. *JAMA.* 2006;296:2832–2838.

17. Mowry EM, Krupp LB, Milazzo M, et al. Vitamin D status is associated with relapse rate in pediatric-onset multiple sclerosis. *Ann Neurol.* 2010;67:618–624.

18. Staples J, Ponsonby AL, Lim L. Low maternal exposure to ultraviolet radiation in pregnancy, month of birth, and risk of multiple sclerosis in offspring: Longitudinal analysis. *BMJ.* 2010;340:c1640.

19. Disanto G, Magalhaes S, Handel AE, et al. HLA-DRB1 confers increased risk of pediatric-onset MS in children with acquired demyelination. *Neurology.* 2011;76:781–786.

20. De Jager PL, Simon KC, Munger KL, et al. Integrating risk factors: HLA-DRB1*1501 and Epstein-Barr virus in multiple sclerosis. *Neurology.* 2008;70:1113–1118.

21. Waubant E, Mowry EM, Krupp L, et al. Common viruses associated with lower pediatric multiple sclerosis risk. *Neurology.* 2011;76:1989–1995.

22. Mikaeloff Y, Caridade G, Tardieu M, Suissa S. Parental smoking at home and the risk of childhood-onset multiple sclerosis in children. *Brain.* 2007;130:2589–2595.

23. Mikaeloff Y, Caridade G, Rossier M, et al. Hepatitis B vaccination and the risk of childhood-onset multiple sclerosis. *Arch Pediatr Adolesc Med.* 2007;161:1176–1182.

24. Bonhomme GR, Waldman AT, Balcer LJ, et al. Pediatric optic neuritis: Brain MRI abnormalities and risk of multiple sclerosis. *Neurology.* 2009;72:881–885.

25. Wilejto M, Shroff M, Buncic JR, et al. The clinical features, MRI findings, and outcome of optic neuritis in children. *Neurology.* 2006;67:258–262.

26. Waldman AT, Gorman MP, Rensel MR, et al. Management of pediatric central nervous system demyelinating disorders: Consensus of United States neurologists. *J Child Neurol.* 2011;26:675–682.

27. Chitnis T, Bar-Or A. Pediatric MS: Biological presentation and research update. In: Chabas D, Waubant EL, eds. *Demyelinating Disorders of the Central Nervous System in Childhood.* New York: Cambridge University Press; 2011.

28. Chabas D, Ness J, Belman A, et al. Younger children with MS have a distinct CSF inflammatory profile at disease onset. *Neurology.* 2010;74:399–405.

29. Bosca I, Magraner MJ, Coret F, et al. The risk of relapse after a clinically isolated syndrome is related to the pattern of oligoclonal bands. *J Neuroimmunol.* 2010;226:143–146.

30. Tintore M, Rovira A, Brieva L, et al. Isolated demyelinating syndromes: Comparison of CSF oligoclonal bands and different MR imaging criteria to predict conversion to CDMS. *Mult Scler.* 2001;7:359–363.

31. Hahn JS, Pohl D, Rensel M, Rao S. Differential diagnosis and evaluation in pediatric multiple sclerosis. *Neurology.* 2007;68:S13–S22.

32. Callen DJ, Shroff MM, Branson HM, et al. MRI in the diagnosis of pediatric multiple sclerosis. *Neurology.* 2009;72:961–967.

33. Ghassemi R, Antel SB, Narayanan S, et al. Lesion distribution in children with clinically isolated syndromes. *Ann Neurol.* 2008;63:401–405.

34. Waubant E, Chabas D, Okuda DT, et al. Difference in disease burden and activity in pediatric patients on brain magnetic resonance imaging at time of multiple sclerosis onset vs adults. *Arch Neurol.* 2009;66:967–971.

35. Chabas D, Castillo-Trivino T, Mowry EM, et al. Vanishing MS T2-bright lesions before puberty: A distinct MRI phenotype? *Neurology.* 2008;71:1090–1093.

36. Hahn CD, Shroff MM, Blaser SI, Banwell BL. MRI criteria for multiple sclerosis: Evaluation in a pediatric cohort. *Neurology.* 2004;62:806–808.

37. Verhey LH, Branson HM, Shroff MM, et al. MRI parameters for prediction of multiple sclerosis diagnosis in children with acute CNS demyelination: A prospective national cohort study. *Lancet Neurol.* 2011;10:1065–1073.

38. Fay AJ, Mowry EM, Strober J, Waubant E. Relapse severity and recovery in early pediatric multiple sclerosis. *Mult Scler.* 2012;18(7):1008–1012.

39. Gorman MP, Healy BC, Polgar-Turcsanyi M, Chitnis T. Increased relapse rate in pediatric-onset compared with adult-onset multiple sclerosis. *Arch Neurol.* 2009;66:54–59.

40. Renoux C, Vukusic S, Mikaeloff Y, et al. Natural history of multiple sclerosis with childhood onset. *N Engl J Med.* 2007;356:2603–2613.

41. Banwell B, Reder AT, Krupp L, et al. Safety and tolerability of interferon beta-1b in pediatric multiple sclerosis. *Neurology.* 2006;66:472–476.

42. Kuntz NL, Chabas D, Weinstock-Guttman B, et al. Treatment of multiple sclerosis in children and adolescents. *Expert Opin Pharmacother.* 2010;11:505–520.

43. Yeh EA, Weinstock-Guttman B. Natalizumab in pediatric multiple sclerosis patients. *Ther Adv Neurol Disord.* 2010;3:293–299.

44. Borriello G, Prosperini L, Luchetti A, Pozzilli C. Natalizumab treatment in pediatric multiple sclerosis: A case report. *Eur J Paediatr Neurol.* 2009;13:67–71.

45. Huppke P, Stark W, Zurcher C, et al. Natalizumab use in pediatric multiple sclerosis. *Arch Neurol.* 2008;65:1655–1658.

46. Amato MP, Goretti B, Ghezzi A, et al. Cognitive and psychosocial features in childhood and juvenile MS: Two-year follow-up. *Neurology.* 2010;75:1134–1140.

47. Amato MP, Goretti B, Ghezzi A, et al. Cognitive and psychosocial features of childhood and juvenile MS. *Neurology.* 2008;70:1891–1897.

48. MacAllister WS, Belman AL, Milazzo M, et al. Cognitive functioning in children and adolescents with multiple sclerosis. *Neurology.* 2005;64:1422–1425.

49. Till C, Ghassemi R, Aubert-Broche B, et al. MRI correlates of cognitive impairment in childhood-onset multiple sclerosis. *Neuropsychology.* 2011;25:319–332.

32

Women's Issues

BRIDGETTE JEANNE BILLIOUX
ELLEN M. MOWRY

KEY POINTS FOR CLINICIANS

- Multiple sclerosis (MS) is more prevalent in women, and the female to male ratios of incident and prevalent MS seem to be increasing.

- Multiple factors likely contribute to the sex differences seen in MS, including genetic, hormonal, and immune factors.

- Sex hormones have effects in the immune system and seem to play a role in MS.

- The premenstrual period is sometimes associated with worsened MS symptoms and may be associated with an increased rate of relapse.

- MS has no effect in and of itself on fertility, although some medications used in the treatment of MS may affect fertility.

- Although it does not affect the overall disease course, pregnancy itself is associated with a decreased rate of relapse, particularly in the third trimester, while there is a rebound increase in the rate of relapse in the first few months postpartum.

- Many medications used to treat MS are contraindicated during pregnancy and should be reviewed if a woman becomes or decides to become pregnant.

- Relapses during pregnancy are often treated with intravenous (IV) steroids, although steroids are ideally avoided during the first trimester.

- Postpartum risk of relapse may be decreased with prophylactic IVIG given intrapartum and postpartum, or postpartum alone.

- Breast-feeding may be associated with a lower risk of relapse postpartum, but studies are conflicting.

- Many MS medications, including disease-modifying therapies, are contraindicated during breast-feeding and should be reviewed if a patient decides to breast-feed.

- Menopause may be associated with worsened symptoms and progression.

- MS patients are at a higher risk for osteoporosis and osteopenia after menopause.

Multiple sclerosis (MS), like many other autoimmune diseases, is well known to be more prevalent in women, particularly those of childbearing age, than men. Many factors, including the neuroendocrine axis and its effects on immunological function, may contribute to these predilections. Given the evidence for hormonal effects on MS, many female hormonal factors have been evaluated for their effect on MS, including the menstrual cycle, oral contraceptive pills, pregnancy, breast-feeding, and menopause.

Pregnancy in MS is a very important topic in the management of the disease, both due to the fact that women of childbearing age are disproportionately affected by the disease, but also because of the many management issues that arise when a person with MS desires to become pregnant. During pregnancy, hormone levels change, impacting the MS relapse rate. Preventing relapses and managing flares and other symptoms can be challenging, as many medications typically used in MS patients are contraindicated during pregnancy. In addition, young women with MS are often concerned about the effects of pregnancy on disease progression; other concerns include the likelihood of passing on MS to offspring and whether, in light of its associated disabilities, MS impacts the ability to become pregnant or to have a safe delivery. This chapter aims to address the many issues pertinent to the management of MS in women.

SEX DIFFERENCES AND HORMONAL INFLUENCE ON MS

MS is well known to have a higher incidence and prevalence in women, with a prevalence approaching 3:1 in comparison to men, and some evidence suggests that this ratio has increased over the past few decades [1]. The most common form of MS, the relapsing-remitting type, has a largely female predominance; primary progressive MS tends to affect males and females equally, with a possible slight male preponderance [2]. Men with MS tend to acquire disability more rapidly compared to women among those with an MS onset between the ages of 16 and 49 years but not when onset occurred at age 50 years or more [3]; they also tend to incur more cognitive disability than women, although this latter result may have been confounded by disease duration or other factors for which statistical analyses did not account [4]. MS also tends to affect women at a slightly younger age than men, with a median difference in onset of 2 to 3 years [5]. Interestingly, there is no documented difference between men and women in response to treatment with disease-modifying therapies (DMTs) [6]. There are likely multiple factors underlying these differences between men and women with MS, including genetic, hormonal, and immune factors.

> There is a disproportionate occurrence of MS in women, which may be further increasing.

There are interesting sex differences in the immune system which likely play a role in the phenotypic differences of MS in men compared to women. Females tend to show a stronger immune response than males; they have higher baseline immunoglobulin levels and CD4+ T cells than males. Females also have a more sustained immunological response to antigenic challenges [7]. In general, autoimmune diseases are much more common in women than men. Interestingly, many of these autoimmune diseases also seem to be affected by hormonal changes, as seen in menstrual cycle fluctuations, pregnancy, and menopause [6]. There are some specific sex differences in the immune systems of patients with MS; for example, women have a greater T-cell response to myelin proteolipid protein, as well as a comparatively increased cytokine secretion in response to lymphocyte stimulation with myelin proteins, than men [8].

Hormonal factors likely play an important role in MS in general. An overwhelming majority of patients are diagnosed between the ages of 15 and 50 years of age. On average, MS typically begins early in the third decade, with less than 1% of MS patients experiencing symptoms prior to onset of puberty. Also, the risk of developing MS declines beyond onset of menopause; these correlations between MS onset and age suggest a role for hormonal factors in MS [6]. Sex hormones, including estrogens, progestins, and androgens, have multiple effects on the nervous system and also act as immunomodulators. Specifically, sex hormones have a significant influence on T-helper lymphocytes. In brief, T-helper (Th) lymphocytes are classified into 2 types: Th1 (proinflammatory) and Th2 (anti-inflammatory) cell types on the basis of their secretion of different cytokines. Th1 cells secrete proinflammatory interleukin (IL)-1, IL-2, IL-12, tumor necrosis factor alpha (TNF alpha), and interferon (IFN) gamma, whereas Th2 cells secrete anti-inflammatory IL-4, IL-5, IL-6, and IL-10 [9]. Estrogen affects levels of these cytokines, largely dependent on the concentration of hormone. With higher concentrations of estrogen (as in pregnancy), TNF alpha levels are decreased and IL-10 levels are increased; conversely, with lower levels of estrogen, TNF alpha levels are increased. Estrogen also stimulates humoral immunity and Th2 cellular function, and it inhibits natural killer cell activity and T suppressor cell activity. Progesterone decreases IL-1 and IFN gamma, and stimulates it IL-4, acting as a relative immunosuppressant [10]. These hormones act synergistically, as well. Testosterone, like progesterone, tends to act as an immunosuppressant [11].

Although these are incompletely understood, there seem to be multiple genetic and epigenetic factors associated with the effect of sex differences in MS. Several studies of half-siblings, avuncular pairs, and extended family pedigrees suggest a maternal parent of origin effect in MS, in which individuals related through the maternal line are more likely to be affected than individuals related through the paternal line [12]. There is also a well-known association of MS with *HLA-DRB1*1501*, which is a specific human leukocyte antigen (HLA) class II allele of the major histocompatibility complex; this association appears stronger in women compared to men [8]. Polymorphisms in apolipoprotein E (APOE) and CD95 genes have been associated in some studies with disease severity in women with MS. Also, a relationship has been reported between MS and polymorphisms in the estrogen receptor gene [11].

SEX HORMONES AND ORAL CONTRACEPTIVE PILLS IN MS

As noted above, estrogens and progesterones shift the immune response from a Th1 to a Th2 pattern and down-regulate proinflammatory cytokines, which would theoretically have a protective role in MS. In animal studies using the MS mouse model, experimental allergic encephalomyelitis, administration of estrogen tends to lessen the severity of disease, and oophorectomy worsens disease [13]. Given these findings in animal models, studies have been conducted with exogenous estriol in female MS patients. While there seemed to be a decrease in inflammatory cytokines and disease activity, there was increased abnormal menstrual bleeding, enlarged uterine fibroids, and increased risk of thrombotic events and gynecological malignancies [14,15]. A randomized clinical trial of estriol is underway (NCT00451204).

> Oral contraceptive pills are safe to use in MS patients, although one must consider the risk of deep vein thrombosis (DVT), particularly in patients with limited mobility.

Oral contraceptives and their potential effects on MS have also been studied. The data are limited and results are conflicting. Some studies suggest that there may be a lower incidence of MS in oral contraceptive pill (OCP) users, while others did not show any significant difference between OCP users and nonusers [16,17]. In general, OCP use is not contraindicated in patients with MS, but caution must be exercised when prescribing these for MS patients with limited mobility due to the increased risk of clotting and thromboembolic events conferred by OCP use.

MENSTRUAL CYCLE AND MS

Many female MS patients report fluctuations in their symptoms corresponding to changes in their menstrual cycle. These symptoms may include fatigue, myalgias, depression, decreased endurance, worsened spasticity, weakness, incoordination, and abnormalities in gait, sensation, vision, or sphincter function [11,18]. Although data on the relationship between the menstrual cycle and MS exacerbations are limited, one questionnaire-based study suggested a higher rate of MS exacerbations occurring in the premenstrual period compared to the rest of the menstrual cycle in a group of premenopausal women with MS [19]. Worsening

of symptoms and exacerbations during the premenstrual period may be explained by the relative drop in estrogen and progesterone, leading to a Th1/Th2 shift [19].

FERTILITY IN MS

MS does not appear to have any direct effect on fertility [5]. One Swedish study suggested that the frequency of infertile women might be higher in the MS population than in the general population [20]. It seems, however, that other factors may influence MS patients' decisions regarding motherhood, such as the influence of disability on parenting or concerns about MS transmission to offspring. In addition, pregnancy is often postponed because of DMT. Although MS does not seem to affect fertility, some medications for MS may have effects on fertility. Specifically, mitoxantrone has been found to cause significantly protracted or even irreversible amenorrhea after prolonged use [21]. Cyclophosphamide exerts a toxic effect on the ovaries and reduces ovarian reserve. Cyclophosphamide also frequently leads to amenorrhea with definitive amenorrhea in up to 33% of female patients receiving pulse dosing for treatment of progressive MS [20]. However, mitoxantrone and cyclophosphamide are not commonly used in the treatment of MS.

> MS has no direct effect on fertility.

PREGNANCY IN MS

Pregnancy is often an important issue for women diagnosed with MS. One issue that arises is whether or not pregnancy affects the overall course of MS, a topic that has been debated widely for years. In the past, MS patients were advised against pregnancy owing to concerns that it worsens prognosis. However, in more recent years it has been found that pregnancy does not seem to have a detrimental effect on the overall disease course. Some studies have suggested that pregnancy actually has a positive effect on MS prognosis, but the veracity of this claim remains unclear [22,23].

> Pregnancy does not seem to have any detrimental effect on the overall disease course.

While it is unclear if pregnancy affects the long-term course of MS, it is well known to affect the course of MS in the short-term. Pregnancy is associated with a decrease in disease activity, particularly in the third trimester, with a rebound increase in risk of relapse in the first few months postpartum [24]. The Pregnancy in Multiple Sclerosis Study (PRIMS), a multicenter European prospective observational study, found that there was a slight reduction in relapse rate during the first 2 trimesters, and a substantial reduction during the third trimester, with an annualized relapse rate of 0.2 during the third trimester compared to 0.7 prior to pregnancy. Post-delivery, there was an increase in annualized relapse rate to 1.2 over the first 3 months postpartum, after which the annualized relapse rate returned to the rate prior to pregnancy [25]. This phenomenon is likely related to the relative immunosuppressive state during pregnancy produced by increases in estrogen, progesterone, and glucocorticoids and other factors leading to a shift toward Th2 responses. Although pregnancy is thought to be protective against MS exacerbations, some underlying MS symptoms may worsen during pregnancy, including fatigue, spasticity, bowel and bladder dysfunction, and difficulty with mobility or ambulation [11].

> Pregnancy is associated with a decrease in disease activity, particularly in the third trimester, with a rebound increase in disease activity postpartum.

MS patients also often have concerns about the potential safety of pregnancy. In general, MS patients show no increase in fetal malformations or spontaneous abortions from the general population [24]. Women with MS also do not seem to have an increase in complications during pregnancy compared to women without MS [26].

Information about genetics is also important to impart to MS patients who are interested in becoming pregnant. While the risk of developing MS in the general population is about 0.2%, the risk increases to 3% to 5% in a child with a parent affected by MS. This risk increases further to 30.5% in the event that both parents are affected by MS [11]. Studies evaluating whether MS transmission is greater depending on which parent is affected have produced conflicting results [27–29].

DMT in Pregnancy

DMT is an important issue during pregnancy. Pregnancy is known to reduce the risk of relapse of patients with MS; however, it does not eliminate the risk. Traditionally, MS patients are counseled to stop DMTs before trying to become pregnant, although clinicians should review the potential risks and benefits of continuing DMTs on a case-by-case basis [30]. The amount of recommended time between stopping a therapy and attempting pregnancy varies by medication and by practitioner. It may be helpful for patients to meet with their obstetrician for help with pregnancy timing and planning so as to minimize the length of time off DMTs. While some of the older DMTs have been studied more extensively, less is known about the safety of the newer therapies during pregnancy, although

> In general, patients are advised to discontinue disease-modifying therapy prior to conception.

teriflunomide is a pregnancy category X medication [31]. Thus, both women and men being treated with teriflunomide must use reliable contraception, and rapid elimination using cholestyramine or activated charcoal for women who wish to conceive or for men whose female partners are planning to conceive is important to prescribe.

In general, the information known about IFN beta and glatiramer acetate is relatively reassuring. The large molecular size of IFN beta may prevent transportation across the placental barrier. Although studies regarding IFN in pregnancy are limited, there is some evidence of decreased birth weight in babies exposed to IFN in utero, and a possible slight increase in rate of spontaneous abortion in women taking IFN during pregnancy. There is no clear evidence of teratogenicity [32,33]. Glatiramer acetate has not been shown to cause birth defects in animal studies. Studies in humans are limited, but glatiramer acetate has been classified as a category B drug by the FDA. However, there may be an increased risk of spontaneous abortion with its use [34]. Newer therapies such as natalizumab and fingolimod have not been well studied in pregnant women and are currently contraindicated during pregnancy (category C) [30]. The DMTs and their respective FDA pregnancy categories are provided in Table 32.1.

Treatment of Exacerbations During Pregnancy

In the event of MS relapse during pregnancy, short doses of high-dose corticosteroids are used, much as in nonpregnant patients. Corticosteroids are known to cross the placenta; however, most of the prednisolone and hydrocortisone that cross to the placenta are converted to less active metabolites by placental syncytiotrophoblasts [30]. Methylprednisolone is typically the preferred agent of treatment, with a 3 to 5 day course being the most common course of treatment with or without a subsequent, short prednisone taper [5,30]. While short-term therapy with glucocorticoids is generally considered safe in pregnant women, there have been some adverse effects described. Studies have reported a possible mild increase in orofacial abnormalities in fetuses exposed to prednisone in the first trimester; hence, high doses of prednisone should ideally be avoided during palate formation in the first trimester [35]. Otherwise, short courses of prednisone and other corticosteroids can be safely tolerated in the second and third trimesters. On the other hand, prolonged tapering courses of corticosteroids are associated with an increased risk of gestational diabetes, hypertension, sodium retention, edema, and premature rupture of membranes, and should hence be avoided during pregnancy [34].

> Short courses of high-dose steroids may be used to treat MS relapses in pregnant women.

Symptomatic Treatment During Pregnancy

Many medications used in the symptomatic treatment of MS (ie, spasticity or urinary dysfunction) are contraindicated

TABLE 32.1
MS Therapies and FDA Pregnancy Categories

DRUG	U.S. FDA PREGNANCY CATEGORY	COMMENT
Dexamethasone	C	Avoid during first trimester
Methylprednisolone	C	Avoid during first trimester
Interferon beta	C	Possible increase in spontaneous abortions
Glatiramer acetate	B	Possible decrease in birth weight
Natalizumab	C	
Fingolimod	C	
Teriflunomide	X	Fetal malformation and embryofetal death in animals
Methotrexate	X	Craniofacial and limb defects, CNS abnormalities, miscarriage
Cyclophosphamide	D	Impaired fetal growth, malformations of skeleton, palate, limbs, and eyes
Azathioprine	D	
Cyclosporine A	C	
Mitoxantrone	D	
Intravenous immunoglobulin	C	Probably safe

Class A: Adequate, well-controlled studies in pregnant women have not shown an increased risk of fetal abnormalities to the fetus in any trimester of pregnancy.
Class B: Animal studies have revealed no evidence of harm to the fetus. However, there are no adequate and well-controlled studies in women. Or animal studies have shown an adverse effect, but adequate and well-controlled studies in pregnant women have failed to demonstrate a risk to the fetus in any trimester.
Class C: Animal studies have shown an adverse effect and there are no adequate and well-controlled studies in pregnant women, or no animal studies and no adequate and well-controlled studies in pregnant women.
Class D: Adequate well-controlled or observational studies in pregnant women showed a risk to the fetus. However, benefits of therapy may outweigh the potential risks. For example, the drug may be acceptable if needed in a life-threatening situation or serious disease for which safer drugs cannot be substituted.
Class X: Adequate well-controlled or observational studies in animals or pregnant women have demonstrated positive evidence of fetal abnormalities or risks. The use of the product is contraindicated in women who are or may become pregnant.
Source: Adapted from [26,34].

during pregnancy [5]. For a listing of commonly used symptomatic medications in MS and their pregnancy classifications, please refer to Table 32.2.

> Many symptomatic therapies are contraindicated during pregnancy.

Delivery in MS
Women with MS do not experience increased obstetrical or neonatal complications than unaffected women [30]. Neither general nor spinal anesthesia is contraindicated in MS, as neither has a particular effect on the disease. Decisions regarding labor and delivery procedures should hence be based entirely on obstetrical evaluation. Although there is no particular increase in the rate of complications in MS patients during delivery, there may be some potential differences from the general population which should be considered. Some MS patients have some degree of pelvic

floor weakness, as well as spasticity and fatigue, which can hamper an efficient abdomen–pelvic push; this may lead to requiring more assistance during delivery. In MS patients with diaphragmatic insufficiency, there may be an increased risk of respiratory failure intra or postpartum, possibly leading to a need for prolonged monitoring. In addition, MS patients on chronic corticosteroid therapy may be at an increased risk of acute adrenocortical failure postpartum and should be closely monitored for such [5].

> In general, delivery is no more complicated in MS patients than in the general population.

Postpartum Relapse and Prevention
While pregnancy confers some protection from MS relapses, there is a higher risk of relapse in the postpartum period. It is generally recommended that patients who were on DMTs prior to pregnancy resume DMTs immediately

TABLE 32.2
Symptomatic MS Treatments and FDA Pregnancy Categories

CATEGORY	DRUGS FOR SYMPTOMATIC TREATMENT
Class B	Oxybutynin
	Cyclobenzaprine
	Tamsulosin
Class C	Baclofen
	Carbamazepine
	Darifenacin
	Dantrolene
	Tizanidine
	Gabapentin
	Dalfampridine
	Amantadine
	Most selective serotonin reuptake inhibitors
	Serotonin-norephinephrine reuptake inhibitors
	Bupropion
	Tolterodine
	Solifenacin
	Trospium
Class D	Most benzodiazepines
	Phenytoin

Source: Adapted from [5,36].

postpartum, unless they plan on breast-feeding. A prophylactic 3 to 5 day course of high-dose steroids may provide up to 4 weeks of protection from relapse and can be used postpartum; steroids are also not contraindicated during breast-feeding, although they must be used cautiously [30]. Intravenous immunoglobulin (IVIG) may also be considered to prevent relapse in the postpartum period; in 1 study, IVIG was found to reduce the relapse rate by 33% [37]. In a study by Achiron et al., IVIG was studied both intrapartum as well as postpartum as prophylaxis against postpartum relapses. Both groups had significantly lower rates of relapse, with the intrapartum IVIG group having a slightly lower rate of relapse compared to the postpartum group [38]. IVIG is also considered to be safe in breast-feeding women [34].

> Unless breastfeeding, DMTs should generally be restarted postpartum.

BREAST-FEEDING IN MS

The effect of breast-feeding on MS is somewhat controversial. Breast-feeding has been shown to hypothetically dampen the proinflammatory response in MS by returning the IFN gamma-producing CD4+ T cells to normal levels [30]. Multiple studies evaluated the effects of breast-feeding on MS. Earlier studies showed conflicting data, with either

no significant difference in relapse rate between patients who breast-fed or bottle fed, or minimal benefit with breast-feeding [5]. More recently, a small prospective cohort of 32 postpartum women with MS found that women who breast-fed exclusively for the first 2 months postpartum were approximately 5 times less likely to have an MS relapse during the first year postpartum when compared to women who did not breast-feed or who supplemented formula with breast-feeding [39]. A larger prospective study of about 300 women by Portaccio et al., however, found no difference in relapse rate profiles between women who breast-fed and those who did not after adjusting for covariates, although the distinction of exclusive breast-feeding was not made in this study [40]. While there may be a relative decrease in relapse rates postpartum in women who breast-feed, this seems to be more evident in women who breast-feed exclusively. In general, there seems to be no significant effect on overall disease progression or evolution in MS patients who have breast-fed [5].

In patients who want to breast-feed, caution must be taken when prescribing medications, as many medications used in MS treatment may be excreted in breast milk. While steroids are known to be transferred to breast milk, infant exposure to corticosteroids from breast milk is thought to be minimal [5]. Nevertheless, overuse of corticosteroids during breast-feeding is not recommended, as they can potentially suppress infant growth. IVIG is generally thought to be safe during lactation [26]. Mitoxantrone, cyclosporine A, cyclophosphamide, and azathioprine should not be used in lactating women, as these agents are secreted in the breast milk. There is some suggestion that IFN beta may not be secreted into breast milk in any significant quantity; however, it is generally not recommended in lactating women [34]. There are insufficient data on glatiramer acetate and breast-feeding at this time [5]. Given the potential risks associated with exposing infants to these medications, DMTs are generally not recommended in breast-feeding patients.

> Breast-feeding may be associated with a decreased relapse rate in the first year postpartum, but this effect seems to be more evident in women who breast-feed exclusively.

> IVIG is safe to use during breast-feeding. Steroids can be used with caution during lactation. DMTs and immunosuppressants are generally contraindicated during breast-feeding.

MENOPAUSE IN MS

There is a relative dearth of information on MS and menopause. In one small study, 54% of postmenopausal patients reported worsening of their MS disability and progressive symptomatology [41]. In addition, menopause is a time during which patients develop other issues, such as osteoporosis and osteopenia. These issues are especially relevant to women with MS, as those who have been treated with high doses of steroids and who have impaired mobility are at an even higher risk of osteoporosis. Bone density scanning should hence be considered in postmenopausal patients. Weight-bearing

> Postmenopausal patients are at a higher risk of osteoporosis or osteopenia.

exercises should also be recommended to all MS patients, unless a contraindication exists. In addition, calcium and vitamin D supplements may be beneficial [11].

KEY POINTS FOR PATIENTS REGARDING PREGNANCY AND LACTATION

- Pregnancy is not contraindicated in patients with MS.
- Notify your care provider if you become pregnant, or plan on becoming pregnant, as some medications used in the treatment of MS may not be safe for use during pregnancy.
- Pregnancy reduces the risk of MS flare, especially in the third trimester.
- Most doctors recommend patients discontinue their DMTs during or prior to pregnancy.
- If you are at a particularly high risk of relapse, your care provider may recommend continuing your DMT during pregnancy.
- If a relapse occurs during pregnancy, a short course of high-dose steroids may be used for management.
- Risk of complications during pregnancy and delivery in MS is the same as the general population.
- General and spinal anesthesia are safe in MS patients during delivery.
- Notify your care provider if you plan on breast-feeding, as some medications used for MS may be secreted in the breast milk and should not be taken if you plan on breast-feeding.

REFERENCES

1. Sellner J, Kraus J, Awad A, et al. The increasing incidence and prevalence of female multiple sclerosis—A critical analysis of potential environmental factors. *Autoimmun Rev.* 2011;10(8): 495–502.

2. Thompson AJ, Polman CH, Miller DH, et al. Primary progressive multiple sclerosis. *Brain.* 1997;120:1085–1096.

3. Tremlett H, Devonshire V. Is late-onset multiple sclerosis associated with a worse outcome? *Neurology.* 2006;67:954–959.

4. Savettieri G, Messina D, Andreoli V, et al. Gender-related effect of clinical and genetic variables on the cognitive impairment in multiple sclerosis. *J Neurol.* 2004;251:1208–1214.

5. Ghezzi A, Zaffaroni M. Female-specific issues in multiple sclerosis. *Expert Rev Neurother.* 2008;8(6):969–977.

6. Coyle PK. Gender issues. *Neural Clin.* 2005;23:39–60.

7. Whitacre C. Sex differences in autoimmune disease. *Nat Immunol.* 2001;2:777–780.

8. Greer J, McCombe P. Role of gender in multiple sclerosis: Clinical effect and potential molecular mechanisms. *J Neuroimmunol.* 2011;234(5):7–18.

9. Sharrief K. Cytokines in multiple sclerosis: Pro-inflammation or pro-remyelination? *Mult Scler.* 1998;4:169–173.

10. Gilmore W, Weiner LP, Correale J. Effect of estradiol on cytokine secretion by proteolipid protein-specific T cell clones isolated from multiple sclerosis patients and normal control subjects. *J Immunol.* 1997;158:446–451.

11. Schwendimann R, Alekseeva N. Gender issues in multiple sclerosis. *Int Rev Neurobiol.* 2007;79:377–392.

12. Ramagopalan S, Knight J, Ebers G. Multiple sclerosis and the major histocompatibility complex. *Curr Opin Neurol.* 2009;22(3):219–225.

13. Jansson L, Olsson T, Holmdahl R. Estrogen induces a potent suppression of experimental autoimmune encephalomyelitis and collagen-induced arthritis in mice. *J Neuroimmunol.* 1994;53: 203–207.

14. Sicotte NL, Live SM, Klutch R, et al. Treatment of multiple sclerosis with the pregnancy hormone estriol. *Ann Neurol.* 2002;52:421–428.

15. Hutchinson M. Oestrogen therapy for multiple sclerosis: Not the way forward. *Int MS J.* 2003;10(3):98.

16. Alonso A, Jick SS, Olek MJ, et al. Recent use of oral contraceptives and the risk of multiple sclerosis. *Arch Neurol.* 2005;62:1362–1365.

17. Thorogood M, Hannaford PC. The influence of oral contraceptives on the risk of multiple sclerosis. *Br J Obstet Gynaecol.* 1998;105:1296–1299.

18. Wilson S, Donnan P, Swingrem R, et al. A serial observational study on hormonal influences in MS symptoms. *Mult Scler.* 2004;SS188–SS189.

19. Zordrager A, DeKeyser J. The premenstrual period and exacerbations in multiple sclerosis. *Eur Neurol.* 2002;48:204–206.

20. Cavalla P, Rovei V, Masera S, et al. Fertility in patients with multiple sclerosis: Current knowledge and future perspectives. *Neurol Sci.* 2006;27:231–239.

21. Cohen BA, Mikol DD. Mitoxantrone treatment of multiple sclerosis: Safety considerations. *Neurology.* 2004;63(Suppl 6):S28–S32.

22. Stenager E, Stenager EN, Jensen K. Effect of pregnancy on the prognosis for multiple sclerosis, a 5-year follow-up and investigation. *Acta Neurol Scand.* 1994;90:305–308.

23. Dwosh E, Guimond C, Duquette P, Sadovnik AD. The interaction of MS and pregnancy: A critical review. *Int MS J.* 2003;10:38–42.

24. Caon C. Pregnancy in MS. In: *Multiple Sclerosis.* Olek MJ, ed. Humana; 2005;145–159.

25. Confavreux C, Hutchinson M, Hours MM, et al. Rate of pregnancy related relapse in multiple sclerosis. *N Engl J Med.* 1998;339(5):285–291.

26. Ferrero S, Pretta S, Ragni N. Multiple sclerosis: Management issues during pregnancy. *Eur J Obstet Gynecol Reprod Biol.* 2004;115:3–9.

27. Hupperts R, Broadley S, Mander A, et al. Patterns of disease in concordant parent-child pairs with multiple sclerosis. *Neurology.* 2001;57:290–295.

28. Kantarci OH, Barcellos LF, Atkinson EJ, et al. Men transmit MS more often to their children vs. women: The Carter effect. *Neurology.* 2006;67:305–310.

29. Herrera BM, Ramagopalan SV, Orton S, et al. Parental transmission of MS in a population-based Canadian cohort. *Neurology.* 2007;69:1208–1212.

30. Tsui A, Lee M. Multiple sclerosis and pregnancy. *Curr Opin Obstet Gynecol.* 2011;23:435–439.

31. www.accessdata.fda.gov/drugsatfda_docs/label/2012/202992 s000lbl.pdf. Accessed 24 November 2012.

32. Sandberg-Wolheim M, Frank D, Goodwin TM, et al. Pregnancy outcomes during treatment with interferon β-1a in patients with multiple sclerosis. *Neurology.* 2005;65(6):802–806.

33. Boskovic R, Wide R, Wolpin J, et al. The reproductive effects of β interferon therapy in pregnancy: A longitudinal cohort. *Neurology.* 2005;65(6):807–811.

34. Ferrero S, Esposito F, Pretta S, Ragni N. Fetal risks related to the treatment of multiple sclerosis during pregnancy and breastfeeding. *Expert Rev Neurother.* 2006;6(12): 1823–1831.

35. Park-Wyllie L, Mazzotta P, Pastuszak A, et al. Birth defects after maternal exposure to corticosteroids: Prospective cohort study and meta-analysis of epidemiological studies. *Teratology.* 2000;62:385–392.

36. *Micromedex® Healthcare Series* [intranet database]. Version 5.1. Greenwood Village, Colo: Thomson Reuters (Healthcare) Inc. Accessed 8 November 2012.

37. Haas J. High dose IVIG in in the postpartum period for prevention of exacerbation of MS. *Mult Scler.* 2000;6(Suppl. 2): S18–S20.

38. Achiron A, Kischner I, Dolev M, et al. Effect of intravenous immunoglobulin treatment on pregnancy and postpartum-related relapses in multiple sclerosis. *J Neurol.* 2004;251(9): 1133–1137.

39. Langer-Gould A, Huang S, Gupta R, et al. Exclusive breastfeeding and the risk of postpartum relapses in women in multiple sclerosis. *Arch Neurol.* 2009;66(8):958–963.

40. Portaccio E, Ghezzi A, Hakiki B, et al. Breastfeeding is not related to postpartum relapses in multiple sclerosis. *Neurology.* 2011;77(2):145–150.

41. Smith R, Studd JW. A pilot study of the effect upon multiple sclerosis of the menopause, hormone replacement therapy and the menstrual cycle. *J R Soc Med.* 1992;85(10):612–613.

33

Multiple Sclerosis and Associated Comorbidities

YUVAL KARMON
BIANCA WEINSTOCK-GUTTMAN

KEY POINTS FOR CLINICIANS

- Several studies have shown an increased rate of vascular comorbidities in multiple sclerosis (MS) patients.

- Presence of vascular comorbidities may delay MS diagnosis and hasten disability progression.

- Smoking was reported to adversely affect the risk for MS disease progression.

- A less favorable lipid profile (high LDL-C) was associated with a worse MS outcome.

- Hypothyroidism is one of the commonest autoimmune comorbidities in MS patients and should always be addressed, especially in interferon-treated patients, as it can affect fatigue, cognitive functions and mood, as well as general well-being.

- Late onset MS can be ascertained in patients over 50 years of age, and is characterized by a lower rate of relapsing disease, usually presenting with a primary progressive course, or an earlier conversion to a secondary progressive course.

COMORBIDITIES IN MS

Comorbidity in general refers to the cumulative burden of illnesses other than the disease of main interest [1]. Comorbidities are not limited to a specific disease or population, and as expected their extent and frequency increase with age, adding to the morbidity associated with the primary condition [1]. Multiple sclerosis (MS) is a chronic disease that affects the central nervous system (CNS), and is considered the second most common cause of disability among young adults after trauma [2]. Comorbid health behaviors and lifestyle factors such as smoking, alcohol intake, and limited physical activity can substantially affect the risk and outcomes of chronic diseases in general, and of MS in particular.

Evidence suggests that comorbidities might:
- delay the time between MS symptom onset and diagnosis;
- affect the clinical phenotype/severity of MS at presentation;
- affect disability progression and health-related quality of life;
- have significant effects on treatment decisions.

Vascular Comorbidities

The existing heterogeneity observed among MS patients may stem from different factors, including underlying comorbidities. A recent study ($n = 8,983$) in the North American Research Committee on Multiple Sclerosis (NARCOMS) registry evaluated the association between disability in MS and the presence of several vascular risk factors [3]. Participants who reported more than 1 vascular comorbidity (diabetes, hypertension, heart disease, hypercholesterolemia, and peripheral vascular disease) at the time of diagnosis had a higher risk of ambulatory disability, and the risk increased with the number of vascular conditions reported (hazard ratio [HR]/condition for early gait disability 1.51; 95% confidence interval [CI] 1.41–1.61). Vascular comorbidities at any point during the disease course also elevated the risk of ambulatory disability (adjusted HR for unilateral walking assistance 1.54; CI 1.44–1.65). This study suggests that outcome in MS might be affected by vascular comorbidities developed at the time of MS symptom onset, or later during the disease course.

In another publication on the same patient sample, the presence of obesity, smoking, and physical or mental comorbidities [4] was associated with a significant delay in diagnosing MS (for up to 11 years from the time of symptom onset). This effect persisted even after accounting for demographic and clinical characteristics. Possible explanations include the presence of a preexisting disease that can mask the symptoms of MS, and new symptoms being mistakenly attributed to the preexisting condition. Moreover, the existing burden of illness could negatively affect the MS outcome.

Further analysis showed that vascular, musculoskeletal, and psychiatric comorbidities, and obesity were associated with more severe disability at the time of diagnosis. After adjustment, the odds ratio (OR) for moderate disability compared with mild disability at diagnosis was 1.51 (CI 1.12–2.05) in participants with a vascular comorbidity and 1.38 (CI 1.02–1.87) in those with obesity. These findings need to be replicated in population-based cohorts but they strongly suggest that comorbidities contribute to the level of disability in MS patients.

A potential approach to slow MS progression may require a more aggressive management of vascular and other comorbidities, including behavioral changes (eg, dietary intervention, active exercise programs, and smoking cessation).

Two nationwide Danish studies evaluating mortality among MS patients reported that patients with MS had a 30% higher risk of death due to cardiovascular disease (CVD), including cerebrovascular disease, compared with the age-matched general population [5,6], while a 6% higher risk of death due to CVD (excluding stroke) was observed in a study from South Wales [7]. Another Danish study [8] showed that the risk of CVD among MS patients is still low, yet higher than in the general population, particularly in the short term correcting for age. The risk of myocardial infarction (MI) was 0.2% among patients with MS (adjusted IRR = 1.84; 95% CI: 1.28–2.65, compared with population cohort members), whereas the 1 year risk of stroke was 0.3% (adjusted IRR = 1.96; 95% CI: 1.42–2.71),

and the IRR for heart failure was 1.92 (95% CI: 1.27–2.90). A possible explanation may be that increased prevalence of CVD is often associated with reduced mobility and ability to exercise, as recently shown in a large cohort of MS patients [9,10].

Hyperlipidemia

The retrospective analysis of NARCOMS registry participants mentioned earlier reported that dyslipidemia was associated with an increased risk for disability progression in MS [3,4]. In a recently published study, our group showed that fasting serum lipid profile evaluated in a group of 492 MS patients (age: 47.1 ± 10.8 years; disease duration: 12.8 ± 10.1 years) followed for approximately 2 years (2.2 ± 1.0 years) correlated with disability and MRI outcomes (quantitative MRI findings at baseline were available for 210 patients). Expanded Disability Status Scale (EDSS) worsening was associated with higher baseline low-density lipoprotein (LDL) ($P = .006$) and total cholesterol ($P = .001$) levels, with trends for higher triglyceride levels ($P = .025$); high-density lipoprotein (HDL) was not associated with clinical disease status. A similar pattern was found for MS Severity Score (MSSS) worsening ($P = .008$ for total cholesterol). However, higher HDL levels ($P < .001$) were associated with lower contrast-enhancing lesion volume. Higher total cholesterol was associated with a trend for lower brain parenchymal fraction ($P = .033$) [11]. Increased total cholesterol was also found to be associated with increases in the number of contrast-enhancing lesions on brain MRI in clinically isolated syndrome (CIS) patients following a first clinical demyelinating event [12].

Dyslipidemia can potentiate inflammatory processes at the vascular endothelium, possibly leading to the induction of adhesion molecules and the recruitment of monocytes [13–15]. Associations between dyslipidemia and increased inflammation are well established in conditions such as atherosclerosis, CVD, metabolic syndrome, and obesity [16]. Similarly, in the context of other autoimmune diseases, a strong association between dyslipidemia and CVD was shown in systemic lupus erythematosus (SLE) [17] and an increased cardiovascular risk and dyslipidemia have been reported in rheumatoid arthritis [18] as well. HDL and LDL also modulate the function and survival of pancreatic beta cells in type 2 diabetes mellitus [19]. Neuromyelitis optica patients were reported to have significantly higher serum cholesterol triglycerides but lower LDL compared to healthy controls [20]. Therefore, a direct influence of hyperlipidemia on the inflammatory and/or neurodegenerative processes in MS (in addition to the known increased risk for cardiovascular pathology) is possible.

Smoking

Smoking was shown to be associated with an increased risk to develop MS [21]. More recently, the relation of smoking to disease progression was also evaluated, the results being still contradictory [22,23]. One study [24] including 780 MS patients who have never smoked, 428 ex-smokers, and 257 who currently smoke, found that current smokers (OR 2.42, 95% CI 1.09–5.35) and ex-smokers (1.91, 1.02–3.58) were more likely to present with primary progressive MS (PPMS) than with relapsing-remitting MS (RRMS). Potential confounders (comorbid obesity or vascular risk factors) were unfortunately not assessed.

Several studies also suggest that smoking is associated with an increased risk of disability progression in patients with MS. In a study using information from the General Practice Research Database [25], smokers with RRMS were 3 times more likely to develop secondary progressive MS (SPMS) than were nonsmokers, whereas only 20 of 179 patients who were never-smokers or ever-smokers had a progressive course. In another study (n = 122) of individuals with newly diagnosed MS, the proportion of patients who developed SPMS after a median follow-up time of 6 years was 72% for ever-smokers who began smoking before the age of 15 years, 40% for ever-smokers who began smoking after the age of 15 years, but only 26% for those who had never smoked [26]. Another study followed 129 patients with a CIS who were at high risk of developing MS on the basis of findings from MRI and CSF examination. After 3 years, 75% of smokers developed MS compared with only 51% of nonsmokers (HR 1.8, 95% CI 1.2–2.8). In 2 studies including the 1 from our group [22,24], smoking was associated with an increased number of gadolinium-enhancing lesions, increased T2-weighted lesion volume, and greater brain atrophy [22]. Neither study included a control group of smokers without MS to assess whether smoking has additive or multiplicative effects on brain imaging measures, such as brain volume.

Anti-Phospholipid Antibodies

Although anti-phospholipid antibody syndrome (APLS) was first described in the context of connective tissue diseases such as SLE, it was soon recognized that the condition can exist as an isolated syndrome. Primary APLS (PAPLS) is an autoimmune disorder characterized by recurrent thrombosis, miscarriages, and thrombocytopenia in the presence of anti-phospholipid antibodies (APLA) and persistently positive (+) anticardiolipin or lupus anticoagulant (LA) tests. It has been established that APLAs are heterogeneous and bind to various antigenic targets [27]. Some studies reported a higher prevalence of various APLAs in MS as compared to other neurological disorders [28]. When MRIs of MS patients were compared to those of PAPLS patients [29], they showed significantly higher T2 and T1 lesion volumes. The same study [30] showed also that APLA+ RRMS and SPMS patients showed significantly higher T2 lesion volume, lower GMF (gray matter fraction), and lower normal-appearing gray matter magnetization transfer ratio (MTR) when compared to APLA–patients. It is possible that APLA mediates heterogeneous cerebral pathology that needs to be further investigated. A recent study from our group suggests that prospectively followed APLA+ RRMS patients treated with interferon (IFN) beta-1a developed more severe MRI and clinical disease activity (relapses and sustained disability progression) as compared with APLA–RRMS patients treated with IFN beta-1a [31] although a decreased effect of IFN cannot be ruled out.

Recently, it was suggested that some phospholipids serve actually as natural anti-inflammatory compounds. Several autoantibodies in MS were found to target a phosphate group in phosphatidylserine and oxidized phosphatidylcholine derivatives (Table 33.1) [32]. The presence of certain anti-phospholipid antibodies therefore, might be a marker for an ongoing systemic underlying inflammatory process. On the other hand, administration of those phospholipids might become an optional therapy in the future.

Other Autoimmune Comorbidities

Several studies investigating the prevalence of other autoimmune comorbidities in MS compared with the general population showed conflicting results [37,42,43], often related to differences in study design [44]. Although the targeted autoimmune diseases were found more frequently in MS patients compared to the general population, their absolute frequency is low, therefore their presence is unlikely to have a substantial effect on MS at the population level, but may have an impact at the individual level (Table 33.1).

In the New York State Multiple Sclerosis Consortium [38] (n = 3,019), 0.8% of patients with MS had comorbid SLE, and an even higher rate of SLE was observed in MS patients' relatives (1.8%). Varying frequencies were also reported for rheumatoid arthritis (RA) [37–39] (0.9%–4.4%). Data from the NY State Consortium revealed a much higher rate of RA, 9.8% in first degree relatives of MS patients compared with the patients (2%) [38]. Thyroid dysfunction was also reported to be more frequent than expected in MS patients, with frequencies of up to 9% in both males and females [40]. This rate was actually found to be significantly higher than a control group only for male MS patients (control group rates: male 1.9%, female 9.2%). Only 2 [40,41] of 4 studies using a control or reference group identified an increased risk. Nevertheless, every MS patient should be screened for thyroid dysfunction (often related to autoimmune thyroiditis), as it could affect energy level, fatigue, mood, and cognitive functions significantly, and proper management should be initiated, because it is easily treatable.

Disease-modifying therapies approved for MS can be also associated with secondary development of autoimmune diseases (see Chapter 13). Interferon beta (IFNb) therapy has been reported to induce antithyroid antibodies and to precipitate thyroid clinical disease in patients with preexisting antibodies [45,46]. Okanoue and colleagues [47] have suggested that IFNb can induce autoimmune disorders including autoimmune thyroiditis, hemolytic anemia, thrombocytopenia, SLE, rheumatoid arthritis, and psoriasis. However, these autoimmune diseases (except for

TABLE 33.1
Evidence Supporting the Role of Comorbidities in MS

COMORBIDITY OR RISK FACTOR	REFERENCE	FINDINGS
CV comorbidity	[4] (NARCOMS registry)	A higher risk to develop ambulatory disability with the presence of more vascular risk factors
	[4]	Median time to disability shortens with presence of vascular risk factors (12.8 vs. 18.8 years)
	[5–8]	Risk of CV death is higher than in general population
Smoking	[21]	Is associated with increased risk to develop MS
	[22–26]	Its association with MS progression is controversial
	[22, 24]	Was associated with more brain atrophy, Gad-positive lesions, and T2-weighted lesion volume
Hyperlipidemia	[4]	Retrospective analysis of NARCOMS registry: dyslipidemia was associated with an increased risk for disability progression in MS
	[11]	Fasting serum lipid profile evaluated in 492 patients correlated with disability and MRI outcomes
	[11]	EDSS worsening was associated with higher baseline LDL and total cholesterol
	[11]	Higher HDL levels were associated with lower contrast-enhancing lesion volume
Anti-phospholipid antibodies	[30]	APLA+ RRMS/SPMS had higher T2 lesion volume, lower GMF, and lower normal-appearing gray matter MTR when compared to APLA– patients
	[31]	APLA+ RRMS patients treated with IFN beta-1a developed more severe MRI and clinical disease activity (relapses, and sustained disability progression) as compared with APLA– RRMS patients treated with IFN beta-1a
	[32]	Administration of phosphatidylserine and oxidized phosphatidylcholine derivatives ameliorated EAE by suppressing activation and inducing apoptosis of autoreactive T cells
Autoimmune comorbidities	[33–36]	Inflammatory bowel disease—questionable association (conflicting results)
	[37–39]	Varying rates for rheumatoid arthritis in MS (0.9–4.4%)
	[40,41]	Hypothyroidism rates are considered to be high in MS male and female patients (up to 9%)

APLA+, anti-phospholipid antibodies positive; APLA–, anti-phospholipid antibodies negative; CV, cardiovascular; EAE, experimental autoimmune encephalomyelitis; EDSS, Expanded Disability Status Scale; GMF, gray matter fraction; HDL, high-density lipoprotein; LDL, low-density lipoprotein; MTR, magnetization transfer ratio; NARCOMS, North American Research Committee on Multiple Sclerosis; RRMS, remitting-relapsing MS; SPMS, secondary progressive MS.

autoimmune thyroiditis), are in general rare events among IFNb therapy users, and may develop at a higher frequency in MS patients in general, as previously mentioned [47]. There are rare reported cases of IFNb-associated SLE in the literature, although subacute cutaneous lupus has been previously reported [48]. Crispin and Diaz-Jouanen have described a female who developed SLE while on continuous therapy with IFN beta-1a for 3 years [49]. Occasional cases of myasthenia gravis [50] following IFNb therapy have also been described. Treatment with glatiramer acetate (GA) was also reported to be associated with autoimmune diseases, such as Crohn's disease, myasthenia gravis, and arthritis [51–54].

New challenges are also envisioned as novel immunologically active agents that are in advanced stages of study completion and/or FDA application will become available. An increased risk for autoimmune diseases was observed in patients treated with alemtuzumab (Campath), a very potent treatment for RRMS. Thyroid disease was seen most frequently, in approximately 20% of treated patients [55], and individual risk was shown to be modified by smoking

and family history of autoimmune diseases, which should be incorporated within the patient counseling process prior to treatment initiation [56].

Other Comorbidities

Physical comorbidities other than autoimmune diseases seem to be common in patients with MS. Additional comorbidities reported in the large NARCOMS registry sample [4], besides the ones already mentioned, include arthritis (16%, excluding RA), irritable bowel syndrome (13%), and chronic lung disease (13%). This list includes 3 of the 5 leading causes of disability in the general population (hypertension, lung disease, arthritis, back or spine problems, and heart disease) [57]. In the parallel self-report from the nationally representative Canadian Community Health Survey [58], 302 respondents with MS reported comorbidities that included back problems (35%), non-food allergies (29%), arthritis (26%), hypertension (17%), and migraine (14%). All these comorbidities have to be assessed, differentiated from MS-related deficits and symptoms, and treated appropriately. Data from several studies have indicated that sleep disorders and related disorders are more common in patients with MS than in the general population [59]. In a large cohort of U.S. veterans with MS (n = 16,074), 940 (6%) had sleep disorders compared with 3% of veterans without MS. Sleep disturbance was defined as the presence of at least 1 abnormal diagnostic polysomnogram or sleep disorder identified during study period [60]. Restless legs syndrome (RLS) was also reported with a frequency ranging from 13.3% to 37.5% depending on the cohort studied [61,62]. In most of these studies, RLS occurred substantially more often in individuals with MS than in the general population. Obesity was found to be as prevalent in MS patients as in the general population (50%) [63].

Comorbidities and Therapeutic Decisions

Comorbidities can affect the treatment of MS, including the selection of whether to initiate treatment, the specific choice of treatment, and its subsequent effectiveness. Severe, uncontrolled depression, for example, is a contraindication for the use of interferon beta [64]. Many clinical trials in patients with MS exclude individuals with severe comorbidities or substance abuse disorders, and therefore may not reflect "real life" results [65]. Consequently, the safety, tolerability, and effectiveness of most drugs are not known in such patients. Depression is known to be seen in higher frequency in MS patients and is also recognized to affect compliance and adherence to disease-modifying therapy [66]. Concurrent ischemic heart disease or hypertension, as well as the use of certain medications (eg, beta- or calcium channel blockers) were found to be associated with a higher risk for developing heart rhythm problems with fingolimod, requiring close monitoring for 24 hours in a hospital setting following the first dose, compared to the usual 6 hour outpatient monitoring for patients without known vascular comorbidities [67]. Previous history of a seizure disorder is usually a contraindication for treatment with 4-aminopyridine (dalfampridine, Ampyra) which was recently approved to improve walking in patients with MS [68].

AGING AND MULTIPLE SCLEROSIS

The assessed prevalence of MS in the United States is about 450,000 (probably underestimated), and about one-half of individuals with MS are over 55 years old. Most neurologists are hesitant to diagnose MS in elderly patients. In fact, previous diagnostic criteria excluded the diagnosis of MS on the basis of age alone [69]. However, population-based studies have shown that the prevalence of late onset MS (above age 50 years) is not rare, ranging between 4.6% and 9.4% of all cases of MS [70]. It is also very likely that patients presenting with a diagnosis after age 50 represent a heterogeneous mixture of patients with true late-onset MS

and those with unrecognized symptoms earlier in life. Of those with MS, about 90% will have a life expectancy similar to their counterparts. This also means that the majority of patients will live with the disease at least 20 years if diagnosed in their late 50s. Few studies have been conducted to evaluate the effects of aging on MS disease course.

A distinction should be made between 2 main groups: those who age with MS while diagnosed at an earlier age, as opposed to the group of patients who are being diagnosed with MS at an older age (late onset MS).

Aging With MS

In a study using hospital discharge notes, older adults with MS experienced more infectious complications, such as pneumonia, urinary tract infection, sepsis, or cellulitis, as compared with their non-MS counterparts who are more likely to have diagnoses of myocardial infarct, congestive heart failure, stroke, angina, diabetes, and lung disease [71]. At the same time, aging individuals with MS have an increased risk for vascular comorbidities as previously mentioned.

In the last 2 decades it has become evident that the underlying MS pathology involves, in addition to the well-known inflammatory process, a significant neurodegenerative component that is primarily responsible for the irreversible neurological clinical progression. This neurodegenerative process probably starts at the very early stages of the disease, but is more prominent in later stages of the disease. Brain parenchymal atrophy, as measured by MRI, represents the best surrogate marker for assessing the associated ongoing neurodegenerative processes in MS, and is considered the best predictor for disability progression [72]. In particular, the thalamus and basal ganglia have been implicated in the process of "central" atrophy. Thalamic atrophy has been reported early on, even in children diagnosed with MS [73], CIS [74], and adult phenotypes of MS, including RRMS, SPMS, and PPMS. The thalamic volume increases in typically developing children [75] and decreases in healthy adults [76]. Accounting for the late development and natural aging changes of the thalamus is important in interpreting the findings in MS, particularly when MS patients include young adults.

A recent study also showed that thalamic volume loss in MS patients correlated with disability after adjusting for natural aging and whole brain lesion volume, suggesting that MS thalamic pathology has a neurodegenerative component independent from the white matter lesions [77]. These findings suggest that thalamic atrophy is a central component in normal aging as well as in MS-associated neurodegeneration. Therefore, it can be anticipated that the aging process in MS patients will have a more deleterious effect than in aging individuals without MS. Accordingly, a similar decline in processing speed was documented in both patients and controls as age increases, indicating that both processes, aging and MS, advance separately but have an additive effect on the overall cognitive status [78].

MS Diagnosed in the Elderly

In a recent work, Bermel et al. [79] described the clinical characteristics of patients diagnosed with MS after the age of 60 years (n = 111). At the time of diagnosis, 8% of patients had a CIS, 33% were in the relapsing-remitting stage, while 23% had a secondary progressive course, and 32% had primary progressive course. Acute partial transverse myelitis was the most common initial clinical presentation (46%), followed by progressive myelopathy (38%). Finally, 46% of patients with RRMS or a CIS exhibited MRI gadolinium enhancement (brain and/or spine). These findings support the opinion that elderly patients, diagnosed after the age of 60 years, can still experience significant inflammatory processes. Another study analyzing time trends and disability milestones among enrollees in a large international database found that the more recent enrollees were significantly older than the earlier enrollees, raising the awareness to what appears as a new trend of relative increase in the age of onset in the MS population [80].

An older age of onset was also shown to be associated with a faster rate of disability decline compared to patients with early age of onset [81]. Similarly, a recent study comparing the outcomes in animal experimental autoimmune encephalomyelitis (EAE) at different ages [82], showed that older age groups developed onset of clinical signs simultaneously with the acute CNS lesions, while the younger mice groups showed some delay in the occurrence of clinical symptoms. This could be explained by a decreased nervous tissue reserve, with shorter time to reach a certain disease progression and/or decreased ability to repair in aging individuals [83]. Myelin repair mechanisms might be impaired in older age groups, as shown in an animal model and attributed to decreased recruitment of oligodendrocyte precursors [84]. An opposite effect of younger age may be responsible for the delay (up to 10 years) in reaching specific progression thresholds as well as conversion to SPMS in pediatric MS patients, compared to adults with MS [83,85].

CONCLUSIONS AND FUTURE DIRECTIONS

There is mounting evidence linking the risk and progression of MS to various environmental risk factors and comorbidities. Heterogeneity in disease severity, including cognition and ambulation, can also be partially attributed to associated vascular risk factors and other comorbidities.

Identifying comorbidities and their impact in MS patients will help in tailoring a more individualized treatment plan. Practice guidelines were implemented in other specialties in the last decade, including the 2003 national hypertension [86] or hyperlipidemia guidelines, that take into account the existence of comorbid conditions (stroke, diabetes mellitus, ischemic heart disease, etc.). Similar therapeutic guidelines will probably be necessary to facilitate a comprehensive management strategy for MS. Further research studies are needed to better understand the incidence and impact of comorbidities and the role of aging on MS.

REFERENCES

1. Gijsen R, Hoeymans N, Schellevis FG, et al. Causes and consequences of comorbidity: A review. *J Clin Epidemiol.* 2001;54(7):661–674.
2. Dean G. How many people in the world have multiple sclerosis? *Neuroepidemiology.* 1994;13(1–2):1–7.
3. Marrie RA, Rudick R, Horwitz R, et al. Vascular comorbidity is associated with more rapid disability progression in multiple sclerosis. *Neurology.* 2010;74(13):1041–1047.
4. Kennedy J, O'Connor P, Sadovnick AD, et al. Age at onset of multiple sclerosis may be influenced by place of residence during childhood rather than ancestry. *Neuroepidemiology.* 2006;26(3):162–167.
5. Bronnum-Hansen H, Koch-Henriksen N, Stenager E. Trends in survival and cause of death in Danish patients with multiple sclerosis. *Brain.* 2004;127(Pt 4):844–850.
6. Koch-Henriksen N, Bronnum-Hansen H, Stenager E. Underlying cause of death in Danish patients with multiple sclerosis: Results from the Danish Multiple Sclerosis Registry. *J Neurol Neurosurg Psychiatry.* 1998;65(1):56–59.
7. Hirst C, Swingler R, Compston DA, et al. Survival and cause of death in multiple sclerosis: A prospective population-based study. *J Neurol Neurosurg Psychiatry.* 2008;79(9):1016–1021.
8. Christiansen CF, Christensen S, Farkas DK, et al. Risk of arterial cardiovascular diseases in patients with multiple sclerosis: A population-based cohort study. *Neuroepidemiology.* 2010;35(4):267–274.
9. Motl RW, Fernhall B, McAuley E, Cutter G. Physical activity and self-reported cardiovascular comorbidities in persons with multiple sclerosis: Evidence from a cross-sectional analysis. *Neuroepidemiology.* 2011;36(3):183–191.
10. Christiansen CF. Risk of vascular disease in patients with multiple sclerosis: A review. *Neurol Res.* 2012;34(8):746–753.
11. Weinstock-Guttman B, Zivadinov R, Mahfooz N, et al. Serum lipid profiles are associated with disability and MRI outcomes in multiple sclerosis. *J Neuroinflammation.* 2011;8:127.
12. Giubilei F, Antonini G, Di Legge S, et al. Blood cholesterol and MRI activity in first clinical episode suggestive of multiple sclerosis. *Acta Neurol Scand.* 2002;106(2):109–112.
13. Cybulsky MI, Gimbrone MA Jr. Endothelial expression of a mononuclear leukocyte adhesion molecule during atherogenesis. *Science.* 1991;251(4995):788–791.
14. Sitia S, Tomasoni L, Atzeni F, et al. From endothelial dysfunction to atherosclerosis. *Autoimmun Rev.* 2010;9(12):830–834.
15. Stokes KY, Calahan L, Hamric CM, et al. CD40/CD40L contributes to hypercholesterolemia-induced microvascular inflammation. *Am J Physiol Heart Circ Physiol.* 2009;296(3):H689–H697.
16. Esteve E, Ricart W, Fernandez-Real JM. Dyslipidemia and inflammation: An evolutionary conserved mechanism. *Clin Nutr.* 2005;24(1):16–31.
17. Torres A, Askari AD, Malemud CJ. Cardiovascular disease complications in systemic lupus erythematosus. *Biomark Med.* 2009;3(3):239–252.
18. Boyer JF, Gourraud PA, Cantagrel A, et al. Traditional cardiovascular risk factors in rheumatoid arthritis: A meta-analysis. *Joint Bone Spine.* 2011;78(2)179–183.
19. von Eckardstein A, Sibler RA. Possible contributions of lipoproteins and cholesterol to the pathogenesis of diabetes mellitus type 2. *Curr Opin Lipidol.* 2011;22(1):26–32.

20. Li Y, Wang H, Hu X, et al. Serum lipoprotein levels in patients with neuromyelitis optica elevated but had little correlation with clinical presentations. *Clin Neurol Neurosurg.* 2010;112(6):478–481.

21. Di Pauli F, Reindl M, Ehling R, et al. Smoking is a risk factor for early conversion to clinically definite multiple sclerosis. *Mult Scler.* 2008;14(8):1026–1030.

22. Zivadinov R, Weinstock-Guttman B, Hashmi K, et al. Smoking is associated with increased lesion volumes and brain atrophy in multiple sclerosis. *Neurology.* 2009;73(7):504–510.

23. Koch M, van Harten A, Uyttenboogaart M, et al. Cigarette smoking and progression in multiple sclerosis. *Neurology.* 2007;69(15):1515–1520.

24. Healy BC, Ali EN, Guttmann CR, et al. Smoking and disease progression in multiple sclerosis. *Arch Neurol.* 2009;66(7):858–864.

25. Hernan MA, Jick SS, Logroscino G, et al. Cigarette smoking and the progression of multiple sclerosis. *Brain.* 2005;128(Pt 6):1461–1465.

26. Sundstrom P, Nystrom L. Smoking worsens the prognosis in multiple sclerosis. *Mult Scler.* 2008;14(8):1031–1035.

27. Horstman LL, Jy W, Bidot CJ, et al. Antiphospholipid antibodies: Paradigm in transition. *J Neuroinflammation.* 2009;6:3.

28. Tourbah A, Clapin A, Gout O, et al. Systemic autoimmune features and multiple sclerosis: A 5-year follow-up study. *Arch Neurol.* 1998;55(4):517–521.

29. Rovaris M, Viti B, Ciboddo G, et al. Brain involvement in systemic immune mediated diseases: Magnetic resonance and magnetisation transfer imaging study. *J Neurol Neurosurg Psychiatry.* 2000;68(2):170–177.

30. Stosic M, Ambrus J, Garg N, et al. MRI characteristics of patients with antiphospholipid syndrome and multiple sclerosis. *J Neurol.* 2010;257(1):63–71.

31. Zivadinov RR, Ramanathan M, Ambrus J, et al. Antiphospholipid antibodies are associated with response to interferon-beta-1a treatment in MS: Results from a 3-year longitudinal study. *Neurol Res.* 2012;34(8):761–769.

32. Ho PP, Kanter JL, Johnson AM, et al. Identification of naturally occurring fatty acids of the myelin sheath that resolve neuroinflammation. *Sci Transl Med.* 2012;4(137):137ra73.

33. Gupta G, Gelfand JM, Lewis JD. Increased risk for demyelinating diseases in patients with inflammatory bowel disease. *Gastroenterology.* 2005;129(3):819–826.

34. Bernstein CN, Wajda A, Blanchard JF. The clustering of other chronic inflammatory diseases in inflammatory bowel disease: A population-based study. *Gastroenterology.* 2005;129(3):827–836.

35. Kimura K, Hunter SF, Thollander MS, et al. Concurrence of inflammatory bowel disease and multiple sclerosis. *Mayo Clin Proc.* 2000;75(8):802–806.

36. Broadley SA, Deans J, Sawcer SJ, et al. Autoimmune disease in first-degree relatives of patients with multiple sclerosis. A UK survey. *Brain.* 2000;123(Pt 6):1102–1111.

37. Seyfert S, Klapps P, Meisel C, et al. Multiple sclerosis and other immunologic diseases. *Acta Neurol Scand.* 1990;81(1):37–42.

38. Jacobs LD, Wende KE, Brownscheidle CM, et al. A profile of multiple sclerosis: The New York State Multiple Sclerosis Consortium. *Mult Scler.* 1999;5(5):369–376.

39. Barcellos LF, Kamdar BB, Ramsay PP, et al. Clustering of autoimmune diseases in families with a high-risk for multiple sclerosis: A descriptive study. *Lancet Neurol.* 2006;5(11):924–931.

40. Niederwieser G, Buchinger W, Bonelli RM, et al. Prevalence of autoimmune thyroiditis and non-immune thyroid disease in multiple sclerosis. *J Neurol.* 2003;250(6):672–675.

41. Sloka JS, Phillips PW, Stefanelli M, Joyce C. Co-occurrence of autoimmune thyroid disease in a multiple sclerosis cohort. *J Autoimmune Dis.* 2005;2:9.

42. Edwards LJ, Constantinescu CS. A prospective study of conditions associated with multiple sclerosis in a cohort of 658 consecutive outpatients attending a multiple sclerosis clinic. *Mult Scler.* 2004;10(5):575–581.

43. Midgard R, Gronning M, Riise T, et al. Multiple sclerosis and chronic inflammatory diseases. A case-control study. *Acta Neurol Scand.* 1996;93(5):322–328.

44. Marrie RA. Autoimmune disease and multiple sclerosis: Methods, methods, methods. *Lancet Neurol.* 2007;6(7):575–576.

45. Durelli L, Ferrero B, Oggero A, et al. Autoimmune events during interferon beta-1b treatment for multiple sclerosis. *J Neurol Sci.* 1999;162(1):74–83.

46. Kreisler A, de Seze J, Stojkovic T, et al. Multiple sclerosis, interferon beta and clinical thyroid dysfunction. *Acta Neurol Scand.* 2003;107(2):154–157.

47. Okanoue T, Itoh Y, Yasui K. Autoimmune disorders in interferon therapy. *Nihon Rinsho.* 1994;52(7):1924–1928.

48. Nousari HC, Kimyai-Asadi A, Tausk FA. Subacute cutaneous lupus erythematosus associated with interferon beta-1a. *Lancet.* 1998;352(9143):1825–1826.

49. Crispin JC, Diaz-Jouanen E. Systemic lupus erythematosus induced by therapy with interferon-beta in a patient with multiple sclerosis. *Lupus.* 2005;14(6):495–496.

50. Dionisiotis J, Zoukos Y, Thomaides T. Development of myasthenia gravis in two patients with multiple sclerosis following interferon beta treatment. *J Neurol Neurosurg Psychiatry.* 2004;75(7):1079.

51. Charach G, Grosskopf I, Weintraub M. Development of Crohn's disease in a patient with multiple sclerosis treated with copaxone. *Digestion.* 2008;77(3–4):198–200.

52. Zheng B, Switzer K, Marinova E, et al. Exacerbation of autoimmune arthritis by copolymer-I through promoting type 1 immune response and autoantibody production. *Autoimmunity.* 2008;41(5):363–371.

53. Frese A, Bethke F, Ludemann P, Stogbauer F. Development of myasthenia gravis in a patient with multiple sclerosis during treatment with glatiramer acetate. *J Neurol.* 2000;247(9):713.

54. Heesen C, Gbadamosi J, Schoser BG, Pohlau D. Autoimmune hyperthyroidism in multiple sclerosis under treatment with glatiramer acetate–a case report. *Eur J Neurol.* 2001;8(2):199.

55. Costelloe L, Jones J, Coles A. Secondary autoimmune diseases following alemtuzumab therapy for multiple sclerosis. *Expert Rev Neurotherap.* 2012;12(3):335–341.

56. Cossburn M, Pace AA, Jones J, et al. Autoimmune disease after alemtuzumab treatment for multiple sclerosis in a multicenter cohort. *Neurology.* 2011;77(6):573–579.

57. Centers for Disease Control and Prevention (CDC). Prevalence of disability and associated health conditions, United States, 1991–1992. *Morb Mortal Wkly Rep.* 1994;40:730–731,7–39.

58. Warren S, Turpin KV, Warren KG. Health-related quality of life in MS: Issues and interventions. *Can J Neurol Sci.* 2009;36(5):540–541.

59. Brass SD, Duquette P, Proulx-Therrien J, Auerbach S. Sleep disorders in patients with multiple sclerosis. *Sleep Med Rev.* 2010;14(2):121–129.

60. Ajayi OF, Chang-McDowell T, Culpepper WJ, et al. High prevalence of sleep disorders in veterans with multiple sclerosis. *Neurology.* 2008;70(Suppl 1):A333.

61. Manconi M, Ferini-Strambi L, Filippi M, et al. Multicenter case-control study on restless legs syndrome in multiple sclerosis: The REMS study. *Sleep.* 2008;31(7):944–952.

62. Gomez-Choco MJ, Iranzo A, Blanco Y, et al. Prevalence of restless legs syndrome and REM sleep behavior disorder in multiple sclerosis. *Mult Scler.* 2007;13(6):805–808.

63. Marrie R, Horwitz R, Cutter G, et al. High frequency of adverse health behaviors in multiple sclerosis. *Mult Scler.* 2009;15(1):105–113.

64. Francis G. Benefit-risk assessment of interferon-beta therapy for relapsing multiple sclerosis. *Expert Opin Drug Saf.* 2004;3(4):289–303.

65. Rudick RA, Stuart WH, Calabresi PA, et al. Natalizumab plus interferon beta-1a for relapsing multiple sclerosis. *N Engl J Med.* 2006;354(9):911–923.

66. Gulick EE. Emotional distress and activities of daily living functioning in persons with multiple sclerosis. *Nurs Res.* 2001;50(3):147–154.

67. US Food and Drug Administration. FDA Drug Safety Communication: Revised recommendations for cardiovascular monitoring and use of multiple sclerosis drug Gilenya (fingolimod). 2012 [updated 05/22/2012]; Available from: www.fda.gov/Drugs/DrugSafety/ucm303192.htm

68. Cornblath DR, Bienen EJ, Blight AR. The safety profile of dalfampridine extended release in multiple sclerosis clinical trials. *Clin Therap.* 2012;34(5):1056–1069.

69. Schumacker GA, Beebe G, Kibler RF, et al. Problems of experimental trials of therapy in multiple sclerosis: Report by the panel on the evaluation of experimental trials of therapy in multiple sclerosis. *Ann NY Acad Sci.* 1965;122:552–568.

70. Polliack ML, Barak Y, Achiron A. Late-onset multiple sclerosis. *J Am Geriatr Soc.* 2001;49(2):168–171.

71. Fleming ST, Blake RL Jr. Patterns of comorbidity in elderly patients with multiple sclerosis. *J Clin Epidemiol.* 1994;47(10):1127–1132.

72. Zivadinov R. Can imaging techniques measure neuroprotection and remyelination in multiple sclerosis? *Neurology.* 2007;68(22 Suppl 3):S72–82; discussion S91–S96.

73. Mesaros S, Rocca MA, Absinta M, et al. Evidence of thalamic gray matter loss in pediatric multiple sclerosis. *Neurology.* 2008;70(13 Pt 2):1107–1112.

74. Henry RG, Shieh M, Amirbekian B, et al. Connecting white matter injury and thalamic atrophy in clinically isolated syndromes. *J Neurol Sci.* 2009;282(1–2):61–66.

75. Ostby Y, Tamnes CK, Fjell AM, et al. Heterogeneity in subcortical brain development: A structural magnetic resonance imaging study of brain maturation from 8 to 30 years. *J Neurosci.* 2009;29(38):11772–11782.

76. Walhovd KB, Westlye LT, Amlien I, et al. Consistent neuroanatomical age-related volume differences across multiple samples. *Neurobiol Aging.* 2011;32(5):916–932.

77. Hasan KM, Walimuni IS, Abid H, et al. Multimodal quantitative magnetic resonance imaging of thalamic development and aging across the human lifespan: Implications to neurodegeneration in multiple sclerosis. *J Neurosci.* 2011;31(46):16826–16832.

78. Bodling AM, Denney DR, Lynch SG. Cognitive aging in patients with multiple sclerosis: A cross-sectional analysis of speeded processing. *Arch Clin Neuropsychol.* 2009;24(8):761–767.

79. Bermel RA, Rae-Grant AD, Fox RJ. Diagnosing multiple sclerosis at a later age: more than just progressive myelopathy. *Mult Scler.* 2010;16(11):1335–1340.

80. Kister I, Chamot E, Cutter G, et al. Increasing age at disability milestones among MS patients in the MSBase Registry. *J Neurol Sci.* 2012;318(1–2):94–99.

81. Trojano M, Liguori M, Bosco Zimatore G, et al. Age-related disability in multiple sclerosis. *Ann Neurol.* 2002;51(4):475–480.

82. Smith ME, Eller NL, McFarland HF, et al. Age dependence of clinical and pathological manifestations of autoimmune demyelination. Implications for multiple sclerosis. *Am J Pathol.* 1999;155(4):1147–1161.

83. Pedre X, Mastronardi F, Bruck W, et al. Changed histone acetylation patterns in normal-appearing white matter and early multiple sclerosis lesions. *J Neurosci.* 2011;31(9):3435–3445.

84. Sim FJ, Zhao C, Penderis J, et al. The age-related decrease in CNS remyelination efficiency is attributable to an impairment of both oligodendrocyte progenitor recruitment and differentiation. *J Neurosci.* 2002;22(7):2451–2459.

85. Kuhlmann T, Miron V, Cui Q, et al. Differentiation block of oligodendroglial progenitor cells as a cause for remyelination failure in chronic multiple sclerosis. *Brain.* 2008;131(Pt 7):1749–1758.

86. Lenfant C, Chobanian AV, Jones DW, Roccella EJ. Seventh report of the Joint National Committee on the Prevention, Detection, Evaluation, and Treatment of High Blood Pressure (JNC 7): Resetting the hypertension sails. *Hypertension.* 2003;41(6):1178–1179.

34

Societal Issues in Multiple Sclerosis

DEBORAH MILLER

KEY POINTS FOR CLINICIANS

- Multiple sclerosis (MS) is often associated with loss of employment.

- Reasons for loss of employment include MS-related symptoms and functional limitations, as well as demographical and environmental factors.

- A multidisciplinary team is needed to help patients maintain or gain employment.

- Social workers are important members of this team as they specialize in helping to connect patients with appropriate resources, whether they seek to maintain employment or become unable to work.

- Issues related to various types of insurance (health, disability, long-term care, and life insurance) must be discussed with MS patients, in order to minimize as much as possible the financial impact of the disease, and to help protect their access to appropriate care.

Multiple sclerosis (MS) is a disease that is typically diagnosed when individuals are between 20 and 40 years of age. It affects physical, cognitive, emotional, and social well-being. One of the most common aspects of social functioning that can be affected is working [1]. Many young to middle aged adults define themselves in terms of the work they do. It provides self-definition, structure to daily life, social interaction, and a means of financial independence for now and the future [2]. Importantly, for persons with a chronic disease including MS, working is a primary source of health, disability, and long-term care insurance. It is well established that persons with MS can be compromised in their ability to work, and the emotional, financial, and social cascade of consequences from loss of work can be devastating. To date, there has been no systematic assessment of the relationship between the use of disease-modifying therapies and job retention.

For all of these reasons, it is essential for MS care specialists to consider with their patients on a regular basis, from the time of diagnosis, how MS is affecting their work lives. It is not expected that health care providers will actively help patients to navigate the complex laws and institutions that are intended to help persons with disabilities maintain employment and manage the consequences of loss of work. However, clinicians do need to understand the factors that influence their patients' ability to work, and be knowledgeable about available resources that can help maintain employment and build a financial safety net, if and when the time comes when employment is no longer feasible.

A key resource within the medical team for addressing these issues is the health social worker. Social workers in health care settings provide a formal psychosocial evaluation of patients and, when indicated, their family members. They will provide essential support by engaging the patient

TABLE 34.1
Factors Associated With Labor Force Participation

FACTOR	COMMENTS
Gender	In general, women have higher rates of unemployment and MS is more common in women
Socioeconomic status	Persons with higher education and less physical work are more likely to remain employed
Age	Generally, older individuals are more likely to be unemployed compared to their younger counterparts, most likely because of the association of increased disability and time since diagnosis
Physiological symptoms	Several reports indicate that exacerbations and symptom severity, especially fatigue, are associated with work discontinuation
Disease course and progression	More aggressive forms of MS and persistence of symptoms make work continuation difficult
Cognitive dysfunction	Perceived cognitive dysfunction is a major predictor of unemployment
Psychological and emotional factors	Research indicates that persons with MS do not commonly attribute loss of work to these symptoms
Variability of symptoms and "invisible disability"	Many of the symptoms of MS are not obvious, yet are disruptive to job performance (eg, fatigue, paresthesias, bladder dysfunction). In addition, the severity of symptoms fluctuates over time
Workplace discrimination	Many individuals worry about the impact of diagnosis disclosure on how they are perceived and treated. While many persons with MS leave the workforce voluntarily, they often report that the departure is the result of both subtle and explicit discrimination by supervisors and coworkers

Source: Adapted from [1].

and family through counseling, advocacy, practical support, and linkages with important community resources. These interventions remove barriers to care, and help patients and family manage distress and successfully negotiate the complex systems that they will have to engage.

Data regarding high unemployment rates for persons with MS is an indication of why this topic is so important. It has been reported that at least 90% of Americans with MS had some work experience at some point [1]; approximately 60% were employed at diagnosis [3], but that only 20% to 30% were employed 15 years beyond diagnosis [4–6]. Rumrill and Nissen note that there are many demographical and environmental factors that affect employment (Table 34.1) [1]. This emphasizes the importance of building a multidisciplinary team, including physicians, advanced practice clinicians, nurses, physical therapists, occupational therapists, social workers, behavioral health psychologists, neuropsychologists, and vocational counselors to help patients maintain employment.

As gaining or maintaining employment is included in the treatment plan, there are several issues that need to be addressed with patients, including issues of disclosing the diagnosis to employers, knowing what resources are available to help gain or maintain employment, and which insurance-related questions they should be asking.

DISCLOSING THE DIAGNOSIS

Persons with MS may be ambivalent about disclosing their diagnosis to an existing or potential employer for fear of losing their job or not being accepted for a position, whether that individual is already employed or seeking a new position. Let us first consider the guidance one might give individuals who are applying for a position with a new company. There is no legal requirement to disclose a chronic condition, or specifics

about it, during the early phases of the interview process. However, as potential employee and employer are in the "post offer" negotiation phases of hiring, potential employers have the right to ask about medical conditions and the potential employee must provide accurate information that is "job-related and consistent with business necessity." Given the subtleties of the different phases of job negotiation, it is important for patients to have an opportunity to discuss with a member of the clinical team how their MS may influence their prospective job responsibilities. For employed individuals who are experiencing MS symptoms that influence their current ability to perform key aspects of their job, it is important to discuss these symptoms and the accommodations that can help lessen their impact with their supervisors. In preparation for this discussion, it is useful to have members of the rehabilitative team assess what accommodations to recommend and to provide documentation of those recommendations. Because there are so many variables that are unique to each work site, it is recommended that each patient develop an appropriate disclosure plan with a social worker, psychologist, or vocational counselor. A list of MS organizations and online resources is provided at the end of this chapter.

GAINING AND MAINTAINING EMPLOYMENT

Vocational Rehabilitation Services

In the United States, there are multiple agencies and legal statutes intended to help individuals with disabilities gain or maintain employment, and to help prevent workplace discrimination. The Rehabilitation Services Administration is a federally mandated agency authorized, in part, to carry out Title V of the Rehabilitation Act of 1973. Their mission is to provide leadership and resources to assist state and other agencies in providing vocational rehabilitation (VR) and other services to individuals with disabilities to maximize their employment, independence, and integration into the community and competitive labor markets [7]. These federally funded services are administered by individual State Vocational Rehabilitation Agencies that are mandated to prioritize services to the most seriously disabled. In addition to these mandated VR agencies, there is a wealth of private and not-for-profit agencies that provide similar services to individuals with disability. Regardless of where they are located, vocational counselors' responsibilities typically include:

- Vocational evaluation to assess interests, abilities, and needed accommodations
- Career counseling
- Training and education
- Development of job-seeking skills
- Assistance with job placement.

There is evidence from at least 1 randomized controlled trial of the effectiveness of individualized rehabilitation programs for persons with MS [8]. However, a comprehensive *Cochrane Review* reveals that there has been little high quality research about the effectiveness of these programs and additional research is recommended [9]. Rumrill and Nissen describe several MS-specific VR programs that are available through Kent State University and the National Multiple Sclerosis Society [1].

Federal Laws That Protect Persons With Disabilities in the Workplace

Important among the legal statutes that protect persons with MS in the workplace are the Americans with Disabilities Act (ADA), which is enforced by the Equal Opportunity Employment Commission, and the Family Medical Leave Act, which is enforced by the Department of Labor. The ADA of 1990 and the ADA Amendments Act of 2008 give civil rights protections to persons with disability in regard to employment, transportation, public accommodations, public services, and telecommunications. Title I of this act addresses employment issues and provides a definition of disability. Under this law, a "qualified individual with disabilities" is an individual who "meets legitimate skill, experience, education, or other requirements of an employment position that s/he holds or seeks, and who can perform the essential functions of the position with or without reasonable accommodation. Requiring the ability to perform 'essential' functions assures that an individual with a disability will not be considered unqualified simply because of inability to perform marginal or incidental job functions" [10]. The law relates to individuals who work for private employers who have 15 or more employees as well as federal and state agencies, employment agencies, and unions. A key interpretation of this law is defining reasonable accommodations that include modifications to the job or work environment, but do not modify the essential functions of the job [11].

The Equal Employment Opportunity Commission (EEOC) is the federal agency that enforces laws prohibiting employment discrimination including Title I of ADA.

A person who believes he or she has been discriminated against generally has 180 days to file a complaint. EEOC becomes involved when a person who believes he or she has been discriminated against files charges either in person, by telephone, or by mail. Once the complaint is received, the EEOC will inform the employer of the complaint and then several different courses of action may occur. It is typical that the EEOC recommends mediation which it helps conduct. If mediation is declined or unsuccessful, the EEOC will investigate the claim in more detail and if it finds merit in the claim, is able to bring suit on behalf of the claimant. If they do not find grounds for discrimination, the claimant may file his own law suit with a private lawyer. Neath and colleagues [12] examined EEOC data regarding 1,028 persons with MS who filed charges with that agency during the period 1992 to 2003. The majority of the "charging parties" (those filing complaints) were women ($n = 687$, 67%) and white ($n = 769$, 76%). The most common allegations made by charging parties with MS included discharge, reasonable accommodation, terms and conditions of employment, and harassment, and two-thirds of those reporting to the EEOC made more than 1 charge at a time. The authors conclude that these are key issues for clinicians to address with their patients so as to position them to be proactive in addressing them.

Another important law is the Family and Medical Leave Act (FMLA) of 1993, a federal law that requires covered employers to provide eligible, covered employees with up to 12 weeks of absence from work that are job-protected and unpaid, and the employee's group health benefits must remain active during the leave. This law is administered by the Employment Standards Administration's Wage and Hour Division of the US Department of Labor. The types of conditions that are covered under this law are less restrictive than those covered by the ADA and include:

1. Birth or placement for foster care or adoption if a child of the employee
2. Care of a spouse, child, or parent who has a serious health problem which may be temporary or permanent
3. Care of an employee's own health problems
4. Specific situation related to the call to active duty of an immediate family member.

This law has important implications for working families living with MS as it allows a person with MS to take FMLA during a worsening of the disease or an extended medical treatment, and also covers employees who need to be away from work in order to care for their immediate family member who has MS. This leave may be taken in 1 block or intermittently over a 12 month period.

Employers who come under the FMLA provision include:

1. Those who participate in the public sector, who engage in commerce or industry affecting commerce and have 50 or more employees each working day during, at minimum, the previous 20 calendar weeks
2. All public agency and education employers regardless of the number of employees.

Employees covered by the FMLA must

1. be employed by a covered employer and work within 75 miles of a worksite that employs at least 50 people,
2. have worked at least 12 months, even if nonconsecutive, for the employer, and
3. worked at least 1,250 hours for the employer before the FMLA begins.

It is likely that a family member living with MS will request documentation from his or her treating physician of the serious medical condition they experience.

INSURANCE

Types of Insurance

There are several types of insurance that are important for patients with MS and their families to have, and it is useful for the clinicians to be familiar with these types of insurance because their terms of coverage will significantly influence the ability to carry out treatment plans for individual patients. The primary types of insurance include health, disability, long-term care, and life. Clinicians should encourage their patients to understand how to obtain, maintain, and afford these insurances and to be familiar with the exact terms of each type of policy. Health insurance covers some portion of the cost of medical and surgical care and may include coverage for prescription, vision, and dental costs as well as durable medical equipment. Disability insurance provides a source of income for individuals who become unable to perform gainful activity. The definition of disability as well as the duration and amount that is paid is highly variable. Long-term care (LTC) insurance covers many of the costs of an extended illness, including help with activities of daily living that are not covered by health insurance. Life insurance provides cash benefits to a named beneficiary (usually a spouse or other family member) in the event of the insured's death. This type of insurance assures a source of income to the beneficiary when the insured is no longer able to provide that support. It is available only if privately purchased.

Health Insurance
Obtaining and maintaining health insurance is a major concern for anyone diagnosed with a chronic illness, including MS, regardless of how minimal their disability. Access to health insurance for individuals with chronic illness has improved greatly with the passage of, and recent Supreme Court decision upholding the Patient Protection and Affordable Care Act (ACA) of 2010. This is a very complex law; as it moves to full enactment in 2020, it will assure that, among its many other provisions, persons with chronic illness cannot be denied health insurance because of a preexisting illness, have insurance coverage withdrawn, or premiums unreasonably increased. Until the ACA is fully enacted, there are 2 existing laws that provide means, although expensive, to continue coverage if a person loses employer-based insurance. The Consolidated Omnibus Budget Reconciliation Act of 1985 (COBRA) offers qualified individuals who lose employment-based group insurance to pay the full cost of the group rate plus an administrative fee for a specified period of time. The Health Insurance and Portability and Accountability Act (HIPAA), among its other provisions, provides protection for individuals participating in group health plans that limit exclusions for preexisting conditions, and provides for individual coverage if no group plan is available, or COBRA has been exhausted. While there are many governmental insurance plans for disabled civilians, federal employees, members of the armed forces, and veterans, we will limit our discussion to the 2 programs for disabled civilians, Medicare and Medicaid. Medicare is typically thought of as the federal government's insurance program for the elderly but it also is the insurance offered to younger age individuals 24 months after they have been determined eligible for Social Security Disability. It is important to understand that this insurance covers many aspects of health care but not all expenses or the cost of long-term care. Medicaid is the federally funded and state-administered medical assistance program for individuals and families with very limited assets and is made available to individuals who receive Supplemental Security Income (see subsequent paragraphs). In addition to providing comprehensive medical and hospital care, unlike Medicare, Medicaid also provides access to long-term care. As this is a state-administered program, the extent of Medicaid coverage varies from state to state. A more exhaustive discussion of the health insurance and related laws can be found elsewhere [13].

Disability Insurance
This insurance is intended to replace wage income for individuals who are disabled. There are private policies that are available through employers or private purchase, and these policies are highly variable in terms of cost and coverage and how long the individual must be unable to work before becoming eligible for the benefit. It is very important to encourage patients to become familiar with the existence and extent of any private disability policy because, if they become totally and permanently disabled under the terms of the Social Security Administration (SSA), this may be their only source of personal income until an SSA determination is made. The SSA administers 2 types of income assistance: Social Security Disability Insurance (SSDI), which is based on prior work history, and Supplemental Security Income (SSI) which is based on significant financial need. Medical determination of eligibility for both of these programs is on the basis of federal criteria that a person is totally and permanently disabled from any type of gainful employment. The criteria for MS are outlined in Table 34.2. Clinicians are involved in the application process by filling out forms and writing letters to demonstrate how the patient's specific symptoms and impairments caused by MS fit these criteria. Although no specific tests are required, obtaining neuropsychological testing or a functional capacity evaluation can help further document cognitive and physical limitations [14].

In order to receive SSDI a person must have earned this insurance by working and paying Federal Social

TABLE 34.2
Social Security Administration Guidelines Pertaining to the Diagnosis of MS

1. "Significant and persistent disorganization of motor function in two extremities, resulting in sustained disturbance of gross and dexterous movements or gait and station. This can be due to MS-related causes, either individually or in combination, of such dysfunction: paresis or paralysis, tremor or other involuntary movements, and caused by cerebral, cerebellar, brainstem, spinal cord or peripheral nerve dysfunction."
2. "Visual impairments with either best corrected vision in the better eye of 20/200 or less, marked contraction of peripheral visual fields to 10 or less from the point of fixation, or visual efficiency in the better eye of 20% or less."
3. "Significant, reproducible fatigue of motor function with substantial motor weakness on repetitive activity, demonstrated on physical examination, resulting from neurological dysfunction in areas of the central nervous system known to be pathologically involved by multiple sclerosis."
4. "Mental Impairment. At least one of the following must be medically documented:

  • Disorientation to time and place
  • Memory impairment (short, immediate or long-term)
  • Perceptual or thinking disturbances
  • Change in personality
  • Disturbance of mood
  • Emotional lability
  • Loss of measured intellectual ability of at least 15 IQ points that results in at least two of the following:
    • Marked restriction in activities in daily living
    • Marked difficulties in maintaining social functioning
    • Marked difficulties in maintaining concentrating, persistence or pace
    • Repeated episodes of decompensation."

Source: [14].

Security Taxes (FICA) for a certain period of time. The work credit requirements are based on the amount earned per year. The criteria for earning credits change from year to year and are dependent on the age of the disabled worker, but generally an individual needs 40 credits, 20 of which were earned in the past 10 years. In addition to the work credit requirements a person will not be eligible to be determined disabled until they have not been "gainfully employed" for 5 months. It typically takes several months to receive a SSDI determination once one becomes not gainfully employed. Given the potential delay between loss of gainful employment and completion of the determination process, the significance of having a private disability policy, if at all possible, becomes clear. There is no similar work credit contributions or wait period to be eligible for SSI but the financial criteria for household income are stringent.

Long-Term Care Insurance
This insurance is intended to cover the medical, social, and personal care services that can be essential for persons living with a chronic progressive disease like MS but are not included in traditional health insurance. The only way that most individuals can access LTC insurance is through the purchase of a private policy through an employer or privately. The younger in life this type of policy is purchased, the less expensive it is. It has proven difficult for persons diagnosed with chronic diseases to purchase such a policy but it may be an important consideration for family members who may have similar needs in the future. For those who are financially indigent and meet criteria for Medicaid, this is a source of LTC insurance.

Life Insurance
There is no federal program that offers this type of coverage; it is available only through private purchase. If patients are exploring this option, it is important for them to work with an independent insurance broker who is aware of their diagnosis and can negotiate with many different insurance providers.

Sources of Insurance

Most individuals in the United States have access to these insurances as group policies through their or a family member's employer. As previously suggested, access to these benefits through work is an important reason to remain employed as long as one is able. If a person becomes unemployed or their employer does not offer these types of coverage, there are often options for continuing health, disability, LTC, or life insurance on a private pay basis but that can prove to be very expensive. For eligible individuals there are federal and state programs that provide for health (Medicare and Medicaid), disability (Social Security Disability and Supplemental Security Income), and LTC (Medicaid).

CONCLUSION

This chapter is intended to be an overview of the work and insurance issues MS patients face. Expertise in this area is not typical of most health care professionals providing MS care. Therefore it is very important to encourage patients to include social workers, lawyers, and financial planners as members of their care team.

KEY MS ORGANIZATIONS RESOURCES FOR CLINICIANS AND FAMILIES REGARDING WORK, INSURANCE, AND DISABILITY ISSUES

Consortium of Multiple Sclerosis Centers (http://www.mscare.org/)
Multiple Sclerosis Association of America (www.msaa.com)
National Multiple Sclerosis Society (www.nationalmssociety.org/index.aspx)

KEY WEB RESOURCES

www.medicaid.gov/Medicaid-CHIP-Program-Information/By-Topics/Eligibility/Eligibility.html
www.nationalmssociety.org/living-with-multiple-sclerosis/employment/knowing-your-rights/index.aspx
www.dol.gov/ebsa/healthreform
www.dol.gov/dol/topic/health-plans/portability.htm
www.dol.gov/ebsa/cobra.html
www.dol.gov/whd/regs/compliance/whdfs28.htm
www.eeoc.gov
www.ssa.gov/pgm/disability.htm
www.ssa.gov/pgm/medicare.htm
www.supremecourt.gov/opinions/11pdf/11-393c3a2.pdf

REFERENCES

1. Rumrill PD, Nissen SW. Employment and career development considerations. In: Giesser BS, ed. *Primer on Multiple Sclerosis.* New York: Oxford; 2011;401–418.

2. Johnson KL, Yorkston KM, Klasner ER, et al. The cost and benefits of employment: A qualitative study of experiences of persons with multiple sclerosis. *Arch Phys Med Rehabil.* 2004;85:201–209.

3. LaRocca NG. *Employment and Multiple Sclerosis. Report.* New York: National Multiple Sclerosis Society; 1995.

4. Fraser R, Clemmons D, Bennet F. *Multiple Sclerosis: Psychosocial and Vocational Interventions.* New York: Demos Medical; 2002.

5. Johnson KL, Fraser RT. Mitigating the impact of multiple sclerosis on employment. *Phys Med Rehabil Clin N Am.* 2005;16: x–xi, 571–582.

6. Roessler RT, Rumrill PD Jr. Multiple sclerosis and employment barriers: A systemic perspective on diagnosis and intervention. *Work.* 2003;21:17–23.

7. Government U. Available at: http://rsa.ed.gov/. Accessed June 22, 2012.

8. Khan F, Pallant JF, Brand C, et al. Effectiveness of rehabilitation intervention in persons with multiple sclerosis: A randomised controlled trial. *J Neurol Neurosurg Psychiatry.* 2008;79: 1230–1235.

9. Khan F, Ng L, Turner-Stokes L. Effectiveness of vocational rehabilitation intervention on the return to work and employment of persons with multiple sclerosis. *Cochrane Database of Syst Rev.* 2009;CD007256.

10. Government U. Available at: www.ada.gov/q%26aeng02.htm. Accessed June 22, 2012.

11. Government U. Available at: www.ada.gov/publicat.htm#Anchor-ADA-44867. Accessed accessed June 22, 2012.

12. Neath J, Roessler RT, McMahon BT, et al. Patterns in perceived employment discrimination for adults with multiple sclerosis. *Work.* 2007;29:255–274.

13. Calder K. Managing the insurance maze. In: Kalb R, ed. *Multiple Sclerosis: The Questions You Have, the Answers You Need.* New York: Demos; 2012:317–333.

14. Sutliff MH, Miller DM, Forwell S. Developing a functional capactiy evalution specific to multiple sclerosis. *Int J MS Care.* 2012;14:17–27.

35

Patient-Oriented Comprehensive Care in Multiple Sclerosis

MARGARET HENNING

SNEHA RAMESH

Over the past few decades, the focus of medical care has shifted from treatment of a disease to treatment of a patient's health and well-being. Effective treatment approaches for many chronic diseases such as diabetes, heart disease, Alzheimer's disease, and multiple sclerosis (MS) now encompass treatment of not just the disease, but also associated symptoms, changes in daily activities, and lifestyle choices.

Few diseases need comprehensive care more than MS [1]. MS is a chronic, incurable disease affecting the brain, spinal cord, and optic nerves. Often starting as an episodic disease with periods of clinical stability, after 10 to 25 years it often transitions into a gradually progressive disorder. All neurological functions can be affected by MS, including cognition, mood, vision, sensation, motor, coordination, sphincter, and sexual function. In the later stages of the disease, progressive impairment can lead to inability to walk or even independent performance of self-care activities. All spheres of life can be affected, including social, professional, and family life. As a result, a large number of health professionals with requisite skills may provide services to patients with MS at various times over the course of the disease [2]. The benefits of these varied services can be tremendous, but also present a challenge for coordination. This chapter focuses on the comprehensive care needed by MS patients and how that care can be delivered in a coordinated fashion.

COMPREHENSIVE CARE

The concept of "comprehensive care" encompasses a wide scope of care activities and is defined by the American Academy of Family Physicians as "the concurrent prevention and management of multiple physical and emotional health problems of a patient over a period of time in relationship to family, life events and environment" [3]. A medical dictionary definition of comprehensive care, also called holistic health care, is "a system of comprehensive or total patient care that considers the physical, emotional, social, economic, and spiritual needs of the person; his or her response to illness; and the effect of the illness on the ability to meet self-care needs" [4]. The needs of individual persons are diverse and with a chronic disease like MS, those needs typically change with disease evolution. A key feature of comprehensive care is tailoring the appropriate care to the needs of the individual person to help manage his or her disease most effectively with minimal suffering (Table 35.1) [2,5].

An important element of comprehensive care is its focus on patient empowerment and wellness [6,7]. The patient is encouraged to be an active participant and is guided with proper resources in a logical, consistent, and efficient manner for the overall treatment and management of the disease [8]. Another important element of comprehensive care is the need for collaborative efforts of multiple health care providers from numerous disciplines [9]. With MS, worsening of disease symptoms may be a result of natural disease progression or may also be triggered by a variety of circumstances, which include changes in comorbid conditions, social changes, including work and family, and emotional changes. Hence, it is essential to discern the causative issue for proper symptom management. A health care system consisting of multiple providers with specialized expertise is better positioned to identify such causative issues, which may go underappreciated and incompletely managed in a care system that relies on a single provider.

Consulting with multiple providers necessitates a structure to ensure proper coordination of appointments and communication between providers, without which there may be fragmented care with duplicated efforts. From a patient's perspective, it can be challenging to follow

TABLE 35.1
The Multiple Sclerosis Comprehensive Care Center

- Patient-focused model with emphasis on self-empowerment and individualized medical services
- Provides a collaborative effort of different care providers to holistically manage the care of a patient with MS through the evolution of the disease
- Offers accessibility to a multitude of disciplines in 1 location that allows for convenience, enhanced communication between providers, and sensitivity for specific needs of patients with MS
- Works to maximize functional ability, coping skills, and symptom control, while minimizing secondary and tertiary complications and symptoms

TABLE 35.2
Potential Barriers to Comprehensive MS Care Centers

- Space limitations
- Provider availability
- Communication among providers
- Traditional health care model, where providers are organized by pedigree specialty rather than disease or service line
- Local patient population may not be sufficient to support a multispecialty MS center
- Payor coverage

complex care plans from different providers. This challenge may be especially difficult for newly diagnosed patients who are frightened by the unpredictable and disabling nature of MS, confused by advice from multiple providers, and overwhelmed with the immense amount of information available about the disease. Recommendations regarding lifestyle adjustments may be met with anger, reluctance, and resistance to change. Providers need to be cognizant of these challenges and nudge uncommitted patients to follow suggestions that are likely to improve their overall health, disease status, and quality of life. It is sometimes beneficial to provide a descriptive guide of symptoms, associated issues, and available treatment options that may arise during the disease course continuum to ensure a smooth navigation through the variable and unpredictable course of disease.

A popular process of delivering comprehensive care is to provide as much of the acute, chronic, preventive, and rehabilitative services within the same facility [8]. Comprehensive MS centers typically offer a variety of care providers, which can include neurologists, advanced practice clinicians (ie, nurse practitioners and physical assistants), physiatrists (specializing in MS rehabilitation), health psychologists, psychiatrists, neuropsychologists, social workers, and occupational and physical therapists. Some also offer onsite MRI, laboratory, and other diagnostic testing facilities, infusion or treatment facilities, as well as educational opportunities and financial counseling [8,10]. Smaller practices (including individual practitioners) may be more practical in urban areas with space constraints in rural areas (Table 35.2). In these smaller practices, MS patients are likely to be referred to other providers to obtain the various requisite services needed by the individual patient. A common complaint from MS patients is the fragmented care that can sometimes arise when services are provided by individual providers or multiple providers with limited interconnection and communication. Intuitively, such disjointed care may occur in individual practices with limited communication with allied care providers, but may also occur in large health care systems that lack effective communication between providers or timely access to care. An open channel of communication that permits constant exchange of information between providers is vital for comprehensive care to succeed [11]. Comprehensive care

can be provided effectively at either a comprehensive care center or at an individual practice if a system (a) is organized to allow timely exchange of information and data between providers, (b) is conveniently located and accessible for the patient, (c) offers access to a wide variety of services, and (d) accommodates appointments as needed by the patient.

Benefits

There are several benefits to comprehensive care received through a multispecialty center. The most obvious benefit is the ease of access to a group of related services at the patient's convenience [12]. An often overlooked secondary benefit of a comprehensive care facility is caregiver support. The waves of setbacks common in MS can be devastating and emotionally draining for both the patient and the support persons (family, significant others, home health caregivers) [13]. During an office appointment, support persons can also be evaluated and if required, receive a referral to a social worker or psychologist who specializes in chronic disease management. Such collaborative care can be immensely beneficial to providers as well. Timely communication between providers from different disciplines allows better insight into a patient's disease status, emotional and social well-being, and enables providers to offer a selection of services that is pertinent to that patient. For instance, an advanced practice clinician could direct an MS patient with walking limitations to a physical therapist familiar with MS, and furnish information pertaining to the patient's disease progression and likely needs in the future. The physical therapist would therefore be able to recommend suitable strategies to cope with the recent walking limitations as well as exercises to minimize the effects of future impending disabilities.

CONTRIBUTORS TO COMPREHENSIVE CARE

The most important members of the comprehensive care team are the patient and the patient's support person(s) (Table 35.3). It is vital for a patient to be actively involved in all treatment decision-making processes as it is crucial to choose a plan of care to which a patient is willing to adhere. Input from the support person is important to gain an

TABLE 35.3
Comprehensive Care Center Team

- **Patient**
  - Family
  - Spouse or significant other
- **Core care team**
  - Neurologists
  - Advanced practice clinicians (nurse practitioners and clinical nurse specialists and physician assistants)
- **Rehabilitation experts**
  - Physiatrists
  - Physical therapists
  - Occupational therapists
  - Speech therapists
- **Mental health experts**
  - Psychiatrists
  - Health psychologists
- **Adjunctive care**
  - Licensed social workers
  - Financial counselors
  - Medical secretaries
- **Testing and diagnostic**
  - Phlebotomists
  - Neuroradiologists/MRI technicians
  - Researchers
- **Infusion center**
  - Nurses
  - Medical assistants

insight into the patient's characteristics and the likelihood of adherence to the plan of care. Support person(s) may often be required to administer medications, assist with daily activities, and provide emotional and financial support to the MS patient; thus their involvement in MS educational sessions and treatment decisions would be critical.

Neurologists and advanced practice clinicians (APCs) serve as the primary contact for an MS patient and are responsible for both MS disease management and symptom control. Spasticity is a common symptom in MS patients and can be one of the more severe symptoms that affect daily life. Physiatrists specializing in the management of spasticity play an important role in the overall MS symptom management. Onsite infusion centers with a dedicated team of nurses administering MS medications are part of most comprehensive care centers. Physical and occupational therapists with expertise in MS issues help with use of appropriate assistive devices and suggest exercises and modifications in performing daily activities to manage functional limitations. The far-reaching physical effects of MS may require services such as neuroophthalmology, urology, gastroenterology, otolaryngology, and a host of other specialties. These particular specialties often require specialized equipment and facilities, thus are not typically located within a comprehensive care facility. Uncertainty about future disability and the entailing effects on patients and their support persons can be particularly challenging. Mental health professionals, such as psychiatrists, psychologists, and counselors are also integral members

of the care team, as their expertise may be essential for some MS patients and their support person(s) to cope with the effects of MS. Services of social workers may also be required to assist some MS patients with daily needs, such as housing, finances, insurance, transportation, and community resources. Involvement of a diverse team of experts for disease management results in a net increase in time spent to understand the patient's disease within the framework of their socioeconomic status which, in turn, lends itself to better disease management and a reduction in possible errors [5]. Often, the services provided by individual providers overlap but the expertise of each is required.

Roles—Primary MS Care Clinicians

A popular delivery method of comprehensive care is to provide most of the necessary services at one outpatient center (Table 35.4). Neurologists and APCs form the core clinical team for MS disease management at many MS centers. Most patients who visit an MS comprehensive care center are either referred for a second opinion or seek assistance in choosing appropriate treatment. Initial consults are typically performed by a neurologist who confirms or refutes an MS diagnosis, or sometimes recommends further testing before a clear diagnosis is made [10,12,14].

APCs include nurse practitioners, clinical nurse specialists, and physician assistants. These clinicians typically hold a masters or doctorate degree in their field and are trained in clinical practice and sometimes research [9,15,16]. Studies have shown that patient outcomes, patient satisfaction, and level of services provided by APCs are of high quality and typically equal that of their physician counterparts [16–19]. Many comprehensive care centers now approach patient visits in a collaborative manner where the roles of the APCs and neurologists have been clearly delineated for effective operations and cost utility.

Routine or urgent office visits typically take 20 to 45 minutes and involve reviewing medical history, medications, treatment adherence, discussing the patient's current disease status and other health issues, and offering suggestions to resolve their concerns. The APC meets with the neurologist to review results from recent diagnostic tests and discuss the patient's disease status and treatment, and if required, the neurologist may also briefly visit the patient to confirm or clarify the evaluation and discuss treatment recommendations. Such a delegation of roles where the APCs carry out most of the routine office visits allows neurologists to reserve their time and expertise to evaluate new patients, yet remain involved in the ongoing care of established patients. Occasionally, patients may feel intimidated or awkward mentioning symptoms or asking certain questions to the neurologist but will feel more at ease confiding their concerns in the APC. Such candid discussions can allow a more accurate evaluation of issues such as treatment adherence, attitudes toward MS, and self-efficacy.

Since APCs frequently triage phone calls and decide upon an action plan to address patient symptoms, medications, or exacerbations, they have more frequent contact with the patient than the physician, which ultimately has a

TABLE 35.4
Patient-Oriented Care in a Comprehensive Care Center

- **General patient care and disease monitoring**
  - Neurologists
    - Initial consult, diagnosis
    - Overseeing disease management
    - Research
    - Education
    - Refills, letters, orders, prior authorizations
  - Advanced practice clinicians
    - Day-to-day management of symptoms
    - Telephone triage
    - Education
    - Procedures: bladder scans, lumbar punctures
    - Refills, letters, orders, prior authorizations
- **Rehabilitation**
  - Rehabilitation consultations
  - Spasticity clinic
    - Medication management
    - Botulinum toxin injections
    - Intrathecal baclofen pump evaluation and management
  - Physical therapy
    - Strengthening, gait training
    - Stretching exercises
    - Evaluation for orthotics, ambulation devices, and wheelchairs
    - Balance, vestibular therapy
    - Aquatherapy
    - Pelvic floor therapy
    - Functional capacity evaluation
  - Occupational therapy
    - Hand, arm strength, and function
    - Truncal stability
    - ADL training
    - Fatigue management (energy conservation strategies)
    - Memory, cognitive training
    - Wheelchair evaluations
    - Driver rehabilitation
  - Speech
    - Dysphagia evaluations and therapy
    - Language, speech, voice therapy
- **Mental health**
  - Psychiatry
    - Initial evaluation for diagnosis
    - Medication management
  - Psychology
    - Adjustment, coping issues
      - Biofeedback, stress reduction
      - Cognitive behavior therapy
    - Family, marital, relationship issues
    - Socialization issues
      - Group therapies
      - Referrals to local resources
    - Chronic pain management
    - NPE
- **Social work**
  - Community resources
  - Financial, housing assistance
  - Assistance with transportation
  - Assistance with medical insurance issues
  - Assistance with benefits (SSI, disability)
  - Contact with charity organizations
  - Assistance with forms: advanced directives, living will, power of attorney

- **Testing and diagnostic facilities**
  - Lab
  - MRI
  - OCT
- **Infusion center**
  - Scheduled and urgent infusions
  - Phlebotomy support
  - Administers medication and monitors MRI sedation patients
- **Additional resources**
  - Primary care physician
    - General health maintenance
  - Gastroenterologists
    - Management of constipation, bowel issues
  - Metabolic bone/orthopedic specialist
    - Bone mineral density testing
    - Management of medications for osteopenia, osteoporosis
    - Management of other musculoskeletal issues
  - Neuroophthalmologists
    - OCT Testing (increasingly utilized within an MS center)
    - Monitoring optic nerve
    - Management of eye health, disease
  - Otolaryngologists
    - Vestibular testing and management
  - Pain management
    - Chronic pain management
  - Sleep medicine
    - Polysomnograms
    - CPAP management
  - Urologists
    - Neurogenic bladder management
    - Urodynamic testing
    - Detrusor botulinum toxin injections
    - Sacral root stimulator
    - Catheters (indwelling, suprapubic, intermittent straight-catheterization)

ADL, activities of daily living; CPAP, continuous positive airway pressure; NPE, neuropsychological evaluation; OCT, optical coherence tomography; SSI, Supplemental Security Income.

positive impact on successful future appointments. These telephone calls also provide additional opportunities for education, such as the common increase in symptoms around the change of seasons (particularly hot weather), and times when people tend to be physically or emotionally stressed (such as holidays).

Roles—Educators

The goal of self-empowerment can only be met by arming the patient and support persons with information [20,21]. Education is essential if patients are expected to make rational, decisive, well-informed decisions regarding treatment and realistic plans for the future. Many patients newly diagnosed with MS have predictably strong emotional reactions to their diagnosis and may not be able to comprehend details of disease information and instructions regarding their medications [22]. Separate, individual education can benefit both patients and their support persons. The focus at such educational sessions should be on the unique challenges faced by MS patients. Symptom management, disease progression and future disability, family and financial planning, and concerns about the ability to continue working, are important topics to cover. All members of the comprehensive MS center are instrumental in educating the patient, the family or support system, the community and other health care professionals on MS-related issues.

Several of the current disease-modifying therapies (DMTs) involve parenteral administration and many pharmaceutical companies provide nurse liaisons who teach injection training in the patient's home. If required, the patient can attend a personalized training session in the office, preferably with a family member or other support person. A few treatments require IV infusions and registered nurses are responsible for running the day-to-day operations of an infusion center. Patients are routinely screened prior to each infusion and new symptoms, contraindications, and other issues requiring attention are reported to the physician or APC. Many of the patients utilizing infusions are seen many times per year (sometimes as often as every 4 weeks) and a relationship between the patient, support person, and nursing staff develop. This is an excellent opportunity to discuss the current treatment, reinforce education, and evaluate changes that may be too subtle for the patient or support person to recognize.

Nontraditional, experimental, and sometimes dangerous treatments purported to be beneficial for MS should be discussed frankly and in detail with the patient so they are well informed about the risks and reported benefits.

Roles—Restoration and Rehabilitation

An important goal of collaborative care is to maximize the functional ability of the patient. Common MS symptoms will often require referral to a group specializing in rehabilitation [23]. Various methods of rehabilitation may be employed depending on the specific issues faced by the patient and support person(s), including individualized exercises, activity modification, and assistive devices. Multidisciplinary rehabilitation teams generally work together focusing on the same issue from different perspectives. For example, an individual who experiences increased difficulty with ambulation will often be referred to physical therapy, but may also require a consult to a physiatrist to help control spasticity that directly affects ambulation. These patients also may benefit from working with occupational therapy because of the limited hand and arm strength required to operate a rollator.

Fatigue is a common MS symptom that can benefit from multidisciplinary management. Fatigue can be a crippling symptom, both in the acute form related to a specific event and in the chronic form that affects patients on a daily basis. Fatigue may be a primary symptom of MS or can be a secondary symptom of another condition such as anemia, thyroid disease, anxiety, or depression. While it is necessary to address the fatigue itself, it is essential that additional contributors to fatigue be investigated and treated [24]. MS

exacerbations, exposure to heat, or a temporary change in the patient's emotional or physical state are just a few of the factors that can contribute to a temporary worsening of fatigue. Some of these factors can be easily corrected in a timely manner. Chronic fatigue states require diagnostic and laboratory testing. Polysomnography can be helpful in detecting obstructive sleep apnea and restless leg syndrome, 2 common contributors to excessive daytime sleepiness and fatigue. Various anemias and deficiencies in vitamin D and thyroid hormones also have been implicated in chronic fatigue states. While these factors can be treated, they usually require a longer course of management. When no factors can be identified, fatigue is assumed to be a primary MS symptom and treatment with symptomatic medications, teaching of energy conservation techniques, and customized exercise programs, are commonly employed.

Roles—Resource Providers

A key feature of comprehensive care is to offer services tailored to meet the needs of the patient along the disease course continuum. Not all specialties can be provided at 1 center. Referrals to specialists in other disciplines such as sleep medicine, pain management, psychiatry, gastroenterology, hematology, and endocrinology are required as dictated by the needs and symptoms of the patient. Identification of clinical providers and centers that are familiar with the challenges that an MS patient experiences and are educated in MS within their particular area will improve the efficiency and effectiveness of referrals.

The persons supporting patients in their homes can have significant anxiety over the care of a disabled spouse, child, family member, or friend. Frustration with the cognitive impairment and resulting strains in interpersonal relationships may need to be addressed as well [13]. Issues that impact patients' lives during the disease course continuum can be identified and addressed by any member of the care team during office visits. Health psychologists and social workers can be very helpful in evaluating the interpersonal strains introduced by MS. While the Internet has become an important source to obtain information related to MS, it is increasingly important to direct patients to reliable Internet sources to obtain truthful and scientifically backed information. Too often, the information shared in blogs or chat rooms can be misleading and frightening for the patient and their support persons.

SUMMARY

MS is a chronic, lifelong disease that can have an impact on a wide number of bodily functions and life roles. The core of MS management arises from the neurologist and APCs directly familiar with the patient's individual disease manifestations and personal circumstances. Many other health care providers contribute with their particular expertise to MS disease and symptom management. Having many of these providers within the same clinical center can improve the speed of referral and the efficiency of care provision, and ultimately improve the quality of care provided to the patient. A network of additional health care providers working in collaboration with the MS center can provide the complement of care needed by MS patients. Patients, their families, and support persons are better served when the care that they receive is collaborative, well organized, easily accessible, and working toward the common goal of patient empowerment and optimal health.

REFERENCES

1. Halper J, Burks JS. Care patterns in multiple sclerosis. *Neuro Rehabil.* 1994;4:67–75.

2. Harris C, Costello K, Halper J, et al. Consortium of multiple sclerosis centers recommendations for care of those affected by multiple sclerosis. *Int J MS Care.* 2003;5:67–78.

3. Comprehensive Care, Definition of. 2012. (Accessed at www.aafp.org/online/en/home/policy/policies/c/comprehensive care2.html)

4. Holistic Health Care. 2012. (Accessed at http://medical-dictionary.thefreedictionary.com/holistic+health+care)

5. Wagner EH, Austin BT, Von Korff M. Organizing care for patients with chronic illness. *Milbank Q.* 1996;74:511–544.

6. Halper J, Holland N. Meeting the challenge of multiple sclerosis. Part II. *Am J Nurs.* 1998;98:39–45; quiz 6.

7. Halper J, Holland N. Meeting the challenge of multiple sclerosis. Part I. Treating the person and the disease. *Am J Nurs.* 1998;98:26–31; quiz 2.

8. Halper J. Comprehensive care in multiple sclerosis – A patient-centered approach. *Eur Neur Rev.* 2009;3:72–74.

9. Aiken LH. Achieving an interdisciplinary workforce in health care. *N Engl J Med.* 2003;348:164–166.

10. The Mellen Center for Multiple Sclerosis, Treatment and Research. Cleveland Clinic, 2012. (Accessed December 16 2012, at http://my.clevelandclinic.org/multiple_sclerosis_center/default.aspx)

11. Smith IJ, ed. *The Joint Commission Guide to Improving Staff Communication.* Oakbrook Terrace, IL: Joint Commission Resources; 2005.

12. Ahearn JP, Schwetz KM. Comprehensive supportive therapy in multiple-sclerosis. *Semin Neurol.* 1985;5:146–154.

13. DesRosier MB, Catanzaro M, Piller J. Living with chronic illness: Social support and the well spouse perspective. *Rehabil Nurs.* 1992;17:87–91.

14. Halper J. *Advanced Concepts in Multiple Sclerosis Nursing Care,* 2nd ed. New York, NY: Demos; 2007.

15. Cooper RA. Health care workforce for the twenty-first century: The impact of nonphysician clinicians. *Annu Rev Med.* 2001;52:51–61.

16. Teske AE. Advanced practice nurses in Ohio community hospitals. *J Nurse Pract.* 2012;8:129–135.

17. Mundinger MO, Kane RL. Health outcomes among patients treated by nurse practitioners or physicians. *JAMA.* 2000;283:2521–2524.

18. Mundinger MO, Kane RL, Lenz ER, et al. Primary care outcomes in patients treated by nurse practitioners or physicians: A randomized trial. *JAMA.* 2000;283:59–68.

19. Bernal EW. The nurse as patient advocate. *Hastings Cent Rep.* 1992;22:18–23.

20. Saunders C, Caon C, Smrtka J, Shoemaker J. Factors that influence adherence and strategies to maintain adherence to injected therapies for patients with multiple sclerosis. *J Neurosci Nurs.* 2010;42:S10–S18.

21. Heesen C, Solari A, Giordano A, et al. Decisions on multiple sclerosis immunotherapy: New treatment complexities urge patient engagement. *J Neurol Sci.* 2011;306:192–197.

22. Comprehensive Care in multiple sclerosis, white paper. 2010. (Accessed December 16, 2012, at www.mscare.org/cmsc/images/pdf/CMSC_WhitePaper_Comprehensive_Care_in_MS.pdf.)

23. Zwibel HL. Contribution of impaired mobility and general symptoms to the burden of multiple sclerosis. *Adv Ther.* 2009;26:1043–1057.

24. Schapiro RT, ed. *Managing the Symptoms of Multiple Sclerosis,* 5th ed. New York: Demos Medical Publishing; 2007.

36

Caregiving in Multiple Sclerosis

AMY BURLESON SULLIVAN

KEY POINTS FOR CLINICIANS

- Caregiving for a loved one with a chronic condition can often be profoundly fulfilling, as many times individuals move closer together when challenges arise.

- Caregiving can become overwhelming, physically and emotionally challenging, and isolating. At times it can be thought of as a burden.

- Caregivers must learn to take care of themselves physically and emotionally.

- The multidisciplinary care model used in the treatment of multiple sclerosis (MS) is important not only for the patient, but also for the caregiver. This care model allows for several practitioners to interact with the caregiver to assess and determine the optional interventions.

- Physical, emotional, and financial abuses secondary to the profound challenges inherent in caring for a relative with a disabling chronic illness are not uncommon. Assessing for abuse is an important component in the clinical management of MS.

Multiple sclerosis (MS) is an unpredictable and progressive neurological disease that most commonly starts in young adulthood [1]. The course of the disease is unpredictable, as is the duration. As the disease progresses, the often numerous and variable symptoms such as fatigue, impaired mobility and vision, bladder and bowel dysfunction, cognitive impairment and depression, can create a need for family members or others to provide care. This responsibility often falls on the partner/spouse or child. Because MS often affects young women, the caregiver, unlike that of caregivers of loved ones with Alzheimer's dementia, stroke, and so on, is often a young parent, with children at home, and who is in the early part of their career development. The long course and duration of MS frequently requires family members to play multiple roles: that of caregiver *and* of assuming the financial and household responsibilities. In most patients, MS does not shorten life span, and so a caregiver's role can encompass a lifetime. Caregiving can be deeply satisfying as partners and family members can be drawn closer together. However, as the demands increase for the person with MS, often less time is available to be devoted to the caregiver's own needs, the children's needs, the home care, or a career. Thus, caregivers often feel a significant demand and burden to their own endurance and coping mechanisms. Caregivers commonly report a plethora of their own physical and psychological symptoms. The aim of this chapter is to review common caregiver challenges and provide suggestions for how caregivers can more effectively care for themselves while maintaining their responsibility to the MS patient.

CAREGIVERS

A *caregiver*, by definition, is an individual who helps with physical and psychological care for a person in need [2]. As is the case for most caregivers, they are often family members (ie, spouse, partner, child, parent) and they are likely unpaid. Caregivers can be called upon to provide a wide variety of assistance with activities of daily living, including bathing, toileting, dressing, transferring, cooking, eating, medications, and managing the home. Demographically, 66% of family caregivers are women, and interestingly, 65% of care recipients are women. In addition, the typical caregiver spends no less than 20 hours per week in a caregiving role [3,4].

> A *caregiver* by definition is an individual who helps with physical and psychological care for a person in need.

Caregiving for a loved one with a chronic condition can be profoundly fulfilling, as individuals often move closer together when challenges arise. However, caregiving can also be daunting, physically and emotionally challenging, and isolating. At times, caregiving may be referred to as *caregiver burden*, which Buhse defines as "a multidimensional response to physical, psychological, emotional, social, and financial stressors associated with the caregiving experience" [5]. The challenges of caregiving are widespread and encompass much more than the care of the recipient, as will be noted here.

> Caregiving can be daunting, physically and emotionally challenging, and isolating.

Economically, many caregivers juggle both work and caregiving, as 58% are currently employed, and the majority of those are men. However, their median incomes are 15% lower than non-caregiving families. In addition, a caregiver is more than 2½ times as likely to live in poverty as non-caregivers; and the average family caregiver spends $5,531 per year on out of pocket expenses, which is 10% of their median family income [3,4].

Caregiving reaches far beyond economics, as it may also have an impact on a caregiver's health. The added stress inherent in caregiving may increase the stress hormone, which can lead to high blood pressure and glucose levels and also by weakening the immune system, making individuals more susceptible to infections [6]. This effect has been seen up to 3 years after the caregiving role has ended, thus putting the individual at an increased risk for chronic illness themselves [6]. Seventy-two percent of family caregivers report not taking care of their own health issues, and frequently forgo their own medical appointments [3,4]. In addition, they report poor eating, self-care, and less routine exercise. Not surprisingly, the extreme stress of caregiving leads to premature aging, and may decrease the caregiver's life expectancy by as much as 10 years [3,4]. Emotionally, caregivers may find themselves with significant depression and anxiety, due to not only the loss of their expectations for their family, but also due to social isolation, lack of support

from coworkers, or participation in previous hobbies or activities [5].

As above, family caregivers have several needs that warrant attention, but are often overlooked because of the care being focused on the MS patient [7]. The rest of the chapter focuses on caregiver issues and gives specific and tangible guidelines for caring not only for the MS patient, but also the caregiver.

STAGES OF CAREGIVING

The natural ebb and flow of life calls for taking care of infants and the elderly, but the care of an adult who suffers a chronic condition is usually unexpected [8]. The course of MS is generally unpredictable, as caregivers are unable to predict a relapse, progression of the disease, and sometimes even a patient's functional ability or emotional response throughout a day. Caregivers may become concerned with both the person with MS and with how the disease has an impact on the caregiver's own life [9].

Caregiving, especially in a disease with an unpredictable course, is a dynamic and ever-changing phenomenon. As each family member presents in the medical team's office, each individual, from the patient to individual family members, will have their own unique reaction to new roles and identity due to the chronic disease. While in the past, the family may have developed a certain identity and rhythm, the development of a disease challenges, and may even disrupt, the family identity. Often, the original family "caregiver" becomes the "caretaker," or the primary "bread winner" no longer holds that role. These new roles can present significant challenges to both individuals.

In many significant ways, a family benefits from progressing through the grieving process of the loss of role and identity and come to some form of acceptance of the disease. Elisabeth Kubler-Ross is widely known for her grief/acceptance model, which she presented in her book *On Death and Dying* [10]. In this model, a person or family who is presented with a major life loss or change engages in a series of emotional reactions. She describes these reactions as shock, denial, anger, bargaining, depression, and acceptance. Each person will engage in their own feelings and reactions and the cycle is not meant to be chronological, but rather a framework for grief and eventual acceptance.

Caregivers themselves also progress through caregiving stages. Lindegren, in 1993, in a study of spouses caring for partners with dementia [11], described "a caregiving career," where the specific stages include the *encounter phase*, wherein the couple confronts the diagnosis, then grieves the loss of their previous life, and acquires the skills necessary to properly care for the family member.

> Caregivers progress through caregiving stages: the *encounter phase*, the *enduring phase*, and the *exit phase*.

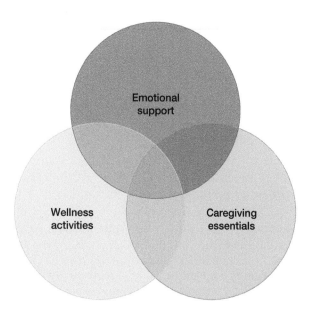

FIGURE 36.1
The trifecta of caregivers' self-care.

In the next phase, the *enduring phase*, the caregiver is submersed in caregiving to a substantial degree, oftentimes to the detriment of their own self-care. In this phase, caregivers must learn to cope with social isolation and their own mental pain. Finally, the *exit phase*, the "caregiving career" is somewhat relinquished because of either death or institutionalization of the patient.

As independent observers, the medical team is in a unique position to identify and discuss these cycles with both the patient and the caregiver. If a member of the medical team becomes aware of a patient or family member's difficulty or if there are unaddressed needs, coordination of care can begin to address these issues.

NEEDS OF THE CAREGIVER

Significant and healthy human relationships are successful only when they are reciprocal and mutual. The MS patient may need a great deal of assistance, but the needs of the caregiver must also be met in order for the relationship to remain healthy. Although several directions could be taken regarding the importance of self-care, this section addresses what one might consider the *trifecta of self-care* (Figure 36.1).

> The MS patient may need a great deal of assistance, but the needs of the caregiver must also be met in order for the relationship to remain healthy.

Emotional Support

Caring for someone with a chronic illness can lead to a decreased quality of life, a decline in psychological health,

increased stress, and depression and anxiety [5,12–14]. Research has clearly demonstrated the negative emotional consequences of caregiving, which can lead to dysfunctional coping skills, strained relationships, and reduced life satisfaction, and emotional and physical sickness [15–17]. In addition, the stress of caregiving can precipitate affective disorders such as anxiety and depression. It is not uncommon for caregivers to identify a need for treatment from a mental health provider, but few actually seek the needed help [18,19]. Recognizing the issue is important, but following through is vital. Failure to seek help has been identified as a factor in caregiver burnout and mental health disorders.

In the proposed medical team model or multidisciplinary model (Figure 36.2), support is built-in. Any member of the team can identify and validate the need for support that can be supplied by the appropriate team member. If practicing outside a Team Model, appropriate referrals can be made.

Mental health practitioners have specific interventions with the aim of reducing caregiver burden and improving mental and physical health. Sharing emotions with others relieves stress and may offer a different perspective on problems. These are helpful steps to improve the emotional and physical health of caregivers. The National MS Society (USA) offers a variety of programs aimed at helping ease the emotional burden such as support groups, psychoeducational programming, referrals to mental health providers, and web chats. When referring to a mental health practitioner, it is important to pick a provider who has extensive experience in chronic disease management and understands the complexities of how MS affects the entire family. Early recognition by a clinician or by the caregiver themselves are linked with successful outcomes [20].

Caregiving Essentials

Caregivers often come into the role of caregiving as a necessity and have no previous knowledge of skill. They may take the "learn as you go" approach, which can create more stress. In addition, oftentimes being the sole care provider comes with additional responsibilities, including, but not limited to, career, parenting, and household chores. As highlighted earlier, the relaying of information and referral to services such at the National MS Society or the Multiple Sclerosis Association of America can be helpful in providing caregivers with useful skills. In addition, please be open to discussing and brainstorming ways to help ease these household task burdens (eg, hired help, enlisting other family members or friends, etc.) [20,21].

Wellness Programs

The behavioral medicine literature is full of studies which show the power of physical activity and wellness in self-care. In general, research has demonstrated that engaging in exercise and physical activity significantly enhances both physiological and psychological health [22–25]. The benefits of exercise and physical activity

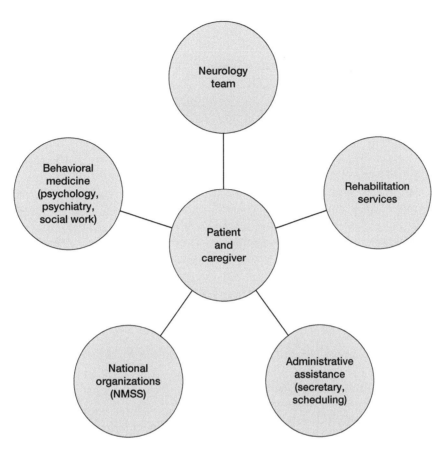

FIGURE 36.2
Patient and caregiver multidisciplinary care model.

have been documented across a wide array of health areas, including chronic disease prevention and control, mental health, and health-related quality of life [22–25]. Many caregivers neglect their own emotional, physical, and spiritual needs. Wellness encompasses healthy all-around living. Some studies suggest eating a balanced diet, getting at least 7 hours of restorative sleep, regular exercise (ie, 30 minutes or aerobic exercise 4 or more days a week), caring for emotional health by way of a mental health provider, maintaining friendships and hobbies, and for those with a spiritual alignment, spending some time on that [20,21].

Within the multidisciplinary team of MS professionals, each and every member should take a moment to assess and address caregiver needs. When assessing a caregiver, "Ten Tips for Caregivers to Avoid Burnout" (Table 36.1) can be helpful.

ABUSE

The physical, financial, and emotional toll brought by caregiving can turn even the most loving family members into individuals who struggle with strong emotions and urges to harm. In people with MS or other disabling conditions, members of the interdisciplinary care team must become comfortable at assessing for abuse by spouse or caregiver, as individuals with disabilities may identify abuse as the most important health issue that they face [26]. In fact, in 2005, the American Medical Association recommended that all patients be screened for domestic violence and safety in their homes [27]. Three types of abuse are described: (a) physical (including sexual and neglect); (b) psychological (including both verbal and non-verbal); and (c) financial. Oftentimes, overlap may occur within the types of abuse.

Physical abuse and emotional abuse are the most common types of abuse in a chronic care population. The care recipient is often frail and becomes an easy target for aggression. Physical abuse generally starts during caregiving. The caregiver can become rough during grooming or transfers. Scratches, bruises, and even the more obvious signs of abuse (eg, black eyes, or broken bones) can be noticed on the person. Neglect is often characterized in terms of physical abuse. This neglect can occur when a caregiver is burned out and decides to forgo on his or her duties to the family members without seeking help outside. A caregiver might leave the care recipient for long periods of time meeting his or her basic needs such as, toileting, eating, transfers. The care recipient may miss appointments or become malnourished, or medications become mismanaged. These signs can be warning signs for the MS professional to seek immediate help. If the abuse happens once, it likely will happen again.

TABLE 36.1
Ten Important Tips for Caregivers to Avoid Burnout

1. **Become Educated About MS.** The more one knows about the disease, the more empowered he or she will feel and the more comfortable he or she will feel with role changes. Ask as many questions as you need when you are in appointments. No question is a stupid question, and all questions are important.

2. **Take Care of Yourself.** As airline stewardesses say, "You must put on your own oxygen mask, before putting on the mask of another," this philosophy stands for caregiving. If you are unhealthy emotionally, physically, or spiritually, you will be of no help to anyone else.

3. **Practice Healthy Living.** One is much more capable of being of help to others when you eat a healthy, balanced diet, you exercise regularly, you are involved with your own interests, and you get enough sleep.

4. **Stay Social.** Connecting with others in similar situations is powerful because you no longer feel isolated and you can learn from others. In addition, make sure you maintain other important relationships such as with children, family members, and close friends.

5. **Accept Help.** As difficult as it is to ask for help from others, realize that you need a break and that others may want to help. You do not have to do it all, nor is it healthy to do it all. The best way to avoid burnout is to accept help. People often want to help, just ask.

6. **Acknowledge Your Emotions.** If you are feeling hopeless, worthless, helpless, sad, anxious or fearful, acknowledge these emotions. These are all normal reactions to your situation.

7. **Allow for Healthy Expression of Your Feelings With Each Other.** Just because you are now a caregiver does not take away that you had a relationship with this person in the past. You are still a spouse, partner, child, and so on and with that comes the responsibility to speak respectfully open. Should difficulties arise, seek couples or family counseling. Your MS neurology team will have a list of qualified mental health professionals.

8. **Allow for Caregiving Holidays.** This simply means take some time away. You will be a better caregiver to your loved one if you take time away.

9. **Encourage Healthy Independence of Your Loved One.** Help your loved one be as independent as he or she can for as long as they can. This may involve assistive devices or new technologies, and so seek these out.

10. **Seek Help Through Your Local Organizations.** Each territory or state has their own MS society which you can find in the United States by calling 1-800-344-4867. The National MS Society has an MS Navigator Program which will help guide you toward available resources for both you and your loved one with MS.

Emotional abuse is often more difficult to detect. It may happen in the home through degrading language, harsh comments, and humiliation. The abuser may control the victim through language and emotional reactions such as ignoring the person, and may cause the victim psychological damage. Emotional abuse may happen when a caregiver is overburdened, overextended, and not taking care of their own emotional needs. Abuse of any kind generally occurs when there is a power differential.

Finally, financial abuse is less likely than the other forms of abuse and generally manifests through exploitation. Examples of this include the abuser improperly, illegally, or without permission, using money or goods that are not their own.

> If abuse of any kind is suspected, referrals should be made through local social services, adult protective services, social work, mental health providers, or the NMSS.

O'Leary and colleagues [28] created "REACH" as an innovative program through their local chapter of the National Multiple Sclerosis Society (NMSS). REACH provides Respite, Education, Awareness, Change, and Hope. This educational and outreach program was designed to help medical providers assess for abuse and provide

subsequent crisis care to those involved. If abuse of any kind is suspected, referrals should be made through local social services, adult protective services, social work, mental health providers, or the NMSS (Table 36.2).

MULTIDISCIPLINARY MEDICAL TEAM

The most efficacious management of chronic disease benefits from access to high quality comprehensive care teams of skilled professionals that include attention to symptom management and quality of life (Figure 36.2). This level of care is not always available and requires a shift from the traditional "medical" model to a more "functional" model of care, incorporating the concerns of patient, family member, and caregiver. Included in a successful multidisciplinary team for the management of MS are the physician, advanced practice clinicians, psychologist, psychiatrist, physical therapist, occupational therapist, social worker, nurses, speech therapist, national associations, and administrative support (Figure 36.1). This model allows for several practitioners, organizations, and even the administrative support to interact with, assess, and determine what types of interventions to recommend for the caregiver. When this type of a team can be assembled, an optimal level of care for both the patient and their family of caretakers can be provided. For those who are unable to practice within a team setting,

TABLE 36.2
Resources

Books

Carter R. *Helping Yourself Help Others: A Book for Caregivers.* Random House/Time Books; 1995
provides basic information for caregivers

Kalb R. *Multiple Sclerosis: A Guide for Families*, 3rd ed. Demos Health; 2006
provides information on a variety of caregiving issues such as emotions, cognitive issues, sexuality, intimacy, and life planning.

Caregiving Support

National MS Society's MS Navigator Program
Tel: 800-344-4867.
www.nationalmssociety.org/living-with-multiple-sclerosis/relationships/carepartners/index.aspx
provides information on educational programs and self-help groups.

Caregiver.com
www.caregiver.com
• is the most visited caregiver site on the internet
• publishes *Today's Caregiver Magazine*
• provides many links to resources and agencies of interest

Today's Caregiver Magazine
Tel: 800-829-2734. www.caregiver.com/magazine
is a bimonthly magazine resource for caregivers.

The Well Spouse Association
63 West Main Street, Suite H, Freehold, NJ 07728
Tel: 800-838-0879. www.wellspouse.org
• advocates and addresses the needs of individuals caring for the chronically ill.
• publishes *Mainstay*, a quarterly newsletter.

National Family Caregivers Association
10400 Connecticut Ave., Suite 500 Kensington, MD 20895
Tel: 800-896-3650. www.thefamilycaregiver.org
educates, supports, and empowers more than 65 million Americans who are caregivers to the chronically ill.

United Way
www.unitedway.org
provides help for individuals and families to achieve their human potential through education, income stability, and healthy lives.

Home Care Agencies/Hiring Help

National Association for Home Care and Hospice
228 Seventh Street, SE, Washington, DC 20003
Tel: 202-547-7424. www.nahc.org
provides referrals to state associations.

Hiring Help at Home
A fact sheet from the National MS Society
Tel: 1-800-344-4867
Adapted from the National MS Society: MS and Carepartners at
www.nationalmssociety.org/living-with-multiple-sclerosis/relationships/carepartners/index.aspx

developing referral listings and partnering with local organizations with the common interest in MS care are highly recommended.

SUMMARY

MS is a chronic, complex illness which can potentially have expansive and profound effects on the entire family. Although caregiving can be greatly rewarding, it also presents challenges. Caregivers can become overburdened with the care of the person with MS and care of the household, finances, and their own self. Caregivers must make it a point to care for themselves emotionally and physically. Although clinical visits are often focused on the MS patient, care providers must make it a point to assess and provide recommendations to the caregiver, particular if that caregiver is experiencing burnout or sometimes even abusing the MS patient (Table 36.2).

KEY POINTS FOR PATIENTS AND FAMILIES

- Caregiving for a loved one with a chronic condition can often be profoundly fulfilling, as many times individuals move closer together when challenges arise.

- Caregiving can become overwhelming, physically and emotionally challenging, and isolating. At times it can be thought of as a burden.

- Caregivers must learn to take care of themselves physically and emotionally.

- The multidisciplinary care model used in the treatment of MS is important not only for the patient, but also for the caregiver. This care model allows for several practitioners to interact with the caregiver to assess and determine the optional interventions.

- Physical, emotional, and financial abuses secondary to the profound challenges inherent in caring for a relative with a disabling chronic illness are not uncommon. Assessing for abuse is an important component in the clinical management of MS.

REFERENCES

1. Frohman EM. Multiple sclerosis. *Med Clin North Am.* 2003;87: 867–897.

2. Hileman J, Lackey N, Hassaneien R. Identifying the needs of home caregivers of patients with cancer. *Oncol Nurs Forum.* 1992;19:771–777.

3. National Family Caregivers Association. Caregiving Statistics. Retrieved June 20, 2012, from: www.thefamilycaregiver.org /who_are_family_caregivers/care_giving_statstics.cfm

4. Pandya S. Caregiving in the United States. Retrieved June 20, 2012, from: http://assets.aarp.org/rgcenter/il/fs111_caregiving .pdf

5. Buhse M. Assessment of caregiver burden in families of persons with multiple sclerosis. *J Neurosci Nurs.* 2008;40(1):25–31.

6. American Psychological Association. The High Cost of Caregiving. Retrieved September 18, 2012, from: www.apa.org /research/action/caregiving.aspx

7. Dewis MEM, Niskala H. Nurturing a valuable resource: Family caregivers in multiple sclerosis. *Axone.* 1992;13:87–94.

8. Bellou M, Vouzavali FJD, Koutroubas A, et al. The 'care' in caregiving: The multiple sclerosis experience for the healthy family members. *Existential Analysis.* 2012;23(1):149–161.

9. McKeown L, Porter-Armstrong A, Baxter G. Caregivers of people with multiple sclerosis: Experiences of support. *Mult Scler.* 2004;10:219–230.

10. Kübler-Ross, E. *On Death and Dying.* Routledge; 1969.

11. Lindgren CL. The caregiver career. *Image J Nurs Sch.* 1993;25: 214–219.

12. Patti F, Amato MP, Battaglia MA, et al. Caregiver quality of life in multiple sclerosis: A multicentre Italian study. *Mult Scler.* 2007;13:412–419.

13. Figved N, Myhr K, Larsen J, et al. Caregiver burden in multiple sclerosis: The impact of neuropsychiatric symptoms. *J Neurol Neurosurg Psychiatry.* 2007;78:1097–1102.

14. Sherman TE, Rapport IJ, Hanks RA, et al. Predictors of well-being among significant others of person with multiple sclerosis. *Mult Scler.* 2007;13:238–249.

15. O'Brien MT. Multiple sclerosis: Stressors and coping strategies in spousal caregivers. *J Community Health Nurs.* 1993;10: 123–135.

16. O'Brien RA, Wineman NM, Nealon NR. Correlates of the caregiving process in multiple sclerosis. *Sch Inq Nurs Pract.* 1995;9:323–338.

17. Gulick EE. Coping among spouses or significant others of persons with multiple sclerosis. *Nurs Res.* 1995;44:220–225.

18. Buchanan RJ, Radin D, Chakravorty B, Tyry T. Informal care giving to more disable people with multiple sclerosis. *Disabil Rehabil.* 2009;31:1244–1256.

19. Buchanan RJ, Radin D, Huang C. Caregiver burden amount informal caregivers assisting people with multiple sclerosis. *Int J MS Care.* 2011;13:76–83.

20. National MS Society. A guide for caregivers: Managing major changes. Retrieved June 10, 2012: www.nationalmssociety.org /search-results/index.aspx?q=caregiver+support&start=0 &num=20

21. Holland NJ, Schneider DM, Rapp R, Kalb RC. Meeting the needs of people with primary progressive multiple sclerosis, their families, and the health-care community. *Int J MS Care.* 2011;13:5–74.

22. Sullivan AB, Covington E, Scheman J. Immediate benefits of a brief 10-minute exercise protocol in a chronic pain population: A pilot study. *Pain Med.* 2010;11(4):524–529.

23. Bouchard C, Shephard RJ, Stephens T. *Physical Activity, Fitness, and Health: International Proceedings and Consensus Statement.* Champaign, IL: Human Kinetics; 1994.

24. Brownell KD, O'Neil PM. Obesity. In: Barlow DH, ed. *Clinical Handbook of Psychological Disorders: A Step-by-Step Treatment Manual,* 2nd ed. New York: Guilford; 1993:318–361.

25. Kirkcaldy BD, Shephard RJ, Siefen RG. The relationship between physical activity and self-image and problem behaviour among adolescents. *Soc Psychiatry Psychiatr Epidemiol.* 2002;37:544–550.

26. Berkeley Planning Associates. *Priorities for Future Research: Results of BPA's Delphi Survey of Disabled Women.* Oakland, CA: Berkley Planning Associates; 1996.

27. *Report 7 of the Council on Scientific Affairs (A-05): Diagnosis and Management of Family Violence.* Chicago, IL: American Medical Association; 2005. Retrieved July 3, 2012: http://www.ama -assn.org/resources/doc/csaph/a05csa7-fulltext.pdf

28. O'Leary M, Lammers S, Mageras A, et al. Relationship between domestic violence and multiple sclerosis. *Int J MS Care.* 2008;10:27–32.

Part VI. Related Diseases

37

Neuromyelitis Optica

MATTHEW S. WEST
JOHN R. CORBOY

Neuromyelitis optica (NMO), also known as Devic's disease, is an inflammatory demyelinating disease of the central nervous system (CNS). Once thought to possibly be a form of multiple sclerosis (MS), NMO has now been defined as a distinct clinical–pathological disorder, although the initial clinical presentation often mimics MS. Clinically, NMO preferentially targets the optic nerves and spinal cord; however, over time, the clinical spectrum has expanded and NMO is now known to affect the brain in a substantial minority of patients. The diagnosis and pathogenesis of NMO have been greatly advanced by the discovery of the NMO-immunoglobulin G (IgG), an antibody directed against, and with high affinity to, the water channel aquaporin-4 (AQP-4) in the CNS. NMO-IgG appears to be pathogenic. Given the clinical aggressiveness of NMO with the associated disability, rapid recognition and diagnosis is important to appropriately tailor both acute and long-term therapies, which are different than therapies for MS and other related disorders.

> NMO is a distinct disease, different than MS.

EPIDEMIOLOGY

Large studies defining the prevalence rate of NMO in populations are lacking. However, data from small epidemiological studies suggest a prevalence rate between 0.52 and 4.4 per 100,000 people in various locations around the world. NMO prevalence is approximately 1% to 2% that of MS in the United States [1]. There is a higher representation of this disease among Asian, West Indian, Afro-Brazilian, Hispanic and other non-white populations [2]. Given this observation, in a patient with a non-white background with severe optic neuritis or myelitis, NMO should be high on the differential diagnosis.

The median age of onset is 39 years old, which is later than MS (Table 37.1), although NMO has been described in both children and the elderly. In the monophasic disease, men and women are affected equally, while the more common relapsing course is 9 times more prevalent in women than men [3].

CLINICAL FEATURES

Although supporting serological and imaging criteria exist, NMO remains a predominantly clinical diagnosis and begins with the recognition of common symptoms. NMO most frequently presents as severe optic neuritis, transverse myelitis, or a combination of both. The diagnosis of NMO should be considered in patients with those presenting syndromes, especially if an MRI of the brain is normal or atypical for MS.

> NMO most often presents as severe optic neuritis, myelitis, or both.

NMO-associated optic neuritis is similar to other inflammatory optic neuritis in clinical presentation. Vision loss typically occurs over hours to days and peaks within 1 to 2 weeks. Ocular pain, often associated with eye movement, is common. Dyschromatopsia (particularly red desaturation), central or paracentral scotoma, and photopsias may also occur. The vision loss in NMO is commonly more severe than in MS. Bilateral simultaneous or rapidly sequential optic neuritis may also be more indicative of NMO.

Transverse myelitis is often severe and complete and can present with a symmetric para, or tetra, paresis, spinal sensory level, and significant sphincter dysfunction early in the course. Myelitis is often heralded by severe spinal pain. In comparison, MS-related myelitis typically has a more mild, unilateral, and asymmetrical clinical presentation (Table 37.1). Approximately one-third of patients have associated Lhermitte's phenomenon, paroxysmal tonic spasms, or radicular pain associated with the myelitis [3].

TABLE 37.1
NMO and MS Comparison

CLINICAL FACTORS	NMO	MS
Average age of onset	Late third to early fourth decade	Second to early third decade
Gender	Relapsing: Female > male Monophasic: Female = male	Female > male
Population prevalence	Higher proportion in non-white populations	Varies geographically, white populations more affected
Clinical features	Primarily severe optic neuritis and myelitis	Dissemination in time and space affecting multiple CNS sites, typically of milder severity
MRI		
Brain	Often normal, may have nonspecific T2 hyperintensities and hypothalamic, periventricular (third/fourth ventricle), or medullary lesions	Lesions are ovoid and periventricular, juxtacortical, callosal, and infratentorial locations
Spine	Lesions typically longitudinally extensive (3 or more vertebral segments), centrally located with cord expansion	1 to 2 vertebral segments, asymmetric, peripheral location
CSF oligoclonal bands	Uncommon (20% to 30%)	Common (90%)
NMO-IgG	Often present	Absent
Secondary progressive course	No	Yes

CNS, central nervous system; CSF, cerebrospinal fluid; NMO-IgG, neuromyelitis optica-immunoglobulin G.

Beyond involvement of the optic nerves and spinal cord, NMO may also present with brain stem symptoms such as intractable nausea and hiccupping (from involvement of the medulla), vertigo, trigeminal neuralgia, diplopia, and nystagmus. Cases have also been described with acute encephalopathy, cognitive changes, and hypothalamic dysfunction such as syndrome of inappropriate antidiuretic hormone secretion (SIADH).

DIAGNOSIS

The diagnosis of NMO is based on clinical features with paraclinical support from neuroimaging and serological testing. NMO should be considered in all patients with severe optic neuritis, longitudinally extensive transverse myelitis (greater than 3 vertebral segments long), recurrent episodes of isolated optic neuritis, or bilateral simultaneous or sequential optic neuritis. Current diagnostic criteria offer guidance, including the revised Mayo Clinic and National MS Society criteria (Table 37.2). Both criteria require both optic neuritis and myelitis for a definitive diagnosis. The supporting features may help establish a diagnosis of NMO spectrum disorder (NMOSD) in patients who do not fulfill required criteria. Sensitivity of the Mayo criteria is 99%, with 90% specificity [4]. Other etiologies of optic neuritis and/or transverse myelitis must be considered and include MS, acute disseminated encephalomyelitis, a systemic vasculitis such as systemic lupus erythematosus (SLE) or Sjögren's syndrome, sarcoidosis, nutritional deficiency such as vitamin B_{12}, and infectious etiologies including neurosyphilis.

NMOSD

Some individuals may not fulfill formal criteria for NMO, but have a limited form with only isolated longitudinally extensive transverse myelitis or bilateral simultaneous or recurrent optic neuritis with positive NMO-IgG. These patients are considered to have NMOSD (Table 37.3).

Approximately 30% to 50% of patients with longitudinally extensive transverse myelitis and up to 25% of bilateral, or recurrent sequential, optic neuritis are NMO-IgG seropositive [6]. About 50% of those seropositive individuals develop a subsequent relapse consistent with the diagnosis of NMO [7]. In Asian opticospinal MS, 1 cohort found 58% of patients with NMO-IgG positivity [6]. NMOSD may also be associated with organ-specific autoimmunity (eg, myasthenia gravis) and non-organ-specific autoimmune disease (eg, SLE and Sjögren's syndrome). Evidence suggests that systemic autoimmune disease coexists with NMO rather than act as a direct cause. Autoantibodies to antinuclear antigen (44%) and Sjögren's syndrome A autoantibody (SSA) (16%) are found more frequently in NMO patients than in seronegative individuals, while no patients with SLE or Sjögren's without manifestations consistent with NMO are NMO-IgG seropositive [9].

LABORATORY STUDIES

The discovery of NMO-IgG directed against aquaporin-4 (AQP-4) has aided in the distinction of NMO from other inflammatory demyelinating disorders. AQP-4 is an osmosis-driven, water-selective transporter expressed on the

TABLE 37.2
NMO Diagnostic Criteria

CRITERIA	REVISED MAYO CLINIC [4]	NATIONAL MS SOCIETY [5]
Required Criteria	Optic neuritis myelitis	Optic neuritis in 1 or 2 eyes myelitis, associated with spinal cord lesion on MRI extending over 3 or more segments on T2-weighted imaging
		No evidence for sarcoidosis, vasculitis, clinically manifest lupus or Sjogren's, or other explanation for symptoms
	AND,	
Supportive Criteria	*At least 2 of the following:* Initial brain MRI not meeting diagnostic criteria for MS	*At least one of the following:* Most recent brain MRI normal or not fulfilling criteria for MS
	Contiguous spinal cord MRI lesion extending Over 3 or more vertebral segments	Positive test in serum or CSF for NMO-IgG/AQP-4 antibodies
	NMO-IgG seropositive	

AQP-4, aquaporin-4; CSF, cerebrospinal fluid; NMO-IgG, neuromyelitis optica-immunoglobulin G.

TABLE 37.3
NMOSD

- Isolated or recurrent longitudinally extensive transverse myelitis (3 or more vertebral segments on MRI)
- Bilateral simultaneous, or isolated recurrent, optic neuritis
- Asian opticospinal MS
- Optic neuritis or longitudinally extensive transverse myelitis associated with systemic autoimmune disease
- Optic neuritis or longitudinally extensive transverse myelitis associated with brain lesions typical of NMO such as hypothalamic, brain stem, and periventricular

astrocytic foot processes throughout the CNS and is involved in water homeostasis, astrocyte migration, neuronal signal transduction, and neuroinflammation. There are high concentrations in subpial, subependymal areas and the hypothalamus, in addition to the optic nerve and spinal cord. The precise role of NMO-IgG has not been fully elucidated; however, there is substantial evidence that AQP-4 antibody has a pathogenic role in NMO [9,10]. The original indirect immunofluorescence assay for NMO-IgG, used with a composite substrate of mouse tissues, identified NMO patients with a sensitivity of 73% and specificity of 91% [6]. Subsequently, a variety of assays based on alternative techniques have been developed. A blinded comparison showed that a combination of cell-based assays and enzyme-linked immunosorbent assay (ELISA) commercial assays was both highly specific (100%) and sensitive (72%) when used in combination. Other currently available techniques, especially when used alone, have a much lower sensitivity and specificity [11]. Additional laboratory studies to help exclude other diagnoses should be based on a patient's clinical characteristics, but often include erythrocyte sedimentation rate (ESR), C-reactive protein (CRP), antinuclear antigen (ANA) with reflexive panel including SSA and anti-Sjögren's syndrome B (SSB) antibodies, angiotensin converting enzyme (ACE) level, vitamin B_{12}, rapid plasma reagin (RPR), and HIV.

NMO-IgG is a highly specific test for NMO.

Cerebrospinal fluid (CSF) abnormalities are common in NMO with an elevation in white blood cells (WBC) noted in approximately 50% and may be greater than 50×10^6 WBC/L, including a high proportion of neutrophils. Oligoclonal bands (OCBs) are present in only 10% to 20%, compared to approximately 90% in MS [3]. The role of testing for NMO-IgG in the CSF is less clear. One study of 26 seronegative NMO patients had 3 patients with CSF positivity [12], while other studies have not supported this finding [9].

IMAGING

MRI Brain

Over time it has been recognized that NMO is not limited to only the optic nerves and spinal cord, and there are reports of both symptomatic and asymptomatic brain lesions on neuroimaging. The lesions are often located within areas of high AQP-4 concentrations such as the hypothalamus, around the third and fourth ventricles, and in the brain stem, particularly the medulla near the area postrema, and are typically distinct from MS lesion appearance. MRI brain early in the disease course is often normal, but up to 60% of NMO patients may develop abnormalities over time, albeit many changes are often nonspecific [13].

MRI Spine

Spinal cord MRI is helpful in patients with signs and symptoms suggestive of a spinal syndrome. NMO affects the cervical and thoracic spine more than lumbar. Lesions are longitudinally extensive (usually greater than 3 vertebral segments in length), centrally located, often occupy more than one-half of the cord area, and are associated with cord expansion and edema (Figure 37.1). T2 hyperintensities are best seen on short tau inversion recovery (STIR) or proton density sequences and may have associated T1 hypointensity. Gadolinium-enhancement is frequently homogenous, involves the central portion of the lesion, and may remain enhancing months after a relapse.

> Spinal cord lesions are typically greater than 3 vertebral segments in length.

CLINICAL COURSE AND PROGNOSIS

Approximately 90% of NMO patients have a relapsing course with further episodes of optic neuritis and/or myelitis, with the remainder being monophasic [2]. In the monophasic disease course, the episodes of optic neuritis and myelitis often occur within days to weeks of each other with no recurrence over time. The sentinel event is typically more severe in monophasic patients; however, greater disability accumulates over time with subsequent attacks in the relapsing form. In relapsing disease, attacks can be separated by months to years at unpredictable intervals. Predictors of a relapsing course includes older age of onset, longer interval between initial clinical attacks, female gender, and less severe motor disability with the index event [14]. Fifty-five percent of relapsing NMO patients have their first relapse within 1 year and 90% within 5 years [15]. Unlike MS, there does not appear to be a secondary or progressive form of NMO.

> Most NMO patients have a relapsing course.

Compared to seronegative patients, NMO-IgG seropositivity is associated with more frequent and severe attacks, coexisting autoimmunity, and higher total spinal cord lesion load. Seronegative patients are more likely to have bilateral optic neuritis, or simultaneous optic neuritis, and myelitis at onset and the disease course is more often monophasic [16].

As in MS, the natural history of NMO is variable between individuals. Some have an aggressive, unrelenting, and ultimately fatal course from the outset, while others have a milder course that stabilizes over time. Overall, prognosis and mortality of untreated patients have generally been poor, and worse than MS. Higher attack frequency within the first 2 years, concomitant autoimmune disease, incomplete

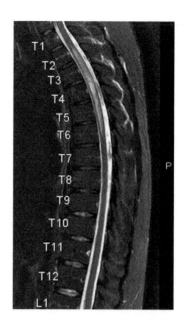

FIGURE 37.1
T2-weighted MRI thoracic spine with longitudinally extensive myelitis.

recovery from the index event, and sphincter signs at onset are associated with poorer outcomes [14]. Without aggressive long-term therapy, 53% of patients presenting with optic neuritis had bilateral vision involvement and 63% were considered blind in 1 eye after 8 years [17]. At 5 years, 65% of patients showed at least moderate disability and 42% require walking assistance [18]. One study in the 1990s found a 5 year survival rate of 68% in relapsing disease with mortality secondary to respiratory failure from high cervical and medullary lesions [3]. It remains to be proven that morbidity and mortality will be diminished substantially with aggressive, early therapy, but this seems likely.

TREATMENT

Acute Relapse

The cornerstone of treatment of acute inflammatory demyelinating disease of the CNS is corticosteroids, and NMO is no different (Table 37.4). Randomized controlled studies of corticosteroids in acute treatment of NMO exacerbations are lacking, and treatment is driven by clinical experience and studies of corticosteroids in MS and optic neuritis. Intravenous (IV) methylprednisolone dosage of 1,000 mg daily for 3 to 5 days, with an optional oral prednisone taper, is most commonly used and up to 80% of patients respond favorably [3]; however, it is not unusual for some patients to have a limited response. In instances of poor response, a repeat course of IV steroids may be considered, but a more beneficial therapy is usually plasma exchange (PLEX).

PLEX has shown efficacy in the treatment of severe relapses of MS, acute myelitis, and acute disseminated encephalomyelitis when not responsive to high-dose steroids. In NMO, treatment with PLEX has been associated with functional improvement in subgroups' analyses of retrospective studies, published case series, and clinical experience. Predictors of favorable response to PLEX include male gender, preserved reflexes at time of diagnosis, and early initiation of treatment [19]. Rescue therapy with early initiation of PLEX is recommended in steroid-unresponsive severe attacks, with 3 to 7 exchanges (commonly 5 exchanges) performed daily to every other day based on tolerance. Clinical improvement may be noticed as early as 1 to 2 exchanges, nonetheless treatment should continue for a full course.

Relapse Prevention

Owing to the relatively low prevalence of NMO, there have been no randomized, double-blinded studies of disease-modifying therapies in this disorder. Given that in NMO, disability is directly related to exacerbations of optic neuritis and myelitis and occurs in a stepwise manner because of incomplete recovery from relapses and additive disability progression, the treatment approach in relapsing NMO is aggressive, early intervention.

Since patients are often initially diagnosed with clinically isolated syndromes (CIS) or MS, many NMO patients have been treated with conventional immunomodulatory therapies such as interferon (IFN) beta and glatiramer acetate (GA). Despite a single case report of GA suggesting benefit, experience suggests these therapies are ineffective, and IFN beta therapy may actually increases relapses and AQP-4 levels [15]. Natalizumab, a common therapy for MS, has also failed to control disease activity in NMO [20].

Clinical experience, further understanding of the pathophysiology of NMO, and increasing clinical study advocates strongly for the use of long-term immunosuppression for relapse prevention. A number of therapies have been considered and include both oral and parenteral options (Table 37.4).

> Prevention of attacks with immunosuppresants is important in relapsing NMO.

Low-Dose Corticosteroids

In a retrospective study of 9 NMO patients, long-term oral prednisolone 5 to 20 mg monotherapy lowered annualized

TABLE 37.4
Treatment Options for NMO

Acute relapse

Medication	Typical dosage	Common or serious side effects
Methylprednisolone	1,000 mg IV daily for 3 to 5 days ±postinfusion oral prednisone taper	Insomnia, irritability, dysphoria, increased appetite, edema, heartburn, hyperglycemia, osteonecrosis
PLEX	3 to 7 exchanges over 1 to 2 weeks	Vagal reaction, hypotension, coagulopathy, hypocalcemia, deep vein thrombosis, infection

Relapse prevention

Medication	Typical dosage	Common or serious side effects
First-line therapy		
Rituximab	1,000 mg IV 2 infusions, 2 weeks apart OR 375 mg/m² weekly for 4 weeks. Repeat infusion about every 6 months, follow CD20 levels	Infusion reaction, infection, leukopenia, progressive multifocal leukoencephalopathy
Azathioprine ±prednisolone	2 to 3 mg/kg per day in divided doses 1 mg/kg per day, begin tapering at 2 to 3 month based on azathioprine effect	Nausea/vomiting, leukopenia, thrombocytopenia hepatotoxicity, infection
Mycophenolate mofetil	1 to 3 g oral per day in divided doses	Nausea/vomiting, diarrhea, peripheral edema, infections elevated blood pressure
Second-line therapy		
Mitoxantrone	12 mg/m² IV monthly for 6 months, then 12 mg/m² every 3 months for 9 months	Nausea, amenorrhea, alopecia, leukopenia, hepatotoxicity, cardiotoxicity, acute leukemia, infection
Cyclophosphamide	500 to 1,000 mg/m² IV monthly for 6 months pretreat with mesna	Nausea, vomiting, amenorrhea, leukopenia, infection, hemorrhagic cystitis, infertility
Methotrexate	50 mg IV weekly plus, prednisone 1 mg/kg per day	Nausea/vomiting, diarrhea, myelosuppression, renal dysfunction, liver dysfunction, infections
Intermittent plasma exchange		

CD20, cluster of differentiation 20; IV, intravenous; PLEX, plasma exchange.

relapse rate (ARR). A dose effect was suggested, as relapses occurred more often in doses less than 10 mg per day [21]. The chronic use of corticosteroids is associated with various adverse effects (Table 37.4), and thus steroid sparing agents are preferred. Those patients maintained on long-term steroids should be treated with gastrointestinal, and osteoporosis, prophylaxis.

Rituximab

If the NMO-IgG is indeed pathogenic, approaches focused on removal of these antibodies, or the cells/precursor cells that produce them, would likely be beneficial. Rituximab is a chimeric anti-CD20 monoclonal antibody that depletes precursor, and eventually mature, antibody-producing plasma cells. Several studies, as well as clinical experience with rituximab, have demonstrated value in NMO. A retrospective study of 25 NMO patients treated with rituximab in doses of either 375 mg/m² once per week for 4 weeks or 1,000 mg for 2 treatments 2 weeks apart, led to a reduction of median ARR from 1.7 to 0 over 19 months, and stabilization, or improvement, in the Expanded Disability Status Scale (EDSS) in 80% [22]. A second study had similar results with reduction in median RR from 1.87 to 0 and stabilization, or improvement, of EDSS in all 23 patients [23]. The onset of depletion of CD20 cells is rapid after starting therapy; however, there is no direct effect on antibody-producing plasma cells; thus, some individuals may experience relapses early in the course of treatment, and there are reports of poor responsiveness to rituximab in more severe cases. A report in 2010 demonstrated that long-term therapy with rituximab in rheumatoid arthritis patients was well tolerated and overall safe [24]. The most common adverse effect is an infusion-related reaction, which can include fever, rash, headache, flu-like symptoms, and bronchospasm. The incidence is highest after the first infusion, occurring in approximately 25% of patients. Prevention of this reaction includes pretreatment with acetaminophen, diphenhydramine, and corticosteroids prior to the infusion. Up to 30% of rituximab-treated patients can develop infections, however only 2% are considered severe [24]. There is a very low, not well-defined, risk of progressive multifocal leukoencephalopathy (PML) in RA and B-cell lymphoma patients treated with rituximab, but there have been no reports of PML in NMO or MS patients treated with rituximab.

Azathioprine

Azathioprine is the prodrug of 6-mercaptopurine (6-MP) and inhibits proliferation of lymphocytes. Treatment dose is 2 to 3 mg/kg per day, often combined with oral prednisone 1 mg/kg per day until peripheral WBC counts are suppresed (approximately 2 months after initiation) at which time the prednisone is slowly tapered. The effect of azathrioprine in NMO has been demonstrated in a small open-label case series and 2 larger studies. One study of 29 Brazilian NMO patients had a 90% reduction in relapse rate and stabilization of EDSS scores over 28 months [25], while a second study of 99 patients showed a reduction of ARR by 76% with 37% of patients being relapse-free over a median of 22 months [26]. Doses less than 2 mg/kg per day have been associated with more frequent relapses. While patients are taking azathioprine, hematological monitoring for pancytopenia is recommended at least monthly initially and then every 2 to 3 months with longer duration of therapy. A small portion of the population have a mutation of thiopurine methyltransferase (TPMT), an enzyme that deactivates 6-MP, which leads to accumulation of 6-MP and increased risk for myelosuppression and infection. TPMT activity can be determined prior to initiating therapy and if suppressed or absent, alternative therapies may be considered. There may be an associated increased risk of cancer, particularly lymphoma, with longer duration and increasing cumulative dosing.

Mycophenolate Mofetil

Oral mycophenolate inhibits proliferation, and transendothelial migration, of B and T lymphocytes. A retrospective study of 24 NMO patients treated with a median dose of 2,000 mg per day led to a lower median ARR in 79% of patients and stabilization or improvement of EDSS in 91% over an average of 27 months [27]. Clinical experience with mycophenolate has led some experts to recommend it as a first-line therapy [2]. Treatment effect may be delayed in mycophenolate, but is thought to be more rapid than azathioprine.

Others

Other immunsuppressant therapies, including mitoxantrone, methotrexate, and cyclophosphamide have less supporting data. Mitoxantrone, an anthracenedione derivative that delays cell-cycle progression, is approved for rapidly progressive relapsing-remitting and secondary progressive MS. An open-label study of 5 patients suggested benefit on relapse rate and disability in NMO [28]. Use, however, is limited by adverse events including cardiomyopathy, treatment-related acute leukemia, and bone marrow suppression, and lifetime dose is limited to 140 mg/m². IV methotrexate 50 mg weekly plus oral prednisone 1 mg/kg per day, showed stabilization of disease in 8 NMO patients [29]. IV cyclophosphamide is an alkylating chemotherapeutic agent with only case reports of effectiveness in NMO patients who also had other autoimmune diseases such as lupus and Sjogren's. A variety of treatment dosages have been used in the literature, however treatment with 1,000 mg/m² monthly for 6 months has been effective in other autoimmune processes such as chronic inflammatory demyelinating polyneuropathy (CIDP), lupus, and MS. Treatment with mesna should be given prior to starting cyclophosphamide to prevent acute hemorrhagic cystitis. Intermittent PLEX in combination with immunosuppressants was shown to reduce relapses in a case report of 2 NMO patients [30]. In the future, treatment may involve the use of recombinant monoclonal anti-AQP-4 antibodies that selectively block NMO-IgG binding, although these therapies are still in development [31]. Use of this therapy would provide a highly specific, nonimmunosuppressive approach to treatment of this challenging disorder.

Treatment Recommendations

Therapies often considered first-line for long-term treatment of NMO include rituximab, azathioprine, and mycophenolate mofetil. The choice of initial therapy must be individualized, weighing the risk and benefits of the medications with each patient. The author's experience with IV rituximab has generally been positive with disease stabilization, limited adverse events, and the benefit of infrequent administration and is often used first-line. Azathioprine or mycophenolate may be considered initially in more mild disease, with transition to rituximab in nonresponders or more aggressive cases.

KEY POINTS FOR PATIENTS AND FAMILIES

- NMO is a different disease process than MS, although the initial clinical presentation may be similar.

- NMO most often affects the optic nerves (causing decrease or loss of vision) and the spinal cord (causing weakness, sensory changes, trouble walking, and bladder/bowel dysfunction).

- The diagnosis is made based on classic clinical symptoms of optic neuritis and myelitis, neuroimaging, and serum testing for NMO antibody.

- Most individuals with NMO have a relapsing course with repeat exacerbations over time.

- Acute treatment for an NMO relapse includes IV steroids and possibly PLEX based on response to steroids and severity of disability.

- Disability appears to be directly related to relapses, so prevention of attacks with either oral or IV immunosuppressive therapies should be started after the diagnosis is made.

- Websites with further information:
  - www.guthyjacksonfoundation.org
  - www.nationalmssociety.org
  - www.msaa.com
  - www.myelitis.org

REFERENCES

1. Mealy MA, Wingerchuk DM, Greenberg BM, et al. Epidemiology of neuromyelitis optica in the United States. *Arch Neurol.* 2012;69(9):1176–1180.

2. Sellner J, Boggild M, Clanet M, et al. EFNS guidelines on diagnosis and management of neuromyelitis optica. *Eur J Neurol.* 2010;17:1019–1032.

3. Wingerchuk DM, Hogancamp WF, O'Brien PC, et al. The clinical course of neuromyelitis optica (Devic's syndrome). *Neurology.* 1999;53(5):1107–1114.

4. Wingerchuk DM, Lennon VA, Pittock SJ, et al. Revised diagnostic criteria for neuromyelitis optica. *Neurology.* May 2006;66:1485–1489.

5. Miller DH, Weinshenker GB, Filippi M, et al. Differential diagnosis of suspected multiple sclerosis: A consensus approach. *Mult Scler.* 2008;14:1157–1174.

6. Lennon VA, Wingerchuk DM, Kryzer TJ, et al. A serum autoantibody marker of neuromyelitis optica: Distinction from multiple sclerosis. *Lancet.* 2004;364:2106–2112.

7. Weinshenker BG, Wingerchuk DM, Vukusic S, et al. Neuromyelitis optica IgG predicts relapse after longitudinally extensive transverse myelitis. *Ann Neurol.* 2006;59:566–569.

8. Pittock SJ, Lennon VA, de Seze J, et al. Neuromyelitis optica and non organ-specific autoimmunity. *Arch Neurol.* 2008;65:78–83.

9. Jarius S, Wildemann B. AQP4 antibodies in neuromyelitis optica: Diagnostic and pathogenetic relevance. *Nat Rev.* 2010;6:383–392.

10. Bennett JL, Lam C, Kalluri SR, et al. Intrathecal pathogenic anti-aquaporin-4 antibodies in early neuromyelitis optica. *Ann Neurol.* 2009 Nov;66(5):617–629.

11. Waters PJ, McKeon A, Leite MI, et al. Serologic diagnosis of NMO: A multicenter comparison of aquaporin-4-IgG assays. *Neurology.* 2012 Feb 28;78(9):665–671.

12. Klawiter EC, Alvarez E, Xu J, et al. NMO-IgG detected in CSF in seronegative neuromyelitis optica. *Neurology.* 2009 Mar 24;72(12):1101–1103.

13. Pittock SJ, Lennon VA, Krecke K, et al. Brain abnormalities in neuromyelitis optica. *Arch Neurol.* 2006;63(3):390–396.

14. Wingerchuk EM, Weinshenker BG. Neuromyelitis optica: Clinical predictors of a relapsing course and survival. *Neurology.* 2003;60:848–853.

15. Kim W, Kim S, Kim HJ. New insights into neuromyelitis optica. *J Clin Neurol.* 2011;7:115–127.

16. Jarius S, Ruprecht K, Wildemann B, et al. Contrasting disease patterns in seropositive and seronegative neuromyelitis optica: A multicentre study of 175 patients. *J Neuroinflammation.* 2012 Jan;9:14.

17. Papais RM, Carellos SC, Alvarenga MP, et al. Clinical course of optic neuritis in NMO. *Arch Ophthalmol.* 2008;126:12–16.

18. Ghezzi A, Bergamaschi R, Martinelli V, et al. Clinical characteristics, course, and prognosis of relapsing Devic's neuromyelitis optica. *J Neurol.* 2004;251:47–52.

19. Keegan M, Pineda AA, McClelland RL, et al. Plasma exchange for severe attacks of CNS demyelination: Predictors of response. *Neurology.* 2002;58:143–146.

20. Kleiter I, Hellwig K, Berthele A, et al. Failure of natalizumab to prevent relapses in neuromyelitis optica. *Arch Neurol.* 2012 Feb;69(2):239–245.

21. Watanabe S, Misu T, Miyazawa I, et al. Low-dose corticosteroids reduce relapses in neuromyelitis optica: A restrospective analysis. *Mult Scler.* 2007;13:968–974.

22. Jacob A, Weinshenker BG, Violich I, et al. Treatment of neuromyelitis optica with rituximab. *Arch Neurol.* 2008;65:1443–1448.

23. Bedi GS, Brown AD, Delgado SR, et al. Impact of rituximab on relapse rate and disability in neuromyelitis optica. *Mult Scler.* 2011;17(10):1225–1230.

24. Van Vollenhoven RF, Emery P, Bingham CO, et al. Longterm safety of patients receiving rituximab in rheumatoid arthritis clinical trials. *J Rheumatol.* 2010;37(3):558–567.

25. Bichuetti DB, Lobato de Oliveira EM, Oliveira DM, et al. Neuromyelitis optica treatment: Analysis of 36 patients. *Arch Neurol.* 2010;67(9):1131–1136.

26. Constanzi C, Matiello M, Lucchinetti CF, et al. Azathioprine: Tolerability, efficacy, and predictors of benefit in neuromyelitis optica. *Neurology.* 2011;77:659–666.

27. Jacob A, Matiello M, Weinshenker BG, et al. Treatment of neuromyelitis optica with mycophenolate mofetil: Retrospective analysis of 24 patients. *Arch Neurol.* 2009;66:1128–1133.

28. Weinstock-Guttman B, Ramanathan M, Lincoff N, et al. Study of mitoxantrone for the treatment of recurrent neuromyelitis optica. *Arch Neurol.* 2006;63:957–963.

29. Minagar A, Sheremata WA. Treatment of Devic's disease with methotrexate and prednisone. *Int J MS Care.* 2000;2:39–43.

30. Miyamoto K, Kusunoki S. Intermittent plasmapheresis prevents recurrence in neuromyelitis optica. *Ther Apher Dial.* 2009;13:505–508.

31. Tradtrantip L, Zhang H, Saadoun S, et al. Anti-aquaporin-4 monoclonal antibody blocker therapy for neuromyelitis optica. *Ann Neurol.* 2012 Mar;71(3):314–322.

38

Acute Disseminated Encephalomyelitis

TIMOTHY WEST

KEY POINTS FOR CLINICIANS

- Acute disseminated encephalomyelitis (ADEM) is a monophasic inflammatory demyelinating disorder of the central nervous system that entails a polysymptomatic clinical presentation and must include encephalopathy.

- ADEM is often preceded by a viral infection or vaccination, and many common infections and vaccines have been associated with ADEM.

- There is no single test that confirms the diagnosis of ADEM. As such, establishing the diagnosis requires both clinical and radiological features and the exclusion of other diseases that resemble ADEM.

- Repeat imaging studies are necessary to evaluate for subsequent demyelinating events, as up to 29% of patients with ADEM go on to develop another demyelinating event within 5 years after the initial attack.

- Acute hemorrhagic encephalomyelitis (AHEM) is a hyperacute variant of ADEM with rapidly progressive, usually fulminant, inflammatory hemorrhagic demyelination in the central nervous system.

- There is no standard therapy for ADEM, but a course of 3 to 5 days of high-dose intravenous methylprednisolone (IVMP) can often provide significant clinical benefit. This is usually followed by a tapering dose of oral corticosteroids over 4 to 6 weeks.

Acute disseminated encephalomyelitis (ADEM) is a monophasic inflammatory demyelinating disorder of the central nervous system (CNS) that is often preceded by an infection, or more rarely a vaccination [1,2]. The hallmark clinical presentation is a multifocal onset with encephalopathy manifesting as behavioral change or alteration in consciousness [1]. ADEM can occur at any age, but tends to affect children more than adults [2], and usually strikes children younger than 10 years of age [3]. There does not appear to be a clear gender predominance [4,5], although a possible increase in risk among males has been reported [2].

> The hallmark clinical presentation for ADEM is a multifocal onset with encephalopathy manifesting as behavioral change or alteration in consciousness.

A challenge in diagnosing and studying ADEM has been the lack of formal diagnostic criteria. In 2007, an international panel of experts was organized by the National Multiple Sclerosis Society. This International Pediatric

Multiple Sclerosis Study Group proposed a consensus definition for demyelinating diseases of childhood [1]. ADEM was defined as a monophasic clinical event with a presumed inflammatory or demyelinating cause affecting multiple areas of the brain [1]. They further clarified that the clinical presentation, "must be polysymptomatic and must include encephalopathy," there can be no other explanation for the symptoms and there cannot be a history of a prior event with clinical features consistent with demyelination [1] (see Table 38.1 for full proposed criteria).

The incidence of ADEM is estimated to be about 0.4 per 100,000 per year among people under 20 years of age [5]. More recent studies have lumped ADEM with other demyelinating diseases in childhood and have reported incidence rates of 0.9 to 1.63 per 100,000 person years [6,7]. The incidence of ADEM does have seasonal peaks in the winter and spring, providing some evidence for an infectious etiology to the disease [4,8]. There are regional cases linked to specific vaccines or infections, but the worldwide distribution of ADEM is not well understood [2]. Reports of a clear illness preceding the onset of symptoms have ranged from 46% to 100% among patients with ADEM [2,5,9].

Many infections have been associated with ADEM. In 1 cohort, nonspecific upper respiratory infections were reported as the most commonly associated infection, accounting for 29% of their cases [9]. Other infectious presentations reported in this cohort were "gastrointestinal disturbance" in 9% of cases and a "nonspecific febrile illness" in 6% of cases. Specific infections were found in relatively few cases but included Varicella (4%), Herpes simplex virus (2%), Mumps (1%) and Rubella (1%) [9].

Similar to infections, many vaccinations have been associated with ADEM including the new H1N1 influenza vaccine [10]. The most common vaccinations to be associated with ADEM are non-neural measles, mumps, and rubella vaccines [11]. Table 38.2 describes the various infections and vaccines that have been linked to ADEM. While many vaccinations have been associated with ADEM,

TABLE 38.1
International Pediatric MS Study Group Consensus Definitions

MONOPHASIC ADEM	RECURRENT ADEM
A first clinical event with a presumed inflammatory or demyelinating cause, with acute or subacute onset that affects multifocal areas of the CNS. The clinical presentation must be polysymptomatic and must include encephalopathy	New event of ADEM with a recurrence of the initial symptoms and signs, 3 or more months after the first ADEM event, without involvement of new clinical areas by history, examination, or neuroimaging
Encephalopathy is defined as:	Event does not occur while on steroids, and occurs at least 1 month after completing therapy
1) Behavioral change 2) Alteration in consciousness	MRI shows no new lesions; original lesions may have enlarged
Event should be followed by improvement, either clinically, on MRI, or both, but there may be residual deficits	No better explanation exists
No history of a clinical episode with features of a prior demyelinating event	**MULTIPHASIC ADEM**
No other etiologies can explain the event	ADEM followed by a new clinical event also meeting criteria for ADEM, but involving new anatomic areas of the CNS as confirmed by history, neurological examination, and neuroimaging
New or fluctuating symptoms, signs, or MRI findings occurring within 3 months of the inciting ADEM event are considered part of the acute event	The subsequent event must occur
Neuroimaging shows focal or multifocal lesion(s), predominantly involving the white matter, without radiological evidence of previous destructive white matter changes:	1) at least 3 months after the onset of the initial ADEM event and
1) Brain MRI, with FLAIR or T2-weighted images, reveals large (more than 1 to 2 cm in size) lesions that are multifocal, hyperintense, and located in the supratentorial or infratentorial white matter regions; gray matter, especially basal ganglia and thalamus, is frequently involved	2) at least 1 month after completing steroid therapy
	The subsequent event must include a polysymptomatic presentation including encephalopathy, with neurological symptoms or signs that differ from the initial event (mental status changes may not differ from the initial event)
2) In rare cases, brain MR images show a large single lesions (more than 1 to 2 cm), predominantly affecting white matter	The brain MRI must show new areas of involvement but also demonstrate complete or partial resolution of those lesions associated with the first ADEM event
3) Spinal cord MR images may show confluent intramedullary lesion(s) with variable enhancement, in addition to abnormal brain MRI findings above specified	

ADEM, acute disseminated encephalomyelitis; CNS, central nervous system; FLAIR, fluid-attenuated inversion recovery.
Source: Adapted from [1].

this is a rare occurrence and only accounts for about 5% to 10% of the cases [5,9]. Unilateral or even bilateral optic neuropathy can occur following vaccination, but most case reports describe either this clinical picture or ADEM, but not both [11]. It is important to realize that while an antecedent infection or vaccination may increase the likelihood of ADEM, it is not required so [12]. Antecedent infection or vaccination may also occur in patients with a first presentation of multiple sclerosis (MS) [13]. As such, antecedent infection or vaccination should not be used as criteria to exclude MS as a diagnostic possibility.

> Antecedent infection or vaccination should not be used as a criterion to exclude multiple sclerosis as a diagnostic possibility.

The proposed pathogenesis of post-vaccinial ADEM was an immune reaction to the viral component of the vaccine. However, it has been recognized that this immune reaction could be caused by contamination of the vaccine (especially with CNS tissue) due to the manner in which it was prepared [15]. This can be likened to the way in which experimental autoimmune encephalomyelitis (EAE) is created in rodents as a model for studying CNS demyelination. When a rodent is inoculated with myelin or myelin antigens, the result is a disease in the rodent that resembles ADEM [11]. It has even been suggested that ADEM following a rabies vaccination is the human form of EAE [4].

EVALUATION

There is no single test that confirms the diagnosis of ADEM. Establishing the diagnosis requires a combination of clinical and radiological features and most importantly, the exclusion of other diseases that resemble ADEM. It is important to recognize that the differential diagnosis of ADEM is broad (see Table 38.3). As such, a thorough work-up should include infectious, immunological, and metabolic tests. Repeating MRI studies to evaluate for progression is also essential. ADEM is by definition monophasic, but MS has been reported to develop out of a single multifocal demyelinating event mimicking ADEM in up to 29% of cases [2]. Importantly, the second demyelinating event can occur years later. One study demonstrated this well as 21% of patients experienced a second attack after only 2.4 years of follow-up, but after 5.6 years of follow-up that number rose to 27% [4].

> Establishing the diagnosis requires a combination of clinical and radiological features and the exclusion of other diseases that resemble ADEM.

TABLE 38.2
Infections and Vaccinations That Have Been Associated With ADEM

VIRUSES	REPORTED FREQUENCY	BACTERIAL	REPORTED FREQUENCY
Coronavirus	Case report	Borrelia Burdoreri	Case report
Coxsackie B	Case report	Chlamydia	Case report
Dengue virus	Case report	Legionella	Case reports
Epstein–Barr virus	Case reports	Mycoplasma Pneumoniae	Case reports
Hepatitis A	Case reports	Rickettsia ricketsii	Case report
Hepatitis C	Case reports	Streptococcus	Case series
Herpes simplex virus	Case series	Tuberculosis	Case report
HIV	Case reports		
Human herpesvirus 6	Case report	**VACCINATIONS**	
Measles	100/100,000	H1N1 influenza	Case reports
Mumps	Case reports	Hepatitis B	Case reports
Parainfluenza virus	Case reports	Japanese B encephalitis	0.2/100,000
Rubella virus	1/10,000–20,000	Measles	0.1/100,000
Varicella-zoster virus	1/20,000–20,000	Mumps	0.06 to 1.4/100,000
		Pertussis	0.9/100,000
OTHER		Polio	Case report
Plasmodium vivax	Case reports	Rabies (live attenuated)	Up to 6/100
Plasmodium falciparum	Case reports	Tetanus	Case report
		Tick-borne encephalitis	Case report

Source: Adapted from [14].

TABLE 38.3
Differential Diagnosis of ADEM [14,16–19]

CNS INFECTIONS	IMMUNE-MEDIATED DISORDERS
Viral encephalitis	Multiple sclerosis
Bacterial encephalitis or abscesses	Neuromyelitis optica
Fungal infection/encephalitis	Behçet's disease
Parasitic encephalitis or CNS infection	Systemic lupus erythmatosus
Rickettsial infection/encephalitis	Primary isolated CNS angiitis
Progressive multifocal leukoencephalopathy	Neurosarcoidosis
	Bickerstaff brain stem encephalitis
METABOLIC LEUKOENCEPHALOPATHIES	Anti-N-methyl-D-aspartate receptor (NMDA-R) encephalitis
Adrenoleukodystrophy	Anti-myelin-oligodendrocyte-glycoprotein (MOG) disease
Adrenomyeloneuropathy	Schilder's myelinoclastic diffuse sclerosis
Metachromatic Leukodystrophy	CNS vasculitis
Mitochodrial encephalomyopathy, lactic acidosis and stroke-like episodes (MELAS)	
OTHER	
Metastatic Neoplasm	

Clinical Features

Distinguishing ADEM from other demyelinating etiologies such as MS can be difficult clinically, but there are a few clinical features that can be helpful. In particular, the presence of fever, seizure, impaired consciousness, or a multifocal onset are more suggestive of ADEM than MS [20–22]. Optic neuritis is common in both ADEM and MS. However, optic neuritis is often bilateral in ADEM, whereas optic neuritis in MS is usually unilateral [22]. The clinical presentation of ADEM can range from an isolated fever of unknown origin [23], to acute onset psychosis [24], but each of these presentations are rare. Table 38.4 shows a breakdown of the commonly reported symptoms at clinical presentation among patients with ADEM.

Though clinical features may be helpful, laboratory and imaging studies are often essential in distinguishing ADEM from other demyelinating diseases.

Imaging Findings

When evaluating for ADEM, it is important to realize that CT scans of the brain are not optimal as they are frequently normal [4,5]. MRI of the brain is the imaging modality of choice. In one ADEM cohort (n = 42), CT scans of the brain were normal in 68%, while 100% of the patients had abnormalities on MRI of the brain or spinal cord [5]. MRI abnormalities are usually noted on the T2-weighted or fluid-attenuated inversion recovery (FLAIR) sequences within the basal ganglia, thalami, brain stem, cerebellum, periventricular white matter or gray–white junction [5]. Contrast (gadolinium) enhancement on T1-weighted images is variable, as it depends on the stage of inflammation at the time of imaging and has been reported in 26% to

TABLE 38.4
Common Symptoms at Clinical Presentation of ADEM [2,5,8,9,16,20,21,25]

CLINICAL FEATURES	% REPORTED
Impaired consciousness/ encephalopathy	33% to 75%*
Fever	39% to 67%
Headache/vomiting	23% to 58%
Motor disturbance/weakness	23% to 85%
Ataxia – cerebellar dysfunction	28% to 65%
Cranial neuropathy	13% to 89%
Seizure	10% to 47%
Meningismus	6% to 43%
Sensory disturbance	2% to 28%
Optic neuritis	13% to 23%
Aphasia/language disturbance	2% to 20%

*Of note, these cohorts were described prior to the proposed consensus definition requiring encephalopathy for a diagnosis of ADEM.

100% of patients with ADEM [2,25]. The pattern of enhancement is also variable and can be complete or incomplete ring-shaped, nodular, gyral, or spotty. In contrast, meningeal enhancement in the brain or spinal cord is unusual [2] (see Figures 38.1 and 38.2).

Computerized Tomography (CT) scans of the brain are frequently normal. MRI of the brain is imaging modality of choice for evaluating ADEM.

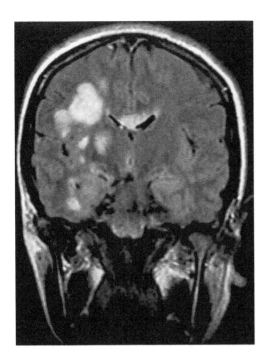

FIGURE 38.1
ADEM—Coronal FLAIR sequences on brain MRI demonstrating T2 abnormal signal within the basal ganglia and periventricular white matter. *Image courtesy of Christopher Hess, MD, PhD. Associate Professor, UC San Francisco.*

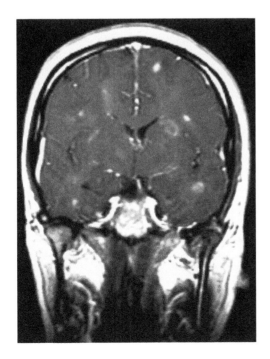

FIGURE 38.2
ADEM—Coronal T1 postcontrast images on brain MRI demonstrating variable Gadolinium contrast enhancement including 1 ring-shaped enhancing lesion. *Image courtesy of Christopher Hess, MD, PhD. Associate Professor, UC San Francisco.*

One of the toughest clinical assessments in ADEM patients is determining the risk of a subsequent demyelinating attack. In 2004, the KIDMUS (Kids with MS) study group proposed new criteria for the diagnosis of MS in children [26]. They found that: (a) lesions radiating perpendicularly to the long axis of the corpus callosum (also known as "Dawson's Fingers") and (b) the sole presence of well-defined lesions, were predictive of further relapses leading to a diagnosis of MS. If both criteria were met, the specificity was 100%, but the sensitivity was only 21% [26]. Then in 2009, Callen et al. proposed new criteria for distinguishing ADEM from MS including: (a) 2 or more periventricular lesions, (b) presence of T1-weighted hypodensities within the white matter or "black holes," (c) an absence of diffuse bilateral lesion distribution pattern. When any 2 out of these 3 Callen MS-ADEM criteria were present, it was predictive of conversion to MS with 95% specificity and 81% sensitivity [27] (see Table 38.5). A recent study testing these 2 criteria head-to-head confirmed that the Callen MS-ADEM criteria had the best combination of sensitivity (75%) and specificity (95%) [28].

Laboratory Findings

In addition to clinical features and radiological findings, some serological markers can be of help in distinguishing ADEM from other demyelinating diseases such as MS. Serum markers such as erythrocyte sedimentation rate (ESR) and white blood cell count (WBC) can be elevated in patients with ADEM, whereas these are usually normal in MS [4,22]. Cerebrospinal fluid (CSF) analysis can also be very helpful in distinguishing ADEM from MS. Many studies have shown that intrathecal synthesis of oligoclonal bands with the absence of these bands in the serum predicts future demyelinating attacks [4,8,9,29,30]. Oligoclonal bands have been reported in 40% to 95% of MS patients and only 0% to 29% of patients with ADEM [4,8,9,30].

> The presence of oligoclonal bands in the CSF with the absence of these bands in the serum predicts future demyelinating attacks.

Neurodiagnostic Studies

Electroencephalography is of limited utility in ADEM. It is often abnormal, demonstrating diffuse slowing indicative of encephalopathy, and epileptiform spikes are rare in ADEM [16]. Visual evoked potentials (VEP) can be helpful if optic neuritis is suspected, but does not distinguish between optic neuritis caused by ADEM and MS [16].

Neuropathological Findings

Patients with ADEM rarely undergo biopsy, and the pathology of ADEM is incompletely understood [16]. The disease

TABLE 38.5
Proposed MRI Criteria for Distinguishing MS From ADEM at the Initial Demyelinating Event

		SPECIFICITY	SENSITIVITY	PPV	NPV
Callen MS-ADEM criteria	2 out of the 3 following: Absence of diffuse bilateral lesion pattern Presence of T1-weighted hypodensities or "black holes" 2 or more periventricular lesions	95%	75%	96%	74%
KIDMUS criteria	1 out of the 2 following: Lesions perpendicular to the long axis of the corpus callosum (Dawson's Fingers) The sole presence of well-defined lesions	95%	57%	94%	63%
	When both criteria are met:	100%	11%	100%	46%

NPV, net present value; PPV, positive predictive value.
Source: Adapted from [28].

is characterized histologically by perivenular infiltrates of T cells and macrophages in association with perivenular demyelination [2]. By contrast, axons are relatively spared [4,9], though axonal degeneration can occur [2]. One case of fatal ADEM in a 5 year old boy demonstrated multifocal perivascular lymphocytic infiltrates associated focally with fibrin deposition within the vascular lumens and adjacent demyelination. In addition, diffuse anoxic ischemic neuronal degeneration and interstitial edema were noted, and no viral, bacterial, fungal, or parasitic infections were found [5]. While ADEM often carries a favorable prognosis with up to 70% of patients experiencing a full recovery [2], this case underscores the need for early diagnosis and treatment as the inflammation and subsequent injury to the CNS can be severe and even fatal.

Variant of ADEM

Acute Hemorrhagic Encephalomyelitis
Acute hemorrhagic leukoencephalitis (AHL), which is also known as acute hemorrhagic encephalomyelitis (AHEM) or acute necrotizing hemorrhagic leukoencephalitis (ANHLE), is considered to be a hyperacute variant of ADEM with rapidly progressive, usually fulminant, inflammatory, hemorrhagic demyelination in the CNS [2]. While ADEM is most commonly seen in children, AHEM is more often diagnosed in adults [31]. Lesions on brain MRI tend to be large with surrounding edema and mass effect [32]. It is often fatal, and death triggered by brain edema is common within 1 week of the onset of encephalopathy [2,31]. Given the rapidly progressive nature of the disease, early and aggressive treatment using various combinations of corticosteroids, immunoglobulin, plasma exchange, and cyclophosphamide is recommended [2,31]. As the level of evidence is limited to case reports, no formal recommendation can be given as to the acute treatment of AHEM. If intracranial pressure is increased, measures such as hyperventilation, mannitol, and even decompressive craniectomy has been reported as a life-saving measure [17,33–36]. At times, corticosteroids are sufficient to arrest the disease [37], but prolonged

immunosuppression with plasmapheresis, steroids, and cyclophosphamide has also been reported to result in a good outcome [36].

TREATMENT

There is no standard therapy for ADEM as there is a lack of evidence-based, prospective clinical trial data for ADEM management [17]. If ADEM is suspected, it is both prudent and the standard of care to pursue empirical antibacterial and antiviral treatment while the work-up for possible infectious encephalitis is ongoing. If seizures are part of the presentation, an antiepileptic medication should also be started. Once a diagnosis of acute demyelinating disease has been established, the most common initial treatment approach for ADEM is high-dose intravenous methylprednisolone (IVMP) at a dosage of 20 to 30 mg/kg per day (maximum 1 g/day) for 3 to 5 days [2,17]. If there is a good response, this is usually then followed by an oral corticosteroid taper over 4 to 6 weeks [17], as there is some suggestion in the literature that corticosteroid taper may protect against recurrent events [4]. The risks and side effects of high-dose corticosteroid treatment should also be managed, including hyperglycemia, hypokalemia, hypertension, facial flushing, and mood disorders [2]. Lastly, it is worth noting that high-dose IVMP is not without risk as rare gastric perforation and death due to gastrointestinal bleeding related to IVMP treatment of ADEM has been reported [38].

> The most common initial treatment approach for ADEM is high-dose intravenous methylprednisolone (IVMP) at a dosage of 20 to 30 mg/kg per day (maximum 1 g/day) for 3 to 5 days.

When treatment response to IVMP is inadequate, or in cases where corticosteroids are contraindicated, there are a few options to consider. Intravenous immunoglobulin G (IVIG) at a dosage of 2 g/kg divided over 2 to 5 days may be the next logical option if the disease is not fulminant or rapidly progressive. IVIG has been used successfully as monotherapy for the treatment of ADEM [39], even when corticosteroids failed [40,41]. When the presentation of ADEM is more severe or life-threatening, plasma exchange should be considered early in the disease course [17]. One case series showed about 40% of patients with ADEM (n = 10) had moderate to marked improvement following plasma exchange [42]. Within that study, early initiation of plasma exchange was associated with better outcome [42]. As with high-dose corticosteroids, there are safety concerns with plasma exchange that need to be taken into consideration. Symptomatic

hypotension, severe anemia, and heparin-induced thrombocytopenia have all been described as possible side effects of plasma exchange [42].

Another treatment option in adults with ADEM is cyclophosphamide. In a case series of 40 patients, 7 patients who had previously failed corticosteroids or had rapid progression who were given cyclophosphamide pulse therapy resulted in clinical improvement [21]. There are no reports within the literature of this medication being used in children [2]. Lastly, decompressive craniectomy has been reported as a life-saving measure after maximal medical treatment in severe cases of ADEM where there is significant edema, mass effect, and intracranial hypertension [17,33–35].

KEY POINTS FOR PATIENTS AND FAMILIES

- ADEM is a rare condition usually seen in children, often after a viral illness or vaccination.

- Symptoms include confusion, unsteadiness, visual blurring, headache, fever, and chills.

- MRI scanning shows changes in the white matter of the brain and spinal fluid shows an increase in white blood cells.

- Treatment is usually IV high-dose steroids for a few days. Sometimes a blood cleaning treatment called plasmapheresis is needed.

- Many patients with ADEM recover but some may be left with residual disability.

- Occasionally, ADEM reoccurs but it is usually a one-time event.

- ADEM and MS may be difficult to tell apart particularly in children.

REFERENCES

1. Krupp LB, Banwell B, Tenembaum S. Consensus definitions proposed for pediatric multiple sclerosis and related disorders. *Neurology.* 2007 Apr 17;68(16 Suppl 2):S7–S12.

2. Tenembaum S, Chitnis T, Ness J, Hahn JS. Acute disseminated encephalomyelitis. *Neurology.* 2007 Apr 17;68(16 Suppl 2):S23–S36.

3. Banwell B, Ghezzi A, Bar-Or A, et al. Multiple sclerosis in children: Clinical diagnosis, therapeutic strategies, and future directions. *Lancet Neurol.* 2007 Oct;6(10):887–902.

4. Dale RC, de Sousa C, Chong WK, et al. Acute disseminated encephalomyelitis, multiphasic disseminated encephalomyelitis and multiple sclerosis in children. *Brain.* 2000 Dec;123 (Pt 12):2407–2422.

5. Leake JA, Albani S, Kao AS, et al. Acute disseminated encephalomyelitis in childhood: Epidemiologic, clinical and laboratory features. *Pediatr Infect Dis J.* 2004 Aug;23(8):756–764.

6. Banwell B, Kennedy J, Sadovnick D, et al. Incidence of acquired demyelination of the CNS in Canadian children. *Neurology.* 2009 Jan 20;72(3):232–239.

7. Langer-Gould A, Zhang JL, Chung J, et al. Incidence of acquired CNS demyelinating syndromes in a multiethnic cohort of children. *Neurology.* 2011 Sep 20;77(12):1143–1148.

8. Hynson JL, Kornberg AJ, Coleman LT, et al. Clinical and neuroradiologic features of acute disseminated encephalomyelitis in children. *Neurology.* 2001 May 22;56(10):1308–1312.

9. Tenembaum S, Chamoles N, Fejerman N. Acute disseminated encephalomyelitis: A long-term follow-up study of 84 pediatric patients. *Neurology.* 2002 Oct 22;59(8):1224–1231.

10. Lee ST, Choe YJ, Moon WJ, et al. An adverse event following 2009 H1N1 influenza vaccination: A case of acute disseminated encephalomyelitis. *Korean J Pediatr.* 2011 Oct;54(10):422–424.

11. Huynh W, Cordato DJ, Kehdi E, et al. Post-vaccination encephalomyelitis: Literature review and illustrative case. *J Clin Neurosci.* 2008 Dec;15(12):1315–1322.

12. Young NP, Weinshenker BG, Lucchinetti CF. Acute disseminated encephalomyelitis: Current understanding and controversies. *Semin Neurol.* 2008 Feb;28(1):84–94.

13. Marrie RA, Wolfson C, Sturkenboom MC, et al. Multiple sclerosis and antecedent infections: A case-control study. *Neurology.* 2000 Jun 27;54(12):2307–2310.

14. Menge T, Hemmer B, Nessler S, et al. Acute disseminated encephalomyelitis: An update. *Arch Neurol.* 2005 Nov;62(11):1673–1680.

15. Bennetto L, Scolding N. Inflammatory/post-infectious encephalomyelitis. *J Neurol Neurosurg Psychiatry.* 2004 Mar;75(Suppl 1):i22–i28.

16. Dale RC. Acute disseminated encephalomyelitis. *Semin Pediatr Infect Dis.* 2003 Apr;14(2):90–95.

17. Pohl D, Tenembaum S. Treatment of acute disseminated encephalomyelitis. *Curr Treat Options Neurol.* 2012 Jun;14(3):264–275.

18. Kennedy PG. Viral encephalitis. *J Neurol.* 2005 Mar;252(3):268–272.

19. Rust RS. Multiple sclerosis, acute disseminated encephalomyelitis, and related conditions. *Semin Pediatr Neurol.* 2000 Jun;7(2):66–90.

20. Atzori M, Battistella PA, Perini P, et al. Clinical and diagnostic aspects of multiple sclerosis and acute monophasic encephalomyelitis in pediatric patients: A single centre prospective study. *Mult Scler.* 2009 Mar;15(3):363–370.

21. Schwarz S, Mohr A, Knauth M, et al. Acute disseminated encephalomyelitis: A follow-up study of 40 adult patients. *Neurology.* 2001 May 22;56(10):1313–1318.

22. Dale RC, Branson JA. Acute disseminated encephalomyelitis or multiple sclerosis: Can the initial presentation help in establishing a correct diagnosis? *Arch Dis Child.* 2005 Jun;90(6):636–639.

23. Costanzo MD, Camarca ME, Colella MG, et al. Acute disseminated encephalomyelitis presenting as fever of unknown origin: Case report. *BMC Pediatr.* 2011;11:103.

24. Nasr JT, Andriola MR, Coyle PK. ADEM: Literature review and case report of acute psychosis presentation. *Pediatr Neurol.* 2000 Jan;22(1):8–18.

25. Davis LE, Booss J. Acute disseminated encephalomyelitis in children: A changing picture. *Pediatr Infect Dis J.* 2003 Sep;22(9):829–831.

26. Mikaeloff Y, Adamsbaum C, Husson B, et al. MRI prognostic factors for relapse after acute CNS inflammatory demyelination in childhood. *Brain.* 2004 Sep;127(Pt 9):1942–1947.

27. Callen DJ, Shroff MM, Branson HM, et al. Role of MRI in the differentiation of ADEM from MS in children. *Neurology.* 2009 Mar 17;72(11):968–973.

28. Ketelslegers IA, Neuteboom RF, Boon M, et al. A comparison of MRI criteria for diagnosing pediatric ADEM and MS. *Neurology.* 2010 May 4;74(18):1412–1415.

29. Tintore M, Rovira A, Rio J, et al. Do oligoclonal bands add information to MRI in first attacks of multiple sclerosis? *Neurology.* 2008 Mar 25;70(13 Pt 2):1079–1083.

30. Mikaeloff Y, Suissa S, Vallee L, et al. First episode of acute CNS inflammatory demyelination in childhood: Prognostic factors for multiple sclerosis and disability. *J Pediatr.* 2004 Feb;144(2):246–252.

31. Borlot F, da Paz JA, Casella EB, Marques-Dias MJ. Acute hemorrhagic encephalomyelitis in childhood: Case report and literature review. *J Pediatr Neurosci.* 2011 Jan;6(1):48–51.

32. Kuperan S, Ostrow P, Landi MK, Bakshi R. Acute hemorrhagic leukoencephalitis vs ADEM: FLAIR MRI and neuropathology findings. *Neurology.* 2003 Feb 25;60(4):721–722.

33. Ahmed AI, Eynon CA, Kinton L, et al. Decompressive craniectomy for acute disseminated encephalomyelitis. *Neurocrit Care.* 2010 Dec;13(3):393–395.

34. Dombrowski KE, Mehta AI, Turner DA, McDonagh DL. Lifesaving hemicraniectomy for fulminant acute disseminated encephalomyelitis. *Br J Neurosurg.* 2011 Apr;25(2):249–252.

35. Refai D, Lee MC, Goldenberg FD, Frank JI. Decompressive hemicraniectomy for acute disseminated encephalomyelitis: Case report. *Neurosurgery.* 2005 Apr;56(4):E872; discussion E1.

36. Seales D, Greer M. Acute hemorrhagic leukoencephalitis. A successful recovery. *Arch Neurol.* 1991 Oct;48(10):1086–1088.

37. Klein CJ, Wijdicks EF, Earnest F. Full recovery after acute hemorrhagic leukoencephalitis (Hurst's disease). *J Neurol.* 2000 Dec;247(12):977–979.

38. Thomas GS, Hussain IH. Acute disseminated encephalomyelitis: A report of six cases. *Med J Malaysia.* 2004 Aug;59(3):342–351.

39. Nishikawa M, Ichiyama T, Hayashi T, et al. Intravenous immunoglobulin therapy in acute disseminated encephalomyelitis. *Pediatr Neurol.* 1999 Aug;21(2):583–586.

40. Marchioni E, Marinou-Aktipi K, Uggetti C, et al. Effectiveness of intravenous immunoglobulin treatment in adult patients with steroid-resistant monophasic or recurrent acute disseminated encephalomyelitis. *J Neurol.* 2002 Jan;249(1):100–104.

41. Pradhan S, Gupta RP, Shashank S, Pandey N. Intravenous immunoglobulin therapy in acute disseminated encephalomyelitis. *J Neurol Sci.* 1999 May 1;165(1):56–61.

42. Keegan M, Pineda AA, McClelland RL, et al. Plasma exchange for severe attacks of CNS demyelination: Predictors of response. *Neurology.* 2002 Jan 8;58(1):143–146.

Index